Paediat
(Healthcare profe

Shout for help

Open airway

NOT BREATHING NORMALLY?

5 rescue breaths

NO SIGNS OF LIFE?

15 chest compressions

2 rescue breaths
15 compressions

Call resuscitation team

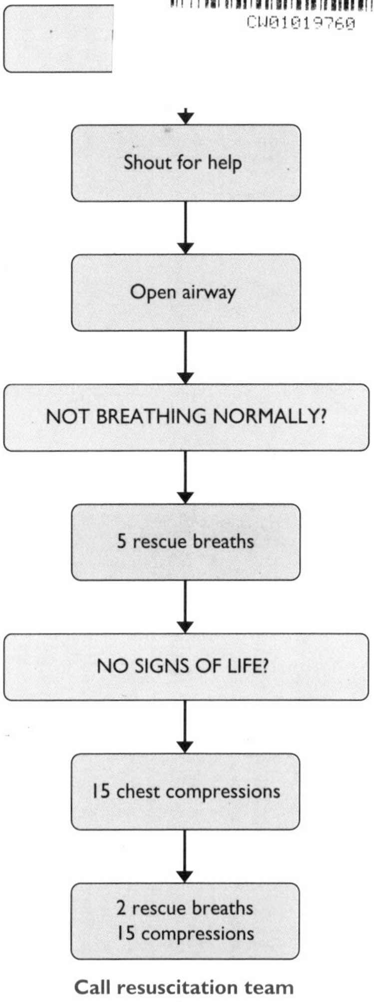

OXFORD MEDICAL PUBLICATIONS

Oxford Handbook of Tropical Medicine

Published and forthcoming Oxford Handbooks

Oxford Handbook for the Foundation Programme 3e
Oxford Handbook of Acute Medicine 3e
Oxford Handbook of Anaesthesia 3e
Oxford Handbook of Applied Dental Sciences
Oxford Handbook of Cardiology 2e
Oxford Handbook of Clinical and Laboratory Investigation 3e
Oxford Handbook of Clinical Dentistry 5e
Oxford Handbook of Clinical Diagnosis 2e
Oxford Handbook of Clinical Examination and Practical Skills
Oxford Handbook of Clinical Haematology 3e
Oxford Handbook of Clinical Immunology and Allergy 3e
Oxford Handbook of Clinical Medicine – Mini Edition 8e
Oxford Handbook of Clinical Medicine 8e
Oxford Handbook of Clinical Pathology
Oxford Handbook of Clinical Pharmacy 2e
Oxford Handbook of Clinical Rehabilitation 2e
Oxford Handbook of Clinical Specialties 9e
Oxford Handbook of Clinical Surgery 4e
Oxford Handbook of Complementary Medicine
Oxford Handbook of Critical Care 3e
Oxford Handbook of Dental Patient Care 2e
Oxford Handbook of Dialysis 3e
Oxford Handbook of Emergency Medicine 4e
Oxford Handbook of Endocrinology and Diabetes 2e
Oxford Handbook of ENT and Head and Neck Surgery
Oxford Handbook of Epidemiology for Clinicians
Oxford Handbook of Expedition and Wilderness Medicine
Oxford Handbook of Gastroenterology & Hepatology 2e
Oxford Handbook of General Practice 3e
Oxford Handbook of Genetics
Oxford Handbook of Genitourinary Medicine, HIV and AIDS 2e
Oxford Handbook of Geriatric Medicine 2e
Oxford Handbook of Infectious Diseases and Microbiology
Oxford Handbook of Key Clinical Evidence
Oxford Handbook of Medical Dermatology
Oxford Handbook of Medical Imaging
Oxford Handbook of Medical Sciences 2e
Oxford Handbook of Medical Statistics
Oxford Handbook of Nephrology and Hypertension
Oxford Handbook of Neurology
Oxford Handbook of Nutrition and Dietetics 2e
Oxford Handbook of Obstetrics and Gynaecology 3e
Oxford Handbook of Occupational Health 2e
Oxford Handbook of Oncology 3e
Oxford Handbook of Ophthalmology 2e
Oxford Handbook of Oral and Maxillofacial Surgery
Oxford Handbook of Paediatrics 2e
Oxford Handbook of Pain Management
Oxford Handbook of Palliative Care 2e
Oxford Handbook of Practical Drug Therapy 2e
Oxford Handbook of Pre-Hospital Care
Oxford Handbook of Psychiatry 3e
Oxford Handbook of Public Health Practice 3e
Oxford Handbook of Reproductive Medicine and Family Planning 2e
Oxford Handbook of Respiratory Medicine 2e
Oxford Handbook of Rheumatology 3e
Oxford Handbook of Sport and Exercise Medicine 2e
Oxford Handbook of Tropical Medicine 4e
Oxford Handbook of Urology 3e

Oxford Handbook of Tropical Medicine

Fourth edition

Edited by

Robert Davidson

Department of Infectious Diseases & Tropical Medicine
Northwick Park Hospital
Harrow, UK

Andrew Brent

Nuffield Department of Clinical Laboratory Sciences
University of Oxford, UK

Anna Seale

Centre for Tropical Medicine
Nuffield Department of Clinical Medicine
University of Oxford, UK;
KEMRI-Wellcome Trust Research Programme
Kilifi, Kenya

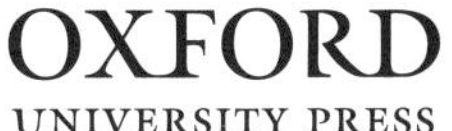
OXFORD
UNIVERSITY PRESS

OXFORD
UNIVERSITY PRESS

Great Clarendon Street, Oxford, OX2 6DP,
United Kingdom

Oxford University Press is a department of the University of Oxford. It furthers the University's objective of excellence in research, scholarship, and education by publishing worldwide. Oxford is a registered trade mark of Oxford University Press in the UK and in certain other countries

First edition published 1999

Second edition published 2005

Third edition published 2008

Fourth edition published 2014

Reprinted 2015

Impression 2

Published in the United States of America by Oxford University Press
198 Madison Avenue, New York, NY 10016, United States of America

British Library Cataloguing in Publication Data
Data available

Library of Congress Control Number: 2013940320

ISBN 978–0–19–969256–9

Printed in China by
C&C Offset Printing Co. Ltd.

Contents

Foreword

Whatever happened to the likely lads?

In my foreword to the second edition in 2005, I recalled how the creators of OHTM had, in vain, sought my support for what I too-readily dismissed as a harebrained Oxford medical students' fancy. Fortunately for OHTM's now global readership, these founders of a new fashion persisted and the rest is history. But what happened to Michael Eddleston and Stephen Pierini? I am delighted to report that both are pursuing successful careers. After spending several years living in Sri Lanka, where he worked on pesticide and plant poisoning, Michael moved to Edinburgh to specialize in toxicology with very much a third world perspective. He was recently appointed full professor and plans to return to clinical research in Asia in the near future. As a medical student, Stephen had an adventurous time exploring by boat the tributaries of the upper Juruá and Purús rivers in Acre, Brazil in search of snake-bites among the rubber tappers and indigenous Amerindians. Nowadays, he is a successful freelance general practitioner with a wide range of medical interests in the Cheltenham area, not far from the rather more prosaic river Severn in an area where snake-bites are rare.

The new edition, NCDs and NTDs

Robert Davidson and Robert Wilkinson joined Michael and Stephen for the 2nd edition while Andrew Brent, another experienced 'Africa hand', replaced Stephen for the 3rd edition. In this current 4th edition, Michael has stepped down as an editor and Anna Seale comes in, strengthening the Oxford link and bringing her special enthusiasm for expedition and wilderness medicine.

The content of the new edition reflects the changes in the pattern of medicine in tropical developing countries. Superficially, medicine in the tropics is becoming less different from what is seen in western temperate countries as the ageing population expands, prevalence of chronic non-communicable diseases (NCDs) increases relentlessly, the importance of psychiatric diseases is better recognized and the burden of infectious diseases is dominated more and more by tuberculosis and HIV/AIDS. However, medical practice in the tropics still demands a range of special attitudes, skills and disciplines that support the continued recognition and use of the term 'tropical medicine'. Much of this is to do with coping with limited resources, employing a wider range of ancillary disciplines, recognizing and treating acutely life-threatening but eminently reversible conditions and an unremitting emphasis on public health and the promotion of prevention through community education. Groups of enthusiastic and dedicated activists and, latterly, the WHO, have established re-prioritisation of a number of key 'neglected tropical diseases' (NTDs) which, although not among the shortlist of causes of 'millions-of-deaths-per-year', are responsible for colossal morbidity and have the enormous attraction of being amenable to control, elimination and even eradication. I applaud

OHTM's strong coverage of the classic tropical diseases, infectious and non-infectious, as well as its systems-based chapters and awareness of the rise in NCDs.

Two special challenges of working in the rural tropics

A fundamental requirement of good medical practice is the ability to communicate with patients. Western doctors working in tropical developing countries may encounter barriers to understanding their patients' complaints and medical needs that far exceed simple linguistic translation. I first encountered this problem when starting work in northern Nigeria in the 1970s. Hausa was not a difficult language (certainly compared to Amharic, with which I had struggled in Ethiopia) and, in any case, professional interpreters were available in Ahmadu Bello University Hospital. The real problem was trying to understand what the expression of a physical symptom implied in the local culture. Luckily, an experienced anthropologist, Murray Last, was living and working with a local Muguzawa community, 2 Hausa-speaking colleagues in the University, Allan Darrah a sociologist and John Froude a physician, produced an invaluable booklet 'Hausa Medicine for Western Doctors' and I had long conversations with a wise old friend in the Emir's court, Madauchi Zazzau. With this considerable help I was able to begin to understand what an ostensibly straightforward symptom, such as feeling cold, might mean and might usefully be interpreted in the process of seeking a diagnosis.

A familiar experience of doctors and other medical staff who work in tropical developing countries is to find themselves, on occasions, confronted with acute medical emergencies far outside their training, experience and competence when there is no expert colleague at hand to help and advise. Mikhail Bulgakov captures the intense feelings of failing professional responsibility, inadequacy and despair created by such situations in his brilliant short story, 'The Blizzard'. With this in mind, I was delighted to find that the new edition now included a chapter on obstetrical emergencies (my greatest nightmare) and more guidance on paediatrics, in addition to its established coverage of trauma and emergency care.

Contributors

Among the 52 authors (9 more than in the last edition), 26 are based in Western countries, 14 in Africa, 5 in Asia and 2 in South America, but all contribute valuable experiences and insights. OHTM remains a uniquely portable, accessible and readable compendium that can quickly provide the practical essentials of tropical medicine when and where they are needed. Grateful reviews from many parts of the world attest to these qualities. The apps for iPhone, Android and Blackberry will be even more convenient for some users although I, personally, will stay with my plastic-bound hard copy, whose pages can be annotated after each new revelation in this most fascinating and rewarding of all medical specialities.

David A. Warrell
Oxford
November 2013

Preface

The 1st edition (1999) of the *Oxford Handbook of Tropical Medicine* was created by Michael Eddleston and Stephen Pierini, to fill a gap between standard handbooks of clinical medicine that were unsuitable for use in resource-poor settings, and WHO guidelines, which were more appropriate, but not available in a collected format. Subsequent editions have evolved, but the vision remains to provide a practical, inexpensive handbook for clinicians working with tropical diseases, especially in low resource settings in the tropics. Anna Seale joins Robert Davidson and Andrew Brent as co-editor of the 4th edition, and a large panel of international experts have once again updated each section. This edition includes new sections on Clinical biochemistry, Obstetric emergencies, Nosocomial infection, Antibiotic prescribing and resistance, and Health emergencies in humanitarian crises, an expanded section on paediatric HIV, and more in-depth coverage of tropical diseases; and additional illustrations. Public health and paediatric-specific issues are highlighted in each section, in recognition of the broad responsibility of many clinicians in low resource settings, and international guidelines from the WHO and other sources are incorporated.

Both the concept and the content of tropical medicine are evolving: in some regions, non-communicable diseases have overtaken traditional tropical infections as major public health challenges. It is impossible for a single book to cater to every continent and context; nevertheless, we hope the book will continue to be a useful resource for doctors, medical assistants, nurses and other healthcare professionals.

We only ask that readers remain critical and selective, deciding what is relevant for their own circumstances and facilities; and that they share their comments and criticisms with the editors to further improve the book for future editions. Comments can be sent via the OUP website: http://ukcatalogue.oup.com/.

Acknowledgements

We would like to thank Professor David Warrell for writing the foreword; Dr Millie Davis for checking drug recommendations and doses; Professor Stan Houston for his detailed review of the previous edition; and Michael Eddleston, without whose initial vision and determination this book would not exist. Finally we would like to extend our sincere thanks to the many expert authors who once again gave of their time and experience in writing and updating each section of the new edition.

Royalties

All royalties from the sale of this book are being donated to Médecins Sans Frontières, earmarked for the clinical tropical diseases programmes administered through Operational Centre Amsterdam.

Symbols and Abbreviations

~	approximately
1°	primary
2°	secondary
3°	tertiary
↑	increased/increasing
↓	decreased/decreasing
→	leads to
+ve	positive
–ve	negative
+/–	with or without
3TC	lamivudine
ABC	airway, breathing, circulation/coma/convulsions
ABCD	airway, breathing, circulation/coma/convulsions, and dehydration
ABCv	abacavir
ABG	arterial blood gases
ACE	angiotensin-converting enzyme
ACh	acetylcholine
AChE	acetylcholinesterase
ACPA	anti-citrullinated peptide antibodies
ACPR	adequate clinical and parasitological response
ACT	artemisinin combination therapies
ACTH	adrenocorticotrophic hormone
AD	auto-destruct
ADA	adenosine deaminase
ADH	anti-diuretic hormone
AF	atrial fibrillation
AFP	acute flaccid paralysis
AIDS	acquired immunodeficiency syndrome
AKI	acute kidney injury
ALA	amoebic liver abscess
ALL	acute lymphoblastic leukaemia
ALP	alkaline phosphatase
ALS	advanced life support
ALT	alanine transaminase
AML	acute myeloid leukaemia

ANA	anti-nuclear antibodies
ANCA	anti-neutrophil cytoplasmic antibody
AP	antibiotic prophylaxis
APBA	allergic bronchopulmonary aspergillosis
APH	antepartum haemorrhage
APTT	activated partial thromboplastin time
AR	atrial regurgitation
ARB	angiotensin receptor blocker
ARDS	acute respiratory distress syndrome
ARI	acute respiratory infection
ART	anti retroviral therapy
ASD	atrial septal defect
ASOT	anti-streptolysin O titre
AST	aspartate transaminase
ATL	adult T-cell leukaemia/lymphoma
ATN	acute tubular necrosis
ATZ	atazanavir
AXR	abdominal X ray
AV	atrio-ventricular
AVPU	alert, voice, pain, unresponsive
AZT	zidovudine
Ba	barium
BA	bacillary angiomatosis
BAL	broncho-alveolar lavage
BCC	basal cell carcinoma
BCG	Bacille Calmette–Guérin vaccine
BCS	Blantyre Coma Scale
bd	twice daily
BHS	β haemolytic streptococcus
BiPAP	bi-level positive airway pressure
BL	Burkitt's lymphoma
BLS	basic life support
BMI	body mass index
BP	blood pressure
BSA	body surface area
BU	Buruli's ulcer
BV	bacterial vaginosis
BVM	bag, valve, and mask
CA	cancer
CABG	coronary artery bypass grafting

CAP	community-acquired pneumonia
CATT	card agglutination trypanosoma test
CCC	chronic Chagas' cardiomyopathy
CCF	congestive cardiac failure
CCS	Canadian Cardiovascular Society
CD	Chagas' disease
CDC	Centers for Disease Control
CDLE	chronic discoid lupus erythematosus
CHB	Chapter 5
CHW	community health worker
CKD	chronic kidney disease
CL	cutaneous leishmaniasis
CLAT	cryptococcal latex agglutination test
CLD	chronic liver disease
CLL	chronic lymphocytic leukaemia
CLO	columnar-lined oesophagus
CM	cerebral malaria
CML	chronic myeloid leukaemia
CMR	crude mortality rate
CMV	cytomegalovirus
CNS	central nervous system
CO	corneal opacity
COPD	chronic obstructive pulmonary disease
CPAP	constant positive airway pressure
CPD	cephalopelvic disproportion
CPK	creatine phosphokinase
CRAG	cryptococcal antigen test
CRF	chronic renal failure
CRP	C-reactive protein
CRT	capillary refill time
CS	caesarean section
CSF	cerebrospinal fluid
CSW	commercial sex workers
CT	computerized tomography
CVP	central venous pressure
CVS	cardiovascular system
CXR	chest X-ray
D&V	diarrhoea and vomiting
d4T	stavudine
DAEC	diffuse-adherent *E. coli*

DC	direct current
DCL	disseminated cutaneous leishmaniasis
DDAVP	desmopressin
ddI	didanosine
DDT	dichlorodiphenyltrichloroethane
DEC	diethylcarbamazine
DEET	diethyltoluamide
DF	dengue fever
DHF	dengue haemorrhagic fever
DI	diabetes insipidus
DIC	disseminated intravascular coagulation
DILI	drug-induced liver injury
DILS	diffuse inflammatory lymphocytosis syndrome
DIP	distal interphalangeal
DKA	diabetic keto-acidosis
DM	diabetes mellitus
DMARDS	disease-modifying anti-rheumatic drugs
DMSA	dimercaptosuccinic acid (in radionuclide scan)
DOT	directly observed therapy
DOTS	directly observed therapy, short-course
DPL	diagnostic peritoneal lavage
DRV	darunavir
DSS	dengue shock syndrome
DT	combination diphtheria toxoid and tetanus toxoid vaccine for use in children <7yrs
dT	combination tetanus toxoid and low dose diphtheria toxoid vaccine for use in individuals >7yrs
DTaP	combination diphtheria toxoid, tetanus toxoid and acellular pertussis vaccine
DTC	diagnostic testing and counselling
DTP	combination diphtheria toxoid, tetanus toxoid and pertussis vaccine
DU	duodenal ulcer
DVT	deep vein thrombosis
DXM	dexamethasone
E	ethambutol
EAEC	enteroaggregative *E. coli*
EBV	Epstein–Barr virus
ECF	extracellular fluid
ECG	electrocardiogram
ECV	extracellular volume

EEG	electroencephalogram
EEV	equine encephalitis virus
EFZ	efavirenz
EHEC	enterohaemorrhagic *E. coli*
EIA	enzyme immunoassay
EIEC	enteroinvasive *E. coli*
ELISA	enzyme-linked immunosorbent assay
EMS	electrolyte/mineral solution
ENL	*Erythema nodosum leprosum*
ENT	ear, nose and throat
EPEC	enteropathogenic *E. coli*
EPI	expanded programme on immunization
ERCP	endoscopic retrograde cholangiopancreatography
ES	encephalopathic syndrome
ESBL	extended-spectrum beta-lactamase
ESR	erythrocyte sedimentation rate
ETAT	Emergency Triage Assessment and Treatment
ETEC	enterotoxigenic *E. coli*
ETF	early treatment failure
ETR	etravirine
FAR	fever, arthralgia and rash
FB	foreign bodies
FBC	full blood count
FDC	fixed drug combination
FDO	fixed-dose combination
FFP	fresh frozen plasma
FHx	family history
FNAC	fine needle aspirate cytology
FPV	fosamprenavir
FSGS	focal segmental glomerulosclerosis
FSH	follicle-stimulating hormone
FTA	fluorescent *Treponema* antibody
FTC	emtricitabine
G6PD	glucose 6-phosphate dehydrogenase
GAHS	Glasgow alcoholic hepatitis score
GAM	global acute malnutrition
GAVI	Global Alliance for Vaccines and Immunisation
GBM	glomerular basement membrane
GBS	Guillain Barré syndrome
GCS	Glasgow Coma Scale

GFD	general food distribution
GFR	glomerular filtration rate
GH	growth hormone
GI	gastrointestinal
GISA	glycopeptide intermediate *Staph. aureus*
GIT	gastrointestinal tract
GKI	glucose -K+-insulin
GlyI	glycaemic index
GMP	good manufacturing practice
GN	glomerulonephritis
GOR	gastro-oesophageal reflux
GORD	gastro-oesophageal reflux disease
GPI	general paralysis of the insane
GTN	glycerol nitrate
GTT	glucose tolerance test
GU	gastric ulcer
H	haemagglutinin
H/A	height for age
HAART	highly active antiretroviral therapy
HAI	hospital-acquired infections
HAT	human African trypanosomiasis
HAV	hepatitis A virus
Hb	haemoglobin
HBsAg	Hepatitis B surface antigen
HBV	hepatitis B virus
HCC	hepatocellular carcinoma
HCG	human chorionic gonadotrophin
HCT	haematocrit
HCV	hepatitis C virus
HCW	healthcare worker
HD	haemodialysis
HDN	haemorrhagic disease of the newborn
HDU	high dependency unit
HDV	hepatitis D
HepB	Hepatitis B vaccine
HELLP	haemolysis, elevated liver enzymes, low platelets
HF	haemorrhagic fever
HHV	human Herpes virus
Hib	*Haemophilus influenzae* type B vaccine

HIE	hypoxic-ischaemic encephalopathy
HIV-	HIV negative/uninfected
HIV	human immunodeficiency virus
HIV+	HIV positive/infected
HIVAN	HIV-associated nephropathy
HL	Hodgkins lymphoma
HMS	hyperreactive malarial splenomegaly
HOCM	hypertrophic obstructive cardiomyopathy
HONK	hyperglycaemic hyperosmolar non-ketotic coma
HPLC	high performance liquid chromatography
HPV	human papillomavirus
HRS	hepatorenal syndrome
HSP	Henoch–Schönlein purpura
HSV	Herpes simplex virus
HT	hypertension
HTLV-1	human T lymphotrophic virus
HUS	haemolytic uraemic syndrome
HW	health worker
IBD	inflammatory bowel disease
ICP	intracranial pressure
ICS	intercostal space
ICU	intensive care unit
ID	intellectual disability
id	intradermal
IDDM	insulin dependent diabetes mellitus
IDPs	internally displaced populations
IDV	indinavir
IE	infective endocarditis
IGRA	interferon gamma release assay
IHD	ischaemic heart disease
IM	intramuscular
IMCI	integrated management of childhood illness
InfM	infectious mononucleosis
INH	isoniazid
INR	international normalized ration
IOL	induction of labour
IOP	intra-ocular pressure
IPC	infection prevention and control
IPSO	iodized poppy seed oil

IPT	intermittent preventive treatment
IPV	injected polio vaccine (Salk vaccine)
IRIS	immune reconstitution inflammatory syndrome
ITP	idiopathic thrombocytopenic purpura
ITU	intensive care unit
IUD	intra-uterine contraceptive device
IUGR	intrauterine growth retardation
IV	intravenous
IVIG	IV immunoglobulins
IVU	intravenous urogram
JE	Japanese encephalitis
JEV	Japanese encephalitis virus
JVP	jugular venous pressure
K	potassium
KMC	Kangaroo mother care
KPC	*Klebsiella pneumoniae* carbapenemase
KS	Kaposi's sarcoma
KSHV	Kaposi sarcoma-associated herpes virus
KUB	kidney-ureters-bladder
LAP	lower abdominal pain
LBRF	louse borne relapsing fever
LBW	low birth weight
LCF	late clinical failure
LDH	lactate dehydrogenase
LFT	liver function tests
LGV	lymphogranuloma venereum
LH	luteinizing hormone
LIF	left iliac fossa
LIP	lymphocytic interstitial pneumonitis
LL	lepromatous
LMN	lower motor neurone
LN	lymph node
LP	lumbar puncture
LPF	late parasitological failure
LPV	lopinavir
LRTI	lower respiratory tract infection
LT	heat-labile enterotoxin
LTB	laryngotracheobronchitis
LTOT	long-term oxygen therapy
LV	left ventricle

LVF	left ventricular failure
LVH	left ventricular hypertrophy
MAC	*Mycobacterium avium* complex
MALT	mucosa-associated lymphoid tissue
MAM	moderate acute malnutrition
MCH	maternal and child health
MCL	mucocutaneous leishmaniasis
MCMD	minor cognitive motor disorder
MCP	metacarpophalangeal
MCTD	mixed connective tissue disease
MCV	mean corpuscular volume
MDR	multi-drug resistant
MHC	major histocompatibility complex
MI	myocardial infarction
MIC	mean inhibitory concentration
MM	multiple myeloma
MMR	combination measles, mumps, and rubella vaccine
MMRV	combination measles, mumps, and rubella, and varicella
MR	combination measles and rubella vaccine
MR	mitral regurgitation
MRI	magnetic resonance imaging
MRSA	methicillin-resistant *Staphylococcus aureus*
MS	mitral stenosis
MSM	men who have sex with men
MSSA	methicillin sensitive *Staphylococcus aureus*
MSU	mid-stream urine
MTB	*Mycobacterium tuberculosis*
MTCT	mother to child transmission
MTP	metatarsophalangeal
MTX	methotrexate
MUAC	mid-upper arm circumference
MV	mitral valve
MVA	motor vehicle accident
MVacA	manual vacuum aspiration
N	neuraminidase
N&V	nausea and vomiting
Na	sodium
NAAT	nucleic acid amplification test
NG(T)	nasogastric (tube)
NGO	non-governmental organization

NGU	non-gonococcal urethritis
NHL	non-Hodgkins lymphoma
NNRTI	non-nucleoside reverse transcriptase inhibitor
NSAID	non-steroidal anti-inflammatory drug
NtRTI/NRTI	nucleotide/nucleoside reverse transcriptase inhibitors
NTS	non-typhi *Salmonella*
NVP	nevirapine
OA	osteoarthritis
OC	oral contraceptive
od	once daily
OI	opportunistic infection
OHL	oral hairy leukoplakia
OP	organophosphates
OPD	outpatient department
OPSI	overwhelming post-splenectomy infection
OPV	oral polio vaccine (Sabin vaccine)
ORS	oral rehydration solution
ORT	oral rehydration therapy
OTP	outpatient therapeutic nutrition programme
$PaCO_2$	arterial partial pressure of carbon dioxide
PAIR	percutaneous aspiration-injection-respiration
PAM	primary amoebic meningoencephalitis
PAN	polyarteritis nodosa
PaO_2	arterial partial pressure of oxygen
PAS	periodic-acid Schiff
PBC	primary biliary cirrhosis
PC	pneumococcal conjugate vaccine
PCI	percutaneous coronary intervention
PCK	polycystic kidneys
PCNSL	primary central nervous system lymphoma
PCP	*Pneumocystis jiroveci* pneumonia, *pneumocystis* pneumonia
PCR	polymerase chain reaction
PCV	packed cell volume
PD	persistent diarrhoea
PE	pulmonary embolism
PEFR	peak expiratory flow rate
PEL	primary effusion lymphoma
PEP	post-exposure prophylaxis
PF	pemphigus foliaceous

PFTs	pulmonary function tests
PGL	persistent generalized lymphadenopathy
PHT	portal hypertension
PI	protease inhibitor
PID	pelvic inflammatory disease
PIM	post-infective malabsorption
PIP	proximal interphalangeal
PJP	*Pneumocystis jiroveci* pneumonia
PKDL	post-kalar dermal leishmaniasis
pLDH	human lactate dehydrogenase
Plt	platelet count
PML	progressive multifocal leukoencephalopathy
PMTCT	prevention of mother to child transmission (of HIV)
po	'per os' (oral)
POC	products of conception
PPE	personal protective equipment
PPH	postpartum haemorrhage
PPI	proton pump inhibitor
PR	pulse rate
pr	per rectum
PT	prothrombin time
PTB	pulmonary TB
PtD	peritoneal dialysis
PTH	parathyroid hormone
PTSD	post-traumatic stress disorder
pv	per vagina
PVD	peripheral vascular disease
PUD	peptic ulcer disease
q4h	every 4 hours
q12h	every 12 hours
qds	four times a day
R	rifampicin
RA	right atrium
RAL	raltegravir
RAST	radioallergosorbent test
RBBB	right bundle branch block
RBC	red blood cells
RCT	randomized controlled trial
RD	respiratory distress
RDA	recommended daily allowance

RDT	rapid diagnostic test
REM	rapid eye movement
RES	reticuloendothelial system
RespR	respiratory rate
RF	rheumatic fever
RhF	rheumatoid factor
RhA	rheumatoid arthritis
RIF	right iliac fossa
RIG	rabies immunoglobulin
RNA	ribonucleic acid
Rota	rotavirus vaccines
RPR	rapid plasma regain
RR	relative risk
RSV	respiratory syncytial virus
RTV	ritonavir
RUSF	ready to use supplementary foods
RUTF	ready to use therapeutic food
RV	right ventricle
RVF	right ventricular failure
Rx	treatment
SAFE	surgery for trichiasis, antibiotics, facial cleanliness and environmental improvement
SAH	subarachnoid haemorrhage
SAM	severe acute malnutrition
SARS	severe acute respiratory syndrome
SBE	subacute bacterial endocarditis
SBP	spontaneous bacterial peritonitis
sc	sub-cutaneous
SCC	short-course chemotherapy
SqCC	squamous cell carcinoma
SCLE	subacute cutaneous lupus erythematosus
SFP	supplementary feeding programme
SGA	small for gestational age
SIADH	syndrome of inappropriate antidiuretic hormone secretion
SIN	squamous intra-epithelial neoplasia
SIRS	systemic inflammatory response syndrome
SJS	Stevens–Johnson syndrome
SLE	systemic lupus erythematosus
SMX	sulfamethoxazole
SOB	short of breath

SOL	space-occupying lesion
SOP	standard operating procedure
SOS	in an emergency
SP	sulfadoxine-pyrimethamine
SQV	saquinavir
SSI	surgical site infections
SSPE	sub-acute sclerosing panencephalitis
SSRI	selective serotonin reuptake inhibitor
STEMI	ST-elevation MI
STI	sexually-transmitted infection
ST	heat-stable enterotoxin
SVT	supraventricular tachycardia
SXR	skull X-ray
TB	tuberculosis
TBd	tuberculoid
TBM	TB meningitis
TBRF	tick-borne relapsing fever
TCA	tricyclic antidepressant
TCBS	thiosulfate-citrate-bile salts-sucrose agar
TDF	tenofovir
tds	three times a day
TEN	toxic epidermal necrolysis
TetT	tetanus toxoid vaccine
TF	trachomatous inflammation—follicular
TFP	therapeutic feeding programme
TFT	thyroid function tests
TI	trachomatous inflammation—intense
TIA	transient ischaemic attack
TIBC	total iron-binding capacity
TIPS	transjugular intrahepatic portosystemic shunting
TMP	trimethoprim
tPA	tissue plasminogen activator
TPE	tropical pulmonary eosinophilia
TPHA	*Treponema pallidum* haemagglutination assay
TR	tricuspid regurgitation
TS	trachomatous scarring
TSH	thyroid-stimulating hormone
TSP	tropical spastic paraparesis
TST	tuberculin skin test
TT	trachomatous trichiasis

TTP	thrombotic thrombocytopenic purpura
U&E	urea & electrolytes
U5MR	under-five mortality rate
ULN	upper limit of normal
UMN	upper motor neurone
UNHCR	United Nations High Commission on Refugees
URTI	upper respiratory tract infection
US	ultrasound
USS	ultrasound scan
UTI	urinary tract infection
UV	ultraviolet
UVC	umbilical vein catheter
VA	Visual acuity
VCT	voluntary counselling and testing
VDRL	syphilis serology (veneral diseases research laboratory)
VF	ventricular fibrillation
VHF	viral haemorrhagic fever
VIM	*Verona imipenemase*
VKDB	vitamin K deficient bleeding
VL	viral load
VMA	vanillyl mandelic acid
VRE	vancomycin resistant enterococcus
VSD	ventriculoseptal defect
VSP	very severe
VSW	visible severe wasting
VT	ventricular tachycardia
VUR	vesico-ureteric reflux
VVM	vaccine vial monitor
VZV	Varicella zoster virus
W/A	weight for age
W/H	weight for height
WBC	white blood cell count
WCC	white cell count
WDM	whole dried milk
WHO	World Health Organization
XDR	extensively drug resistant
YF	yellow fever
Z	pyrazinamide
ZN	Ziehl–Nielsen (stain for acid fast bacilli)

Contributors

Dwomoa Adu (Chapter 9)
Department of Medicine and Therapeutics
University of Ghana Medical School, Accra, Ghana

Alexander Aiken (Chapter 25)
Department of Infectious Disease Epidemiology
London School of Hygiene and Tropical Medicine
London, UK;
KEMRI-Wellcome Trust Research Programme, Nairobi, Kenya

Samuel Akech (Chapter 1)
KEMRI-Wellcome Trust Research Programme, Kilifi, Kenya

Theresa Allain (Chapter 12)
Department of Medicine
College of Medicine
University of Malawi
Blantyre, Malawi

Tania C. Araujo-Jorge (Chapter 18)
Instituto Oswaldo Cruz,
Rio de Janeiro, Brazil

James A. Berkley (Chapters 1 and 17)
Nuffield Department of Medicine
University of Oxford, UK;
KEMRI-Wellcome Trust Research Programme
Kilifi, Kenya

Bernadette E. Brent (Chapter 1)
Department of Paediatrics,
St Mary's Hospital
London, UK; KEMRI-Wellcome Trust Research Programme
Kilifi, Kenya

Subarna Chakravorty (Chapter 11)
Department of Paediatric Haematology, Imperial College Healthcare NHS Trust,
London, UK

François Chappuis (Chapter 18)
International and Humanitarian Medicine
Department of Community Medicine and Primary Care
Geneva University Hospitals
Geneva, Switzerland

Cecilia Chung (Chapter 18)
Division of Rheumatology
Department of Medicine
Vanderbilt University
Nashville, USA

Nick Day (Chapter 2)
Oxford University Clinical Research Unit, Wellcome Trust Major Overseas Programme, Vietnam; Hospital for Tropical Diseases, Ho Chi Minh City, Vietnam;
Centre for Tropical Medicine, University of Oxford, UK

Michael Eddleston (Chapter 21)
Clinical Pharmacology Unit
University of Edinburgh, UK;
Department of International Health, Immunology and Microbiology
University of Copenhagen, Denmark

Lee Fairlie (Chapter 3)
Wits Reproductive Health and HIV Institute
University of the Witwatersrand
Johannesburg, South Africa

Jeremy Farrar (Chapter 10)
Oxford University Clinical Research Unit
Vietnam Hospital for Tropical Diseases;
South East Asia Infectious Diseases Clinical Research Network;
Global Scholar Princeton University, USA;
London School of Hygiene and Tropical Medicine;
Hospital for Tropical Diseases
Ho Chi Minh City, Vietnam

John Frean (Chapter 18)
Centre for Opportunistic, Tropical and Hospital Infections
National Institute for Communicable Diseases
Johannesburg, South Africa;
School of Pathology
University of the Witwatersrand
Johannesburg, South Africa

Sara Ghorashian (Chapter 11)
London, UK

Stephen Gordon (Chapter 5)
Respiratory Medicine & ARI
Liverpool School of Tropical Medicine, Liverpool, UK

Kevin Griffith (Chapter 18)
Centers for Disease Control & Prevention Atlanta, Georgia, USA

Sally Hamour (Chapter 9)
Imperial College London, UK

Charlotte Hanlon (Chapter 19)
Department of Psychiatry
School of Medicine
College of Health Sciences
Addis Ababa University
Ethiopia;
Institute of Psychiatry
King's College London, UK

Bryn Kemp (Chapter 24)
New Training Building
KEMRI-Wellcome Trust
CGMR—Coast
Kilifi, Kenya

Angela Koech (Chapter 24)
KEMRI-Wellcome Trust Research Programme, Kilifi, Kenya

Diana Lockwood (Chapter 10)
London School of Hygiene & Tropical Medicine
London, UK

Bongani Mayosi (Chapter 8)
Department of Medicine
University of Cape Town
Groote Schuur Hospital
Cape Town, South Africa

Marc Mendelson (Chapter 7)
Division of Infectious Diseases and HIV Medicine
University of Cape Town
Groote Schuur Hospital
Cape Town, South Africa

Graeme Meintjes (Chapter 3)
Institute of Infectious Diseases and Molecular Medicine
Observatory, Cape Town
South Africa

Susan Morpeth (Chapter 25)
KEMRI-Wellcome Trust Research Programme
Kilifi, Kenya;
Nuffield Department of Clinical Medicine
University of Oxford, UK

Ben Naafs (Chapter 14)
Nuffield Department of Obstetrics and Gynaecology
University of Oxford, UK;
KEMRI-Wellcome Trust Research Programme, Kilifi, Kenya

Charles Newton (Chapter 10)
Department of Psychiatry
University of Oxford, UK

Marc Nicol (Chapter 18)
University of Cape Town
Groote Schuur Hospital
Cape Town, South Africa

Sam Nightingale (Chapter 18)
Department of Neurological Science and Institute of Infection and Global Health, University of Liverpool, UK

Andy Parrish (Chapter 3)
Department of Internal Medicine
Walter Sisulu University
Umtata, South Africa;
Department of Internal Medicine
East London Hospital Complex
Eastern Cape Province, South Africa

Chris Parry (Chapter 18)
Mahidol Oxford Tropical Medicine Research Unit
Faculty of Tropical Medicine
Mahidol University
Bangkok, Thailand;
Centre for Tropical Medicine
Nuffield Department of Medicine
Churchill Hospital
University of Oxford, UK

Vikram Patel (Chapter 19)
London School of Hygiene and Tropical Medicine
Sangath, India;
Public Health Foundation of India
Sangath Centre, Goa, India

Sharon Peacock (Chapter 18)
University of Cambridge, UK

Mary E. Penny (Chapter 6)
Instituto de Investigación Nutricional, Lima, Peru;
Lecturer on Pediatrics,
Harvard University, Boston, USA

Erwan Piriou (Chapter 18)
Public Health Department
Médecins Sans Frontières
Amsterdam, The Netherlands

Koert Ritmeijer (Chapter 23)
Public Health Department
Médecins Sans Frontières
Amsterdam, The Netherlands

Fulton P. Rivera (Chapter 6)
Instituto de Medicina Tropical Alexander von Humboldt,
Universidad Peruana Cayetano Heredia, Lima, Peru

Matthew D. Snape (Chapter 22)
Oxford University Hospitals NHS Trust
Oxford Biomedical Research Centre
Oxford Vaccine Group
Department of Paediatrics
University of Oxford, UK

Tom Solomon (Chapter 18)
Neurological Science
Liverpool Brain Infections Group
Institute of Infection and Global Health
University of Liverpool, UK

Robert Spencer (Chapter 18)
HPA Regional Laboratory
Bristol Royal Infirmary,
Bristol, UK

Charles M. Stein (Chapter 18)
Division of Clinical Pharmacology
Vanderbilt Medical School
Nashville, USA

Yupin Suputtamongkol (Chapter 18)
Division of Infectious Diseases and Tropical Medicine
Department of Medicine, Faculty of Medicine
Siriraj Hospital, Mahidol University
Bangkok, Thailand

Nguyen Thi Hoang Mai (Chapter 10)
Oxford University Clinical Research Unit & Hospital for Tropical Diseases, Ho Chi Minh City, Vietnam

Jenny Thompson (Chapter 20)
John Radcliffe Hospital
Oxford, UK

Jonathan Underwood (Chapter 15)
Department of Infectious Diseases & Tropical Medicine
Northwick Park Hospital
London, UK

Colette van Hees (Chapter 14)
Department of Dermatology
Erasmus Medical Centre
Rotterdam, The Netherlands

David Warrell (Chapters 10 and 21)
University of Oxford, UK;
Royal College of Physicians, London, UK

Douglas A. Wilkinson (Chapter 20)
Nuffield Department of Anaesthetics
University of Oxford, UK

Robert J. Wilkinson (Chapter 4)
National Institute for Medical Research UK
Imperial College London, UK;
Wolfson Pavilion
Institute of Infectious Diseases and Molecular Medicine
University of Cape Town
Cape Town, South Africa

Henrietta Williams (Chapter 16)
Melbourne Sexual Health Centre Alfred Health, and Sexual Health Unit, Melbourne School of Population Health, University of Melbourne, Victoria, Australia

David Yorston (Chapter 13)
Gartnavel Hospital
Glasgow, UK

Chapter 1

Management of the sick child

Invited authors

Samuel Akech

Bernadette E. Brent

James A. Berkley

Introduction

Of the 9 million deaths/yr that occur in children <5yrs, 3.6 million occur in the 1st month of life and 70% of the others are caused by acute respiratory infections, diarrhoea, measles, and malaria, +/– malnutrition. Most very sick children present with clinical features of more than one diagnosis; ∴ a single diagnosis at admission is often impossible. In many low-resource settings, there may be no paediatrician and sick children are managed by non-specialists.

Deaths in hospitals often occur within the first 24h, so sick children need to be identified on arrival, and appropriate treatment instituted. The Emergency Triage Assessment and Treatment (ETAT) strategy, advocated by WHO, is a rapid screening process to identify children who require immediate treatment to avert death and long-term morbidity. Treatment of sick children must never be on a 'first come, first served' basis. WHO has published guidelines for the management of common childhood illnesses (second edition 2013), available online (see Box 1.1).

Box 1.1 WHO online paediatric publications

- *Pocket book of hospital care for children: guidelines for the management of common illnesses with limited resources.* Available at: http://www.who.int/maternal_child_adolescent/documents/child_hospital_care/en/index.html
- *Emergency triage, assessment and treatment: manual for participants.* Available at: http://www.who.int/maternal_child_adolescent/documents/9241546875/en/
    - Developed by the World Health Organization (WHO), for rapid screening of sick children to identify those with emergency, priority, or non-urgent signs (triage), and to instigate immediate treatment for children with emergency signs.
    - Children should be prioritized on presence of emergency signs, rather than on a 'first come first served' basis.
    - All health workers should triage and follow ABCD approach (airway, breathing, circulation/coma/convulsions, and dehydration).
    - Disease-specific treatment should be started after managing ABCD.
- *Integrated management of childhood illness (IMCI).* Available at: http://www.who.int/maternal_child_adolescent/documents/imci/en/
    - IMCI uses a syndromic approach, combining management of individual diseases with nutrition, immunization, and maternal health. It aims to improve the skills of healthcare workers (HCWs).
    - 'Danger signs' are first identified. Children are then assigned defined clinical syndromes on the basis of simple questions and a basic clinical examination; more than one syndrome may be assigned.
- The severity of each syndrome is defined and management directed: either urgent referral to a secondary care facility, treatment, and advice, or advice to the parent/caregiver for home management.
- IMCI is targeted at HCWs in health centres and outpatient departments of small hospitals. This can be extended to include community health workers, shopkeepers, and pharmacists, who are often the first port of call for medical advice.
- IMCI has improved healthcare seeking behaviour, rational prescribing, immunization coverage, and availability of basic equipment, and has also reduced costs.
- Bigger reductions in mortality should result from combining IMCI with key programmes, such as the WHO pneumonia and diarrhoea case management strategies.

Emergency triage assessment

Immediately on presentation to a health facility (i.e. *before* joining a queue), children should be rapidly triaged to identify those with:

- *Emergency signs:* require immediate treatment to prevent death (see Box 1.2; 📖 Emergency management of the sick child—ABC, p. 8).
- *Priority signs:* should be assessed and treated without delay (Box 1.3).
- *Non-urgent cases* that have neither emergency nor priority signs who should follow the regular queue.

Triage should be carried out at the first point of contact; this may be at the outpatient clinic, the emergency room, or even in a hospital paediatric ward. All children must be assessed for these signs *before* any routine procedures like registration and weighing.

Assess airway and breathing

- Look, listen, and feel for chest movement, exhaled air, and breathing sounds by placing your ear close to the child's nostrils.
- Check for respiratory distress and signs of airway obstruction (Box 1.4).
- Check the tongue and buccal mucosa for central cyanosis.
- Do not move neck if cervical injury is possible, e.g. following trauma. Use jaw thrust manoeuvre to open the airway if needed.

Box 1.2 Emergency signs

- Central cyanosis.
- Severe respiratory distress.
- Obstructed breathing.
- Altered level of consciousness.
- Convulsions.
- Signs of shock.
- Signs of severe dehydration in a child with diarrhoea.

Box 1.3 Priority signs

- Any sick child aged <2mths.
- Visible severe wasting; oedema affecting both feet.
- *High fever:* temperature >38.5°C.
- Irritability, restlessness, lethargy.
- Severe palmar pallor.
- Major burns.
- Any respiratory distress.
- Child with urgent referral note from the health facility.
- Trauma or urgent surgical condition.
- Poisoning.
- Severe pain.

Box 1.4 Signs of severe respiratory distress

- Lower chest wall indrawing (Fig. 1.1).
- Grunting.
- Inability to speak, drink, or feed due to respiratory distress.
- Head nodding/use of accessory muscles of respiration.

Other signs of respiratory distress

- *Fast breathing:* ≥60 breaths/min in infants <2mths; ≥50/min in children 2–11mths; ≥40/min in children 12mths to 5yr.
- Nasal flaring.

Signs of obstructed breathing

- Stridor.
- Weak cough.
- Drooling.
- Inability to speak.
- Splinted chest.

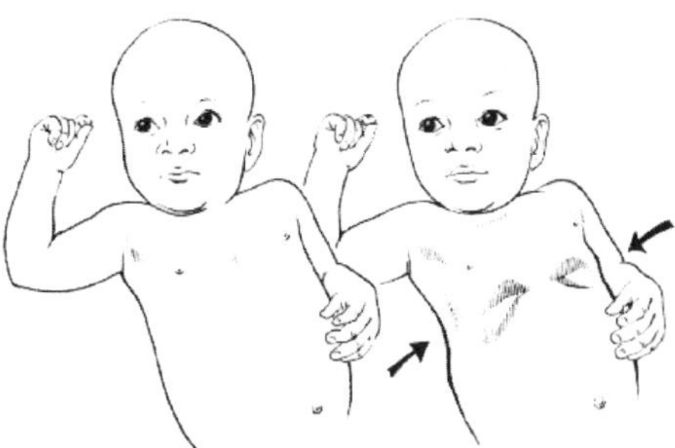

Fig. 1.1 Lower chest wall indrawing: with inspiration the lower chest wall moves in. (Note the distinction between lower chest wall *indrawing* and *intercostal recession*, in which the soft tissue between the ribs is sucked inwards on inspiration. Although intercostal recession may occur in respiratory distress, alone, it is not a sign of severe respiratory distress.)

Reproduced from World Health Organization, *Pocket Book of Hospital Care for Children*, 2005: 74, with permission of WHO.

Assess circulation for signs of shock

- Check if child's hands are cold.
- *Assess capillary refill time (CRT):* apply pressure to whiten nail of thumb or big toe for 5s. Release pressure and note how long it takes nail bed to refill and turn pink; CRT ≥3s usually a sign of shock or dehydration.
- *Check pulse:* if radial pulse not palpable, feel for brachial or femoral pulse in infant, or carotid pulse in older children. In hypovolaemic shock, central pulses may be weak and rapid, or absent. In septic (distributive) shock you may find warm peripheries, CRT <1s and bounding pulse.

- *Blood pressure:* if able to measure blood pressure (BP) you may see a wide pulse pressure, but measurement of BP is difficult in children (important to have correct cuff size), and low BP is a late clinical sign.
- WHO definition of shock is given in Box 1.5.

Assess for coma, convulsions, or other abnormal mental status

- Check for continued irritability, restlessness, lethargy, or convulsions.
- Assess level of consciousness using AVPU scale (Box 1.6) or Blantyre Coma Scale.

Assess for severe dehydration if child has diarrhoea

- Check with mother if the child's eyes are unusually sunken.
- Assess skin turgor by pinching skin of abdomen halfway between umbilicus and flank. Pinch for 1s and observe how the skin returns. >2s implies marked loss of skin turgor.
- Severe dehydration is defined as ≥2 of the following: lethargy or unconsciousness; sunken eyes; marked loss of skin turgor; inability to drink or drinking poorly.
- Signs of severe dehydration are unreliable in children with severe malnutrition and management should be guided by a history of diarrhoea or change in appearance.
- See Box 1.7 for calculation of maintenance fluids.

Assess for signs of severe malnutrition

- Examine for severe muscle wasting, especially around ribs, shoulders, arms, buttocks, and thighs.
- Assess mid-upper arm circumference (MUAC): if <11.5cm (age 6mths–6yr) or bilateral pedal oedema +/– other signs of kwashiorkor. Treat as severe malnutrition.

Assess for severe anaemia

Compare the colour of the child's palm with yours: if the skin is very pale or so pale that it looks white, the child has severe palmar pallor.

Assess for a major burn

See 📖 Burns, p. 868.

Assess for other priority indicators

- All sick infants <2mths.
- All children referred from another health facility.

Box 1.5 WHO defined shock

Cold hands *and* CRT >3s, *and* weak, fast pulse.

Signs of hypovolaemic shock (e.g. due to dehydration)

- Temperature gradient (peripheries much colder than trunk).
- CRT >3s.
- Fast, weak pulse.

Signs of distributive shock (e.g. due to sepsis)

- Warm hands and feet: no temperature gradient.
- CRT <1s.
- Bounding pulses.
- Large pulse pressure with low diastolic pressure.

Also note

- Anuria.
- Hypotension is a late sign in children.
- Altered level of consciousness.
- Acidotic (Kussmaul) breathing 2° to poor tissue perfusion.

Box 1.6 AVPU scale

The AVPU scale is a quick and approximate way of rating a person's level of consciousness:

- **A** Alert.
- **V** Responds to verbal commands.
- **P** Responds to painful stimulus. Press down firmly on the middle fingernail with a pen, or rub your knuckles on the sternum.
- **U** Unconscious.

Box 1.7 Calculating maintenance fluids in children

- If oral or NG feeds are tolerated, these are usually preferable to giving intravenous (IV) fluids.
- For children, total daily maintenance IV fluid requirement is calculated with the following formula:
  - 100mL/kg for the first 10kg.
  - 50mL/kg for the next 10kg.
  - 25mL/kg for each subsequent kg.
- For example, a 6-kg infant receives 6 × 100mL = 600mL/day, an 18-kg child (10 × 100) + (8 × 50) = 1400mL/day.
- An alternative formula is to use 4mL/kg/h for the first 10kg, 2mL/kg/h for the second 10kg and 1mL/kg/h for each subsequent kg. For example, a 6-kg infant receives 6 × 4mL/h = 24mL/h, an 18-kg child (4 × 10) + (2 × 8) = 56mL/h.
- For neonates, see feed and fluid requirements (📖 Fluid requirements, p. 20). Fluid requirements may be higher in febrile children, and in hot environments.

Emergency management of the sick child—ABC

If emergency signs are present, call for help and give emergency treatment:

Airway and breathing

- Severe respiratory distress, obstructed breathing, or central cyanosis is an emergency.
- If there is a history or evidence of foreign body aspiration, manage as for a choking child (see 🕮 Foreign body aspiration in an unconscious child, p. 9).
- Open airway using head tilt and chin lift: in infants the 'tilt' should be to the neutral position to avoid obstruction of the airway due to hyperextension. In older children, tilt the head to the 'sniffing' position (see Fig. 1.2).
- If this fails to open the airway (or if you suspect cervical spine injury), use the jaw thrust manoeuvre to open the airway: place the first two fingers of each hand behind each side of the child's mandible and push the jaw forward.
- Inspect the mouth and remove any visible foreign body.
- Clear secretions from oropharynx (use suction if available).
- If inadequate or no spontaneous respiratory effort, use bag, valve, and mask (BVM) ventilation: 40–60 breaths/min in newborns and a slower rate in older children.
- Where expertise/facilities exist, endotracheal intubation should be performed. However, attempted intubation by the inexperienced must not compromise adequate BVM ventilation.

Foreign body aspiration in a choking, conscious child

- If the child has an effective cough, encourage coughing and continually reassess for clinical deterioration or relief of the obstruction.
- If NO effective cough, or there is severe respiratory distress, obstructed breathing, or central cyanosis, manage as for choking child.
- Position infant head down and give up to 5 sharp back blows between the shoulder blades using the heel of the hand as shown in Fig. 1.3.
- If obstruction persists:
  - If <1yr, give five chest thrusts using two fingers (Fig. 1.3), similar to chest compressions, but sharper and at a slower rate.
  - If >1yr, if obstruction persists, perform the Heimlich manoeuvre (Fig. 1.3): stand behind the child and form a fist below the sternum with one hand. Place other hand over fist and pull both hands backwards and upwards. Repeat manoeuvre 5 times.
  - If obstruction persists, check infant's mouth for any obstruction that can be removed and repeat this sequence, starting with back blows.

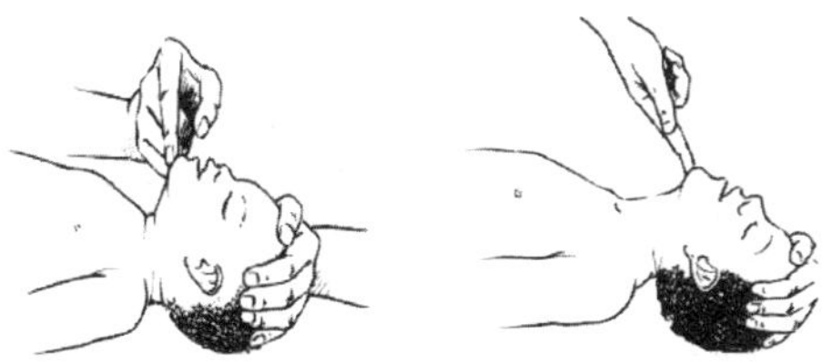

Fig. 1.2 (A) Neutral position in infants (B) 'Sniffing' position in older child.
Reproduced from World Health Organization, *Pocket Book of Hospital Care for Children* 2005: 8, with permission of WHO.

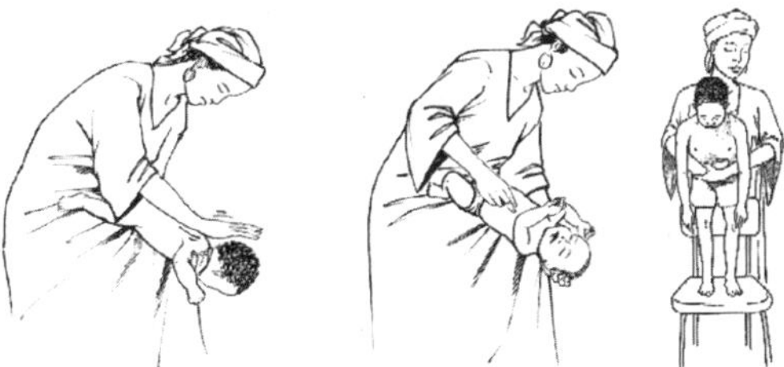

Fig. 1.3 Back blows and chest thrusts to relieve airway obstruction in a choking infant. Heimlich manoeuvre in an older choking child.
Reproduced from World Health Organization, *Pocket Book of Hospital Care for Children* 2005: 6–7, with permission of WHO.

Foreign body aspiration in an unconscious child

If infant/child with a foreign body aspiration is or becomes unconscious, call for help, place on a flat surface, and proceed with airway, breathing, circulation/coma/convulsions (ABC). Open the airway and remove any visible object and attempt 5 rescue breaths. If no response, proceed with chest compressions as detailed on 📖 Foreign body aspiration in a choking, conscious child, p. 8. When you re-assess A, check for any removable foreign body. If obstruction has been relieved, continue giving rescue breaths until the child is breathing spontaneously.

Circulation and shock

- Remember ABC and give oxygen; **shock is an emergency** (Box 1.8).
- Assess for WHO defined shock (cold hands *and* CRT >3s, *and* weak, fast pulse). ❗ This is a contentious area: see Box 1.5 for children who do not fulfil WHO definition of shock.
- Insert IV line (blood for Hb/haematocrit, glucose and cross-match).
- If unable to establish peripheral IV access quickly, insert external jugular or intraosseous line (Fig. 1.4), whichever is quicker.
- Fluid resuscitate for WHO defined shock according to guidelines listed below, unless severely malnourished, which is managed differently (see 🕮 Management of shock in children with severe malnutrition, p. 12).
- Stop bleeding; look for severe palmar pallor (severe anaemia, Box 1.9).
- Ensure child is warm.
- Monitor blood glucose levels whilst fluid resuscitating.

Management of shock in children who fulfil WHO definition of shock and are NOT severely malnourished

Fluid resuscitate rapidly

- Give 20mL/kg bolus (normal saline or Ringer's lactate) as rapidly as possible, then reassess.
- If no improvement, give a second 20mL/kg fluid bolus (blood 20mL/kg over 30min if child is bleeding and it is available) then reassess.
- If still no improvement and signs of dehydration or septic shock, give a third 20mL/kg bolus as rapidly as possible. Otherwise management is guided by the working diagnosis.

If improvement occurs at any stage (pulse slower, CRT faster)

- Assess need for rehydration.
- If no rehydration needed, give maintenance IV fluids.
- If dehydrated or history of profuse diarrhoea, give 70mL/kg Ringer's lactate or normal saline over 5h if <12mths and over 2.5h if 12mths–5yr.
- Continue to assess the child every 1–2h. Some children may deteriorate after initial recovery.
- Give oral rehydration solution (🕮 ORS, p. 279) 5mL/kg/h as soon as child can drink.
- Follow appropriate treatment plan A, B, or C for dehydration (see 🕮 Diarrhoeal diseases, p. 233) based on this assessment.

Box 1.8 Treatment of shock

A recent large randomized controlled trial (RCT) comparing fluid bolus resuscitation to IV maintenance fluid in children in Africa with clinical features of shock, showed increased mortality in those treated with fluid boluses. The study did not include children with hypotension, severe acute malnutrition or gastroenteritis. The study also showed that WHO defined shock is rare in the population studied and did not demonstrate evidence for harm in children with WHO defined shock.

Children with WHO defined shock should be resuscitated according to WHO guidelines (p. 10). For children with gastroenteritis, rehydrate according to WHO guidelines (General management of dehydration, p. 272) and for children with severe acute malnutrition (SAM) treat shock as per WHO guideline (Management of shock in children with severe malnutrition, p. 12). In children with some features of shock, but not fulfilling the WHO definition, treatment of their underlying condition is the priority. Maintenance fluids should be given, and giving additional fluids cannot be recommended.

Maitland K, Kiguli S, Opoka RO, *et al.* Mortality after fluid bolus in African children with severe infection. *N Engl J Med* 2011; **364**(26): 2483–95. Available at: http://www.nejm.org/doi/full/10.1056/NEJMoa1101549

Box 1.9 Children with severe anaemia and shock

Do not delay fluid resuscitation, resuscitate as required per guidelines on p. 10, while awaiting blood for transfusion.

- Obtain blood for Hb/haematocrit, cross-match (and malaria slide in endemic areas) in all children with severe palmar pallor.
- If Hb <4g/dL, or haematocrit <12%, or Hb result not available quickly and clinical signs of severe anaemia, transfuse 20mL/kg whole blood.
- *In the presence of very severe palmar pallor and shock*, consider urgent transfusion with O -ve blood.

Box 1.10 Cardiac arrest

Unlike in adults, most arrests in young children are 1° respiratory arrests +/– 2° cardiac arrest. As a result, adequate ventilation alone is sufficient to maintain cardiac output in most cases, while the cause of the arrest is identified and treated.

If there is also cardiac arrest requiring chest compressions:

- Give ratio 3:1 compressions to breaths in neonates.
- Give a ratio of 15:2 in infants and children.

Drugs

If no response after 2min, administer IV or intraosseous adrenaline 0.1mL/kg of 1:10 000 solution (10microgram/kg) and continue chest compressions and ventilation. This may be repeated after 3–5min if there is no response. In newborns the preferred access is through an umbilical vein catheter (UVC).

Management of shock in children with severe malnutrition

WHO recommended treatment for children with severe malnutrition, signs of shock and who are lethargic or have lost consciousness. See 📖 Nutrition, p. 683, for treatment of dehydration in severe acute malnutrition.

- Signs of shock and dehydration are less reliable in children with severe malnutrition.
- Types of fluid, volumes, and rates of administration are different to those used in well-nourished children.
- 💣 Giving too much IV fluid can → overload if cardiac output is impaired. They cannot excrete Na^+ load. This is a contentious area and further studies are awaited.
- Never use diuretics to treat the oedema of kwashiorkor as this will extract fluid from the intravascular space only.

At the start of treatment

- Weigh the child (or estimate weight) to calculate fluid requirements.
- Record pulse rate (PR) and respiratory rate (RR).
- Assess and treat hypoglycaemia (5mL/kg of 10% dextrose). If unable to measure glucose, assume there is hypoglycaemia.
- *For WHO-defined shock:* infuse 15mL/kg IV fluid over 1h. Use (in order of preference) Ringer's lactate with 5% glucose, half-normal saline with 5% glucose, or half-strength Darrow's solution with 5% glucose. Use Ringer's lactate if these are not available.
- Monitor PR and RR every 5–10min.
- If child deteriorates during IV rehydration (RR ↑ by 5/min or PR ↑ by 15/min or ↑ oedema or facial puffiness), stop the infusion.

If there are signs of improvement (PR & RR ↓)

- Repeat 15mL/kg IV bolus over 1h.
- Then switch to oral or NG feeds if not comatose. Give hourly feeds, 10mL/kg/h alternating ReSoMal with F75.
- Assess 2–3-h hydration status and continue the hourly rehydration to a maximum of 10h (be careful not to overload).
- Continue feeding with F75.

If there are still no signs of improvement

- Give maintenance IV fluids while waiting for blood.
- Transfuse 10mL/kg fresh whole blood slowly over 3h; give packed cells if fluid overload/heart failure; consider furosemide during transfusion.
- Start frequent small feeds with F75, or alternative low lactose and low osmolarity preparation (📖 Nutrition, p. 683).

In all cases, proceed to full assessment and management of severe malnutrition, including broad-spectrum antibiotic therapy (📖 Diarrhoeal diseases, p. 233).

Box 1.11 Intraosseous needle insertion

Intraosseous infusion is a quick, safe, and reliable method of giving fluid, blood and drugs when it is not possible to establish peripheral venous access. The usual site of insertion is the proximal tibia (Fig. 1.4):

- Place padding under child's knee so that it is flexed ~30° from the straight position with the heel resting on the bed.
- Identify the insertion site 1–2cm below the tibial tuberosity, midway between the anterior ridge of the tibia and its medial edge.
- Use a dedicated intraosseous or bone marrow aspiration needle (15–18 gauge or, if not available, 21 gauge); if neither available, a large bore hypodermic needle may be used in young children.
- Clean the skin with antiseptic solution.
- Stabilize the leg, grasping thigh and knee above and lateral to the cannulation site with non-dominant hand, taking care to keep hand away from cannulation site to avoid needle-stick injury.
- Using aseptic technique, insert needle with point angled slightly away from the joint space and bevel pointing towards foot.
- Advance needle using a gentle, but firm twisting or drilling motion, until there is a sudden ↓ in resistance as it enters marrow cavity; needle should sit firmly in the bone.
- Remove the stylet, attach a syringe, aspirate marrow contents (looks like blood), and flush with normal saline to confirm needle is in marrow cavity. Blood from marrow aspirate may be sent for full blood count (FBC), biochemistry, malaria slide, and cross-match.
- Apply dressing and secure needle in place. It is now ready to use.
- Stop the intraosseous infusion as soon as venous access is available.

Contraindications

Infection at the insertion site; fracture of the bone.

Alternative sites of insertion

Distal femur, 2cm above the lateral condyle (~ 1–2cm proximal to the superior border of the patella), slightly lateral to anterior ridge.

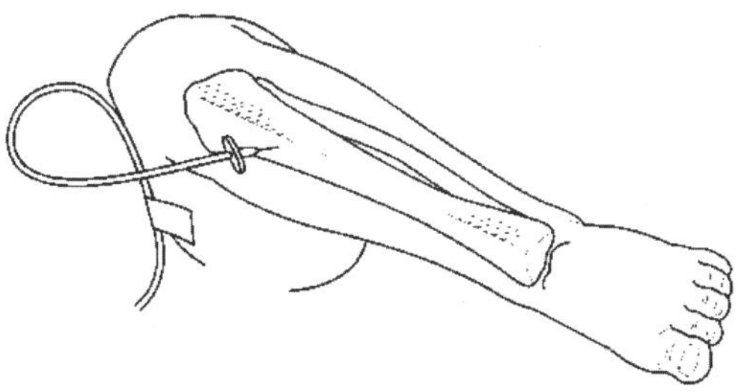

Fig. 1.4 Intraosseous needle insertion.

Reproduced from World Health Organization, *Pocket Book of Hospital Care for Children* 2005: 311, with permission of WHO.

Coma and convulsions

The presence of coma or convulsions is an emergency.

Manage airway, breathing and circulation

See 📖 Emergency management of the sick child—ABC, p. 8), assess and treat hypoglycaemia.

If convulsing

- Give diazepam 0.5mg/kg rectally or midazolam (buccal) 0.3mg/kg (1–6mth), 2.5mg (6mth–1yr), 5mg (1–5yr).
- If still convulsing after 10 min, give 2nd dose of diazepam or midazolam, or if IV access: diazepam 0.25mg/kg IV.
- If still convulsing after a further 10min, give paraldehyde 0.3–0.4mL/kg rectally, or phenobarbital 15mg/kg IV (as slow infusion over 20min) or IM (*Note:* peak concentration reached 1–4h after intramuscular (IM) administration). In infants <2wks old, give phenobarbital 20mg/kg as slow IV infusion.
- To prevent aspiration, avoid oral medications until the convulsions have terminated and the child is alert.

Note: seizures, especially in children with malaria, may be very subtle, comprising one or more of irregular respiration, nystagmus, or twitching of extremities or lips.

If unconscious

- Position in the left lateral 'recovery' position. If head or neck trauma is suspected, stabilize the neck first and keep the child lying on the back.
- Tepid sponge and administer antipyretics if high fever.
- Assess and treat the treatable: hypoglycaemia, poisoning, diabetes mellitus, septicaemia/meningitis, herpes simplex encephalitis.

Hypoglycaemia

Assess and treat hypoglycaemia

- If lethargic or unconscious, measure blood glucose.
- If unable to measure glucose quickly, or if blood glucose <2.5mmol/L in a well-nourished child (<3mmol/L in severe malnutrition), give 5mL/kg 10% glucose rapidly IV.
- If alert, treat hypoglycaemia with 10mL/kg milk or 10% glucose by mouth or NG tube (NGT).
- Recheck blood glucose level after 2 hours.

Nutritional status

Assess and treat severe malnutrition 📖 Nutrition, p. 683.

Further assessment and diagnosis

After triage assessment complete clinical assessment. Common acute problems in children are:

- Lethargy, ↓ level of consciousness, or convulsions.
- Cough, wheeze, or difficulty breathing.
- Diarrhoea.
- Fever.

Common problems that present less acutely include:
- Chronic cough ≥30 days.
- Fever lasting >7 days.

Major differential diagnoses for each clinical presentation

Causes of lethargy, impaired consciousness, or convulsions
- Meningitis 🕮 Neurology, p. 429.
- Cerebral malaria 🕮 Malaria, p. 33.
- Febrile convulsions (see Box 1.12).
- Hypoglycaemia (see 🕮 Hypoglycaemia, p. 14).
- Head injury 🕮 Neurology, p. 429.
- Poisoning/overdose 🕮 Poisoning and envenoming, p. 871.
- Sepsis (unlikely to cause convulsions unless meningitis).
- Shock (unlikely to cause convulsions).
- Acute glomerulonephritis with encephalopathy 🕮 Renal medicine, p. 403.
- Diabetic ketoacidosis 🕮 Endocrinology and biochemistry, p. 537.

Causes of difficulty breathing +/– cough
- Pneumonia 🕮 Chest medicine, p. 180.
- Severe anaemia.
- Malaria 🕮 Malaria, p. 33.
- Cardiac failure 🕮 Cardiovascular medicine, p. 365.
- Congenital heart disease.
- Inhaled foreign body (see 🕮 Emergency management of the sick child—ABC, p. 8).
- Tuberculosis 🕮 Tuberculosis, p. 151.
- Pertussis 🕮 Chest medicine, p. 200.
- Prematurity 🕮 Surfactant deficiency.

Causes of wheeze
- Asthma 🕮 Chest medicine, p. 214.
- Bronchiolitis 🕮 Chest medicine, p. 197.
- Viral upper respiratory tract infection (URTI).
- Pneumonia 🕮 Chest medicine, p. 180.
- Inhaled foreign body (🕮 Emergency management of the sick child—ABC, p. 8).

Causes of diarrhoea See 🕮 Diarrhoeal diseases, p. 233.
- *Infections:* viral, bacterial, and parasitic.
- Severe malnutrition.
- Malabsorption.
- Antibiotic related diarrhoea.
- Intussusception (Box 1.13).

Causes of fever without localizing signs
In most children with fever, cause is clinically apparent. Examine upper airways (viral URTI, otitis media, tonsillitis) and joints (septic arthritis), as well as the major systems (pneumonia, meningitis). Examine skin for infection or a rash (e.g. measles). In absence of localizing signs, consider:
- Malaria 🕮 Malaria, p. 33.
- Sepsis bacteraemia/septicaemia (see Box 1.14).

- Urinary tract infection (UTI).
- Typhoid.

Causes of chronic cough

- Tuberculosis 📖 Tuberculosis, p. 151.
- Asthma 📖 Chest medicine, p. 214.
- Persistent infection e.g. Pertussis 📖 Chest medicine, p. 200.
- Inhaled foreign body 📖 Chest medicine, p. 175.
- Bronchiectasis 📖 Chest medicine, p. 222.
- Lung abscess 📖 Chest medicine, p. 204.
- Recurrent pneumonia or HIV-associated lung disease 📖 HIV/AIDS, p. 185.
- Recurrent aspiration.

Differential diagnosis of fever lasting >7 days

Diagnosis is often difficult. Many children will have already been empirically treated and diagnostic facilities may be limited. A detailed clinical assessment is essential. Causes will vary in different regions. A carefully considered trial of treatment for the most likely cause may be necessary if a secure diagnosis cannot be made.

Consider

- Partly treated, drug-resistant malaria.
- Occult abscess (e.g. subphrenic, psoas, retroperitoneal, lung).
- Typhoid and non-typhi *Salmonella* infection (see Box 1.14).
- Infective endocarditis 📖 Cardiovascular medicine, p. 394.
- Rheumatic fever 📖 Cardiovascular medicine, p. 392.
- Tuberculosis 📖 Tuberculosis, p. 151.
- Brucellosis (in endemic areas) 📖 Multi-system diseases and infections, p. 768.
- Visceral leishmaniasis (in endemic areas) 📖 Multi-system diseases and infections, p. 794.

Box 1.12 Febrile convulsions

- Occur in children aged 6mths–6yr.
- Generalized tonic or tonic-clonic seizure lasting up to 5min during a febrile illness.
- Full neurological recovery.
- Generally benign.
- May have a family history.
- In a minority of children may recur in the same or subsequent illness.

More serious cause (e.g. meningitis, cerebral malaria, encephalitis, brain abscess) suggested by:

- Prolonged seizures (>30min).
- Multiple or focal seizures.
- Impaired consciousness or neurological abnormalities.
- Age <6mths or >6yrs.

If in doubt, perform full septic screen including lumbar puncture (LP).

Box 1.13 Intussusception

- Invagination of part of intestine into lumen of adjoining bowel.
- Important cause of intestinal obstruction in children aged 2mths–5yr (peak incidence 4–10mths).
- Classically presents with recurrent, colicky, abdominal pain, vomiting, and bloody 'redcurrant jelly' stool; may palpate a sausage-shaped abdominal mass.
- Abdominal X-ray (AXR) may show soft tissue mass displacing loops of bowel; barium enema, a filling defect; and ultrasound (US) scan, a 'target lesion'.
- Urgent intervention can prevent bowel ischaemia and perforation: reduce with air/contrast enema; if this fails, operate.
- Treat shock, sepsis, or electrolyte derangement.

Box 1.14 Bacteraemia and septicaemia

- Common among children in the tropics.
- Under-diagnosed where there are no facilities for blood culture.
- Often there is a focus of infection (e.g. pneumonia, meningitis, soft tissue infection), but may occur without a focus, or a focus may develop later.
- Typhoid and non-typhoid *Salmonella* infections are a cause of sepsis without localizing signs; a similar syndrome may occur with many other organisms, especially in children with severe malnutrition or HIV.
- All children with sepsis should be admitted and started on empiric antibiotics, e.g. ampicillin (or benzylpenicillin) and gentamicin (ideally after blood cultures), during investigations. Note that malaria may be accompanied by bacterial sepsis.

Non-typhi Salmonella (NTS) infection

- NTS infections are a common cause of childhood bacteraemia. Risk factors include malnutrition, malaria, HIV, and sickle cell disease.
- Children may present with acute infection, or sub-acute or prolonged fever without localizing signs, but focal signs and/or diarrhoea occur; splenomegaly is common.
- Some first line antibiotics (e.g. penicillin) do not cover NTS. Treatment is with chloramphenicol, co-trimoxazole, or ampicillin, but multi-drug resistance is an increasing problem. Alternatives are ciprofloxacin (resistance emerging) or ceftriaxone.

The sick young infant

Infants <2mths are vulnerable, and their illnesses may rapidly → death. All sick young infants should, therefore, be given priority, even in the absence of emergency signs.

Assessment of the sick young infant

Symptoms and signs of illness in young infants are often subtle and non-specific and more than one illness may co-exist.

Check for the danger signs (see Box 1.15), these indicate possible septicaemia, pneumonia, or meningitis requiring immediate treatment.

- *Check for focal signs of infection:* including joint/limb swelling, ↓ limb movement, or tenderness (osteomyelitis or septic arthritis); peri-umbilical hyperaemia +/– purulent discharge; purulent ear discharge; skin infection. Suspect meningitis if child has convulsions or is irritable with high pitched cry, ↓ feeding, lethargy/unconscious, or bulging/tense anterior fontanelle. *Note:* neck stiffness is a rare sign of meningitis in young infants.
- *Check for feeding problems and weight:* check if sucking well and weight adequate for age. Refusal of feeds or inability to suck may be due to sepsis, cardiac or respiratory problems, or oral thrush. In an infant who feeds well, but has low weight for age, look for underlying problems, e.g. metabolic disorders or congenital heart disease.
- *Check for signs of dehydration* (📖 p. 6). ↓ Intake, ↑ fluid loss from diarrhoea, vomiting or tachypnoea may → dehydration. Diarrhoea is uncommon in breastfed infants of this age except as a sign of sepsis.
- *Check immunization status:* ensure that child is up to date with immunization according to the national schedule.
- Check for congenital malformations.

Box 1.15 Danger signs in young infants

- ↓ Activity or lethargy.
- Poor feeding.
- Vomiting.
- Convulsions, usually subtle or focal.
- Bloody diarrhoea.
- Fever (axillary temp >37.5°C, or rectal >38°C), less common in this age group, but may indicate serious bacterial infection.
- Hypothermia (axillary <35.5°C or rectal <36°C).
- Pallor, jaundice, or cyanosis.
- Tachypnoea (RR ≥60 breaths/min) or ↓ RR (<20/min) or apnoea (no breathing for >15s).
- Severe chest wall indrawing (minimal intercostal indrawing may be normal in young infants in absence of other respiratory signs).
- Nasal flaring and grunting.
- Irregular respiration.
- Bulging/tense fontanelle when not crying.

Emergency treatment of the sick young infant

Establish regular respiration and heart rate. Resuscitation is usually successful if promptly performed:

Airway

Ensure patent airway by careful suctioning and correct positioning of the neck: place a towel under the shoulders to allow the neck to drop to a neutral position or just minimal extension with chin lift; do not hyperextend the neck (Fig. 1.5).

Breathing

Look, listen, and feel for 10s. If breathing is irregular, shallow, or absent, commence BVM ventilation with O_2, ensuring mask covers nose and mouth. Check pulse every 2min. Use room air if O_2 is not available. If the child is breathing, but cyanosed or RR >60/min, give O_2.

Circulation

Check for brachial pulse for no longer than 10s. If PR <60/min, absent, or not sure, commence chest compressions. After 2min give adrenaline if no cardiac output (see Box 1.10). Combine chest compressions with ventilation in cycles of 15 compressions to 2 breaths (30:2 if there is no assistance). Use two finger tips over lower third of sternum or both thumbs with hand encircling chest and compress 1/3 of antero-posterior diameter. Aim for 90 compressions and 10 breaths/min. *For neonates*, give 3 compressions for 1 breath every 2s (90 compressions and 30 breaths/min) see algorithm for newborns (Fig 1.7).

General measures in the management of sick young infants

Young infants with signs of serious illness (📖 p. 18) require admission to prevent complications and rapid deterioration. Treatment, including

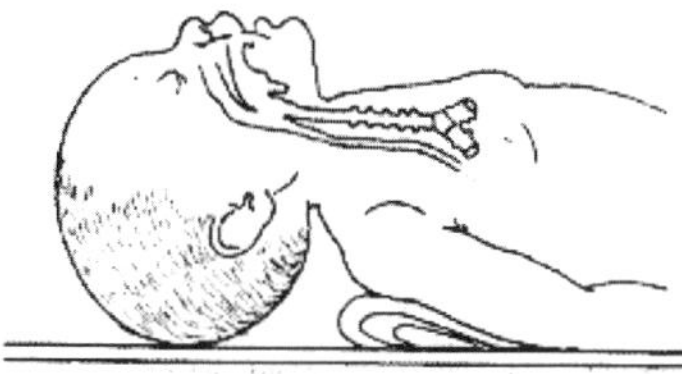

Fig. 1.5 Correct position of the neck for ventilation.

Reproduced from World Health Organization, *Pocket Book of Hospital Care for Children* 2005: 44, with permission of WHO.

antibiotics (see Box 1.16), will be directed at the specific clinical syndrome. In addition, all young infants require ongoing supportive care, which is crucial to survival even after recovery from the acute illness.

Feeding

Ensure continued regular feeding. Express breastmilk and give by NGT if infant is unable to suck, or by cup and spoon as soon as infant is able to take oral feeds. Oral intake should be stopped if there is abdominal distention, severe vomiting, frequent convulsions, or respiratory distress. Treat hypoglycaemia with IV 10% dextrose 5mL/kg or 10mL/kg via nasogastric tube and continue regular feeds or IV fluids.

Fluid requirements

Total amount, given as oral or IV in neonates with feeding difficulties: Day 1 (60mL/kg/day), Day 2 (90mL/kg/day), Day 3 (120mL/kg/day), thereafter (150mL/kg/day). May ↑ to 180mL/kg/day). If on phototherapy, increase ×1.2–1.5.

Fluid therapy

Assess hydration status and give oral rehydration solution (ORS) or IV fluids according to WHO guidelines (📖 Diarrhoeal diseases, p. 233).

Temperature control

Keep infant dry and well dressed/wrapped, including bonnet and booties. Maintain environmental temperature of at least 25°C. Avoid excessive exposure during examination and procedures as this may → chilling. Use incubators when available to allow easy observation with minimal handling of baby in addition to thermal control. Direct skin to skin care (Kangaroo mother care (KMC) see Box 1.17) may be used when the infant is stable. If there is fever, remove clothes and expose, but do not give antipyretics.

Oxygen therapy

Indications for O_2 therapy include: central cyanosis, grunting, severe lower chest wall indrawing, difficulty in feeding due to respiratory distress, and head nodding. Stop O_2 if saturations>90% in room air.

Treatment of convulsions

Neonates (<2wks old)

IM phenobarbital 20mg/kg stat; if maintenance is required, give 5mg/kg/day oral/IV.

Infants 2 wks–2mths old

Rectal diazepam 0.5mg/kg, repeat rectal diazepam at 10min if convulsions persist (or IV diazepam 0.25mg/kg). If still convulsing after another 10min give third dose of diazepam or rectal paraldehyde 0.3–0.4mL/kg may be given.

Monitoring

It is essential to observe infant at least every 6h for improvement or deterioration.

Outpatient treatment

Infants with non-bloody diarrhoea, and some or no signs of dehydration (📖 Assessment of dehydration in children with diarrhoea, p. 277), or poor weight gain due to feeding mismanagement, may be treated as outpatients. However, the mother should be informed of danger signs that require urgent review. Local bacterial infections without constitutional symptoms are common and may be treated as an outpatient, with follow-up at short intervals because of the risk of rapid progression to septicaemia. These include omphalitis (*without* hyperaemia of surrounding skin), skin sepsis (if only a few skin pustules), paronychia, and mild conjunctivitis.

Box 1.16 Antibiotic therapy of infections in young infants

When chosing antibiotics be aware of local data of prevailing organisms and antibiotic sensitivities.

- *Sepsis or pneumonia:* give ampicillin 50mg/kg IV/IM qds* (or benzyl-penicillin 50 000U/kg qds*) plus gentamicin 7.5mg/kg* IV/IM od. Cefotaxime 50mg/kg IV/IM qds* or ceftriaxone 80mg/kg IV/IM od*† are alternatives. If S. *aureus* infection suspected (e.g. nosocomial sepsis, soft tissue infection), give cloxacillin 50mg/kg IV qds* or cefuroxime 25mg/kg tds, plus gentamicin. Treat until child has remained well for 4 days.
- *Meningitis:* give ampicillin 50mg/kg IV/IM qds*, plus gentamicin 7.5mg/kg*. Treat for a minimum of 14 days, or 21 days if Gram –ve bacterial meningitis proven or suspected. Alternatives are cefotaxime 50mg/kg IV/IM qds* or ceftriaxone 100mg/kg IV/IM od.*†
- *Focal bacterial infections:* co-trimoxazole, amoxicillin, or a cephalosporin.
- Conjunctivitis: teach mother to clean eyes with saline or clean water +/– apply topical antibiotic. Review child after 2 days.
  - *Ophthalmia neonatorum*(📖 Conjunctivitis, p. 578; 📖 Gonorrhoea, p. 670)— a severe, suppurative conjunctivitis, often with associated blepharitis, that occurs in neonates, particularly in the first week of life, and may → permanent blindness if not treated. Caused by *N. gonorrhoea* or *C. trachomatis* perinatally; other organisms include *S. aureus*. Gram stain of the discharge may demonstrate Gram +ve diplococci (*N. gonorrhoea*). If so, give ceftriaxone 50mg/kg IM as a single dose, treat the parents presumptively for *N. gonorrhoea* (📖 Gonorrhoea, p. 670).

* Doses in first week of life as follows: ampicillin 50mg/kg bd; benzylpenicillin 50 000U/kg bd; gentamicin 5mg/kg od if normal birth weight, 3mg/kg od if low birth weight; cefotaxime 50mg/kg tds in term neonates, bd in premature neonates; cloxacillin 25–50mg/kg bd.

† Avoid ceftriaxone in neonatal jaundice as the drug may displace bilirubin from albumin, increasing the risk of kernicterus.

Neonatal notes

Newborns and neonates (<28 days) have some special considerations beyond those of the sick young infant (Fig. 1.7). Resuscitation at birth differs from young infants, in particular with the need for inflation breaths (can be undertaken with air) after delivery. See summary diagram for special features; 📖 Newborn life support, p. 23.

A common complication is perinatal asphyxia (Box 1.19) in resource-poor settings where access to emergency obstetric care may be limited. Fig. 1.6 shows a traditional birth attendant kit for home deliveries. Care after delivery is also important and KMC (see Box 1.17) can help with this. Most at risk are those with low birth weight (LBW) or preterm delivery. Common problems are sepsis (see Box 1.16 for antibiobiotic therapy), jaundice, hypothermia and hypoglycaemia.

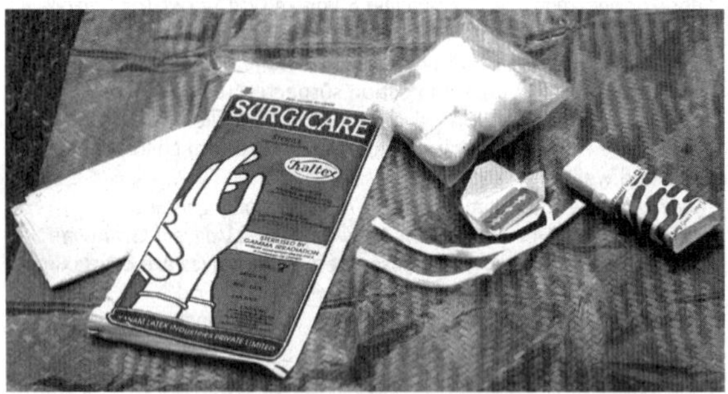

Fig. 1.6 Traditional birth attendant kit for home deliveries. As well as illustrated instructions, the kit contains (all sterile) plastic sheet for delivery, soap, towels, gloves, cotton wool, umbilical cord ties, and razor blade.

Reproduced from the Kenya Ministry of Health, with permission.

Box 1.17 Kangaroo mother care (KMC)

Direct skin-to-skin care of the infant. Baby is placed naked (except for nappy) directly on mother's bare chest, and strapped in place to get warmth, while the mother goes about her regular activity. KMC is an alternative to an incubator and may reduce hospital stay, help early establishment of breastfeeding, and promote mother/child bonding. Close family members, including the father, can also provide KMC.

Newborn life support

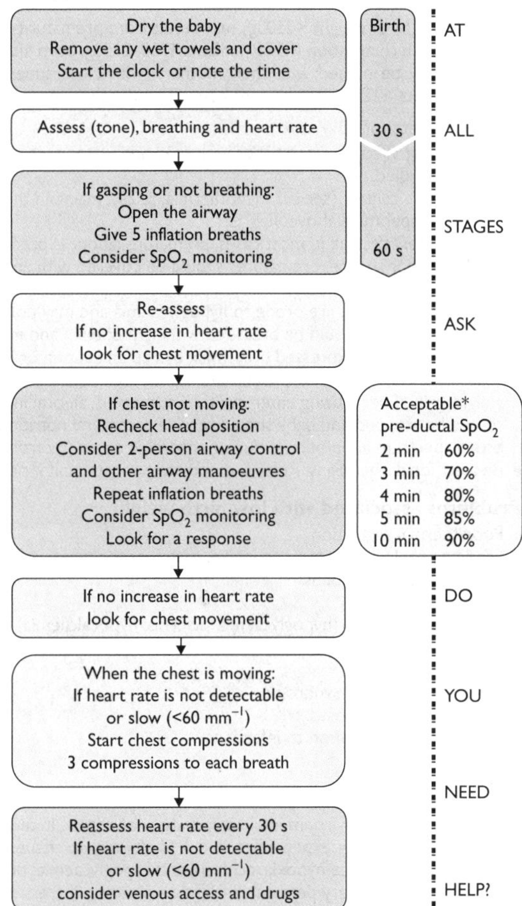

*Dawson JA, Kamlin CO, Vento M, et al. Defining the reference range for oxygen saturation for infants after birth. *Pediatrics 2010* 125:e1340–7.

Fig. 1.7 Newborn life support. Note that there are special situations (e.g. meconium at delivery, preterm delivery). See http://www.resus.org.uk/pages/GL2010.pdf for more information.

Reproduced from the Resuscitation Council Guidelines (2010), with permission from the Resuscitation Council UK.

Low birth weight and prematurity

LBW infants (birth weight <2500g) may result from prematurity or intra-uterine growth retardation (IUGR). Infants 1750–2250g, born after 34wks' gestation may be nursed with their mothers, with close supervision, in nursery. Infants >2250g may be sent home if no danger signs.

Essential aspects of LBW care

- *Prevention of infection:* wash hands with soap and water each time infant is to be handled.
- *Temperature control:* (see 🕮 Hypothermia, p. 24): maintain the infant's axillary temperature above 36.5°C.
- *Treatment of infection:* In most cases, premature labour is precipitated by an infection, hence, prematures should be covered with ampicillin and gentamicin empirically.
- *Feeding:* LBW babies are prone to hypoglycaemia and may not suck adequately. They should be breastfed within 1h of birth and may require additional expressed breastmilk by cup and spoon or via NGT. Mothers should be shown proper latching-on techniques. Monitor weight gain. If necrotizing enterocolitis is suspected, all oral intake should be stopped and baby should receive parenteral nutrition, and broad spectrum antibiotics, including anaerobic cover (metronidazole)
- Be alert for danger signs: Refer promptly to neonatal unit if present.

Problems associated with low birth weight

- Poor thermal regulation.
- Feeding problems (inadequate intake, gastro-oesophageal reflux).
- Necrotizing enterocolitis.
- Neonatal jaundice.
- Metabolic problems (hypoglycaemia, acidosis, hypocalcaemia, fluid, and electrolyte imbalance).
- Apnoea.
- Respiratory distress syndrome.
- Patent ductus arteriosus.
- Increased predisposition to infections.

Hypothermia

Hypothermia (body temp <36°C) is a common problem of LBW infants, resulting from low environmental temperature or sepsis. It causes ↑ O_2 consumption, ↑ energy expenditure, and ↓ O_2 delivery to tissues.

- *Complications:* include hypoxia, acidosis, and hypoglycaemia; poor weight gain; ↑ capillary permeability; and respiratory distress due to ↓ surfactant production.
- *Treatment:* re-warm infant using warm clothing, incubator preheated to 35–36°C, heated mattress, or skin-to-skin care. Exclude sepsis.
- *Prevention:* nurse infants in warm environments. Avoid wet clothes and do not place infant on cold surfaces, e.g. X-ray plates and weighing scales.

Apnoea

Apnoeic episodes are common in LBW infants. May be accompanied by bradycardia if prolonged. Gentle physical stimulation often stimulates breathing, but respiratory stimulants (caffeine or theophylline) and occasionally ventilatory support, may be required. Seek underlying causes: infection, hypoxia, metabolic derangement, anaemia, or subtle seizures.

Neonatal jaundice

Jaundice occurs in >50% neonates and is more common in LBW infants. Jaundice may be a sign of serious disease (e.g. infection; see Box 1.18), especially if it occurs on day 1, is associated with fever, is deep (involves palms and soles), or lasts >14 days (>21 days if premature). Jaundice is also commonly physiological, but other causes should be first considered.

Severe jaundice may → *kernicterus* (neurotoxicity). In its mild form, there is lethargy and reduced feeding. Severe kernicterus → irritability, hypertonia +/– opisthotonos, and long-term neurological sequelae.

Investigations for abnormal jaundice

Consider (if available) total serum bilirubin and conjugated/unconjugated bilirubin, FBC, maternal and infant blood group, Coombs test, G6PD screen, thyroid function, syphilis serology, and abdominal US scan.

Management of jaundice

- Ensure adequate hydration.
- Exclude serious causes (see Box 1.15).
- Treat severe jaundice to prevent kernicterus (see Table 1.1).
- *Phototherapy:* reduces jaundice by using ultraviolet light → photodegradation of bilirubin in the skin. Protect infant's eyes. Beware of dehydration, hypothermia, or hyperthermia. Other complications include diarrhoea and rash.
- *Exchange blood transfusion:* may be required for severe jaundice. Twice the infant's blood volume (i.e. 2 × 80mL/kg) is exchanged for fresh donor blood in 10–20mL aliquots via UVC. Low, but definite risk attached to procedure.

Box 1.18 Common causes of neonatal jaundice

Jaundice starting <24h after birth

- Haemolysis (e.g. Rhesus or ABO incompatibility; G6PD or pyruvate kinase deficiency; congenital spherocytosis).
- Infection (TORCH* organisms).

Jaundice starting from day 2 to week 2 after birth

- Physiological jaundice.
- Breastmilk jaundice.
- Severe bruising.
- Infection.
- Haemolysis.

Jaundice persisting for >2wks after birth

- Biliary atresia.
- Neonatal hepatitis.
- Haemolysis.
- Congenital hypothyroidism.
- Infection.
- May also be persistence of breastmilk or physiological jaundice.

*Toxoplasma; syphilis, Varicella zoster virus (VZV), measles; rubella; CMV; Herpes simplex.

Table 1.1 Indications for treatment of neonatal jaundice according to serum bilirubin concentration

	Phototherapy				Exchange Transfusion			
	Healthy term baby		Preterm or risk factors		Healthy term baby		Preterm or risk factors	
	mg/day	µmol/L	mg/dL	µmol/L	mg/dL	µmol/L	mg/dL	µmol/L
Day 1	Any visible jaundice				15	260	13	220
Day 2	15	260	13	220	25	425	15	260
Day 3	18	310	16	270	30	510	20	340
≥ Day 4	20	340	17	290	30	510	20	340

Reproduced from World Health Organization, *Pocket Book of Hospital Care for Children* 2005: 58, with permission of WHO.

Perinatal asphyxia/hypoxic ischaemic encephalopathy

In perinatal asphyxia there is hypoxia, acidosis, and CO_2 accumulation around time of delivery, which may → hypoxic-ischaemic encephalopathy (HIE). It accounts for much neonatal mortality and long-term morbidity, especially in low-resource settings. Largely preventable with improved obstetric care, prompt resuscitation, and supportive care of the neonate.

Assessment

Risk factors for the development of asphyxia are listed in Box 1.19. Prenatal and intrapartum parameters can indicate asphyxia and the following are indicators of asphyxia at birth:

- Apgar scores ≤5 at 10min (see Table 1.2).
- Resuscitation >10min before spontaneous respiration.
- Cord blood pH <7 or base excess >12mmol/L.

Prevention

Monitoring the mother in pregnancy and labour helps to predict infants at risk of asphyxia. However, some babies who present with birth asphyxia have not been exposed to known risk factors. Everyone involved in the delivery of babies should be skilled in newborn resuscitation in order to ↓ morbidity and mortality associated with asphyxia.

Classification of HIE

HIE is used to describe the clinical manifestation of brain injury starting immediately or up to 48h after hypoxic insult (asphyxia) in a term baby. It can be graded into;

- *Mild:* baby is irritable and responds excessively to stimulation, may have feeding difficulties, hyperventilation, or staring eyes.
- *Moderate:* baby shows abnormal tone and movements, cannot feed and may have convulsions.
- *Severe:* baby has no spontaneous movements or response to pain; tone in limbs may fluctuate between hypotonia and hypertonia. Convulsions may be prolonged and often not respond to treatment. Multi-organ failure is present.

Prognosis of HIE

- *Mild HIE:* complete recovery can be expected.
- *Moderate HIE:* if fully recovered by day 7, excellent long-term prognosis, but if abnormalities persist >day 10, full recovery becomes unlikely.
- *Severe HIE:* has a mortality of 30–40%; 80% of survivors have neurodevelopmental disabilities, in particular cerebral palsy.

Table 1.2 APGAR score

	Score=0	**Score=1**	**Score=2**
Appearance (colour)	Pale/blue	Blue extremities	Completely pink
Pulse rate	Absent	<100/min	>100/min
Respiration	Absent	Slow, irregular	Regular, crying
Reflexes (grimace)	No response to stimulation	Grimace/feeble cry on stimulation	Cry/pull away when stimulated
Activity (muscle tone)	None/flaccid	Some flexion	Well flexed and legs resist extension

Treatment

- *In resource-poor settings:* this is primarily treatment of symptoms and supportive care.
- *In resource-rich settings:* therapeutic cooling of term babies in intensive care settings with rigorous protocols has proven effective in reducing morbidity from perinatal asphyxia. Safety and applicability of this has not been established in resource-poor settings and more research is needed before it could be recommended.

Box 1.19 Risk factors for perinatal asphyxia

- *Maternal medical or obstetric factors:* hyper- or hypotension, heart failure, diabetes, severe anaemia, haemoglobinopathies, infections, respiratory illness (e.g. pneumonia, asthma), smoking, alcoholism, pre-eclampsia/eclampsia, primigravidity or grandmultiparity, induction of labour, sedation, analgesia, prolonged rupture of membranes, prolonged labour.
- *Foetal factors:* multiple gestation, prematurity or post-term, IUGR or large for gestational age, intrauterine infections, abnormal presentation, congenital abnormalities.
- *Placental factors: abruptio placenta*, placenta praevia, placental insufficiency, cord compression.

Complications of asphyxia and their management

Asphyxia may → multi-organ dysfunction.

- *Respiratory system:* persistent pulmonary hypertension and respiratory distress syndrome. Ensure good oxygenation.
- *Cardiovascular system:* myocardial damage → poor cardiac output. Monitor capillary refill and BP. Avoid fluid overload and give inotropes if necessary.
- *Gastrointestinal system:* risk of necrotizing enterocolitis. Avoid enteral feeding in first 24–48h (beware hypoglycaemia!). With introduction of feeds, avoid hyperosmolar feeds and stasis.
- *Metabolic:* hypoglycaemia or hyperglycaemia may worsen hypoxic damage to the brain. Hyponatraemia, hyperkalaemia, hypocalcaemia or acidosis may result; monitor blood glucose and electrolytes.
- *Renal function:* ↑ risk of urinary retention and renal failure. Monitor fluid intake, urine output, and urine specific gravity. Catheterize to differentiate between failure to produce or void urine.
- *Haematologic:* bone marrow suppression, neutrophil dysfunction, and coagulopathies. Monitor FBC for evidence of bleeding.
- *Brain:* encephalopathy results from hypoxia, cerebral oedema, ↑ intracranial pressure (ICP). Look for ↓ reflexes, abnormal muscle tone, seizures, varying degrees of altered consciousness, and long-term neurological sequelae.

Other general measures: ensure thermoneutral environment, adequate calories, and hydration, and treat neonatal jaundice.

Neonatal tetanus

This frequently fatal, preventable condition remains common in some resource-poor countries. *Clostridium tetani* usually infects the infant through the umbilical stump (due to poor hygiene or a tradition of applying dung to the stump) or unsterile circumcision. The pathogenesis of tetanus is described in 📖 Neurology, p. 454.

Clinical features

Usually presents at 2–14 days, but may occur later.

- Inability to open mouth.
- Refusal of feeds.
- Excessive crying.
- *Muscle rigidity and spasms:* provoked and spontaneous.
- Fever.
- Intact consciousness.

Diagnosis

Mainly clinical.

Treatment

- *Muscle relaxants:* oral diazepam 5mg/kg/day in divided doses via NGT.
- *For difficult to control spasms:*
  - IV diazepam 0.1–0.3mg/kg every 1–4h titrated to spasm frequency.
  - IV midazolam 0.06mg/kg/h is a suitable, but expensive alternative.
  - IV magnesium sulphate may also be useful.
- IM tetanus immune globulin 500U or equine anti-tetanus serum 10 000U single dose.
- Tetanus toxoid (in a different site) if >6wks old.
- *Antibiotics:*
  - Metronidazole (drug of choice) or penicillin or erythromycin.
  - Add broad-spectrum antibiotics (e.g. ceftriaxone if sepsis suspected).
- *Supportive care:*
  - Nutritional support.
  - Nurse in quiet, dark environment to prevent provoked spasms
  - (but ensure adequate clinical supervision).
  - Ensure clear airway and give ventilatory support if needed.

Poor prognostic factors

- Incubation period <7 days.
- Period of onset <24h.
- Associated pneumonia.

Public health note: prevention of neonatal tetanus

- Maternal education.
- Maternal tetanus toxoid immunization.
- Hygienic delivery and cord care practices.
- Immunization of all women in childbearing age with tetanus toxoid.

Chapter 2
Malaria

Invited author **Nick Day**

Introduction

Malaria, a protozoan infection transmitted by anopheline mosquitoes, is the most important parasitic disease of humans. Around 3.3 billion people in endemic areas are at risk of malaria and ~250 million clinical cases occur annually. Nearly 1 million die annually, largely African infants and young children. There are four human malaria parasite species (*Plasmodium falciparum, P. vivax, P. ovale, and P. malariae*), and human infection with the macaque malaria species *P. knowlesi* is increasingly recognized in Southeast Asia. The clinical manifestations of malaria vary greatly, depending on a number of factors including the infecting malaria species (*P. falciparum* causing the vast majority of severe disease), transmission intensity, and the degree of resistance, acquired and genetic, of the host.

Life cycle and transmission

The life cycle of the malarial parasite alternates between the sexual cycle in the invertebrate host (the female *Anopheles* mosquito) and the asexual cycle in the vertebrate host (in this case, human).

- Transmission occurs when the mosquito, requiring blood for the development of her eggs, bites the human host and injects motile sporozoites (see Fig. 2.1) into the bloodstream, which then invade hepatocytes, where they develop into liver schizonts.
- When each schizont ruptures, thousands of merozoites are released that invade red cells and initiate that part of the cycle responsible for all the clinical manifestations of the disease.
- Either immediately after release from the liver or (in the case of *P. falciparum*) after several asexual cycles, some parasites develop into longer-lived, morphologically distinct sexual forms, gametocytes.
- Male and female gametocytes ingested by mosquitoes taking a blood meal combine to form a zygote, which matures into an ookinete that encysts in the gut wall.
- There an oocyst develops, expanding by asexual division until it bursts, releasing numerous sporozoites that migrate to the salivary glands. These await inoculation into a human host when the mosquito next feeds.

Incubation periods

- *P. falciparum* 7–14d usually, but may be longer (up to 6wks) in those with partial immunity or those on inadequate prophylaxis.
- *P. vivax* 12–17d, but may relapse months or years later as a result of the reactivation of a dormant form in the liver called the hypnozoite.
- *P. ovale* 15–18d but may relapse months or years later as a result of the hypnozoite.
- *P. malariae* 18-40d and has no hypnozoite form.

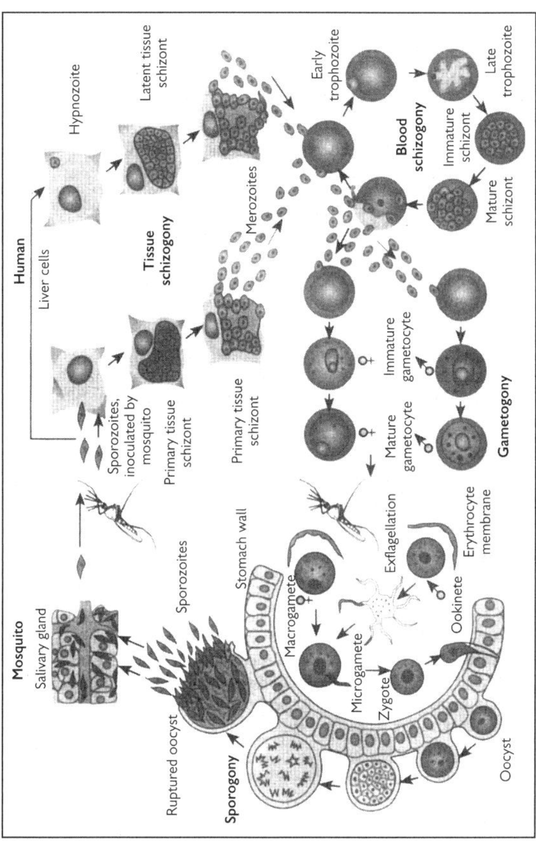

Fig. 2.1 The malaria life cycle (hypnozoite stage is limited to *P. vivax* and *P. ovale*)

Epidemiology

Malarial transmission depends upon a number of factors including:

- Mosquito longevity (lifespan).
- Ambient temperature (shortens the cycle in the mosquito).
- Population density of both mosquito and humans.
- Mosquito's human-biting habit.
- Host immune response.
- Whether the drugs used in treatment have any activity against gametocytes.

In endemic areas (see Fig. 2.2), the entomological inoculation rate is used as an indicator of transmission intensity. Transmission may be estimated clinically using the parasite rate (% of the population who are +ve for malarial parasites on blood film), or the spleen rate (% of population with splenomegaly), although the latter is less reliable since an enlarged spleen may be a result of other diseases.

Two distinct patterns of malarial transmission emerge, which represent extremes:

- Stable malaria, where there is intense all year round transmission. The disease predominantly affects young children and pregnant women. Adults might be +ve on blood film, but are rarely ill with malaria.
- Unstable malaria, in which the disease affects all ages and occurs in areas of seasonal or low transmission.

There is a concern that malaria control interventions in stable areas that ↓ transmission, but do not eradicate the disease, may impair the development of naturally acquired immunity in the population, resulting in a pattern of unstable disease.

Protection against malaria

Many innate factors of resistance against infection were first identified in *P. falciparum* malaria. Acquired resistance to malaria is slow to develop and the immune mechanisms involved are still unclear.

Innate immunity

Falciparum malaria remains the best example of a selective agent that results in genetic polymorphisms in the host that might provide partial protection against severe disease. Certain genetic variants of the red cell, notably sickle cell trait, glucose 6-phosphate dehydrogenase (G6PD)-deficiency, thalassaemia trait, and ovalocytosis, may partially protect against severe disease. The lack of Duffy antigen (the receptor for merozoites of *P. vivax*) on red cells in most West Africans may account for their relative protection against this infection.

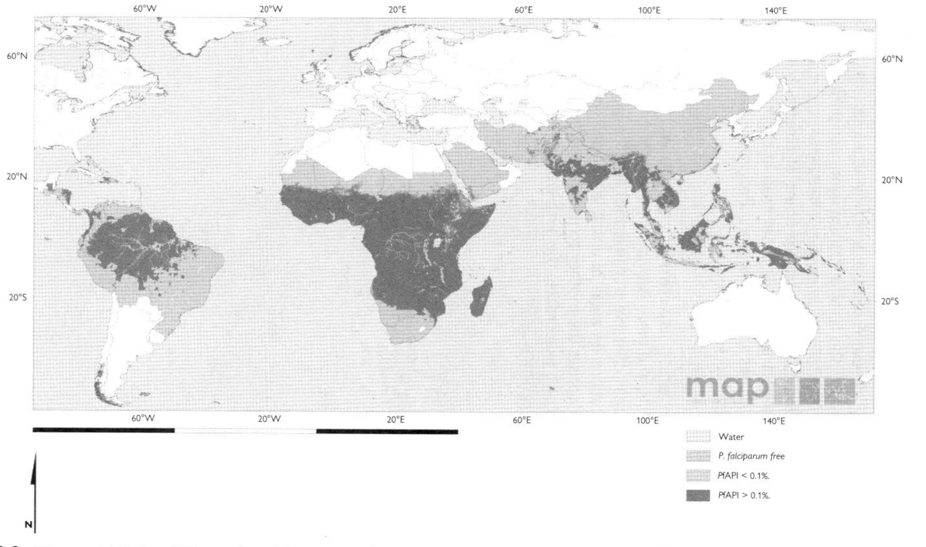

Fig. 2.2 The spatial limits of *Plasmodium falciparum* malaria transmission in 2010 (Available at: http://www.map.ox.ac.uk/browse-resources/transmission-limits/Pf_limits/world/)

Acquired immunity

Believed to require repeated exposure to malarial infection, possibly with differing genetic variants of parasite. In areas of intense, stable transmission, neonates are usually protected by maternal antibodies for first ~6mths of life, followed by a period of ↑ susceptibility, during which it is thought that immunity to severe disease is slowly acquired (*anti-disease immunity*). Depending upon the level of transmission, *anti-parasite immunity* appears later, at ~10yrs of age, when the parasitaemia rate may be as high as 50%. Adults tend to get less severe bouts of disease, but when they do, parasite densities are generally lower than in children. Without re-infection, immunity wanes after a few years. Pregnancy, severe illness, and surgery may also lead to ↓ immunity.

HIV infection

A complex interaction exists between HIV and malaria. Malaria ↑ viral loads in HIV+ individuals, and there is evidence that HIV ↑ both the incidence of malaria (in areas of stable transmission) and the occurrence of severe malaria complications (in areas of unstable transmission; Box 2.1). In pregnancy, HIV predisposes the mother to malaria and the newborn to congenital malaria. HIV also exacerbates the birth weight reduction associated with malaria in pregnancy.

Box 2.1 Complications of malaria

Falciparum malaria

- Falciparum malaria may → to severe disease and death (see 📖 Severe malaria, p. 42).
- In endemic areas where parasites persist after treatment or patients are soon re-infected, anaemia is common and further attacks, due to recrudescence of blood forms, may occur.
- In some countries, 30% of patients with falciparum malaria develop symptomatic *P. vivax* infection within 2mths without re-exposure to parasites, implying an initial mixed infection or activation of existing hypnozoites in the liver.

The benign malarias

- *P. vivax:* a rare complication of this infection is splenic rupture (mortality 80%). It results from acute enlargement with or without trauma and presents with sudden and persistent abdominal pain, guarding, fever, shock, and a ↓ haemocrit. Recent clinical epidemiological studies from Southeast Asia suggest that vivax infection may be responsible for a higher mortality than previously recognized.
- *Relapses: P. vivax* and *P. ovale* may relapse from 30d to 5yrs after initial infection despite treatment that eliminates all blood forms, due to latent liver hypnozoites undergoing schizogony and re-entering the blood stream—a true relapse (as opposed to recrudescence).
- *P. malariae:* persistent parasites may cause recurrent fevers when infection recrudesces, even decades after 1° infection. Fevers ↓ in frequency and severity over time. Anaemia and splenomegaly may occur.

Clinical features

P. falciparum infection, if treated promptly and appropriately, generally follows a relatively mild course. However, without effective therapy it can become life-threatening, especially in young children and non-immune adults.

P. ovale, *P. malaria*, and *P. vivax* infection are much less likely to → severe disease or death, although recent reports from Southeast Asia indicate that vivax infection may be less benign than previously thought. Chronic infection or infection of pregnant women with these 'benign' species may lead to marked morbidity, e.g. anaemia and ↓ birth weight.

Two important features distinguish falciparum infection from the other malarias and account for the differences in severity:

- Only *P. falciparum* malaria → high blood parasite densities.
- Only *P. falciparum* demonstrates 'sequestration' in the microvasculature of red cells containing mature parasites.

Sequestration results mainly from cyto-adherence of parasitized red cells to endothelial cells in the post-capillary venules of critical organs including the brain, although other factors, such as ↓ deformability of both parasitized and unparasitized red cells, autoagglutination of parasitized cells, and adherence of unparasitized to parasitized red cells (rosetting) may play a role.

Acute malaria

The clinical presentation of acute malaria in adults with rigors is well known. There is usually a history of travel to or residence in an endemic area. Even the best compliance with the most effective antimalarial chemoprophylaxis cannot exclude malaria. There may be a prodromal period of tiredness and aching. The features of a classical paroxysm are:

- An abrupt onset of an initial 'cold stage' associated with a dramatic rigor (paroxysm) in which the patient visibly shakes.
- An ensuing 'hot stage' during which the patient may have a temperature >40°C, be restless and excitable, and vomit.
- Finally, the sweating stage, during which the patient's temperature returns to normal (defervesces) and sleep may ensue.

Such a paroxysm can last 6–10h; a prolonged asymptomatic period may follow lasting 38–42h in the case of vivax and ovale malaria ('tertian' fever) and 62–66h in *P. malariae* infections ('quartan' fever; see Box 2.2).

In falciparum malaria, the periodicity of fever is less predictable and the fever may be continuous. There may be an accompanying headache, cough, myalgia (flu-like symptoms), diarrhoea, and mild jaundice.

Malaria is rarely, if ever, the cause of lymphadenopathy, pharyngitis, or a rash, and alternative diagnoses need to be considered for these symptoms. In children, the presentation may be non-specific and misleading with fever, early cough, diarrhoea and vomiting (D&V), anaemia, and hypoglycaemia. Jaundice, pulmonary oedema, and renal failure are rarer in children than adults, although progression to other severe complications is usually faster (1–2d) in children.

Box 2.2 Chronic malaria

The persistence of low-level parasitaemia in the blood may lead to 'chronic' malaria. Symptoms include recurrent acute attacks of malaria, anaemia, hepatosplenomegaly, diarrhoea, ↓ weight, and ↑ incidence of other infections. Chronic malaria may resolve, with the onset of partial immunity, or progress, with 2° complications.

Burkitt's lymphoma

A childhood tumour common in areas of high falciparum malaria transmission. It is thought to be due to Epstein–Barr virus infection in the setting of impaired T-cell immunity associated with repeated malaria infections (📖 Infectious mononucleosis, p. 798 and Burkitt's lymphoma, p. 524).

Hyperreactive malarial splenomegaly

Formerly called tropical splenomegaly syndrome. May develop with recurrent infections. It is characterized by massive splenomegaly, profound anaemia, 2° bacterial infections, fever, and (occasionally) jaundice. There is hypersplenism with pancytopenia, hypergammaglobulinaemia, and a lymphocytic infiltrate in the liver. There is marked ↑ serum IgM. Although malarial parasites are seldom found in the blood, the condition responds to prolonged courses of antimalarial prophylaxis.

Quartan malarial nephropathy

P. malariae infection appears to be a cause of nephrotic syndrome, particularly in West and East Africa. Malarial antigens are found in the renal glomerular basement membrane. Unfortunately, the condition does not respond to antimalarial treatment, glucocorticoids, or cytotoxic drugs but is becoming less common.

Pregnancy

Pregnancy ↑ risk of contracting falciparum malaria in all levels of endemicity.

- In areas of high, stable transmission, despite higher parasite burdens, most infections are asymptomatic, but result in ↓ in birth weight, with consequent ↑ infant morbidity and mortality. The effect is greater in primagravidae and (independently) in younger women.
- In areas of unstable transmission, pregnancy causes more severe malaria, particularly anaemia, hypoglycaemia, and acute pulmonary oedema. Fetal distress, premature labour, and stillbirth occur and low birth weight is common. In severe malaria, foetal death is the usual outcome.
- *P. vivax* malaria in pregnancy is also associated with a ↓ in birth weight, although to a lesser extent than *P. falciparum*. The effect is ↑ in multigravidae compared with primagravidae.

Congenital malaria has a very variable incidence. In some high transmission areas, parasitaemia in the newborn is >50%, but symptomatic disease rare.

Severe malaria

Severe malaria is a serious multisystem disease. The onset can be rapid, with death (particularly in children) occurring in a matter of hours. In travellers from endemic regions, it is most frequently observed when the diagnosis of malaria is made late and treatment delayed (see Box 2.3).

Cerebral malaria

Is the most important complication of falciparum malaria; it is uniformly fatal if untreated and has a ~20% treated mortality. It most often occurs in non-immune adults and in children. Cerebral malaria (CM) is 'unrousable coma in the presence of peripheral parasitaemia where other causes of encephalopathy have been excluded'. However, any alteration in consciousness in the context of falciparum malaria should be taken seriously. Neck rigidity and photophobia are not usually seen and Kernig's sign is –ve. There may be one or more of: diffuse cerebral dysfunction with coma, generalized convulsions (~50%), focal neurological signs, and brainstem signs such as abnormal doll's eye or oculovestibular reflexes. Retinal haemorrhages are seen in ~15% of cases, ↑ to ~40% if pupillary dilatation and indirect ophthalmoscopy are used. Neurological sequelae are found in ~5% of survivors (10% in children) and include hemiparesis, cerebellar ataxia, cortical blindness, hypotonia, and mental retardation. In children, CM carries 10–40% mortality, most deaths occurring within the first 24h.

Reduced Glasgow coma score (GCS) can also be caused by hypoglycaemia, which must be excluded. Malarial convulsions can occur at any temperature and post-ictal coma may last several hours. In deep coma, abnormalities of posture and muscle tone are frequently seen. For young children use the Blantyre Coma Scale (BCS; see Box 2.4) to grade the coma.

Respiratory distress

Is manifest by rapid, laboured breathing, sometimes with abnormal rhythms of respiration. In children, there may be intercostal recession, use of the accessory muscles of respiration and nasal flaring, which is difficult to differentiate from an acute respiratory infection. Respiratory distress (RD) in patients with malaria can result from a number of pathologies; each requires different treatment:

- In most cases, particularly in children, RD represents respiratory compensation for a profound metabolic acidosis. Severe metabolic acidosis (base deficit >12mmol/L) is associated with an 8-fold ↑ risk of death in children.
- Acute respiratory distress syndrome (ARDS) caused by direct alveolar capillary damage by parasites and neutrophils; worsened by hypoalbuminaemia and iatrogenic fluid overload.
- A lung infection because of the immunosuppression caused by malaria.
- Air hunger as a result of severe anaemia.

Box 2.3 WHO criteria for severe malaria

One or more of the following clinical or laboratory features:

Clinical manifestations

- Impaired consciousness.
- Respiratory distress (acidotic breathing).
- Multiple convulsions.
- Circulatory collapse.
- Pulmonary oedema (radiological).
- Abnormal bleeding.
- Jaundice.
- Haemoglobinuria.

Laboratory tests

- Severe anaemia.
- Hypoglycaemia.
- Acidosis.
- Renal impairment.
- Hyperlactataemia.
- Hyperparasitaemia.

Adapted from *WHO Guidelines for the Treatment of Malaria*. Geneva: WHO, 2010.

Box 2.4 Blantyre Coma Scale

To obtain 'coma score' add the scores from each section.

Best motor response	
• Localizes painful stimulus*	2
• Withdraws limb from painful stimulus**	1
• No response or inappropriate response	0
Best verbal response	
• Cries appropriately with painful stimulus, or if verbal, speaks	2
• Moan or abnormal cry with painful stimulus	1
• No vocal response to painful stimulus	0
Eye movements	
• Watches or follows (e.g. mother's face)	1
• Fails to watch or follow	0

*Pressure with blunt end of pencil on sternum/supraorbital ridge.

**Pressure with horizontal pencil on nail bed of finger or toe.

Reproduced from Molyneux, ME, *et al. Q J Med* 1989; **71**: 265, 451–9, with permission from Oxford University Press.

Anaemia

All patients with malaria will have some ↓ in Hb level. The anaemia is normocytic. Severe anaemia with haematocrit <15% (or Hb <5g/dL) in the presence of parasitaemia >10 000/μL (about 0.2% of red cells infected) is a common presentation in African children. Pallor, breathlessness, gallop rhythm, RD, pulmonary oedema, and neurological signs are common features of severe anaemia. Anaemia is exacerbated by 2° bacterial infections, haemorrhage, and pregnancy. Hyperparasitaemia and/or G6PD deficiency can result in massive intravascular haemolysis. In children, repeated episodes of otherwise uncomplicated malaria may lead to chronic normochromic anaemia with dyserythropoeitic changes in the bone marrow.

Jaundice

Common in adult patients and results from several mechanisms:

- Haemolysis.
- Hepatocellular damage.
- Cholestasis.

Both unconjugated and conjugated bilirubin may be >50μmol/L (3.0mg/dL). Clinical signs of liver failure very rare unless there is concomitant viral hepatitis.

Renal impairment

May be pre-renal or renal in origin, usually occurs in adults, and is characterized by a ↑ serum Cr (>265μmol/L or 3mg/dL) and ↑ urea, with oliguria (<400 ml urine/24 h in an adult) or anuria due to acute tubular injury. Renal impairment may occur at the time of maximal parasitaemia or even when the parasites have been cleared. In some cases, there is polyuria. Renal failure (anuria) in malaria has a poor prognosis (~45% die) unless acute dialysis or haemofiltration can be provided, in which case, good recovery of renal function is expected within 1–2wks.

Blackwater fever

Massive haemoglobinuria (urine becomes very dark, like Coca Cola) in context of malaria. Urine is +ve for blood (Hb) on dipsticks, but no red cells are seen on microscopy. Cause is not completely characterized, but in some cases it follows treatment with quinine, or treatment or prophylaxis with oxidant drugs, such as primaquine. More common in patients with G6PD deficiency or other red cell enzyme deficiencies (e.g. pyruvate kinase). In colonial times, blackwater fever was more common and mortality much higher.

Hypoglycaemia

Whole blood glucose (<2.2mmol/L, 40mg/dL) may be due to ↓ liver function or quinine/quinidine-induced hyperinsulinaemia (pregnant women are particularly prone). It presents with anxiety, sweating, breathlessness, dilated pupils, oliguria, hypothermia, tachycardia, and light-headedness, eventually → ↓ consciousness, convulsions, and coma. However, it can easily be missed in patients with disturbed conscious level. In a fasting adult, hepatic glycogen stores last ~2d; in a child ~12h. Hence, hypoglycaemia is common in 1–3-yr-olds (especially those with CM, hyperparasitaemia, or convulsions). It is also more common in pregnant women. Hypoglycaemia indicates a poor prognosis and is a risk factor for neurological sequelae. It is not associated with signs of malnutrition (Box 2.5).

Box 2.5 Indicators of a poor prognosis

Clinical

- Marked agitation.
- Hyperventilation (respiratory distress).
- Hypothermia (<36.5°C).
- Deep coma.
- Repeated convulsions.
- Bleeding.
- Anuria.
- Haemodynamic shock.

Laboratory

- Blood film showing hyperparasitemia >100 000/μL (about 2% of cells infected) in low transmission areas or >250 000/μL (about 5%) in high transmission areas.
- Blood film showing >20% of parasites to be 'late stages' (pigment-containing trophozoites and schizonts).
- Blood film showing >5% of neutrophils with visible pigment.
- Hypoglycaemia (<2.2mmol/L).
- Hyperlactataemia (>5mmol/L).
- Acidosis (arterial pH <7.3, serum HCO_3 <15mmol/L).
- Elevated serum creatinine (>265μmol/L).
- Elevated total bilirubin >50μmol/L.
- Leucocytosis (>12 000/μL).
- Severe anaemia (packed cell volume (PCV) <15%).
- Coagulopathy:
  - decreased platelet count (<50,000/μL)
  - prolonged prothrombin time (PT)
  - decreased fibrinogen (<200mg/dL).

Lactic acidosis

pH <7.3, or ↑ plasma and CSF lactate levels (plasma >5mmol/L) and a low plasma HCO_3^- (<15mmol/L) carry a poor prognosis in both adults and children. Acidosis is a major contributor to RD, especially in children.

Fluid and electrolyte disturbances

Hypovolaemia and dehydration are thought to be common, although recently this has become controversial. Low Na+, Cl–, PO4– , Ca2+, Mg2+, and endocrine dysfunction also occur, but seldom have major clinical implications except in the severely ill.

Acute respiratory distress syndrome

Carries 50% mortality and may occur even when the patient is otherwise improving. Excessive IV fluid replacement exacerbates this complication and is suggested by ↑ respiratory rate (exclude aspiration or acidosis). Predisposing causes include hyperparasitaemia, renal failure, and pregnancy (may occur suddenly after delivery). Hypoxia may → convulsions and death within a few hours.

Shock (algid malaria)

- Cold, clammy cyanotic skin.
- Weak rapid pulses.
- Prolonged capillary refill time in children (>3s).
- Supine systolic BP <70mmHg (<50mmHg in children) suggests circulatory collapse.
- Shock in malaria is commonly associated with 2° bacterial infection, metabolic acidosis, pulmonary oedema, dehydration, or a gastrointestinal (GI) bleed.

Give empiric parenteral antibiotics for bacteraemia, e.g. IV ceftriaxone.

Disseminated intravascular coagulation

Is due to pathological activation of the coagulation cascade. Disseminated intravascular coagulation (DIC) may manifest with bleeding gums, epistaxis, petechiae, haematemesis, and/or melaena with significant blood loss. DIC occurs in <10% of patients, but is more common in non-immune people (especially travellers). Blood film shows thrombocytopenia and schistocytes (damaged red cells). There is ↑ PT and ↓ plasma fibrinogen (note that thrombocytopenia alone may be present in about half of all cases of malaria and does not, by itself, indicate DIC).

Hyperparasitaemia

A parasite density >100 000 parasites/μL (about 2% of cells infected) is associated with ↑ mortality, although non-immune patients may die with much lower counts and, in highly endemic areas, individuals may tolerate greater densities without accompanying clinical features. Parasitaemias of >500 000 parasites/μL (>10% red cells infected) carries a 50% case fatality.

Gastrointestinal symptoms

Common in children. Nausea, vomiting, abdominal pain, and diarhoea without blood or pus are frequently seen. Persistent vomiting requires urgent parenteral drug administration.

Secondary infection

With septicaemia, pneumonia (e.g. following aspiration), UTI (following catheterization) and post-partum sepsis are common. Gram –ve septicaemia may occur without any focus of infection.

Differential diagnosis

Differential diagnosis of malaria

Malaria is a great mimic and must enter the differential diagnosis of several clinical presentations.

- The presentation of fever needs to be differentiated from common viral and bacterial infections, as well as other endemic diseases, such as typhoid and rickettsial infections, viral illnesses; such as dengue fever and influenza, brucellosis, and respiratory and UTIs. Less common causes of tropical fevers include visceral leishmaniasis, trypanosomiasis, and relapsing fevers.
- The coma of CM needs to be differentiated from meningitis (including tuberculous meningitis), encephalitis, enteric fevers, trypanosomiasis, brain abscess, and other causes of coma.
- The anaemia of malaria can be confused with other common causes of haemolytic anaemia in the tropics, such as that due to the haemoglobinopathies. The anaemia of malaria must be differentiated from that of iron, folate, or vitamin B12 deficiency.
- The renal failure of malaria must be distinguished from massive intravascular haemolysis, sickle cell disease, leptospirosis, snake envenoming, use of traditional herbal medicines, and chronic renal disease resulting from glomerulonephritis and hypertension.
- The jaundice and hepatomegaly of malaria must be distinguished from that of viral hepatitis (A, B, and E, cytomegalovirus, and Epstein–Barr virus infections), leptospirosis, yellow fever, biliary disease, and drug-induced disease including alcohol.

Clinical diagnosis on its own is notoriously inaccurate in the diagnosis of malaria and a blood film or rapid diagnostic test (RDT) is essential (see 🕮 Diagnosis, p. 48). Malaria cannot be diagnosed without a +ve blood film or RDT. However, in areas of stable transmission with high population parasite rates a +ve test can be non-specific. In seriously ill patients empiric antibiotic treatment should be given alongside antimalarial drugs.

Diagnosis

WHO now recommends that, wherever possible, a +ve diagnosis of malaria (or at least the presence of malaria parasites) be made in all cases using either high-quality microscopy of peripheral blood film or, if unavailable, RDTs. Presumptive treatment without a diagnosis should be avoided wherever possible.

Even when using RDTs or blood smears, in high transmission areas, where asymptomatic parasitaemia is common, over-diagnosis of malaria is a major problem. This can lead to under-treatment of the real cause of the symptoms, particularly when this is a bacterial infection. In these areas, cases of 'severe malaria' should routinely be treated with presumptive antibiotics, as well as antimalarials.

Nucleic acid detection tests using polymerase chain reaction (PCR) are extremely sensitive, highly accurate in speciation, and can be used to identify drug resistance mutations. However, they are technologically complex and, hence at present, not applicable to routine diagnosis.

Blood films

See Fig. 2.3 for blood film diagrams and Fig. 2.4 for thick/thin film methodology. Thin films are basically peripheral blood smears; thick films are more sensitive since they enable examination of a larger quantity of blood per microscopic field, but require more expertise to read.

Maintain a high index of suspicion and carry out ≥3 blood films (or RDTs) if the fever does not resolve. Malaria infection may exceptionally occur via transfusion, needlestick injury, IV drug abuse, and during brief airport stopovers in endemic areas or when infected mosquitoes 'alight' from airplane flights from endemic areas and bite individuals ('airport' malaria). In falciparum malaria, the presence of schizonts in peripheral blood samples may indicate severe infection as these forms would normally sequester.

Pitfalls of blood films

- Expertise is required for preparation and accurate interpretation of blood films; this is often lacking in clinical setting and quality control.
- A single –ve film does not exclude malaria. Repeat on three occasions at intervals. Blood films do not have to be taken at times of fever spikes. The patient may have been partially treated, suppressing patent infection. Malaria prophylaxis should be stopped whilst investigating for active infection.
- In endemic areas, a +ve film does not prove that malaria is responsible for the current symptoms.
- Correlation between parasite density and disease severity may be poor. Patients with a low parasitaemia may be very ill, whilst semi immunes may harbour high parasitaemias with relatively few symptoms.
- Platelets, cell fragments, and impurities in the stain can be mistaken for malarial parasites.

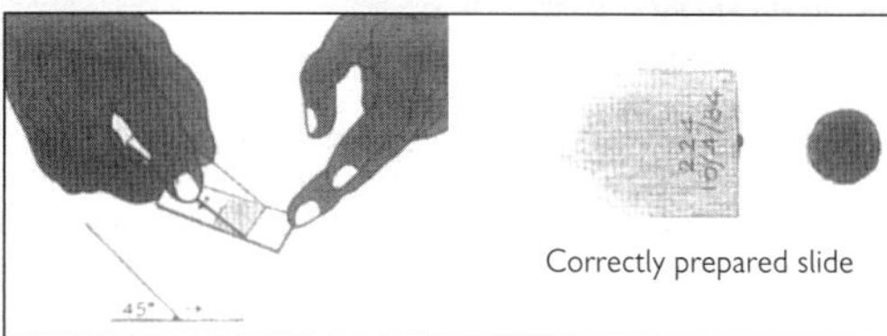

Fig. 2.3 Preparing blood film.

- Clean the tip of the patient's left index finger.
- Pierce the pulp of the fingertip with a sterile lancet or needle.
- Squeeze the finger until a droplet of blood forms and place it onto the middle of a clean slide (holding the slide by the edges). This is for the thin film.
- Place a further 3 droplets of blood onto the slide at a point to one side of the first droplet. These are for the thick film.
- Using a second clean slide as a spreader, touch the first, small drop with the edge and allow the blood to run along its edge. With the spreading slide at 45°, push the spreader forwards slowly, ensuring even contact, so that the blood is spread as a thin film over the surface of the slide (see Fig. 2.3).
- Using the corner of the spreading slide, amalgamate three drops of blood on the other half of the slide into a single small, denser film about 1cm in diameter.
- Label the slide with a pencil and allow to dry horizontally.

Problems

Badly-positioned blood droplets, too much or too little blood, using a greasy slide, a chipped edge of the spreader slide.

Staining Consult a laboratory manual for more details.

Giemsa stain

May be used for both films, but is costly and difficult to do. It should be filtered before use. Thin films must first be fixed in anhydrous methanol then dipped in 10% Giemsa for 20–30min; thick films are unfixed, stain with 5% solution for 30mins.

Field's stain

Uses 2 solutions, A and B, that are cheaper and more suited to rapid bulk staining. Thin films should be fixed in methanol, thick films are unfixed. For thick films, dip dried slides into solution A for 5s, avoiding agitation. Wash in tap water (preferably neutral pH) for 5s, avoiding washing unfixed smear off slide. Then dip into solution B for 3s. Wash again in water for 5s, then allow to dry vertically. The centre of the film may not be stained, but optimal parasite staining occurs at the edges of the film. For thin films, use solution B before solution A.

Rapid diagnostic tests

- There are numerous RDTs, which are antigen capture tests using a monoclonal antibody to detect the histidine-rich protein II (HRP2) of *P. falciparum*. These require minimal expertise to perform. Their main limitations are that they are non-quantitative, their sensitivity is ↓ at low parasitaemias and they cannot be used to monitor treatment response, as they remain +ve for some time after clearance of parasitaemia.
- Other tests detect parasite, rather than human, lactate dehydrogenase (pLDH); or parasite aldolase. pLDH and aldolase are +ve in all malaria species (pan-specific).
- In most tests, HRP2 detection is combined with pan-LDH or pan-aldolase. ∴ Detection can diagnose all species with good sensitivity (>95%), and distinguish *P. falciparum* from non-falciparum malaria infections.

	Early trophozoite (ring form)	Mature trophozoite
Plasmodium vivax	Thick rings, 1/3–1/2 the diameter of the red cell 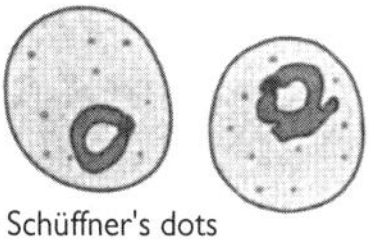 A few Schüffner's dots Accolé (shoulder) forms and double dots less common than with *P. falciparum*	Ameboid rings, 1/2–2/3 the diameter of the red cell Pale blue or lilac parasite with prominent central vacuole 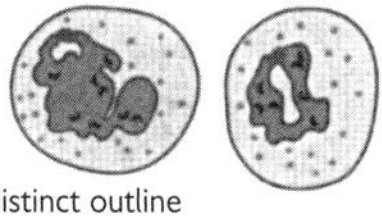 Indistinct outline Scattered fine yellowish-brown pigment granules or rods
Plasmodium ovale	Thick, compact rings, 1/3–1/2 the diameter of the red cell 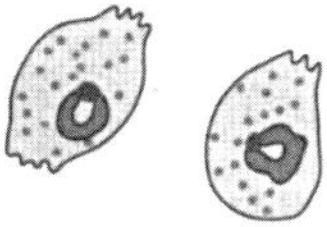 Numerous Schüffner's dots but paler than with *P. vivax*	Thick rings, less irregular than those of *P. vivax*, 1/3–1/2 the diameter of the red cell 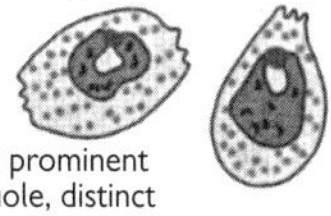 Less prominent vacuole, distinct outline. Yellowish brown pigment which is coarser and darker than that of *P. vivax* Schüffner's dots prominent
Plasmodium falciparum	Delicate rings, 1/6–1/4 the diameter of the red cell 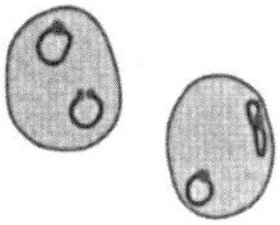 Double dots and Accolé forms common	Fairly delicate rings, 1/3–1/2 the diameter of the red cell 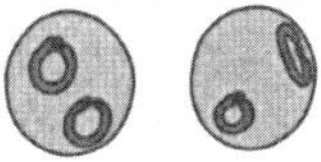 Red-mauve stippling (Maurer's dots or clefts) may be present Mature trophozoites are less often present in peripheral blood than ring forms
Plasmodium malariae	Small, thick, compact rings Small chromatin dot which may be inside the ring 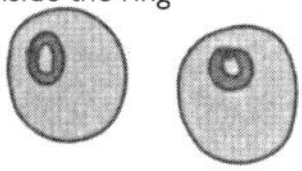 Double dots and Accolé forms rare	Amoeboid form more compact than *P. vivax* Sometimes angular or band forms 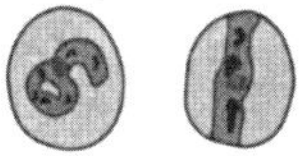 Heavy, dark-yellow-brown pigment No stippling unless overstained

Fig. 2.4 Diagrams of malarial blood cells.

	Early trophozoite (ring form)	Mature trophozoite
Plasmodium vivax	Thick rings, 1/3–1/2 the diameter of the red cell 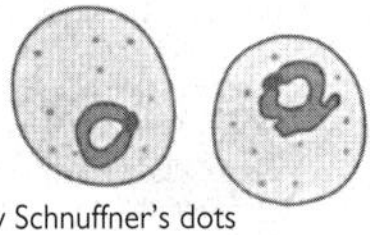 A few Schnuffner's dots Accolé (Shoulder) forms and double dots less common than with *P. falciparum*	Ameboid rings, 1/2–2/3 the diameter of the red cell Pale blue or lilac parasite with prominent central valuole 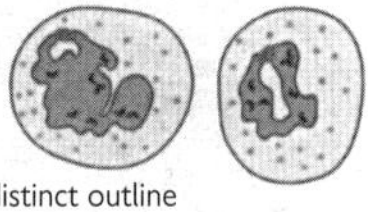 Indistinct outline Scattered fine yellowish-brown pigment granules or rods
Plasmodium ovale	Thick, compact rings, 1/3–1/2 the diameter of the red cell 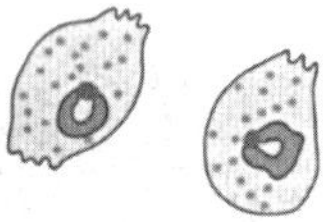 Numerous Schuffner's dots but paler than with *P. vivax*	Thick rings, less irregular than those of *P. vivax*, 1/3–1/2 the diameter of the red cell 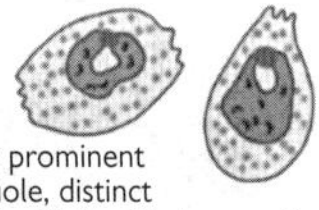 Less prominent vacuole, distinct outline Yellowish brown pigment which is coarser and darker than that of *P. vivax* Schuffner's dots prominent
Plasmodium falciparum	Delicate rings, 1/6–1/4 the diameter of the red cell 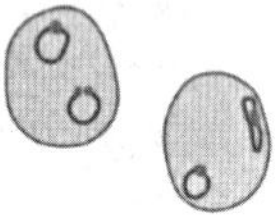 Double dots and Accolé forms common	Fairly delicate rings, 1/3–1/2 the diameter of the red cell 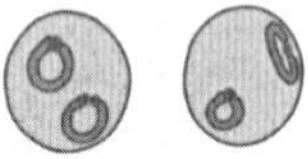 Red-mauve stippling (Maurer's dots or clefts) may be present Mature trophozoites are less often present in peripheral blood than ring forms
Plasmodium malariae	Small, thick, compact rings Small chromatin dot which may be inside the ring 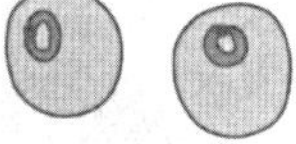 Double dots and Accolé forms rare	Ameboid form more compact than *P. vivax* Sometimes angular or band forms 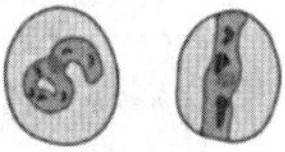 Heavy, dark-yellow-brown pigment No stippling unless ovestained

Fig. 2.4 (Continued).

	Early schizont	Late schizont
Plasmodium vivax	Rounded or irregular Amoeboid Loose central mass of fine yellowish-brown pigment 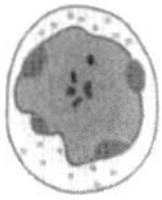 Schizont almost fills cell Schüffner's dots	12–24 (usually 16–24) medium-sized merozoites 1–2 clumps of peripheral pigment 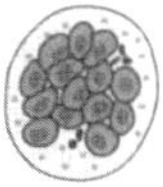 Schizont almost fills cell Schüffner's dots
Plasmodium ovale	Round, compact Darkish brown pigment, heavier and coarser than that of *P. vivax* 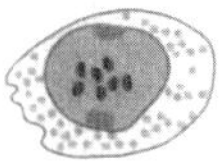 Schüffner's dots	6–12 (usually 8) large merozoites arranged irregularly like a bunch of grapes 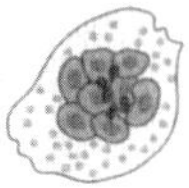 Central pigment Schüffner's dots
Plasmodium falciparum	Not usually seen in blood Very small, amoeboid Scattered light-brown to black pigment	Not usually seen in blood 8–32 (usually few) very small merozoites; grouped irregularly Peripheral clump of coarse dark brown pigment
Plasmodium malariae	Compact, round, fills red cell 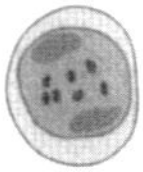 Coarse dark yellow-brown pigment	6–12 (usually 8–10) large merozoites, arranged symmetrically, often in a rosette or daisy head formation 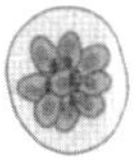 Central coarse dark yellowish-brown pigment

Fig. 2.4 (Continued). Reproduced with permission from Bain BJ *Blood Cells. A Practical Guide*. Oxford: Blackwell Science 1995.

General management

Once a diagnosis of malaria is made, preferably with laboratory support, assess the patient for the presence of features of severe malaria (see 📖 Severe malaria, p. 42). If a laboratory diagnosis cannot be made quickly or is not available, patients with suspected severe malaria should be treated empirically without delay.

Basic rules

- In many instances, especially in endemic areas, uncomplicated malaria can be treated on an outpatient basis.
- Advise patients to return promptly if symptoms worsen or do not improve within 48h.
- Beware of sending home patients who have mild symptoms, but high levels of parasitaemia, since they may deteriorate rapidly.

All patients will require antimalarial chemotherapy

Antimalarial treatment with appropriate antimalarial drugs should be started immediately, usually following national guidelines (see Box 2.6). Choose parenteral therapy in severely ill patients or those unable to tolerate oral medication.

Many patients will need analgesics

If fever causes distress, an analgesic/antipyretic should be given orally or by suppository. In two studies, paracetamol has been shown to prolong parasite clearance, although clinical significance of this is unclear. Several studies demonstrated a greater antipyretic effect with ibuprofen, which should be considered if there are no contraindications. Avoid aspirin in children, because of Reye's syndrome and because aspirin can ↑ acidosis.

Management

- *Assess the airway, breathing, and circulation:* intervene where necessary. Record vital signs: temperature, pulse, BP respiratory rate and capillary refill time (in children).
- *Obtain reliable venous access:* take blood for investigations including blood film, Hb or haematocrit, blood glucose, blood group and crossmatch. If available, do blood culture, biochemistry (electrolytes, renal and liver function), arterial blood gases (ABG) analysis, and coagulation studies.
- *Treat hypoglycaemia (blood glucose <2.2 mmol) if present:* give 20% glucose 50mL, retest and repeat if necessary. 50% solutions have been used, but there is ↑ risk of extravasation injury and these should be given very carefully. In children give 10% glucose 5mL/kg by slow IV bolus.
- Follow bolus treatment with 10% glucose infusion (0.1mL/kg/h). Monitor blood glucose levels frequently, especially following quinine infusion.

Box 2.6 *WHO Guidelines for the Treatment of Malaria* 2nd edn, 2010 (revised 2011)

The WHO guidelines encompass all the recent important developments in the treatment of malaria, both uncomplicated and severe. The guidelines are evidence-based, a valuable resource on all aspects of treatment and discuss in detail two major recent developments:

- The wide acceptance and recommendation of artemisinin-based combination therapy (ACT) as treatment of choice for uncomplicated falciparum malaria. The main clinical advantages of ACTs are a rapid therapeutic response and rapid initial ↓ in parasite numbers; in addition, they ↓ chance of drug resistance emerging and spreading and may, through their gametocytocidal effect, interfere with transmission.
- The recommendation that artesunate, the most rapidly acting parenteral antimalarial, is now the drug of choice in preference to quinine for the treatment of severe malaria. It can be used in the 2nd and 3rd trimesters of pregnancy, and is a drug of choice alongside quinine in the 1st trimester.

The complete guidelines can be downloaded in PDF format from the WHO website at: http://whqlibdoc.who.int/publications/2010/9789241547925_eng.pdf and http://www.who.int/malaria/publications/atoz/mal_treatchild_revised.pdf

- *Weigh patient and initiate antimalarial therapy:* see Antimalarial chemotherapy, p. 58.
- *Consider empirical broad-spectrum antibiotic therapy:* e.g. IV ceftriaxone if hypotensive or suspicion of bacterial infection (in Kenya bacteraemia occurs in 8–12% of children with severe malaria).
- *Lumbar puncture:* patients with ↓ levels of consciousness should have a lumbar puncture to exclude bacterial meningitis. If there is concern about ↑ intracranial pressure (ICP), if the patient is too unwell for the procedure, or if platelets count too low, LP can be delayed, but antibiotic cover should be given.
- *Assess hydration:* consider urinary catheterization. Rehydration may be required, particularly if diarrhoea and vomiting are present. Adults with severe falciparum malaria usually require 1–3L of isotonic saline over the first 24h. However, avoid overhydration. In children rapid fluid resuscitation may be associated with ↑ mortality, see notes of use of fluids in the sick child, Treatment of shock, p. 11.
- *Monitor renal output and BP hourly:* aim to keep CVP (if available) in the low–normal range.
- *Blood transfusion:* with pathogen-free, compatible fresh blood or packed cells should be considered in patients with a haematocrit <15% or Hb <5g/dL. Transfusion should be given urgently in children with a Hb <4g/dL or a Hb <5g/dL with respiratory distress or acidosis or parasitaemia >10%; in such cases, give blood 10mL/kg over 30min, then a further 10mL/kg over 2–3h without diuretics. In DIC, fresh blood, clotting factors (FFP), and/or platelets should be given as required.

- *Exchange transfusion:* has not been subject to a randomized controlled trial (RCT). It has been rarely carried out since the use of artesunate, with its rapid and reliable action, became established.
- *Dialysis if patient develops renal failure:* haemofiltration or haemodialysis may be indicated. Peritoneal dialysis should be used if these are unavailable but is less effective.
- *Oxygen and mechanical ventilation:* may be required for patients with respiratory distress or significantly ↑ ICP. If distress is due to pulmonary oedema, the patient should be nursed at 45° and IV diuretics given. Haemofiltration may be used if available.
- *Inotropes:* e.g. dopamine may be given, preferably through a central line, if hypotension does not respond to volume expansion. Adrenaline should be avoided as it can exacerbate acidosis.

Box 2.7 Cerebral malaria

Treat as in 📖 General management, p. 54 with the following additional specific measures:

- Nurse the patient on her side to avoid aspiration of vomit. Turn every 2h.
- The patient should be catheterized and have temperature, heart rate and RR, BP, and fluid balance measured regularly.
- Consciousness must be assessed regularly with the GCS or BCS (see 📖 p. 433).
- Hypoglycaemia must be treated promptly, but is very difficult to detect in an unconscious patient. Blood sugar should be actively monitored at least 4–6-hourly and whenever there is any deterioration in the patient's clinical condition.
- *If convulsions arise:* be alert, since they may be subtle. Treat with diazepam (10mg in adults) by slow IV, repeat once if necessary. An alternative is diazepam 10–20mg rectally, repeated after 10–15min if required.
- Corticosteroids, mannitol, or other ancillary agents for cerebral oedema are of no proven benefit.

Antimalarial chemotherapy

There have been recent major changes in the treatment of malaria, particularly the use of ACTs for treatment of uncomplicated falciparum malaria and emergence of parenteral artesunate as the drug of choice for severe malaria.

Resistance to many antimalarial drugs is an increasing problem worldwide and it is important to have up-to-date information on local resistance patterns. Chloroquine, for example, can no longer be used to treat falciparum malaria in most parts of the world. Resistance to the artemisinin derivatives has been described in Southeast Asia and, resistance to partner drugs in the ACT combinations is a major problem in many areas.

Artemisinin-based combination therapies

Combination therapy is simultaneous use of two or more drugs with independent modes of action. The aim is to ↓ the spread of resistance, with the two components protecting each other. This principle has been widely applied in the treatment of human immunodeficiency virus (HIV)/ acquired immunodeficiency syndrome (AIDS) and tuberculosis (TB). In ACTs, one of these agents is an artemisinin derivative, the most rapidly acting class of antimalarial. This ensures a rapid fall in parasitaemia, which ↓ the risk of developing resistance. Artemisinin derivatives are also gametocytocidal and thus may ↓ malaria transmission. Partial courses of ACTs should not be given, even when patients are considered to be semi-immune or the diagnosis is uncertain. This may encourage the development of resistance. For non-artemisinin based treatment see comments in 🕮 Box 2.9: Non-artemisinin based combination therapies, p. 621.

Treatment of uncomplicated *P. falciparum* malaria

- The aim is to ↓ parasitaemia as quickly as possible and to prevent recrudescence of the infection. Antimalarial drugs are given orally if tolerated. If the species is unknown or there is mixed infection, treat as falciparum malaria.
- ACTs are the recommended treatment of choice for uncomplicated falciparum malaria worldwide. Monotherapy is specifically discouraged.
- Be aware of local patterns of resistance, particularly to the artemisinin derivative partner drug. These will influence the 1st line ACT for the area (Box 2.8).
- Treatment failures within 14d of receiving an ACT should be treated with a 2nd line antimalarial (see 🕮 Currently recommended ACTs, p. 59).
- Treatment failures (recurrent parasitaemia) after 14d can be retreated with the original 1st line ACT. However, retreatment with mefloquine within 28d is associated with an ↑ risk of neuropsychiatric disorder, so if the 1st line ACT was artesunate + mefloquine, a 2nd line antimalarial should be given.

Box 2.8 Treatment of the 'benign' malarias

- The standard treatment is chloroquine 25mg base/kg divided over 3 days (e.g. 10mg base/kg followed by 5mg base/kg at 6, 24, and 48h).
- *P. malariae* does not produce hypnozoite forms, so chloroquine is curative.
- Hypnozoite stages of *P. ovale* and *P. vivax* are not affected by blood schizonticides, such as chloroquine, so to prevent relapses and effect a 'radical cure', primaquine (a liver schizonticide) must be given as well (0.25mg base/kg daily for 14d (0.375–0.5mg base/kg daily in Southeast Asia and Oceania, where relatively primaquine-resistant strains occur). Primaquine can cause GI symptoms; should be given with food.
- Primaquine is an oxidant and causes haemolysis in G6PD-deficient individuals. Screening is generally unavailable, but in areas where mild to moderate G6PD deficiency is the common variant, primaquine in weekly doses of 0.75mg base/kg for 8 wks is better tolerated. Primaquine should not be given in severe G6PD deficiency. It should also not be given to pregnant women.
- Chloroquine-resistant *P. vivax* is increasingly a problem (particularly in Oceania, Indonesia, and Peru), and can be treated with an ACT combined with primaquine.
- The benign malarias are susceptible to all ACTs (the exception being *P. vivax* and artesunate + sulfadoxine-pyrimethamine (SP), since *P. vivax* responds poorly to SP in many areas). Primaquine is still required for radical cure.

Currently recommended ACTs

Artemether + lumefantrine

(For comments on second line antimalarials for falciparum malaria see 📖 Box 2.10, p. 62 and for Pregnant and lactating women see Box 2.11, p. 62.) Fixed-dose combination (artemether 20mg/lumefantrine 120mg in each tablet) suitable for use in areas of multidrug resistance (Southeast Asia), as well as worldwide. Six doses over 3d. Should be taken with milk or fat-containing food.

Adult dose (wt >35kg): 4 tablets at 0, 8, 24, 36, 48, and 60 h.

Paediatric dose

Recommended for children ≥5kg. Reduce number of tablets at each dose—body wt 25–34kg, 3 tabs/dose; 15–24kg, 2 per dose; 5–14kg, 1 per dose. This is the equivalent of 1.7/12mg/kg body weight of artemether and lumefantrine, respectively, per dose, given bd for 3d, with a therapeutic dose range of 1.4–4mg/kg of artemether and 10–16mg/kg of lumefantrine.

Artesunate + mefloquine

The prototype ACT, with a fixed-dose combination is in an advanced stage of development. Suitable for use in areas of multidrug resistance (Southeast Asia); effective elsewhere, but expensive. Currently available as separate scored artesunate (50mg) and mefloquine (250mg base) tablets. 3-d course.

Dose

Artesunate 4mg/kg on days 1, 2, and 3; mefloquine 15mg/kg on day 2 and 10mg/kg on day 3. Alternatively as 8.3mg/kg/day od for 3 days. The therapeutic dose range is between 2–10mg/kg/dose/d of artesunate and 7–11mg/kg/dose/d of mefloquine.

Artesunate + sulfadoxine-pyrimethamine (SP)

Currently available as separate scored artesunate (50mg) and SP (500/25mg) tablets. Only suitable for areas where SP monotherapy 28d cure rates >80%. Useful in some parts of Africa, but these are diminishing rapidly.

Dose

A target of 4mg/kg/d artesunate given od for 3d and a single administration of 25/1.25mg/kg SP on day 1, with a therapeutic dose range between 2–10 mg/kg/d artesunate and 25–70/1.25–3.5mg/kg SP.

Artesunate + amodiaquine

Now available as a fixed-dose combination (three tablet sizes containing artesunate/amodiaquine 100/270, 50/135, and 25/67.5mg). Only suitable for areas where amodiaquine monotherapy 28-d cure rates exceed 80% (mainly West Africa).

Dose

A target of 4mg/kg/day artesunate and 10mg/kg/day amodiaquine od for 3d, with a therapeutic dose range between 2–10mg/kg/day artesunate and 7.5–15mg/kg/dose amodiaquine.

Dihydroartemisinin + piperaquine

Currently available as a fixed-dose combination with tablets containing dihydroartemisinin 40mg and piperaquine 320mg.

Dose

Administered once a day for 3 days, dose varying with body weight: 5–7.9kg, ½ tablet/day; 8–9.9kg, 0.75 tablets/day; 10–14.9kg, 1 tablet/day; 15–20.9kg, 1.5 tablets/day; 21–29.9kg, 2.0 tablets/day; 30–39.9kg, 2.5 tablets/day; 40–50.9kg, 3 tablets per day; and ≥51kg, 4 tablets/day.

Artesunate plus tetracycline or doxycycline or clindamycin

There are no blister co-packaged forms of any of these combination options. They are reserved for very rare occasions of treatment failures to recommended ACTs and in some special groups, e.g. pregnant women failing ACT treatment (Box 2.11). Should only be used in a hospital setting.

Dose

Artesunate (2mg/kg od) plus tetracycline (4mg/kg qid) or doxycycline (3.5mg/kg od) or clindamycin (10mg/kg bd). These combinations should be given for 7d.

Box 2.9 Non-artemisinin based combination therapies

SP + chloroquine is not recommended, as resistance to both components is already widespread and no synergy has been demonstrated. SP + amodiaquine in areas of parasite sensitivity may be more effective than either drug alone but less rapidly acting than ACTs. ∴ Only recommended when ACTs are unavailable. Atovaquone + proguanil (malarone) has been used to treat uncomplicated malaria in the context of artemisinin resistant malaria, but this use is controversial because of the high risk of the development of resistance.

Box 2.10 Second line antimalarials for falciparum malaria

Used in cases of treatment failure <14d after receiving an ACT.
In order of preference they are:

- An alternative ACT known to be effective in the region (generally a 3d course).
- Artesunate (2mg/kg od) plus either tetracycline (4mg/kg qds) or doxycycline (3.5mg/kg od) or clindamycin (10mg/kg bd).
- Quinine (10mg salt/kg tid) plus either tetracycline (4mg/kg qds) or doxycycline (3.5mg/kg od) or clindamycin (10mg/kg bd).

Regimens 2 and 3 should be given for 7d. The quinine regimens are poorly tolerated and adherence is often poor. Doxycycline and tetracycline should not be used in pregnancy or in children <8yr.

Box 2.11 Pregnant and lactating women

- First trimester: quinine and clindamycin (see doses in 📖 Currently recommended ACTs, p. 59) given for 7d. If clindamycin is unavailable, give quinine monotherapy. Treatment failures should be treated with 7d of artesunate + clindamycin (see 📖 Currently recommended ACTs, p. 59). Use an ACT as 1st line treatment if it is the only effective treatment available.
- Second and third trimesters: an ACT that is known to be effective in the region, or artesunate + clindamycin (7d) or quinine + clindamycin (7d).
- Lactation: lactating women should in general be given standard antimalarial treatment, including ACTs, but should not receive dapsone, primaquine, or doxycycline/tetracycline.

Treatment of severe malaria

General management of the severely ill patient and of complications are covered in 📖 General Management, p. 54. Severe malaria is a medical emergency. Full doses of parenteral antimalarial therapy should be started immediately and continued until the patient is well enough to take oral follow-on treatment (see Box 2.12).

Drugs currently in use

Artesunate

2.4mg/kg IV or IM at 0, 12, and 24h, then od. Artesunate is the WHO recommended therapy for the treatment of severe malaria in both low and high transmission settings. It is 1st line treatment for severe malaria in the 2nd and 3rd trimesters of pregnancy (Boxes 2.13 and 2.14).

- In two multi-country studies of severe malaria, IV artesunate was associated with a 35% ↓ in mortality compared with IV quinine in Asian adults and children, and a 22.5% ↓ in mortality in African children.
- The currently available formulation of artesunate is non-GMP, although it is this formulation that has demonstrated superior efficacy over quinine in low transmission areas. A good manufacturing practice (GMP) formulation is being developed.

Artemether

IM injection into the anterior thigh, 3.2mg/kg then 1.6mg/kg/d. Artemether absorption from IM injection is erratic, especially in very ill patients. It is a WHO recommended therapy if artesunate is unavailable.

Quinine

Is no longer recommended by WHO as 1st line treatment for severe malaria, but remains recommended when artesunate and artemether are unavailable and is an option in the 1st trimester of pregnancy. A loading dose 20mg quinine salt/kg should be given on admission, then 10mg quinine salt/kg tds thereafter, each dose given by rate-controlled IV infusion over 4h or by divided IM injection (rate should NOT exceed 5mg/kg/h).

- For IV infusion, quinine must be diluted in 5–10mL/kg body weight of glucose or saline solution. For IM use, quinine should be diluted in normal saline to 60mg/mL and half the dose given in each anterior thigh. IM injection can cause abscess formation.
- Quinine can cause severe hyperinsulinaemic hypoglycaemia, particularly in pregnant women.
- In acute renal failure or hepatic dysfunction, the dose should be reduced by one-third after 48h to prevent accumulation and resulting toxicity. Dose adjustment in renal failure is unnecessary if the patient is receiving haemofiltration or haemodialysis.
- The 1st dose can be reduced to 10mg salt/kg if there is certainty that the patient has received adequate pre-treatment with quinine before presentation. If in doubt, give the loading dose.

Quinidine

If the other, recommended, parenteral antimalarials are unavailable (e.g. in the USA), the anti-arrhythmic drug quinidine (an enantiomer of quinine) may be used. Give 15mg base/kg infused IV over 4h, followed by 7.5mg base/kg over 4h q8h. Cardiac monitoring is required. Dose adjustments are necessary in renal failure and hepatic impairment as for quinine. Convert to oral therapy as soon as possible.

Box 2.12 Follow-on treatment

Following initial parenteral therapy, when the patient is well enough to take oral medication, a full course of an ACT known to be effective in the region should be given. Either 3 days of artesunate + amodiaquine or artemether + lumefantrine or completion of 7d treatment with oral artesunate + 7 days of doxycycline or clindamycin (in children and pregnant women).

Box 2.13 Pregnancy

Give the parenteral antimalarial used locally for severe malaria in full doses. Because quinine causes severe recurrent hypoglycaemia, where available, artesunate is the first choice and artemether the second choice in the 2nd and 3rd trimesters. As little evidence is available in the 1st trimester, artesunate, quinine, and artemether may all be considered options.

Box 2.14 Pre-referral treatment

Rectal artesunate is well absorbed and is an option to start treatment and prevent progression of severe disease while referral to a health care facility capable of giving parenteral treatment is made. Quinine can also be given intra-rectally in such circumstances.

Box 2.15 Artemisinin resistance

Resistance to the artemisinin drugs has been described recently in Southeast Asia. This was seen initially in Western Cambodia, but is now also a problem on the Thai-Myanmar border. Artemisinin resistance is characterized by prolonged parasite clearance and an increase in treatment failures. It is regarded as the single biggest global threat to malaria control and elimination programmes. See http://www.wwarn.org/resistance/malaria and http://www.who.int/malaria/areas/drug_resistance/updates/en/index.html for the latest information.

Prevention

Prevention against malaria includes both chemoprophylaxis and measures taken to ↓ the number of mosquito bites. Insect repellents containing DEET (10–50%) or picardin (7%) should be used, and insecticide-treated bed nets in areas where anophelene mosquitoes bite indoors at night. Individuals should be aware of malarial symptoms, which may be non-specific, and report early for a blood film or RDT if malaria is suspected. Malaria vaccines are currently in clinical trials and may offer protection in the future (see 📖 Public health note: malaria control, p. 67).

Travellers to malarial areas

Should preferably begin prophylaxis 1wk (2–3wks in case of mefloquine) before arrival, and must continue for 4wks after departure, except in cases of atovaquone-proguanil and primaquine, where prophylaxis may be commenced 1d before entry into malarial area and end 7d after return.

Any febrile illness occurring <1yr of travel could be malaria. For long-term, non-immune residents, there is a balance between the risks of infection and side-effects of chemoprophylaxis. It may be possible to target prophylaxis during the transmission season alone.

Malaria endemic areas

Antimalarial prophylaxis is not logistically or financially feasible for the entire population, but has been used in those at highest risk, young children and pregnant women, in endemic areas. Intermittent preventive treatment (IPT) is an alternative that shows some promise and may work at least partly through its prophylactic effects.

Drugs used in prophylaxis

Atovaquone-proguanil, mefloquine, doxycycline, and primaquine can all be used as prophylaxis throughout the malaria endemic world, whereas the usefulness of chloroquine and proguanil has been severely restricted by resistance.

Atovaquone-proguanil

Well-tolerated, once-daily, fixed-dose combination effective against all types of malaria, including multidrug-resistant falciparum malaria. Should be taken with food and a milky drink to improve absorption. There is insufficient data to recommend its use in pregnancy, and it is very expensive. Dose in children best adjusted to weight.

Dose Adult daily dose atovaquone 250mg/proguanil 100mg.

Mefloquine

Nausea, dizziness, and vivid dreams are common side-effects, and approximately 1 in 10 000 recipients develops an acute reversible neuropsychiatric reaction. Mefloquine is not recommended in neonates, but has been used for prophylaxis in pregnancy.

Dose 250mg oral weekly in adults and children >45kg (62.5mg wkly in children 6–16kg; 125mg for 16–25kg, 187.5mg for 25–45kg).

Doxycycline

Useful as an alternate to mefloquine. Side effects include GI (nausea, diarrhoea) and photosensitivity.

Dose

Adults and children >12yr, 100mg od oral; children >8yr, 1.5mg/kg oral od, to a max 100mg. Do not use in children <8yr and in pregnant and lactating women.

Primaquine

Has proven in adults to be effective and safe against drug-resistant *P. falciparum* and *P. vivax*. Should be taken with food to reduce GI side-effects. Should not be given to G6PD-deficient individuals or pregnant women.

Dose

0.5 base mg/kg daily for children; 30mg od as daily adult dose.

Proguanil

Used for prophylaxis in pregnant women and non-immune people in areas of low risk only. It is more commonly used in combination with chloroquine (see 📖 Chloroquine, below). Of limited use now due to resistance.

Dose

200mg oral od in adults, including pregnant women. Children <12wks 25mg/d; 12wks–1yr 50mg/d; 1–4yr 75mg/d; 4–8yr 100mg/d, and 8–13yr 150mg/d.

A folic acid supplement should be taken during pregnancy.

Chloroquine

Is used in combination with proguanil in low-risk areas, in pregnant women and individuals who cannot tolerate other antimalarials. Not effective against most *P. falciparum* strains world-wide; resistance in *P. vivax* is ↑.

Dose

300mg (base) oral weekly in adults, including pregnant women. Child dose chloroquine base: <12wks, 37.5mg once weekly; 12wks–1yr, 75mg weekly; 1–4yr, 112.5mg weekly; 4–8yr, 150mg weekly, and 8–13yr, 225mg weekly.

Monitoring antimalarial drug resistance

With the rapid recent spread of drug resistance, there is an increased need to monitor the current levels of resistance to provide evidence to inform choice of antimalarial drug therapy and ensure proper management of clinical cases. A number of monitoring systems are available.

Therapeutic efficacy testing

The WHO has developed a protocol for in vivo testing of the efficacy of antimalarial drugs against *P. falciparum* in the field (http://whqlibdoc.who.int/publications/2009/9789241597531_eng.pdf). It is a simple one-arm trial, with the treatment outcomes divided into a number of classes.

Early treatment failure (ETF)

- Development of danger signs or severe malaria on days 1–3 in the presence of parasitaemia.
- Parasitaemia on day 2 higher than the day 0 count, irrespective of axillary temperature.
- Parasitaemia on day 3 with axillary temperature ≥37.5°C.
- Parasitaemia on day 3 that is ≥25% of count on day 0.

Late clinical failure (LCF)

- Development of danger signs or severe malaria after day 3 in the presence of parasitaemia, without previously meeting any ETF criteria.
- Presence of parasitaemia and axillary temperature ≥37.5°C on any day from days 4 to 28, without previously meeting any ETF criteria.

Late parasitological failure (LPF)

Presence of parasitaemia on any day from days 7 to 28, and axillary temperature <37.5°C, without previously meeting any of the criteria of ETF or LCF.

Adequate clinical and parasitological response (ACPR)

- Absence of parasitaemia on day 28 irrespective of axillary temperature without previously meeting any of the criteria of ETF, LCF, or LPF.
- 'Clinical failure' can be summarized as ETF + LCF.
- 'Total failure' can be summarized as ETF + LCF + LPF.

In vitro resistance tests

Technologically demanding and limited by exclusion of host factors and parasite factors unrelated to resistance. These tests are useful for providing additional information to support clinical efficacy data.

Molecular markers

If the molecular basis for resistance is known, these techniques can provide early warning of the presence of resistance to a range of antimalarial tests in a parasite population and guide therapeutic choices in epidemic situations.

See http://www.wwarn.org/resistance/malaria for information on areas with resistant malaria.

Public health note: malaria control

The three main components of malaria control are:

- Effective antimalarial drug treatment to ↓ mortality and morbidity, particularly with ACTs, which may ↓ transmission through their gametocytocidal effect. The addition of a single dose of primaquine to ACT treatment may also decrease transmission of falciparum malaria by killing mature gametocytes.
- Personal protection with insecticide-impregnated materials, such as bed nets and curtains.
- Vector control by insecticide spraying, particularly indoors, and possibly, in selected ecologic circumstances, larval control measures.

Education of the population on the importance and practical application of all three of these is a pre-requisite for success.

The resources to apply these principles have benefitted through major investment from, e.g. Global Fund for HIV/AIDS, Malaria & Tuberculosis, the Roll Back Malaria Initiative, and the President's Malaria Initiative. Since the Gates Malaria Forum of October 2007 malaria eradication has been back on the table as a viable long term objective. Increasingly the explicit aim of malaria control efforts are local elimination. This is particularly the case in areas of low transmission, which are also usually the areas with the most antimalarial drug resistance. For example, the best hope of preventing the spread of artimisinin resistance to Africa is thought to lie in elimination of artemisinin resistant parasites within Southeast Asia.

A malaria vaccine has been the holy grail of malaria researchers for decades, but while there have been major recent advances, an effective, deployable vaccine is not yet available. The RTS,S vaccine has had the most promising results to date, but there are uncertainties, including duration of protection.

Further research is needed into the biology of the vector and the parasite, and their interaction with the human host, the pathophysiology of the disease process, and the socio-cultural factors that determine health-seeking behaviour and compliance with drug regimens.

There is an urgent need to discover and develop novel classes of antimalarial drug if we are not to face a malaria control catastrophe if and when the parasite develops resistance to the artemisinin derivatives.

Chapter 3

HIV/AIDS

Invited authors (adult) **Andy Parrish**
Graeme Meintjes
Invited author (paediatric) **Lee Fairlie**

Epidemiology of HIV

The human immunodeficiency viruses are the cause of the AIDS global pandemic.

AIDS was first recognized in the USA in 1981 and cumulative global mortality from HIV infection to date is >25 million. There are ~33.3 million people living with HIV infection worldwide, including 2.5 million children <15yr. Of those with HIV infection, ~68% live in sub-Saharan Africa, where 5% of the adult population is HIV+. Seroprevalence rates among pregnant women are 30–40% in parts of southern Africa. There are also rapidly growing HIV epidemics in eastern Europe and in Central and East Asia.

Transmission

Potentially infectious body fluids are: blood, serous effusions, CSF, semen, vaginal fluid, and breastmilk. Urine, vomitus, and saliva are non-infectious unless they are contaminated with blood. The virus survives poorly in the environment; no cases of environmental (e.g. discarded needles) or insect transmission are documented.

The main routes of HIV transmission are:

- *Unprotected sexual intercourse* (both heterosexual and homosexual): sexually-transmitted infections (STIs), particularly those that cause genital ulceration, ↑ the risk of sexual transmission. In resource-poor regions, heterosexual intercourse is the major mode of transmission for adults.
- *Mother to child transmission* (MTCT): the highest risk is at time of delivery, but transmission may also occur during the pregnancy or via breastmilk. In the absence of preventative strategies, the risk of transmission in non-breastfeeding populations is 15–30%, but increases to 20–45% in breastfeeding women.
- Receipt of infected blood products (screening of blood products minimizes this risk).
- Sharing of needles or equipment during injecting drug use.
- Injections or treatments with unsterile needles, syringes, surgical apparatus, or skin-piercing instruments.
- Needle stick injuries to health care workers. The risk is estimated to be 0.3% if no post-exposure prophylaxis (PEP) is administered.

Virology and immunology

HIV virology

- *Genus:* Lentivirus. *Family:* Retroviridae.
- Enveloped RNA virus (two identical RNA copies of genome in each virus).
- Spherical and measures 80–100nm in diameter (see Fig 3.1).
- Contains 3 enzymes: reverse transcriptase, integrase, and protease.
- Two types of HIV are recognized: HIV-1 and HIV-2.

HIV-1 accounts for ~99% of cases in the global pandemic. HIV-1 is divided into four groups: M, O, N, and P. Group M accounts for the majority of infections worldwide, and is itself divided into clades (e.g. clade C, the predominant circulating clade in southern Africa; see Table 3.1).

HIV-2 affects <0.5 million people. It is found mainly in West Africa and in people from that region. HIV-2 is a zoonotic virus of primates, which has 40–60% genetic homology with HIV-1. HIV-2 is less transmissible and is associated with a ↓ rate of CD4 and clinical decline. Many patients with HIV-2 are co-infected with HIV-1. Third generation ELISAs will diagnose both HIV-1 and 2, whereas earlier generation ELISAs and some of the rapid tests only diagnose HIV-1. HIV-1 viral load assays will not detect HIV-2. HIV-2 is intrinsically resistant to non-nucleoside reverse transcriptase inhibitors (NNRTIs) and may carry pre-existing protease inhibitor (PI) mutations.

Once HIV infects a human it attaches to and enters immune cells that bear the CD4 protein on their surface—mainly CD4 T-lymphocytes and macrophages. Within these cells, the virus replicates using viral enzymes, such as reverse transcriptase and protease, as well as hijacking human cellular mechanisms for RNA and protein production. During this process, copies of viral DNA are inserted into the chromosomal DNA of the host cell. Billions of new HIV particles are formed daily in this way in an infected person. The immune system responds by destroying the formed viruses, keeping circulating virus at a constant or 'setpoint'. This → a state of immune activation that persists for many years, during which the CD4 count ↓ from the normal count of 500–1400cells/mm^3 at a rate that varies widely between individuals. CD4 T-lymphocytes coordinate the body's immune response and, when CD4 cell numbers are profoundly depleted in the late stages of HIV infection, profound immunosuppression (AIDS) results. This predisposes to a variety of infections that would not normally cause disease in an immunocompetent person—so-called 'opportunistic' infections. The specific opportunistic infections (OIs) that occur depend on both the geographical area and the patient's degree of immunosuppression. Certain tumours associated with viruses, are more common in AIDS patients: lymphomas (mainly due to Epstein–Barr virus (EBV), see 📖 Infectious mononucleosis, p. 796) and Kaposi sarcoma-associated herpes virus (KSHV or HHV-8). AIDS-related conditions usually occur when the CD4 is <200cells/mm^3.The risk of certain infections, such as pneumococcal disease and TB, which are capable of causing disease in immunocompetent hosts, is dramatically ↑ in the presence of immunosuppression due to HIV.

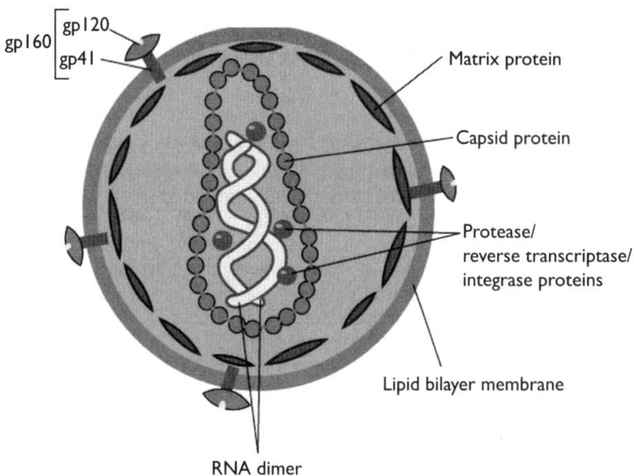

Fig. 3.1 HIV-1 virus structure.

Reproduced from Torok E, Moran E, and Cooke F, *Oxford Handbook of Infectious Disease and Microbiology* (2009) with permission from Oxford University Press.

Table 3.1 HIV statistics for high burden regions (WHO estimates for 2009) Source: UNAIDS Report on the Global AIDS Epidemic, 2010

Region	**Adults and children living with HIV (million)**	**Adults and children newly infected with HIV**	**% Adult HIV prevalence (15–49yrs)**
Sub-Saharan Africa	22.5	1 800 000	5
South and Southeast Asia	4.1	270 000	0.3
North America	1.5	70 000	0.5
Central and South America	1.4	92 000	0.5
Eastern Europe and Central Asia	1.4	130 000	0.8

Source: http://www.unaids.org/globalreport/global_report.htm

Natural history of HIV infection

HIV infection progresses from a seroconversion illness soon after infection → a long asymptomatic period → symptomatic disease → AIDS (see Fig. 3.2).

Acute retroviral illness

An acute retroviral illness occurs in ~50% of patients 2–5wks after infection, lasting 3–21d. The underlying HIV aetiology is recognized only in a minority of cases at this time. It is clinically similar to infectious mononucleosis (see 🕮 Infectious mononucleosis, p. 798) with variable signs and symptoms that include malaise, fever, sore throat, myalgia, anorexia, arthralgia, headache, diarrhoea, nausea, generalized lymphadenopathy, and a maculo-papular eruption involving the trunk and arms. It is often clinically misdiagnosed as another intercurrent illness (e.g. influenza). Rare complications include aseptic meningoencephalitis and mono/polyneuritis. Atypical lymphocytes may be seen in the blood film. There may be significant temporary immunosuppression during the acute infection with OIs reported during this period and serological antibody tests for HIV are -ve or indeterminate. There appears to be some correlation between severity of seroconversion illness and speed → HIV disease progression.

Asymptomatic HIV infection

Seroconversion is followed by an asymptomatic stage, during which the body's immune system attempts to control the virus. HIV is not latent at this stage, but is in balance with the immune system. Billions of HIV virions are produced and destroyed each day. The only sign of infection during this period may be persistent generalized lymphadenopathy (PGL), but a high proportion of patients have no abnormalities on physical examination. The asymptomatic stage varies in length, but ends when immune system dysfunction produces symptoms.

Symptomatic HIV infection

Symptoms are often absent or non-specific until the immune system's function becomes significantly compromised. These symptoms may initially be mild, such as skin rashes (especially seborrhoeic dermatitis, papular pruritic eruption or shingles) or oral candidiasis, but later the patient suffers from OIs, as well as the direct effects of HIV. ↓ Weight, weakness, ↓ functional capacity, diarrhoea, and peripheral neuropathy are common. OIs attack multiple systems. Certain OIs become more common as the CD4 count falls, and this is reflected in the WHO's staging system. TB is a very common presenting illness irrespective of CD4 count.

In the absence of anti retroviral therapy (ART), the average time course from infection → AIDS is 9yrs. Some patients are rapid progressors and may develop AIDS just a few years after infection. Typically, these patients have ↑ viral load setpoints with ↑ CD4 decline (see Table 3.2). Other patients may be slow progressors with slow CD4 and clinical decline. OIs, in particular TB, may ↑ HIV disease progression by ↑ viral replication and the viral setpoint 2° to immune cell activation.

Table 3.2 CD4 count and HIV complications

CD4 count	Complications
>500/mm^3	Acute retroviral syndrome, candida vaginitis, PGL, Guillain–Barré syndrome (GBS), myopathy, aseptic meningitis, TB
200–500/mm^3	Pneumococcal and other bacterial pneumonia, pulmonary tuberculosis, herpes zoster, oropharyngeal candidiasis, cryptosporidiosis, Kaposi's sarcoma, oral hairy leukoplakia, cervical intra-epithelial neoplasia, cervical cancer, B-cell lymphoma, anaemia, mononeuritis multiplex, idiopathic thrombocytopenic purpura (ITP), Hodgkin's lymphoma, lymphocytic interstitial pneumonitis (LIP)
<200/mm^3	*Pneumocystis carinii* pneumonia (PCP), disseminated histoplasmosis, disseminated coccidioidomycosis, miliary/extrapulmonary TB, progressive multifocal leucoencephalopathy (PML), wasting syndrome, peripheral neuropathy, HIV-associated dementia, cardiomyopathy, vacuolar myopathy, progressive radiculopathy, non-Hodgkin's lymphoma (NHL)
<100/mm^3	Disseminated herpes simplex, toxoplasmosis, cryptococcosis, chronic cryptosporidiosis, microsporidiosis, oesophageal candidiasis
<50/mm^3	Disseminated cytomegalovirus (CMV), disseminated *Mycobacterium avium* complex (MAC), primary central nervous system lymphoma (PCNSL)

There is no vaccine and no cure for HIV infection. Good therapies have been developed, however, for many OIs. Combination ART can control viral replication, and allow a considerable and durable restoration of immune function.

WHO clinical staging system for HIV infection and disease

This staging system (see Box 3.1) was developed for epidemiological purposes. It is useful for estimating progression of HIV-related immunosuppression and assisting in making decisions about the need for co-trimoxazole prophylaxis and starting ART. The presence of any of these manifestations in a previously healthy adult should suggest HIV infection.

Box 3.1 WHO clinical staging system (2006)

Clinical stage 1

- Asymptomatic.
- PGL.

Clinical stage 2

- Weight loss <10% of body weight.
- Minor mucocutaneous lesions (seborrhoeic dermatitis, papular pruritic eruptions, fungal nail infection, recurrent oral ulceration, angular cheilitis).
- Herpes zoster.
- Recurrent URTI.

Clinical stage 3

- Weight loss >10% of body weight.
- Unexplained chronic diarrhoea for >1mth.
- Unexplained prolonged fever for >1mth.
- Oral candidiasis, chronic vaginal candida.
- Oral hairy leukoplakia.
- Pulmonary TB.
- Severe bacterial infections (pneumonia, pyomyositis, empyema).
- Acute necrotizing ulcerative oral disease.
- Unexplained anaemia (<8g/dL), neutropenia (<0.5 × 10^9/L) and/or chronic thrombocytopenia (<50 × 10^9/L).

Clinical stage 4

- HIV wasting syndrome*.
- PCP.
- Central nervous system (CNS) toxoplasmosis.
- Chronic cryptosporidiosis.
- Chronic isosporiasis.
- Cryptococcosis (extrapulmonary).
- CMV infection (retinitis or other organs).
- Chronic Herpes simplex virus (HSV) infection of >1mth or visceral.
- PML.
- Candidiasis of the oesophagus, trachea, bronchi, or lungs.
- Disseminated non-tuberculous mycobacterial infection.
- Recurrent septicaemia including non-typhoid *Salmonella*.
- Extrapulmonary TB.
- Lymphoma (cerebral or B cell NHL).
- Kaposi sarcoma (KS).
- HIV encephalopathy.
- Invasive cervical cancer.
- Recurrent severe bacterial pneumonia.
- Disseminated mycosis (histoplasmosis or coccidioidomycosis).
- Atypical disseminated leishmaniasis.
- Symptomatic HIV nephropathy or cardiomyopathy.

*HIV wasting syndrome is defined as weight loss of >10%, plus either unexplained diarrhoea (lasting >1mth) or chronic weakness and unexplained fever for >1mth.

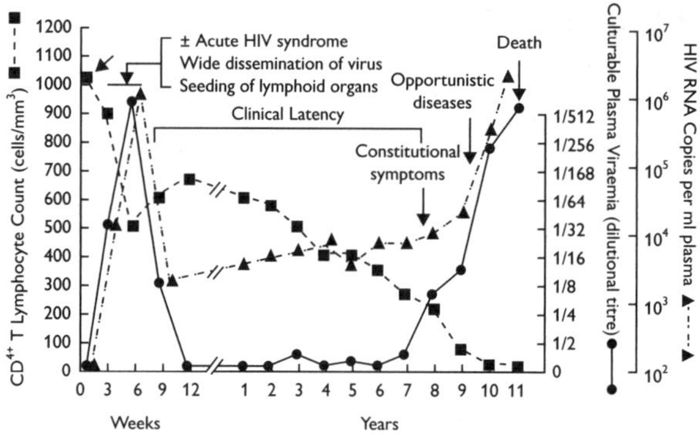

Fig. 3.2 Course of untreated HIV infection in adults.

Adapted with permission from Pantaleo G, *et al.* The immunopathogenesis of human immunodeficiency virus infection. *N Engl J Med* 1993; 328(5): 327–35.

HIV diagnosis

HIV antibody testing may be performed in the following situations:

- *Transfusion/transplant safety:* screening of donated blood and organs to prevent HIV transmission.
- *Surveillance:* unlinked and anonymous testing to monitor prevalence and trends in HIV infection in a given population.
- *Diagnostic Testing and Counselling* (DTC): diagnostic testing should be offered in all patients who present with features of HIV disease. Consideration should be given to offering testing to all patients, particularly those who are admitted, with appropriate counselling using an 'opt-out' model.
- *Voluntary counselling and testing* (VCT): voluntary testing of asymptomatic persons in the community who wish to know their status. Expanding VCT and DTC will allow more people to know their status, ↑ access to treatment, and may prevent transmission.
- All pregnant women should be tested to allow for interventions to prevent vertical transmission among those who are HIV+.

The diagnosis of HIV can be made by the detection of HIV itself or the detection of antibodies to HIV.

Direct detection of virus (these tests may not be available in resource limited settings due to cost):

- HIV viral RNA PCR.
- Integrated HIV viral DNA PCR.
- P24 antigen enzyme-linked immunosorbent assay (ELISA).

Tests for antibodies to the virus (serological tests):

- 1st, 2nd, 3rd generation ELISA.
- *rapid tests*—point-of-care tests are similar to ELISAs; they have sensitivity and specificity similar to ELISA when performed by appropriately trained operators.
- Western blot.
- 4th generation combo-ELISA able to detect antibodies and p24.

All tests have a '*window period*' (interval between initial infection of patient and test becoming +ve). Important *average* window periods are: HIV RNA PCR, 10d; p24 antigen, 17 days; 3rd generation ELISA, 22 days. There is wide inter-individual variation in any window period. Antibody tests are +ve in virtually 100% of patients by 3mths, unless post-exposure prophylaxis was taken that may delay seroconversion.

In most settings, antibody tests are used for diagnosis of HIV. An exception is testing infants for HIV. Infants exposed to HIV will have +ve antibody tests that might not represent infection, but only placental passive transfer of maternal IgG. Thus, HIV-exposed infants should be tested with an HIV DNA PCR to establish infection (this is usually done at 4–6wks of age). A +ve antibody test beyond 18mths of age is diagnostic of infection. A single test for HIV infection should never be considered +ve, and the patient informed, until it has been confirmed by a second test. The 1st screening test may be an ELISA or a rapid test and should have high sensitivity to avoid false –ves. The 2nd or confirmatory test should be different: a 2nd ELISA, a 2nd rapid test, or a Western blot. The 2nd test should have high specificity to avoid false +ves. Two separate blood specimens should be used to prevent laboratory error. The 2nd rapid test should use different antigen specificity or a different platform.

Quantitative HIV viral load (HIV-1 RNA)

(Copies/mL) determines the amount of virus circulating in blood. A higher viral load → more rapid progression and ↑ risk of transmission.

CD4 T-lymphocyte count

Is measured by flow cytometry. It is used to assess the degree of immunosuppression and decide on the need for OI prophylaxis and ART. New and simpler methodologies for CD4 count testing have been developed that allow testing closer to the point of care.

Importance of counselling

Pre-test counselling

Whether testing is initiated by the patient or the health worker, the patient should receive information about HIV infection and the test, have an opportunity to ask questions and agree to testing.

Pre-test information could include (depending on the patient's needs and level of knowledge):

- Information about who will have access to the test results.
- Exploration of the patient's knowledge and beliefs regarding HIV.
- Education around HIV, its transmission, prevention, clinical course, and treatment. Discuss the 'window period'.
- Discussion regarding benefits of testing (OI prophylaxis, ART, prevention of transmission to sexual partner).
- Exploration of consequences of +ve and –ve test. Discuss patient's support systems and coping strategies.
- Discussion of issues of disclosure of +ve result and obligation to inform sexual partners.
- Documentation of consent (written or verbal).
- The testing process must include an assurance of confidentiality and an arrangement of follow-up for result unless a rapid test is used.

Post-test counselling

Post-test counselling for a +ve result ideally should consist of two or more sessions. Many patients will be in a state of shock when first told the result and 'information overload' should be avoided in the 1st session. The session(s) should:

- Include feedback about the result.
- Allow expression of emotions and discussion about them.
- Identify immediate concerns and plans.
- Discuss prognosis and potential benefits of ART.
- Identify supports and include discussion of disclosure, especially to sexual partner.
- Include talk about safe sex and other risk reduction, healthy lifestyle, treatment, and prophylaxis of opportunistic infections and ART.
- Arrange follow-up and/or referral for appropriate HIV/ART care.
- If necessary, offer psychological or psychiatric referral, since some patients become depressed after a +ve result.

If the result is -ve, post-test counselling should focus on a discussion of the 'window period' and the need for a repeat test in 3mths and reinforce prevention messages. The emphasis should be on the person staying –ve.

Management of asymptomatic HIV infection

Explain the aim of promoting and maintaining optimal psychological and physical health among HIV+ people, their partners, relatives, and caregivers. The prevention of transmission of HIV to others should also be discussed.

Medical management

- Detect and treat early HIV-associated disease.
- Prescribe primary prophylaxis when indicated (see Table 3.3).
- Determine the appropriate time to start ART.

The CD4 count is of value when interpreting symptoms and signs, and in deciding when to start 1° prophylaxis and ART.

All HIV+ individuals are at ↑ risk of developing TB. On presentation, and at all subsequent visits, ask about TB contacts and symptoms of cough, fever, night sweats, and weight loss. Weight loss between visits, or any concerning symptoms, should prompt focused examination (particularly looking for new adenopathy or respiratory findings) and may warrant further investigation, such as a sputum for TB testing and CXR.

Physical examination

Should include:

- *General:* ↓ weight, fever.
- *Neurological system:* peripheral neuropathy, cognitive disorders.
- *Skin:* herpes zoster or simplex, folliculitis, tinea, KS, papular pruritic eruption, seborrhoeic dermatitis, psoriasis.
- *Mouth:* thrush, 'hairy' leukoplakia, gingivitis, KS.
- *Eyes:* fundoscopy (CMV).
- Lymph nodes (see 📖 Lymphadenopathy, p.85).
- *Lungs:* consolidation signs, crackles, or pleural effusion.
- *Abdomen:* liver enlargement or tenderness, splenomegaly.
- *Genitalia:* ulceration or genital warts.
- *Anus:* ulceration or warts.

Investigations (depending on local resources)

- CD4 count (transiently suppressed by intercurrent infections).
- Serum creatinine (urea and electrolytes and glucose).
- FBC.
- Serology for syphilis and hepatitis B (HBV).
- Cervical smear in women.
- Liver enzymes: e.g. AST or ALT and ALP or GGT.
- Serum cryptococcal antigen test (in those with CD4 count <100). If this is +ve, patients should have an LP to exclude meningitis (essential if neurological symptoms). If no neurological symptoms and LP not possible, treat pre-emptively with fluconazole.

Serial viral RNA measurements prior to initiating ART add very little to management. Other investigations should be directed by clinical problems.

Drug therapy

Co-trimoxazole 1° prophylaxis should be considered in all individuals with a CD4 count <350 or WHO stage 3 or 4 disease. The WHO also advises co-trimoxazole prophylaxis in stage 2 disease when CD4 counts are unavailable. This therapy provides a modest survival advantage, probably by its effect on bacterial infections, malaria in endemic areas, pneumocystis and toxoplasmosis.

Table 3.3 Primary prophylaxis

Condition	Medication	When to stop	Efficacy
Pneumocystis	Co-trimoxazole 2 tabs daily*	CD4 >200 on ART	NNT (mortality) = 15
Tuberculosis	INH 300mg/d for 6mths if no clinical evidence of TB, +ve tuberculin skin test (TST), and well-functioningTB programme	Usually 6mths; may be additional benefit when given for 36mths	Reduces new cases of TB** in patients with +ve TST (NNT 22)
Pneumococcal infections	Pneumococcal vaccine is of unclear value		

*Co-trimoxazole single strength contains 80mg trimethoprim and 400mg of sulfamethoxazole. Dose may be reduced to 480mg (1 tablet) daily to improve tolerance.

**Defined as 'confirmed, probable, or possible active TB'. If given regardless of TST status, if TST not known, and if used the stricter definition of 'confirmed or probable TB' the NNT is about 50. (NNT is the number needed to treat for 6mths.)

Symptomatic HIV infection

Fever Infections common in a particular geographical area are often more frequent and severe in HIV+. HIV-related OIs may also vary by region (e.g. penicilliosis is common in parts of Southeast Asia and China). Always consider TB as a cause of systemic illness in HIV+ individuals.

History

- Duration may be difficult to determine, but if hours or days, it suggests a septicaemic process, and if days or weeks, chronic infections, such as TB, are more likely.
- *Localizing symptoms:* cough, dyspnoea, headache, diarrhoea, dysuria, genital discharge may → a particular organ system.
- Weight loss may suggest a more chronic infection unless due to GI fluid loss.
- Take a travel history.

Examine for cause of fever in HIV positive individuals

- *Mouth:* candidiasis? Tonsillitis or retropharyngeal abscess?
- *Lymph nodes*: particularly in the neck, axillae, and groin.
- *Chest:* dullness, crackles, bronchial breathing.
- *Heart:* is there a pericardial rub, muffled sounds or abnormal dullness on percussion suggesting a pericardial effusion? ↑ Jugular venous pressure (JVP) or pulsus paradoxus indicating tamponade? Is there a murmur or other features of endocarditis?
- *CNS:* neck stiffness suggesting meningitis (or local cervical sepsis), focal neurological signs suggesting brain mass or encephalitis, or cord signs suggestive of subdural or epidural pus. Is there local facial tenderness suggesting sinusitis?
- *Abdomen:* tenderness over liver or appendix, renal angle, or suprapubic tenderness. Is the spleen palpable?
- *Skin:* is there evidence of local infection, particularly in the axillae, groin, or ischiorectal area? Is there a skin rash?
- *Musculoskeletal:* is there arthritis? Is there localized muscle tenderness suggestive of pyomyositis?
- *Pelvic examination in women:* ?PID.

Investigations

Consider:

- CD4 (influences differential diagnosis).
- Blood culture.
- Urine dipsticks, and if +ve, microscopy and culture.
- Stool microscopy and culture (if diarrhoea).
- Sputum and other specimens (e.g. induced sputum or early morning urine) for TB microscopy and culture.
- Needle aspiration of nodes >2cm.

- Malaria smears in endemic areas or traveller from endemic area.
- Bone marrow biopsy if pancytopenic.
- LP if headache (to exclude bacterial, cryptococcal, or TB meningitis).
- Aspirate pleural or pericardial effusions for bacterial and TB microscopy and culture.
- Skin biopsy of a rash may be helpful (e.g. disseminated histoplasmosis).
- Chest radiograph.
- US abdomen and pericardium (pericardial effusion, abdominal adenopathy, splenic hypodensities, or ascites are suggestive of TB in endemic areas and, less commonly, fungal infection or lymphoma).

Viral illnesses may also present with fever and other features, such as coryza, pharyngitis, and cough with central chest pain, but are less likely to have a ↑ white cell count (WCC) or ↑ markers of inflammation (e.g. ↑ C-reactive protein (CRP)).

Immune reconstitution inflammatory syndrome (IRIS) may present with fever after ART is started (see 📖 Immune reconstitution inflammatory syndrome, p. 128). Also consider non-infective causes of fever such as deep vein thrombosis (DVT) and drug fever.

Lymphadenopathy

Consider:

- TB
- Syphilis (papulosquamous rash +/– recent genital ulcer).
- Fungal (histoplasmosis, cryptococcosis).
- *Malignancy:* KS (not always with obvious cutaneous KS), lymphoma.
- *Dermatological conditions:* seborrhoeic dermatitis, chronic pyoderma.
- *Local infection that might explain the lymphadenopathy.*

Persistent generalized lymphadenopathy (PGL) of HIV itself is common. It is defined as follows:

- >3 separate lymph node groups affected.
- At least 2 nodes >1.5cm in diameter at each site.
- Duration of >1mth.
- No local infection that might explain the lymphadenopathy.

PGL also tends to involve lymph node regions symmetrically and nodes are seldom >2cm in diameter and are non-tender. PGL lymph nodes are not visible on CXR as enlarged hila.

If nodes are rapidly enlarging or asymmetrical or there are systemic signs, a lymph node aspiration should be performed. If this is not diagnostic, a formal full node biopsy should be considered to exclude TB, lymphoma, KS, and fungal infection.

Wasting syndrome and malnutrition Patients should be weighed at each outpatient visit and weight recorded in a prominent place in the case notes.

Management

- Investigate for, and treat underlying chronic infections, such as TB.
- Manage chronic diarrhoea if present (📖 Management of persistent diarrhoea, p. 284).
- Consider issues such as depression, poor diet (often due to loss of income) and ↓ appetite. May be iatrogenic contribution (iron tablets, antibiotics, such as erythromycin and metronidazole, and even milk-based nutritional supplements in individuals with lactose intolerance).
- Having excluded obvious causes, consider starting ART in HIV+ individuals with significant weight loss.

Nutrition

Good nutrition is essential in order to maintain immune competence and strength, and minimize the impact of infection (see 📖 Recipes and formulas for management of ill and severely malnourished children, p. 712).

Multivitamins

This should include the recommended daily allowance (RDA) of vitamins A, B, C, E, and minerals. Most multivitamin preparations contain only normal RDAs of vitamins and these may be inappropriate for the correction of severe deficiencies—use single agents in appropriate doses e.g. nicotinamide for pellagra, thiamine for beriberi, ascorbic acid for scurvy (doses see 📖 Nutrition, p. 683).

Skin and oral disease

Itchy rashes

Pruritic rashes are common. Consider treating for scabies even if distribution atypical as treatment is cheap and safe. Drug reactions are often itchy, but in the absence of a clear drug aetiology, generalized itchy, fine, papular eruptions may be due to the so-called papular dermatitis of HIV ('itchy bump disease' or 'papular pruritic eruption'). This may respond to topical 0.1% betamethasone valerate (1% hydrocortisone for the face).

Herpes zoster

- A vesicular eruption typically in a unilateral dermatomal distribution.
- If started <72h of onset of blistering, aciclovir (800 mg 5× daily for 7d) or valaciclovir (1g 3× daily for 7d) may ↓ rash duration and ↓ risk of post-herpetic neuralgia.
- Zoster involving the eye should be treated with topical aciclovir ophthalmic ointment—if possible, refer to an ophthalmologist.
- Give analgesia, e.g. paracetamol 1g qds (max per 24h) +/– amitriptyline 10–25mg at night (initially 10mg nocte usually); occasionally opiates may be required.

Crusted (Norwegian) scabies

- A hyperkeratotic form of scabies seen in immunocompromised persons.
- Extensive crusting in areas accessible to scratching, with sparing of less accessible areas, such as the middle of the back.
- The scalp is usually involved.
- *Treatment:* see 📖 Skin infestations, p. 590.

Cutaneous cryptococcosis

- Vesicular or papular rash which mimics molluscum contagiosum, although umbilication is less common.
- Diagnosis by either aspiration (India ink stain or culture) or skin biopsy or serum cryptococcal antigen test.
- Manage like cryptococcal meningitis.

Penicillium marneffei

- Common in Southeast Asia.
- Similar skin findings to cryptococcosis
- Initial treatment with amphotericin, but itraconazole thereafter until CD4 count >100 for 6mths.

Histoplasmosis

- This may present with mucocutaneous ulceration, but a more chronic form presents with a generalized crusting rash, which may resemble 'chronic' impetigo.
- Diagnosis by blood culture, or skin biopsy, or serum/urine antigen.
- Therapeutic alternatives are amphotericin and itraconazole.

Drug rashes

- Drug rashes vary from mild papular eruptions to Stevens–Johnson syndrome.
- Common causes include co-trimoxazole, anti-TB drugs, and NNRTIs, but practically any drug can be involved.
- Danger signs are an absolute indication to stop all drugs that could possibly be causative: fever, new adenopathy, facial swelling, mucosal involvement, blistering, eosinophilia, or ↑ liver enzymes (any ↑ ALT with symptoms of hepatitis, or ALT >5× upper limit of normal even if asymptomatic).
- Do not use drugs to treat a drug-induced skin disease—once the drug is stopped it will improve with time and supportive measures.
- Self-limiting rashes are relatively common with the NNRTIs. In patients with only mild reactions (none of the above danger signs present), it may be reasonable to consider continuing 'essential' drugs under close supervision.

Gingivostomatitis

- This may be due to Candida or Herpes simplex (📖 Herpes simplex virus, p. 615).
- Major aphthous ulceration is a disabling gingivostomatitis with extensive ulceration and necrosis.
- Consider topical therapy (e.g. povidone iodine mouthwashes) and oral amoxicillin plus metronidazole.
- In refractory cases with persistent ulceration, biopsy to exclude TB and syphilis.
- Persistent symptoms without an easily identifiable cause are an indication for considering antiretroviral therapy.

Vaginal candidiasis

See 📖 Candida vaginitis, p. 680.

Kaposi's sarcoma

See 📖 HIV-related malignancy, p. 108.

Seborrhoeic dermatitis

See 📖 Dermatology, p. 587.

Bacillary angiomatosis

See section on 📖 Bartonella, p. 758.

Respiratory disease

See Table 3.4 for overview.

Community-acquired pneumonia

- Acute presentation (hours–days), with fever, pleuritic chest pain, and cough with muco-purulent sputum.
- Signs may be less marked in patients with ↓ immunity.
- Common differential diagnoses include atypical TB or PCP, as well as organisms also found in HIV –ve individuals (e.g. *Strep. pneumoniae*).
- Treat ill immunosuppressed patients with IV ceftriaxone 1–2g od or, if not available, IV ampicillin 1g qds. In severe cases, add cover for atypical pneumonia (doxycycline 100mg bd or macrolide). Search for TB if poor treatment response. Parenteral therapy can be changed to oral once there is clinical response.

Pneumocystis carinii pneumonia

- Dry cough and ↑ dyspnoea for days → week or longer.
- Few physical signs on respiratory examination, in the presence of quite marked hypoxia (cyanosis and tachypnoea).
- CXR typically shows a diffuse ('ground glass') interstitial infiltrate without effusion or adenopathy. Patient tends to be worse clinically than the CXR would suggest.
- Sputum induced by 10min of nebulization with hypertonic saline may be +ve on microscopy.
- Treatment is usually initiated on clinical and radiographic grounds in the absence of laboratory confirmation.
- Treat with co-trimoxazole (trimethoprim/sulfamethoxazole 480mg) 4 tablets qds for 21d. If <60kg—the majority of adult patients—reduce to 3 tablets qds. ↑ serum K+ and creatinine are common on this regimen.
- If hypoxic, add prednisolne 40mg bd for 5d; then 40mg od for 5d; then 20mg od for 10d. Start as soon as hypoxia noted, do not wait for patient to deteriorate.
- Response is not always dramatic and some patients may take > a week to start to improve. After treatment, give prophylaxis with co-trimoxazole 960mg daily.

Chronic cough

- Cough associated with ↓ weight should prompt a search for an underlying chest infection, usually TB.
- Extrinsic bronchial compression from lymphadenopathy (TB, lymphoma, KS).
- Parenchymal lung diseases presenting atypically, without major clinical or radiological manifestations e.g. PCP and lymphocytic interstitial pneumonia (LIP).
- Bronchiectasis may be present with few radiological signs.
- Pulmonary KS is uncommon, typically presenting with nodular opacities, hilar adenopathy, and pleural effusions. It may mimic TB. Skin or oral Kaposi's lesions are often present.
- HIV+ individuals can also suffer from all the diseases of HIV –ve individuals, e.g. late onset asthma, drug side-effects (e.g. angiotensin converting enzyme inhibitors) and foreign bodies.

Table 3.4 Respiratory infection in HIV+ individuals

Feature	Bacterial pneumonia	Pulmonary tuberculosis	Pneumocystis pneumonia
Duration of symptoms	hours or days	days or weeks	days or weeks
Loss of weight	If present, due to something else	Usually present	If present, due to something else
Purulent sputum	Occurs in 1/2 patients	Occurs in 1/3 patients	Very rare—small amounts of white sputum occasionally
Chest pain	Poor discriminator, although the chest discomfort in PCP is classically described as central and non-pleuritic		
Hypoxia	Variable	Uncommon unless severe TB	Common, can be very severe
Chest signs	Variable	Often unimpressive	Usually unimpressive
Chest X-ray	May show lobar pattern	Typically hilar and upper mediastinal adenopathy with lower zone non-cavitating infiltrate (cavitation may be present if ↑ CD4)	Diffuse bilateral infiltrate. Effusion or adenopathy make PCP unlikely (but consider dual pathology)
Serum lactate dehydrogenase	Only helpful in discriminating between pneumocystis and suspected viral pneumonias		
Sputum induction	Rarely diagnostic	Helpful	Helpful
Fine–needle node aspiration (peripheral lymph nodes)		Frequently diagnostic	

Gastrointestinal disease in HIV

Acute diarrhoea (short history or abrupt deterioration)

- *Assess hydration:* pulse and BP lying and standing or sitting, urine specific gravity, and laboratory measurement of serum K+, Na+, urea, and creatinine if available.
- Signs of dehydration can be misleading in severely malnourished patients who commonly have sunken eyes and ↓ skin turgor and fluid resuscitation guidelines are different (📖 Dehydration, p. 696).
- If IV therapy necessary (ongoing vomiting or severe dehydration) give 5% glucose-saline, 1L 4–6-hourly adjusted according to clinical response.
- As most patients are hypokalaemic, start replacement with IV K+ 20mmol/L, unless the patient is anuric at presentation, in which case wait for a laboratory K+ result. Oral K+ tablets may ↑ nausea and vomiting; fruit or fruit juice contains K+ in a palatable form.
- In febrile patients with colitis (bloody diarrhoea with abdominal tenderness over the colon) or who do not respond to fluid resuscitation, Gram –ve septicaemia is a possibility; e.g. give IV ceftriaxone—it has activity against *Salmonella* and *Shigella* (check local susceptibility patterns); if amoebiasis endemic, add metronidazole. If possible, take blood culture before giving antibiotics.

Chronic diarrhoea

Consider:

- *Infective causes:*
  - Protozoal (e.g. *Giardia, Isospora, Cyclospora, Cryptosporidia, Microsporidia, Entamoeba*).
  - Viruses (e.g. CMV).
  - Bacteria (e.g. TB, MAC).
- *Medications:* e.g. protease inhibitors, excess Vitamin C, medications or food supplements containing sorbitol or lactose.
- *HIV enteropathy:* generally a diagnosis of exclusion.

History

Diarrhoea can wax and wane, creating the illusion of response to symptomatic therapy and antibiotic cocktails.

- Nausea, bloating, and cramps suggests stomach or small intestinal involvement by protozoa.
- Tenesmus or fresh blood rectally suggests colitis/dysentery, e.g. CMV, *Shigella, Campylobacter, Clostridium difficile.*

Examination

- Look for cervical or local abdominal adenopathy suggestive of TB.
- Tenderness on palpation over the colon suggests large bowel pathogens as mentioned above.
- A review of weight charts usually reveals significant weight loss.

Investigation

- Stool microscopy for ova and parasites. Special Ziehl–Neelsen (ZN) stain required to identify coccidian parasites such as *Isospora*.
- Stool culture, +/– *C. difficile* toxin.
- Sigmoidoscopy and biopsy may be of value in diagnosing CMV.

Management

- For general management of diarrhoea see 📖 Management of persistent diarrhoea. p. 284.
- See below for summary of management of diarrhoea in HIV.

The majority of organisms, e.g. *Cryptosporidium* respond poorly, if at all, to specific medical therapy. Important to assess for ART, 2° ↑ immunity usually cures the diarrhoea. Empiric antibiotic treatment common, on assumption that offending organism has been missed on culture. Choices include ciprofloxacin for undiagnosed *Salmonella* infection, and metronidazole for *Giardia, Entamoeba*, and *Clostridium difficile*. Efficacy of this practice unclear. Isosporiasis may respond to co-trimoxazole 960mg qds for 10d followed by 960mg bd for 3wks. Maintenance therapy may be needed to prevent relapses. Also limited evidence for efficacy of albendazole 400mg bd oral for a month in patients with microsporidia. In afebrile patients where no infecting organism has been found, and inflammatory markers and examination do not suggest infection, anti-peristaltic agents, e.g. loperamide 2mg oral tds may be considered for symptom control, particularly if the diarrhoea is affecting nutritional status.

Abdominal pain

Usual differential of acute abdomen is applicable in HIV, and recovery rate after surgery is similar to HIV-uninfected people. Also consider:

- *Salmonella typhi* and its complications.
- *Abdominal TB:* may be accompanied by ascites and retroperitoneal adenopathy. Splenic hypodensities on USS is suggestive of TB.
- CMV colitis or oesophagitis is sometimes associated with vasculitis and severe episodic pain. Negative CMV IgG makes the diagnosis less likely. Confirmation of CMV is by biopsy; in some settings, CMV serum viral load is available.
- *Pancreatitis:* may be due to CMV, TB, or associated with ART use (stavudine (d4T) or didanosine (ddI)). Isoniazid (INH) and co-trimoxazole are also recognized causes.
- Hepatitis (see 📖 Liver disease, HIV cholangiopathy, p. 96).
- Hepatic steatosis (non-alcoholic steatohepatitis) associated with ART (particularly d4T).
- Lactic acidosis (due to ART such as d4T and ddI).
- Herbal enema usage.
- 'Pus anywhere', e.g. subphrenic abscess, liver abscess, pelvic inflammatory disease (PID; tubo-ovarian collections), psoas abscess.
- *Neuropathic pain:* zoster without the rash yet (it appears the next day, or may never develop, but dermatomal distribution is suggestive).
- Gastritis related to medication.
- Pyelonephritis and cystitis (check the urine) or PID.
- Pregnancy complication (urine pregnancy test).

Odynophagia and dysphagia

Oral causes

Usually due to *Candida* infection. Candidiasis can present with:

- White plaques which can be scraped off the mucosa.
- Ulceration.
- Generalized erythema of the buccal mucosa and tongue (often painful).
- Circumoral dermatitis or angular cheilitis.

Topical antifungals are usually effective, e.g. nystatin 100 000U swirled around in the mouth and swallowed, every 6h for 1 wk. Other choices include clotrimazole.

Major aphthous ulceration

See 📖 Skin and oral disease, p. 88. May be due to polymicrobial bacterial infection and is sometimes associated with perineal disease.

Herpetic ulcers (due to HSV)

Have a typical clinical appearance and are usually self-limiting; aciclovir 400mg tds or valaciclovir 500mg bd for 5d may help; analgesia important. If severe oral pain, lidocaine gel (as used for urinary catheterization) may be self-applied for short-term relief.

Oesophageal causes

Pain or discomfort in the chest or lower neck is likely an oesophageal problem. *Candida* is the commonest cause and there is usually oral candidiasis visible, although oesophagitis can sometimes be present without this, e.g. if topical nystatin has been used. Treat oesophagitis with oral fluconazole 200mg od for 10–21d. Severe discomfort may make swallowing tablets impossible, necessitating parenteral treatment with amphotericin 0.5–1mg/kg/day IV for 7d (IV fluconazole is an alternative). If no visible *Candida* or no response to systemic anti-fungal therapy (fluconazole for 3wks), then oesophagoscopy with biopsy is usually indicated, and may establish a diagnosis of CMV or herpes oesophagitis or apthous ulceration.

Perianal pathology

- Often very painful.
- Consider and treat *Candida* infection.
- Consider STIs and check syphilis serology.
- Non-specific painful ulceration is common.
- Investigations depend on clinical presentation and available resources. Cultures of superficial swabs are seldom helpful. In refractory cases or if there is evidence of fistula formation, a biopsy may reveal treatable disease, e.g. TB or CMV.
- Consider early treatment with specific therapy for *Herpes* infection (e.g. aciclovir or valaciclovir) or a trial of antibiotics, which include anaerobic cover (e.g. co-amoxiclav) for infected-looking lesions.
- Topical therapy for pain, e.g. lignocaine gel, varies in efficacy.

Liver disease

Asymptomatic ↑ liver enzymes is common in HIV+ individuals, often reflecting systemic illness or drug reactions.

Viral hepatitis

- Commonly due to HBV infection, although CMV, HSV, and hepatitis A are sometimes responsible. HCV is an important cause of chronic hepatitis and cirrhosis in injecting drug users.
- HBV morbidity and mortality is ↑ in HIV+ patients.
- Patients started on ART may develop an immune reconstitution response (IRIS, see 📖 Immune reconstitution inflammatory syndrome, p. 128) against quiescent HBV, theoretically partially ameliorated by using drugs with activity against HBV (e.g. lamivudine and tenofovir.)
- An ART combination containing both tenofovir and lamivudine is preferable in HBV co-infected patients. Discontinuation of such a regimen can cause HBV to flare. In patients with HBV co-infection it is advised that tenofovir plus lamivudine (or emtricitabine (FTC)) be continued throughout in their ART regimens to maintain HBV suppression, together with the additional drugs necessary to maintain HIV suppression.

Drug-induced liver injury (DILI)

- Common causes are TB drugs and ART, but almost any drug can be responsible. Nevirapine is commonly associated with hepatitis. Stavudine is a common cause of fatty liver and another drug should be used in patients who develop fatty liver.
- Minor ↑ in transaminases (ALT <3× upper limit of normal) with drug therapy (e.g. anti-TB medication) in an asymptomatic patient can be managed by repetition of the test a week later; if there is no ↑ trend, continue therapy.
- Because the recognition of drug-induced hepatitis is often delayed, patients may present with severe liver dysfunction, and it is usually advisable to stop all medication initially—especially if alanine transaminase (ALT) rise is >5× upper limit of normal (ULN), or if there is vomiting, anorexia, fever, leukocytosis or an associated rash.
- In patients who develop DILI after starting ART, principles of management are early recognition (also consider HBV or hepatitis C virus (HCV) flare as part of IRIS); assessment of severity; and evaluation of the importance of the drug to the patient's treatment. In severe cases the culprit ART drug should be substituted with an alternative after interruption, provided the liver functions have improved (e.g. switch nevirapine to efavirenz).
- There are many approaches to managing patients who develop DILI while simultaneously on ART and TB treatment. In general, if the hepatitis is severe (ALT > 5 × ULN, particularly if there is jaundice, coagulopathy or encephalopathy) drugs should be stopped, alternative TB treatment (e.g. streptomycin, quinolone, and ethambutol) could be substituted once the liver function tests (LFTs) are improving. When the LFTs have normalized the drugs should be rechallenged, starting

first with the TB drugs (rifampicin then INH; if these are successfully reintroduced, do not re-start pyrazinamide) and then ART. ALT should be monitored closely. If patients have had life threatening liver failure (encephalopathy and coagulopathy) it is advisable to use an alternative TB regimen, rather than rechallenging rifampicin and INH, but without rifampicin/INH, TB treatment needs to be prolonged for 18mths.

HIV cholangiopathy

Patients with late-stage HIV disease may develop right upper quadrant discomfort and a cholestatic (↑ ALP and ↑ GGT) LFT profile. In the absence of gallstones (US) or features of disseminated tuberculosis, low-grade cholangitis should be considered; this may progress to resemble sclerosing cholangitis on endoscopic retrograde cholangiopancreatography (ERCP). A wide range of potential pathogens (e.g. *Salmonella* spp., *Toxoplasma* sp., CMVs, and *Cryptosporidium*) have been implicated, but response to specific therapy is generally poor. Consider ART.

Hepatomegaly

- Cardiac causes (cardiomyopathies, pericardial disease).
- Infections, e.g. TB, leishmaniasis.
- Infiltrates (e.g. lymphoma).
- Medication-associated steatohepatitis and malnutrition.

Cardiac disease

HIV-associated cardiomyopathy

- Usually due to HIV itself, but cardiotropic viruses and OIs may also be implicated. Typically presents with dilated cardiomyopathy in patients with a CD4 count <100/mm^3. Anecdotal reports of some improvement on starting ART, but management is generally the same as that for dilated cardiomyopathy in HIV– individuals, plus ART.
- Consider thiamine deficiency.
- Daunorubicin/doxorubicin to treat KS is another potential cause.

Pericardial disease

- In areas with high TB prevalence, >85% of pericardial effusions in HIV+ patients are tuberculous.
- A presumptive diagnosis of TB pericarditis may be made without diagnostic pericardiocentesis in high prevalence settings and/or in patients in whom there is a high clinical suspicion of TB.
- Also consider bacterial (e.g. *Salmonella*), fungal, malignant (KS, lymphoma), or idiopathic pericardial effusions.
- Pericardiocentesis is warranted for tamponade or in patients who fail to settle on TB therapy, and in patients where a pyogenic infection is suspected (acute sepsis presentation). Where possible, all patients with pericardial effusion should have blood culture performed for bacteraemia (e.g. *Staphylococcus* sp., non-typhi *Salmonella*).

HIV-associated vasculopathy

- Wide range of presentation, including coronary artery disease, cerebrovascular disease, aneurysms, peripheral vascular disease, and small vessel vasculitis.
- Aneurysmal dilatation is rare and may involve any vessel.
- Pulmonary hypertension often presents late, with right heart failure, and carries a poor prognosis even with ART.
- The incidence of coronary artery disease is ↑ in patients on protease inhibitors (PIs) due to their adverse effect on lipid and glucose metabolism.

Renal disease

Acute renal failure

- Renal failure due to sepsis or dehydration is common.
- Renal function usually recovers with rehydration, but may be delayed for several weeks if acute tubular necrosis occurs—short-term dialysis may be required.
- Interstitial nephritis 2° to medication (e.g. rifampicin) should be considered.
- Other medications well recognized to be associated with renal dysfunction include co-trimoxazole, tenofovir, and amphotericin.

HIV-associated nephropathy

- HIV-associated nephropathy (HIVAN) manifests initially with proteinuria, which may → nephrotic syndrome → progressive renal dysfunction → end-stage renal failure over several months.
- Patients are typically not oedematous or hypertensive because the condition is salt-wasting.
- Histology of HIVAN shows focal segmental glomerulosclerosis (FSGS), as well as tubular disease. The pathology results from direct infection of renal epithelial cells by HIV.
- Treatment includes angiotensin converting enzyme (ACE) inhibitors and ART. ART may stabilize or improve milder cases but, if patients have lost significant renal function, the condition progresses despite ART.
- Other forms of glomerulonephritis, such as post-infectious, may also occur in HIV+ individuals. Thus, it is always preferable to confirm the diagnosis with renal biopsy if available. An immune complex mediated nephritis, distinct from FSGS, has been described in association with HIV.

Neurological disease

Headache

Any new headache should always be taken seriously in HIV+ individuals. Fever and meningeal irritation may be absent in lymphocytic meningitis, and frontal lobe mass lesions may have little in the way of localizing signs until late. Consider:

- Meningitis (bacterial, TB, cryptococcosis, syphilis).
- Sinusitis +/– subdural empyema.
- Space-occupying lesions (toxoplasmosis, tuberculoma, lymphoma).

Drugs (co-trimoxazole can rarely cause a sterile meningitis; zidovudine (AZT) and efavirenz cause various CNS symptoms, including headache).

Meningitis

Any HIV+ individual with a new headache or unexplained fever should be considered to have meningitis. Signs of meningism may not be present so absence of neck stiffness does not exclude the diagnosis. The variability in physical signs and CSF findings reflect the degree of immunocompromise and pattern of the associated meningeal process (see Table 3.5).

Cryptococcal meningitis

- Due to infection by *Cryptococcus neoformans*, carried by birds (especially pigeons) and excreted in avian faeces.
- Infection follows inhalation of *Cryptococcus neoformans*.
- Disseminated cryptococcosis may occur, involving almost any organ including skin, mucosae, and bones.

Clinical features

Insidious onset of headache, malaise, low-grade fever, +/– altered mental state.

Diagnosis

- Often only a few cells in the CSF.
- India ink staining of CSF may show characteristic capsulated yeast cells (capsule seen as a clear halo around the yeast); sensitivity 80–90%.
- Fungal culture highly sensitive, but requires a good laboratory.
- CLAT (cryptococcal latex agglutination test) is highly sensitive and specific in both blood and CSF.

Treatment

This is for life, unless immunity is restored with ART. There are three phases.

- *Initial intensive phase:* amphotericin B (1mg/kg/d diluted in 1000mL 5% glucose in water infused over 4h) od for 14d. This should be combined with flucytosine (100mg/kg/d, seldom available in resource limited settings, reduced dosage in renal impairment). Test doses of amphotericin are unnecessary. Severe allergic reactions in amphotericin-naïve patients are rare. Amphotericin is best avoided in renal failure. Renal impairment can be largely avoided if patients are given adequate hydration (prehydrate with 1000mL normal saline with 20mmol KCl over 2h). Monitor K+ as life-threatening hypokalaemia may occur and pre-emptive K+ supplementation is advised.

- *Consolidation phase:* fluconazole 400–800mg od for 2mths.
- *Long-term low dose maintenance (2° prophylaxis):* fluconazole 200mg od for life, or until CD4 >200 for 6mths on ART and at least 12mths antifungal therapy in total.
- If ongoing headache or drowsiness, consider repeat LP with CSF manometry: if pressure >30cm CSF, remove sufficient CSF to reduce to <20cm CSF. This often leads to dramatic symptomatic relief but may need to be repeated if symptoms recur.
- Monitor haemoglobin as amphotericin B → anaemia.

Table 3.5 Differences between forms of meningitis in HIV infection

Feature	Pyogenic	Tuberculous	Cryptococcal
Symptom duration	Hours or days	Days or weeks	Days or weeks
Headache	Usually	Usually, but not invariable	Usually, but not invariable
Neck stiffness	Variable	Variable	Usually absent (80%)
Fever	Usually	Variable	Variable
Chest signs (and CXR)	Rare	May have features of pulmonary TB	Usually normal, but pulmonary disease possible
CSF opening pressure	Variable	↑ in 75%, but an unreliable differentiator	
CSF glucose	Low	Usually low	Normal in 50%
CSF protein	Usually ↑	Often markedly ↑	May be normal, but usually mildly ↑
Cell count	Usually moderately or extremely ↑	Usually modestly ↑	Normal in about 1/3 of patients
Cell type in CSF	Predominantly neutrophils	Lymphocytes or may have early neutrophil predominance	If any cells, usually lymphocytes
Gram stain	May show organisms	–ve (ZN rarely +ve)	–ve; sometimes reported 'fungal elements present'
Indian ink	–ve	–ve	80–90% +ve
Cryptococcal CSF antigen test	–ve	–ve	95–100% +ve
CSF culture	Often +ve unless prior antibiotics	Often +ve, but takes 4–6wks	Almost always +ve, but usually unnecessary

Space-occupying lesions in the brain

- Present with one or more of: headache, focal neurological signs, or seizures (see 📖 Space occupying lesions, p. 469). Frontal lobe lesions may → personality changes.
- Careful neurological examination for focal signs and ↑ ICP.
- Where facilities allow, diagnosis and treatment should be based on investigations including serology (*Toxoplasma* IgG, serum cryptococcal antigen, and syphilis), brain imaging (CT or MRI), CSF examination (if LP not contra-indicated), and brain biopsy.
- Most common finding on brain imaging is a contrast-enhancing mass lesion with surrounding oedema.
- Single lesions with considerable basal contrast enhancement and an abnormal CXR (particularly hilar adenopathy, lower zone infiltrate, or a miliary pattern) suggest TB. Other causes include primary CNS lymphoma (rare), pyogenic brain abscess, cryptococcoma, and syphilitic gumma; consider neurocysticercosis in endemic areas.
- Multiple lesions in a patient with a CD4 count <50 are more likely due to toxoplasmosis (see 📖 Toxoplasmosis, p. 103).

Management

In resource-poor environments and the absence of a specific diagnosis, the following is a pragmatic approach:

- If evidence of TB elsewhere (lymphadenopathy, CXR, abdominal US showing splenic hypodensities or adenopathy), treat for TB initially.
- In the absence of features suggesting TB, treat for toxoplasmosis initially, as therapy is less arduous and response can be assessed within 1–2wks. (If this approach is followed, avoid corticosteroids, as they will cause many patients to improve both clinically and radiologically.)
- If there is no response to treatment for toxoplasmosis by 2wks, and no other diagnostic pointers, it is common practice to commence therapy for TB. Where there is access to a neurosurgical service, consultation with a view to brain biopsy is desirable.
- In patients who respond partially, there is no simple answer. It is usually preferable to treat for TB, as well, but the previously listed differential diagnosis should be re-scrutinized at this stage.
- In patients who present with life-threatening neurological deterioration (e.g. severe cerebral oedema complicating SOL) this staged approach is not appropriate, such patients may require initial treatment for toxoplasmosis and tuberculomas plus corticosteroids (as well as serological screening for the other causes listed).

Seizures

Causes include those common to HIV– individuals, but in HIV+ individuals attention should be taken to exclude SOLs and chronic meningitides. In HIV+ individuals with very low CD4 counts, HIV encephalopathy may itself cause seizures.

- Doses of anticonvulsants may need adjusting for the reduced weight of patients, bearing in mind that the liver induction due to other medications may counterbalance this.

- In patients on ART, or in whom ART is being contemplated, the drug interactions with phenytoin, carbamazepine, and phenobarbitone lead to inadequate levels of some NNRTIs and PIs, and a switch of anticonvulsant to valproate or lamotrigine is necessary.

Toxoplasmosis

Toxoplasma gondii is an obligate intracellular parasite. Cats are the definitive host.

Transmission occurs by eating food contaminated with oocytes from cat faeces or from tissue cysts in undercooked meat from domesticated animals. Asymptomatic infection is common in immunocompetent adults (20–50% normal adults are IgG seropositive).

Latent infection (reflected by +ve IgG in serum) may become reactivated in immunocompromised patients, → severe disease involving brain, lungs, heart, and choroid/retina. Cerebral toxoplasmosis is common in AIDS.

Clinical features

For cerebral toxoplasmosis these include headache, focal neurological signs, an altered mental state, and coma. Diffuse cerebral involvement may present as an altered mental state without focal signs. Toxoplasma pneumonitis manifests as fever with cough and dyspnoea; chorioretinitis is uncommon.

Diagnosis

Diagnosis of cerebral toxoplasmosis is clinical, supported by serology and brain imaging (MRI) or CT. Typically, it presents with multiple ring-enhancing brain lesions on CT; CD4 count is usually <50 and serum toxoplasma IgG is +ve. Toxoplasmosis is less likely with a CD4 count >150, if IgG is –ve, or if patient is on co-trimoxazole prophylaxis. Brain biopsy may be helpful in atypical presentations.

Management

1st line therapy

With pyrimethamine plus sulphadiazine (or clindamycin) for 6wks. Pyrimethamine is a folate antagonist (can lead to bone marrow suppression), so folinic acid is also given:

- Pyrimethamine 200mg oral loading dose, then if <60kg, 50mg oral od, if >60kg, 75mg oral od *plus*
- Folinic acid 10mg daily, *plus*
- *either* sulfadiazine if <60kg 1g oral tds, if >60kg 1.5g oral qds
- *or* clindamycin 600mg oral qds.

Maintenance therapy should then continue until CD4 > 200 for > 6mths on ART with: pyrimethamine 25–50mg oral od plus folinic acid 10mg daily plus sulfadiazine 0.5–1g qds.

Alternative regimen

Where above regimen unavailable, there is preliminary evidence that 480mg co-trimoxazole 4 tablets bd for 4wks, followed by 2 tablets bd for 3mths, is adequate. Secondary prophylaxis after that should continue for life (or until immune reconstitution on ART) with 2 tablets od.

Not all patients treated with co-trimoxazole will demonstrate a complete clinical response, particularly if there is an associated infarct.

HIV encephalopathy and progressive multifocal leukoencephalopathy

HIV is a neurotropic virus that can cause a slowly progressive (months) dementing illness characterized by forgetfulness and minor motor apraxias. Minor cognitive-motor disorder (MCMD) is a pre-dementia manifestation. Vacuolar myelopathy is a variant where the subcortical changes are preceded by a progressive spastic weakness. Always exclude Vitamin B12 deficiency in the latter.

Progressive multifocal leukoencephalopathy (PML) is a white matter illness due to JC virus infection, which presents with focal signs, speech, and cognition difficulties. ART is always worth attempting in dementing patients who have adequate home resources to ensure adherence—some patients may respond well to ART. A response in PML less often occurs, but ART may prevent deterioration and improves survival.

HIV-associated dementia

- A slow onset process characterized by motor apraxia and mental slowing with forgetfulness.
- Is an indication for ART so early identification is important.
- Standard mini-mental tests are designed to screen for the predominantly cortical lesions of Alzheimer's disease, so alternative screening tools that also evaluate subcortical function have been proposed. One scale (see Table 3.6) consists of three components—a memory test, a psychomotor component, and a motor component.

Psychosis

This is often multifactorial, consider:

- *Acute situational stressors:* reactions to learning HIV status, often in the face of inadequate counselling.
- *Opportunistic CNS infections:* chronic meningitides, frontal space-occupying lesions, and severe OIs elsewhere.
- *Metabolic disorders:* hyponatraemia, dehydration, and uraemia.
- *Medications:* e.g. efavirenz, isoniazid.
- *Nutritional deficiencies of thiamine or niacin:* these may be worth treating empirically even if merely suspected (see 🕮 Vitamin B1 (thiamine) deficiency: beriberi, p. 716). Vitamin B12 deficiency is another potential cause for abnormal mentation.
- Use of neuroleptic agents in frail, thin HIV+ individuals should be cautious—often tiny doses (e.g. haloperidol 0.5mg bd) may be adequate.

Stroke

The abrupt onset of focal neurological signs is a devastating event for young HIV+ individuals, particularly if the resultant disability impacts on activities of daily living and ability to look after children.

Table 3.6 Rapid screening test for HIV dementia

Item	Description	Outcome	Score
Motor	Tap together finger and thumb of non-dominant hand as many times as possible in 5s	>15 × in 5s	4
		11–14	3
		7–10	2
		3–6	1
		0–2	0
Psychomotor	Repeat the following sequence of placement of the non-dominant hand on a flat surface as often as possible in 10s: 1. Clenched fist. 2. Open hand, palm down 3. Ulnar surface of open hand down	≥4 repeats	4
		3	3
		2	2
		1	1
		Cannot perform	0
Memory	Before doing the previous two components, give the patient four words to remember (dog, hat, bean, red) and after finishing the other components, ask what they were	Each word spontaneously recalled	1
		Each word recalled after prompting	0.5
Total score	Add together scores from each of the three components	Max 12. <10 should prompt more formal evaluation for dementia	

Reproduced from Sacktor NC, *et al.* The International HIV Dementia Scale: a new rapid screening test for HIV dementia. *AIDS* 2005; **19**: 1367–74.

Causes

- Blood, e.g. hyperviscosity syndromes, disseminated intravascular coagulation (DIC), antiphospholipid antibody syndromes, acquired protein C, protein S, or antithrombin III deficiency, or thrombotic thrombocytopenic purpura.
- *Blood pressure:* hypertension (e.g. due to HIV nephropathy) or hypotension (septicaemia, dehydration).
- *Embolic:* infective endocarditis related either to previous rheumatic heart disease, or IV drug use.
- *Vessel wall:* infective vasculitis (meningitis—TB, syphilis, cryptococcal, CMV, herpes zoster, toxoplasmosis), autoimmune vasculitis.
- Haemorrhage (mycotic aneurysm, intracerebral KS).
- HIV vasculopathy (discussed in 📖 HIV-associated vasculopathy, p. 98).

Diagnosis

Look for clinical signs of embolic source; FBC, blood film, urea & electrolytes (U&E), CRP, syphilis serology, total serum protein (?hyperviscosity), +/– thrombophilia screen (PT, anticardiolipin antibodies, protein C, protein S, and antithrombin III levels); brain imaging (CT or MRI).

Management

Involves treatment of any identified underlying cause and counselling about the condition and expected prognosis, physiotherapy, attention to nutrition (able to swallow, adequate hydration plan?), and urine and bowel care plans (decisions about catheter versus nappies/linen savers if incontinent.) In the absence of any identified remediable cause, give aspirin 75–150mg daily as 2° prophylaxis, although evidence of benefit in this patient population has not been established.

Peripheral neuropathy

Consider:

- HIV neuropathy.
- Medication (INH, stavudine, didanosine).
- CMV (often painful).
- Nutritional deficiencies (thiamine, niacin, pyridoxine, vitamin B12).
- Vasculitic neuropathy (stepwise progression).
- Acute and chronic inflammatory demyelinating polyneuropathies (Guillain–Barré syndrome) present in the same way as in HIV– individuals, and a few cells in the CSF should not exclude the diagnosis if the clinical picture is correct. Steroids are often given in the chronic form but, as with the acute form, are probably of little value, and in patients with the asymmetrical pure motor form in fact do harm.

Mononeuropathies

The most common mononeuropathy is an isolated VIIth nerve paralysis (Bell's palsy), but practically any cranial nerve can be involved. The natural history of a VIIth nerve palsy is similar to that in HIV– individuals. The importance is recognizing the lower motor neurone nature of the lesion, which makes intracranial pathology unlikely.

Paraparesis

Patients with weak legs can have any of the causes of peripheral neuropathy; also consider intrinsic cord disease if upper motor neurone signs are present. TB and syphilitic myelo-radiculitis are sometimes associated with dermatomal pain at the level of the lesion, and CMV infection may classically present with lumbosacral pain.

Depression

Depression in HIV+ individuals is under-recognized. It may be situational or due to medication, intercurrent illness, or organic brain disease. Depressed people adjust poorly to new disease and therapeutic challenges, and adherence may be affected. Antidepressant medication and PIs may interact; interactions with NNRTIs are less significant.

Eye disease

See 📖 HIV infection and the eye, p. 585.

HIV-related malignancy

Kaposi sarcoma

- A tumour of lymphatic endothelial cells, caused by the KSHV (also known as human herpesvirus-8, HHV-8).
- KSHV is sexually-transmitted; its seroprevalence in healthy adults varies from <5% (Europe) to >50% (commonest in West Africa).
- Presents with lesions of the skin, oral cavity, and, in some cases, the viscera.
- Incidence of KS in HIV+ populations is closely related to background seroprevalence of KSHV.

Clinical features

- Single or multiple papular or nodular hyperpigmented lesions.
- Appear black on black skin and purple on pale skin.
- Early lesions may look like bruises and be difficult to recognize.
- May become painful or ulcerate, but are often asymptomatic until late.
- Can occur on all parts of body, not just skin. Rarely limited to one anatomical region. Lesions on face, legs, and in mouth are common.
- Visceral disease may occur without skin involvement—the only visible lesion may be in the mouth. Oral lesions are often not raised and are usually asymptomatic but may → bleeding, pain, and dysphagia.
- KS commonly involves lymph nodes (characteristically → lymphoedema), the GI tract (→ bleeding and anaemia), and lungs (→ dyspnoea, cough).
- Patients with extensive KS may have ↓ weight and fever.

Diagnosis

- Clinical in most cases. The major differential diagnosis is bacillary angiomatosis, particularly if the lesions grow rapidly.
- Skin biopsy shows characteristic histology; KSHV immunostaining +ve.
- Pulmonary involvement → characteristic CXR changes (flame-shaped linear and nodular infiltrates spreading from the hila) and may be accompanied by a blood-stained pleural effusion.
- Gastrointestinal tract (GIT) and pulmonary involvement can be confirmed on endoscopy or bronchoscopy.

Management:

ART is the 1st line of therapy. Limited skin and oral KS may regress with ART alone. If there is progression on ART, chemotherapy is considered. Patients with visceral involvement or extensive disease (many lesions or lymphoedema) usually require ART plus chemotherapy from the start. The common regimen used in resource-poor settings is a combination of doxorubicin, bleomycin, and vincristine. Radiation or topical liquid nitrogen can be used for localized lesions.

Lymphoma

Lymphomas typically present with chronic symptoms, including wasting, fever, and symptoms related to location of disease. Common forms in HIV+ individuals:

- NHL.
- Primary CNS lymphoma.
- Primary effusion lymphoma (PEL).

Patients may have adenopathy and/or GI, hepatic, pulmonary, bone marrow, and CNS involvement. Diagnosis is confirmed by lymph node excision biopsy, bone marrow biopsy, or biopsy of other involved organs. Immunoblastic or Burkitt's lymphoma are the most common histologies and most are B cell in origin.

Management

Combination chemotherapy (e.g. CHOP—cyclophosphamide, doxorubicin, vincristine and prednisolone); ART is essential and prevents relapses.

NHL: far more common than in the general population and usually related to underlying oncogenic EBV infection.

Primary CNS lymphoma: causes focal signs and SOLs on CT and is EBV related: a +ve EBV PCR in CSF supports diagnosis. Prognosis is poor even with chemotherapy, radiotherapy, and ART.

PEL: presents with lymphomatous serous effusions in the absence of mass lesions. It is related to KSHV. It is diagnosed by pleural biopsy. Treatment is with chemotherapy and ART.

Cervical cancer

HIV infection in women is associated with a higher rate of cervical squamous intra-epithelial neoplasia (SIN) and a modest ↑ risk of cervical cancer. This is closely related to infection with certain oncogenic types of human papillomavirus (HPV, for which vaccines now exist see 📖 Immunization, p. 910). Invasive cervical carcinoma is a WHO stage 4 condition. HIV+ women should be screened annually with cervical smears (frequency of screening may be less in resource limited settings due to programmatic limitations). If high-grade SIN is present, then colposcopy and biopsy is indicated. Cervical cancer is treated with surgery and/or radiotherapy.

Prevention of opportunistic infections

Opportunistic infections should be prevented through 1° prophylaxis (see Table 3.3) and 2° prophylaxis, as summarized in Table 3.7.

Table 3.7 2° Prophylaxis prevention of opportunistic infections

Condition	Medication	When to stop
Cryptococcal meningitis	Fluconazole 200mg od	On ART with CD4 >200 for 6mths (total >12mths)
Toxoplasmosis	Co-trimoxazole 2 tabs daily	On ART with CD4 >200 for 6mths
Non-typhi *Salmonellae*	Ciprofloxacin 500mg bd	After 4wks
Pneumocystis	Co-trimoxazole 2 tabs od	On ART with CD4 >200 for 6mths
Mycobacterium avium complex	Ethambutol and azithromycin	Stop when CD4 >100 for 6mths and at least 12mths of MAC treatment
Leishmaniasis	Amphotericin B	CD4 >200 for 6mths
Penicilliosis	Itraconazole	CD4 >100 for 6mths CD4 >200 for 6mths
Isosporiasis	Co-trimoxazole 2–4 tabs daily	

Antiretroviral therapy

Preparing patients for antiretroviral therapy

Prior to ART being commenced, the patient should be medically and psychosocially prepared. The following issues need to be addressed.

Screen for opportunistic infections

- Ask about cough, night sweats, and recent ↓ weight— if any of these present, investigate for TB.
- *Ask about visual disturbances:* if present, examine for CMV retinitis.
- Screen for peripheral neuropathy (symptoms and signs).
- Use WHO clinical staging system to classify each patient (📖 HIV/AIDS, WHO clinical staging system for HIV infection and disease p. 76).
- Treat all active OIs before starting ART; patients should be on appropriate 1° and 2° prophylaxis.

Baseline blood tests

Depending on availability, these should include:

- FBC, LFTs (ALT is a useful screen), creatinine.
- CD4 count, HIV viral load.
- Syphilis serology (veneral diseases research laboratory, VDRL), hepatitis B surface antigen (HBsAg), HCV antibody, and cryptocccal antigen (the latter in patients with CD4 < 100cells/mm^3).
- Lack of access to these investigations should not be a barrier to ART initiation, e.g. in community or rural programmes.

Potential drug interactions

Ensure there will be no significant drug interactions between drugs patient is taking and ART to be started. Adjustments of medication or doses may be required.

Counselling

These issues should be addressed before patient commences ART:

- HIV transmission and disease progression.
- Safe sex and other prevention messages (provide condoms).
- Understanding of CD4 count (and viral load if available).
- Benefits of therapy (treatment is not a cure).
- Side-effects and monitoring of treatment.
- Adherence and resistance.
- Family disclosure.
- Integrating treatment into daily life.
- Drug interactions (including alternative therapies).
- Dealing with drug side effects.

Other issues

- *Substance abuse* should be addressed (counselling and referral) before ART is started.
- *Depression* should also be treated before starting ART (counselling +/– antidepressants).
- Patients with food shortages should be referred for appropriate support if this is available.

Disclosure of HIV status

- Patients should be encouraged to disclose their status to sexual partners (and household members). Non-disclosure compromises adherence. There are, however, potential risks associated with disclosure particularly for women (partner violence and being thrown out of the home) and this issue needs to be handled sensitively and flexibly.
- Partners should be offered HIV testing.
- If possible, patients should bring in a treatment supporter (friend, partner, or family member) who can also be educated about HIV and ART, and remind and motivate the patient about their therapy. Other adherence tools may include alarms, pillboxes, tick sheets, and reminders sent by mobile phone.

Monitoring prior to ART

- If patients do not yet meet the criteria for commencing ART, they should be followed up and assessed at intervals.
- CD4 count should be repeated at 6mths intervals.
- Prior to starting ART, clinical staging and/or CD4 count are the best monitoring tools.

Antiretroviral drugs

Act by inhibiting various steps in the replication cycle of HIV.

- Non-nucleoside reverse transcriptase inhibitors (NNRTI) and nucleoside/nucleotide reverse transciptase inhibitors (NRTI/NtRTI) inhibit the viral enzyme reverse transcriptase.
- Protease inhibitors inhibit the viral enzyme protease.
- Integrase inhibitors inhibit the viral enzyme integrase.
- CCR5 blockers inhibit the entry of CCR5-tropic viruses into CD4 cells by blocking the CCR5 co-receptor on the host cell.

The goal of therapy is to combine ART drugs, usually ≥3, into a regimen sufficiently potent to inhibit all viral replication and thereby prevent the emergence of resistant mutants—this is known as highly active antiretroviral therapy (HAART or ART).

With ART, it is possible to suppress the viral load below the limit of detection (usually <50copies/mL) indefinitely, provided patients adhere correctly. There are differing levels of adherence needed to maintain virological suppression, depending on the ART used. The adherence level needed for unboosted PIs has been established as >95% of doses taken correctly, but >80% adherence to boosted PIs or NNRTIs may be sufficient. Virological suppression allows CD4 count to recover—on average 75cells/mm^3 in the 1st month and 75cells/mm^3/yr thereafter, although this response is widely variable. With the ↑ CD4 count, patients experience immune restoration. Opportunistic infections occur with ↓ incidence, some OIs regress without specific therapy (e.g. *Cryptosporidium*), and patients are generally able to stop preventative therapies when CD4 counts >200cells/mm^3 for sustained periods. This → ↓ progression to AIDS, ↑ in quality of life, and ↑ survival. Individuals whose viraemia is suppressed are markedly less infectious.

Treatment is life long, and adherence with therapy is critical. Patients taking ART should be counselled before starting therapy. Patients need to have full insight into their disease, the drugs, need for strict adherence, side-effects, and OI prevention. Missing doses → inadequate viral suppression → selection of mutations in the virus → resistance to the drugs (HIV mutates rapidly). This → sequential loss of drugs in a regimen due to the development of resistance, and patients require a change of regimen to attain viral suppression again. Over time, it is possible for patients to develop resistance to all classes of antiretrovirals making viral suppression impossible (MDR HIV).

Starting therapy

The WHO recommendations regarding when to start ART are shown in Table 3.8. In general, all patients with clinically advanced disease and/or CD4 ≤350/mm^3 or a diagnosis of TB require ART initiation. AIDS-defining illnesses (except TB) are uncommon with a CD4 count >200/mm^3.

In patients with TB, ART should be started 2–8wks after diagnosis of TB. In patients with advanced immunosuppression (CD4 <50) and TB, starting ART 2wks after TB treatment improves outcome—such patients should be prioritized for early ART.

Table 3.8 Criteria for ART initiation in specific populations, WHO guidelines 2010

Target population	Clinical condition	Recommendation
Asymptomatic individuals (incl. pregnant women)	WHO clinical stage 1	Start if CD4 ≤350
Symptomatic individuals (incl. pregnant women)	WHO clinical stage 2	Start if CD4 ≤350
	WHO clinical stage 3/4	Start irrespective of CD4 cell count
TB or HBV co-infections	Active TB disease	Start irrespective of CD4 cell count
	HBV infection requiring treatment	Start irrespective of CD4 cell count

Source: World Health Organization. Antiretroviral therapy for HIV infection in adults and adolescents. Recommendations for a public health approach, 2010 revision. WHO: Geneva, 2010. http://whqlibdoc.who.int/publications/2010/9789241599764_eng.pdf

In patients with OIs such as PCP, clinicians should aim to start ART within 2wks of OI diagnosis. In cryptococcal meningitis ART should be started 4 to 6 weeks after diagnosis.

In addition to medical criteria, patients must be psychosocially ready to commence lifelong daily therapy. This involves addressing issues such as substance abuse, depression, disclosure, and family relationships before starting. Also useful for patient to have treatment supporter from their household or friend to motivate and remind them.

First-line therapy

First-line therapy involves three drugs. Common choices are one of tenofovir (TDF)/zidovudine (AZT)/abacavir (ABCv) + one of lamivudine (3TC)/emtricitabine (FTC) + one of efavirenz (EFV)/nevirapine (NVP); (see Table 3.9 for drug names, classes and doses).

For example, two common 1st line regimens are:

- TDF + 3TC + EFV.
- TDF + FTC + EFV (which is also available as a once daily fixed dose combination (FDC)).

Where resources permit, 1st line therapy regimens may also include PI or integrase inhibitor (either of which is combined with 2 NRTI drugs).

The following simple rules help decide which drug combination to use:

- Avoid AZT in patients with anaemia/neutropenia as AZT bone marrow suppression is more likely if pre-existing problems.
- Avoid TDF in patients with renal dysfunction (calculated creatinine clearance < 50mL/min).
- Avoid stavudine (d4T) unless there are no other alternatives (either because of supply or patient has anaemia and renal impairment and ABC is unavailable). Very important to avoid d4T and didanosine (ddI) combination (severe mitochondrial toxicity).

- Never use d4T and AZT together as they are antagonistic.
- Avoid combination of TDF and ddI (potentiates toxicity and worse virological and CD4 responses).
- Avoid NVP in patients with underlying liver disease, those with CD4>250 in women or >400 in men (↑ risk of hepatitis/rash) and those on TB treatment (shared toxicities and drug interactions).

Table 3.9 ART doses and adverse effects

Nucleoside reverse transcriptase inhibitors (NRTIs)		
Abacavir (ABC)	300mg bd	Hypersensitivity (may be fatal) in 4–8% (risk lower in those of African ethnicity): fever, rash, GI. *Do not re-challenge*
ddI	400mg od (250mg if <60kg)	Take on empty stomach (1h before or 2h after food). Peripheral neuropathy, pancreatitis, GI; rarely lactic acidosis, hepatic steatosis
FTC	200mg od	Minimal. Palmar hyperpigmentation
3TC	150mg bd or 300mg od	Minimal. Red cell aplasia (rare). Pancreatitis reported in children
d4T	30mg bd	Peripheral neuropathy, lipoatrophy, pancreatitis, lactic acidosis, hepatic steatosis
AZT	250–300mg bd	Bone marrow suppression (anaemia, neutropenia), myopathy; rarely lactic acidosis, hepatic steatosis
Nucleotide reverse transcriptase inhibitors (NtRTIs)		
TDF	300mg od	Renal insufficiency, tubular wasting, GI side effects, ↓ bone mineral density
Non-nucleoside reverse transcriptase inhibitors (NNRTIs)		
EFZ	600mg od[1]	CNS effects (advise to take at night), hepatitis, rash
NVP	200mg bd	Initially 200mg daily, ↑ to 200mg bd after 2wks. Rash, Stevens–Johnson syndrome, hepatitis
Etravirine (ETR)	200mg bd	Hepatitis, rash. CNS effects less common than with EFZ

Table 3.9 (*Continued*)

Protease inhibitors (PIs)		
Where a ritonavir-boosted PI regimen is used (📖 p. 119), the dose given in brackets is used.		
Atazanavir (ATZ)	400mg daily[300mg od]	Take with food. ↑ Bilirubin, cardiac conduction defect (prolonged PR interval) hepatitis. Less effect on lipids
Darunavir (DRV)	[600mg bd or 800mg od if naïve]	GI, hepatitis, rash. Contains sulphonamide moiety. Lipid abnormalities
Fosamprenavir (FPV)	1400mg bd [700mg bd]	GI, rash, hepatitis, lipid abnormalities
Indinavir (IDV)	800mg tds [800mg bd]	Nephrolithiasis, GI, ↑ bilirubin, hepatitis. Lipid abnormalities and insulin resistance
		Fluid intake 2L daily
Lopinavir (LPV)	[400mg bd]	Take with food
		GI, hepatitis, lipid abnormalities. Cardiac conduction defects
Nelfinavir (NFV)	1250mg bd or 750mg tds	Take with food. Diarrhoea, hepatitis. Lipid abnormalities
Saquinavir (SQV)	[1000mg bd][2]	GI, hepatitis, lipid abnormalities
Integrase inhibitor (II)		
Raltegravir (RAL)	400mg bd	Rash
Combined preparations		
Combivir®		1 tablet bd, contains AZT 300mg + 3TC 150 mg
Trizivir®		1 tablet bd, contains AZT 300mg + 3TC 150mg + ABCv 300mg
Truvada®		1 tablet od, contains TDF 245mg + FTC 200mg
Kivexa®		1 tablet od, contains ABCv 600mg + 3TC 300mg
Kaletra® (also known as Aluvia®)		2 tablets bd; 1 tablet contains LPV 200mg + RTV 50mg. 100+25mg tablets also available
Atripla®		1 tablet nocte, contains TDF 245mg + FTC 200mg + EFV 600mg

[1]Consider ↓ dose to 400mg if <40kg.

[2]Alternative boosted PI regimen: SQV 400mg bd + RTV 400mg bd.

Table adapted with permission from Pattman R, Sankar N, Elawad B, et *al. Oxford Handbook of Genitourinary Medicine, HIV and AIDS*. Oxford: Oxford University Press 2005. All doses are for adults.

Monitoring treatment response

Monitor for adherence to therapy (e.g. self-reporting, identifying tablets on a chart, pill counts, pharmacy refills); adverse effects (clinically, FBC, LFTs); new OIs and IRIS; CD4 and viral load where available. Viral load is the best method to monitor therapy. If viral load is undetectable, CD4 lymphocyte counts rarely alter management except to guide when to discontinue prophylaxis for OIs.

Treatment failure

This can be:

- Virological (virus detected in plasma repeatedly).
- Immunological (no CD4 response or CD4 decline).
- Clinical (new WHO stage 3 or 4 events).

There is ↑ evidence that clinical and CD4 count monitoring are inadequate because they do not correlate closely with virological response, and there is a time lag between virological failure and CD4 fall or clinical failure. However, there is no realistic alternative in settings where viral load is currently unavailable. Consider changing to 2nd line regimen in the following settings:

- *Virological failure:* patients should be switched when viral load is persistently above a certain threshold (e.g. >1000copies/mL on two occasions) despite adequate adherence interventions. Where viral loads are available this is the only guide that should direct decisions regarding the need for switching.
- *Immunological failure (CD4 count but not viral load available):*
  - ↓ CD4 count to pre-therapy baseline (or below) *or*
  - 50% fall from the on-treatment peak value *or*
  - persistent CD4 count <100cells/mm^3 (without concomitant infection to cause transient CD4 cell ↓).
- *Clinical failure* (if CD4 count/viral load not available): development of new or recurrent WHO stage 4 condition (excluding IRIS).
- Most cases of virological failure are the result of inadequate adherence → accumulation of drug resistant mutations. A minority of cases are due to 1° drug resistant (the patient was infected with resistant HIV). It is expected that the latter will become more frequent as ART programmes mature.

Second-line therapy

Will successfully re-suppress HIV replication in most patients. However, patients who have failed once, most commonly due to poor adherence, are at risk for poor adherence in the future. Second line therapy includes a ritonavir-boosted protease inhibitor (see 📖 Boosted protease inhibitor (PI) regimens, p. 119) and two NRTIs (at least one of which has not been used previously). The decision regarding which regimen to use will depend on what drugs were used in the first line, available alternatives, and the national programme, and may need to be discussed with an experienced physician. For example, in a patient who fails first line of TDF/3TC/NVP then second line could be AZT/3TC/lopinavir-ritonavir.

Boosted PI regimens

Combining PIs with a small dose of ritonavir significantly improves the PI's pharmacokinetic profile, 'boosting' its concentration. 'Boosted PI' regimens utilize this by combining ritonavir 100mg bd with a second PI (e.g. lopinavir 400mg + ritonavir 100mg bd, co-formulated as Kaletra®).

ART dose adjustments in renal impairment

Table 3.10 gives a simple summary of some suggested ART dose adjustments in renal impairment. For a more detailed breakdown of ART doses by creatinine clearance, consult more specialist texts, or http://cid.oxfordjournals.org/content/40/11/1559.full.pdf.

Table 3.10 ART dose adjustments in renal failure

Drug	Creatinine clearance 10–50mL/min	Creatinine clearance <10mL/min
AZT	Unchanged	300mg daily
ddI	>60kg 150–200mg daily	>60kg 100mg daily
	<60kg 100–150mg daily	<60kg 75mg daily
3TC	100–150mg daily	50mg daily
d4T	15mg 12-hourly	15mg daily
ABC	Unchanged	Unchanged
Tenofovir	*avoid**	*avoid**
PIs	Unchanged	Unchanged
NNRTIs	Unchanged	Unchanged

Sources: adapted from Bartlett JG. *Medical Care of Patients with HIV Infection* 2003; and *The Sanford Guide to Antimicrobial Therapy* 2003.

*There are tenofovir dosing adjustment guidelines for renal impairment in the package insert. However, it is advised tenofovir is avoided in renal impairment because of ↑ risk of nephrotoxicity. In situations where tenofovir use cannot be avoided (e.g. hepatitis B co-infection) then tenofovir could be used with dose adjustment according to package insert and with closer monitoring of creatinine.

Antiretroviral therapy side-effects

Many patients commencing ART will experience side-effects, especially in the first few weeks (see Table 3.11). Most will be mild and resolve spontaneously, e.g. abdominal discomfort, nausea and vomiting (ddI and AZT), diarrhoea (PIs), headaches, and fatigue (AZT). Warn patients these may occur. Management then involves excluding serious side-effects (e.g. hepatitis if nausea or vomiting), reassurance, and symptomatic therapy (e.g. antiemetic). More serious side-effects may also occur, with potentially life-threatening/long-term consequences:

Peripheral neuropathy

Due to d4T or ddI. Peripheral sensory neuropathy initially, but may → motor involvement. Patients first complain of pain and paraesthesia in the feet.

Management Exclude other causes; amitriptyline 10mg nocte, increased if necessary max 75mg; switch ART drugs if possible (e.g. d4T to AZT).

Drug-induced hepatitis and/or skin rash

NVP (and less commonly EFV or ETR) may cause this, usually within 3mths of starting treatment. Women, and particularly those with CD4 >250mm^3 are most at risk. Hepatitis may be asymptomatic. In those with ↑ ALT and symptoms, or those asymptomatic but with ALT >200units/L, NVP should be switched to an alternative drug (e.g. EFV or PI). If the hepatitis is severe (e.g. complicated by liver failure) ART should be temporarily stopped before starting the new regimen. The allergic rash is macular-papular, but may → Stevens–Johnson syndrome. If mild, drugs can be continued with close monitoring. However, if severe (extensive rash, angioedema, desquamation or blistering, any mucous membrane or systemic involvement such as fever or associated hepatitis)—NVP should be switched to EFV or a PI. In the case of life-threatening NVP-induced hepatitis or rash it is best to avoid EFV in future regimens as cross-reactivity is described.

Mitochondrial toxicity

Is the underlying mechanism for many NRTI side-effects—neuropathy, fatty liver, pancreatitis, hyperlacattaemia/lactic acidosis. Combinations of d4T and ddI (the most significant causes) should ∴ be avoided.

Hyperlactataemia and lactic acidosis

NRTIs (d4T > ddI > AZT > others) may cause build-up of lactate as a consequence of mitochondrial toxicity. Severe lactic acidosis carries a high mortality (>50% in some studies). About a quarter of patients on these drugs will have a mildly ↑ lactate and be asymptomatic with no adverse consequences. Symptomatic hyperlactataemia is heralded by abdominal discomfort, nausea and vomiting, and ↓ weight. It usually occurs after patients have been on ART for several months (median 9mths). In severe lactic acidosis, patients may present in a critical condition with Kussmaul breathing +/– circulatory collapse.

Management: Early detection of hyperlactataemia is critical. Check lactate and bicarbonate in symptomatic patients. If lactate ↑ (normal venous lactate <2.5mmol/L) drugs should be stopped and a safer combination started once lactate has normalized (usually takes 2–3mths). (Clinicians may choose to keep patient on an NNRTI + boosted-PI regimen permanently or until lactate has normalized, rather than interrupting ART completely.) Patients who are acidotic should be admitted for IV fluids and vitamins. Sepsis may mimic lactic acidosis so it is often prudent to add a broad-spectrum antibiotic. Patients with symptomatic hyperlactataemia or lactic acidosis should never receive d4T or ddI again.

Fatty liver: steatohepatitis

Is also caused by NRTIs and is commonly associated with hyperlactataemia. Management principles are similar. Patients present with RUQ discomfort, firm hepatomegaly, and ↑ LFTs.

Pancreatitis

Is a complication of ddI > d4T.

Management Involves stopping ART, admission and treatment for acute pancreatitis. Once resolved, ART can be recommenced with a regimen excluding these 2 drugs.

Bone marrow suppression

AZT may cause anaemia and neutropenia, usually in the first 3mths of therapy. AZT causes macrocytosis. Patients with underlying marrow compromise (e.g. nutritional or TB) are at ↑ risk.

Management Involves blood transfusions and neutropenic support if required. AZT should be switched to an alternative drug (e.g. d4T), especially if Hb < 6.5g/dL and neutrophil <500/mm^3.

Lipid and glucose abnormalities

Some PIs may → 2° hypercholesterolaemia and glucose intolerance (risk factors for cardiovascular disease) and hypertriglyceridaemia (which may → pancreatitis). Patients on PIs should ↓ other cardiovascular risk factors (e.g. stop smoking, control BP) and all should be advised on a low-fat diet. Check lipids annually in patients on PIs if practicable. Hypertriglyceridaemia >10mmol/L should be treated with dietary advice and a fibrate. In patients with hypercholesterolaemia and additional cardiovascular risk factors dietary advice and consider therapy with a fibrate or a statin. Use atorvastatin. Certain statins (e.g. simvastatin) are contra-indicated with PIs.

Lipodystrophy: fat redistribution

Is a consequence of long-term ART therapy. NRTIs (d4T > AZT) result in lipoatrophy (loss of facial and limb fat). Lipohypertrophy (central obesity and dorsocervical fat accumulation) was previously thought to be a complication of PI therapy, but evidence now shows that it may occur on any ART, unrelated to any specific class of drugs.

Management Involves switching to alternative agents for lipoatrophy if possible, but reversal is slow and incomplete.

Renal disease

TDF is associated with renal dysfunction and Fanconi's syndrome (a syndrome of renal tubular wasting of glucose, protein, phosphate, and other substances) in a minority of patients, particularly those with pre-existing renal dysfunction. TDF should be avoided in patients with estimated creatinine clearance < 50mL/min. Creatinine should be monitored in those on TDF. Avoid concomitant nephrotoxins (e.g. if a patient needs prolonged aminoglycoside treatment for MDR TB. Consider switching TDF to alternative for this period.). IDV, and less commonly ATZ may → renal stones, particularly if a good fluid intake is not maintained.

Abacavir hypersensitivity

Occurs in 4–8% patients (much less frequent in Africans). Associated with major histocompatibility complex (MHC) class I allele *HLA-B*5701* haplotype (ideal is to test for *HLA B*5701* before use of ABCv). Clinical features include flu-like symptoms, rash, fever and hepatitis; may be life-threatening with continued use.

Management Stop ABCv; do not re-challenge.

Neuropsychiatric

Side-effects occur with EFV, including dizziness, inattention, vivid dreams, sleep disturbance, dysphoria, and occasionally acute psychosis. These side-effects occur early and resolve in the majority within a few weeks. Advise patients to take EFV at night.

AZT-induced myopathy

Is described, usually after prolonged therapy, but is rare.

Table 3.11 Side-effects of antiretroviral therapy

Severe ART toxicities	Most likely candidates
Anaemia/neutropenia	AZT (especially with co-trimoxazole)
Neuropathy	d4T, ddl
Pancreatitis	ddl, d4T
Hepatic steatosis	d4T, ddl
Lactic acidosis	d4T, ddl > AZT > other NRTIs
Hypersensitivity	ABCv (life-threatening, do not re-challenge)
Renal impairment	Tenofovir
Stevens–Johnson syndrome	Nevirapine > EFZ
Hypersensitivity hepatitis	Nevirapine > EFZ. Also ABC, ETR
Psychiatric	EFZ > ETR
Nephrolithiasis	IDV (less commonly ATZ)
Diarrhoea	PI
Hyperlipidaemia	PI
Lipoatrophy	Nucleoside analogues, d4T > AZT
Insulin resistance	Some PIs

Antiretroviral therapy metabolism and interactions

NNRTIs and PIs have a number of important drug interactions (see Table 3.12). These result from the fact that they are substrates of the cytochrome P450 enzyme system in the liver and intestine. The PIs are generally inhibitors of these enzymes, nevirapine is an inducer, and EFZ may be an inducer or inhibitor. Exceptions do, however, occur. Drugs that are commonly involved in these interactions are:

Inducers Carbamazepine, phenytoin, phenobarbital, rifampicin.

Inhibitors Macrolides (e.g. erythromycin), cimetidine, azoles (e.g. fluconazole).

Substrates

- Warfarin.
- Carbamazepine, phenytoin, phenobarbital.
- Oral contraceptive.
- Statins.
- Certain benzodiazepines (e.g. midazolam).
- Ergot alkaloids.
- Macrolides.
- Calcium channel blockers.
- Azoles.

When prescribing other drugs with ART it is important to check for interactions. A useful source of ART drug interaction information is: 🖱 www.hiv-druginteractions.org

Some combinations are contraindicated (e.g. ergotamine and PI) and in others, dose adjustments are required (e.g. warfarin and nevirapine guided by international normalized ration (INR)). The interactions may be bi-directional, e.g. carbamazepine and nevirapine may ↓ each other's levels. Other drug combinations share toxicities and should not be used together, e.g. ganciclovir and AZT because both drugs are bone marrow suppressants.

NRTIs are not metabolized by the cytochrome P450 system, but are renally excreted. Certain interactions occur at this level, e.g. tenofovir ↑ didanosine levels and thus ↑ toxicity. For this reason (and also because this combination is less potent than other NRTI combinations), these two drugs should not be used together. If renal function is impaired, it is important to ↓ the dose of NRTI drugs (see Table 3.10).

Table 3.12 Common ART drug interactions and how to manage these

Interacting drugs	Effect	Management
R (rifampicin) and EFZ	R ↓ EFZ levels moderately (22%)	Standard-dose EFZ
R and nevirapine	R ↓ nevirapine levels more substantially (37%) and these drugs have common toxicities	Preferably avoid nevirapine, but if it is started in patients on rifampicin do not use lead-in dose (i.e. commence treatment with 200mg bd)
R and LPV/ritonavir	Marked ↓ in LPV level (75%)	In patients on R, use LPV/ritonavir 4 tablets bd (i.e. double dose); monitor LFTs
NNRTI or PI and warfarin	Warfarin levels ↑ or ↓ and INR control disturbed	Monitor INR closely when starting, switching, or stopping ART and adjust warfarin dose accordingly
Phenytoin, phenobarbital, or carbamazepine and NNRTI	Bidirectional inter-action: levels of both these anticonvulsants and the NNRTI are ↓	Avoid if possible—use amitriptyline, rather than carbamazepine for neuropathic pain and valproate or lamotrigine for epilepsy
EFZ and oral contraception	Levels of ethinyl oestradiol are ↑	Avoid high-dose oral contraceptive (OC)—low-dose oral or injectable contraceptive or IUD are alternatives. A barrier method must also be used
PIs or nevirapine and oral contraceptives	Levels of ethinyl oestradiol are ↓	Avoid low-dose OC—high-dose oral or injectable contraceptive or IUD are alternatives. A barrier method must also be used
PIs and midazolam or triazolam	Levels of benzodiazepines ↑ with risk of sedation	*Avoid*
PIs and ergot alkaloids	Substantial ↑ in levels of ergot alkaloids leading to vasospastic crises	*Avoid*

Antiretroviral therapy resistance

ART drugs taken with inadequate adherence or in a regimen that is sub-optimal will select out viruses in the viral population that have resistance mutations.

- These are point substitutions in the sequence of reverse transcriptase, protease or integrase genes that reduce binding of drugs to their target and thereby reduce their suppressive effect.
- There may be cross-resistance between drugs for certain mutational patterns.
- Genotypic resistance testing is costly and is unavailable in most resource limited settings. It detects resistant mutants if the viral load (VL) >1000copies/mL and they are present in >20% of viral population (patient must be on ART when test is done).
- Mutations are annotated with the position in the protein sequence represented by a number, the wild type amino acid at that position precedes the number and the mutant is after it (e.g. the 3TC mutation is M184V, which is a methionine to valine substitution at position 184 in reverse transcriptase enzyme).
- Certain drugs require a single mutation to confer high level resistance (e.g. 3TC), whereas other drugs require several mutations for high level resistance and are said to have a high barrier to resistance (e.g. boosted PIs).
- The first line ART mutations are shown in Table 3.13.

Programmatic guidelines for second line ART regimens in resource limited settings take into account what are the likely mutations that occur on the first line and advise a second line that will predictably re-suppress viral load for the majority of patients if adherence is adequate. The ritonavir-boosted PI used in second line is robust and provides reliable suppression particularly when at least one new NRTI is used with it. In patients who fail second line rapidly the majority do not have resistance and would suppress if adherence improved. For these reasons, in the majority of patients in resource limited settings resistance testing is not an essential aspect of management (adherence interventions are far more critical to treatment success).

Table 3.13 First line ART mutations

Drugs	Resistance mutations selected
3TC or FTC	M184V
EFV or NVP (there is cross-resistance between these 2 drugs)	One or more of several NNRTI resistance mutations (e.g. K103N, Y181C)
d4T or AZT (these 2 drugs select similar mutations)	Thymidine analogue mutations (TAMs - M41L, D67N, K70R, L210W, T215Y/F, K219Q/E/N). If several TAMs present may cause cross-resistance to most drugs in the NRTI class
TDF	K65R (TAMs are not selected by TDF, but certain pre-existing TAMs will compromise TDF efficacy)

Immune reconstitution inflammatory syndrome

After ART is commenced, there is rapid ↓ viral load, slower ↑ CD4 count, and restoration of pathogen-specific immunity. Dysregulated immune responses may → immunopathological reactions in days to months after starting ART, often in response to high burden of microbial antigen related to OI present prior to ART, termed IRIS (Box 3.2).

Box 3.2 Definition of IRIS

- HIV+ patient receiving ART with ↓ viral load and ↑ CD4 count (which may lag behind the fall in viral load) *and*
- Clinical features consistent with inflammatory process (e.g. lymphadenitis or pulmonary infiltrate on CXR) *and*
- Clinical course not consistent with expected course of either a previously diagnosed OI or newly-diagnosed OI or drug toxicity.

Several forms of IRIS are described:

- '*Unmasking*' *IRIS*: an inflammatory and often atypical presentation, soon after starting ART, of an OI that was unsuspected prior to ART.
- *Paradoxical reactions*: recurrence or worsening of OI symptoms and signs after starting ART despite being on appropriate OI treatment. The reaction here is thought to result from an ↑ immune response directed towards residual antigen.
- KS may worsen with an ↑ in lesions or inflammation of existing lesions (most KS lesions regress on ART).

IRIS occurs mainly in patients with low pre-treatment CD4 cells counts (<200cells/mm^3) and in association with OI such as TB, cryptococcosis, MAC, CMV, and HBV. An example of a CMV 'unmasking' IRIS is a patient with an inflammatory CMV uveitis after starting ART. TB paradoxical reactions are seen in up to 45% of patients starting ART, while on TB treatment, manifesting as recurrence of fever and other TB symptoms, enlarging lymphadenopathy, or recurrent pulmonary infiltrates early after starting ART. Dermatological manifestations (e.g. flare of acne) are also seen.

Management

IRIS can be challenging, but is rarely fatal and with careful clinical management there is rarely a need to interrupt ART.

- Diagnose the OI and exclude additional OIs or antimicrobial resistance (such as MDR TB).
- In most cases, continue ART and effective OI therapy.
- In certain severe cases of mycobacterial or fungal IRIS, steroids (e.g. prednisolone 1mg/kg/d, duration dependent on response) should be considered.

In paradoxical TB-IRIS prednisolone starting at 1.5mg/kg/d → more rapid symptom improvement, but should only be prescribed when alternative reasons for clinical deterioration are excluded. If the reaction is life-threatening (e.g. CNS involvement) and not responding to steroids, it may be necessary to interrupt ART.

Special aspects of paediatric HIV/AIDS

Diagnosis (WHO guidelines)

Early diagnosis and treatment is the key to effective management of HIV in children. HIV+ adults should be encouraged to get their children tested, and in areas where the prevalence of paediatric HIV is high, HIV testing should become a routine part of inpatient care and not merely reserved for children with signs of advanced HIV/AIDS (Box 3.3).

In children > 18mths Diagnosis is as for adults (Box 3.1).

In children < 18mths Diagnosis is based on:

- Positive virological test for HIV, ideally an HIV DNA PCR (qualitative) performed at 4–6wks of age. A +ve result may be confirmed by a second virological test, an HIV RNA PCR (quantitative), also called HIV viral load or a repeat HIV DNA PCR obtained from a separate sample.
- Antibody testing is *not recommended* for definitive or confirmatory diagnosis of HIV infection in children until 18mths as it merely indicates transfer of maternal HIV antibodies, and not infection. Antibody testing in this age group may be used as a screen for HIV exposure in cases where the mother's status is unknown.
- *HIV infection in a child <18mths:* suspect if the following are present:
  - the infant is HIV antibody +ve and
  - an AIDS-defining illness is present (WHO stage IV condition including disseminated TB, cryptococcal disease, severe wasting) or
  - the infant has >2 symptoms of: oral thrush, severe pneumonia or severe sepsis.

However, confirmation of the diagnosis should be sought as soon as possible as other diseases, such as TB and cancers, e.g. lymphoma may present similarly to HIV.

In children started presumptively on ART, based on a +ve serological test at <18mths, an HIV antibody test should be repeated at 18mths to confirm the diagnosis, provided the child is no longer exposed to HIV antibodies through breastfeeding.

Effects on growth and development

- Poor growth is one of the most sensitive indicators of HIV progression. From birth, HIV+ infants are often smaller and have lower birth weight than uninfected children born to HIV+ women.
- *Causes of poor growth include:* alterations in GI function, chronic or recurrent infections, alterations in metabolic and endocrine function, and side effects of medication for HIV (including exposure to ART in utero) and OI. Pubertal delay is common, especially among boys.
- The use of effective ART leads to improvements in growth indices. Growth monitoring on ART is essential in children and children on ART require dose adjustments with ↑ weight. This may also alert the clinician to ART disease effects, such as fat redistribution syndrome caused by NRTI's such as stavudine (or *less commonly*, didanosine and zidovudine).

Prevention of opportunistic infections in children

Pneumocystis carinii pneumonia

- *Co-trimoxazole (trimethoprim-sulfamethoxazole (TMP-SMX)):* prophylaxis halves all-cause mortality, including prevention of other bacterial infections such as *Salmonella* and is recommended for all HIV+ children.
- *Dose:* TMP 5mg/kg/day and SMX 25mg/kg/day in two divided doses.
- *Alternative is dapsone:* 2/3 of children intolerant of TMP-SMX will tolerate dapsone at a dose of 2mg/kg/day (max 100mg daily).

TB

HIV+ children with household TB contacts and those stable on HAART should receive INH prophylaxis if active TB disease has been excluded. 1° INH preventive therapy is also associated with an all-cause mortality benefit and, although optimal duration of therapy is unknown, 6mths of INH 10mg/kg daily to max. 300mg daily is currently recommended by WHO.

Therapy of opportunistic infections in children

Whilst many of the principles required to recognize, diagnose and manage OI in children are similar to those in adults there are important differences, e.g. higher incidence of some OIs in children and the problems posed by drug therapy. The notes on the following pages emphasize management and are not exhaustive. They are based on a comprehensive CDC review: http://www.cdc.gov/mmwr/preview/mmwrhtml/rr5811a1.htm#tab4

Box 3.3 WHO clinical staging for HIV/AIDS in children with confirmed HIV infection (2010)

Clinical stage 1

- Asymptomatic.
- PGL.

Clinical stage 2

- Unexplained persistent hepatomegaly.
- Papular pruritic eruption.
- Extensive wart virus infection.
- Extensive molluscum contagiosum.
- Recurrent oral ulcerations.
- Unexplained persistent parotid enlargement.
- Linear gingival erythema.
- Herpes zoster.
- Recurrent/chronic URTIs (otitis media, otorrhoea, sinusitis, tonsillitis).
- Fungal nail infections.

Clinical stage 3

- Unexplained moderate malnutrition not adequately responding to standard therapy.
- Unexplained persistent diarrhoea for >14 d.
- Unexplained persistent fever for >1mth.
- Persistent oral candidiasis (after 6wks of life).
- Oral hairy leukoplakia.
- Acute necrotizing gingivitis/periodontitis.
- Pulmonary TB.

Box 3.3 (*Continued*)

- Lymph node TB.
- Severe recurrent bacterial pneumonia.
- Symptomatic lymphoid interstitial pneumonitis.
- Chronic HIV-associated lung disease incl. bronchiectasis.
- Unexplained anaemia (<8g/dL), neutropenia (<0.5 × 10^9/L) and/or chronic thrombocytopenia (<50 × 10^9/L).

Clinical stage 4

- Unexplained severe malnutrition. No response to standard therapy.
- *Pneumocystis carinii* pneumonia (PCP).
- Recurrent severe bacterial infection (e.g. empyema, pyomyositis, bone or joint infection, meningitis, but excluding pneumonia.
- Chronic HSV infection (orolabial or cutaneous of > 1mth duration or visceral at any site.
- Extrapulmonary TB.
- KS.
- Oesophageal candidiasis (or candidiasis of trachea, bronchi, or lungs).
- CNS toxoplasmosis (after 1mth of life).
- HIV encephalopathy.
- Cytomegalovirus (CMV) infection, retinitis or CMV infection involving any other organ with onset after 1mth of life.
- Extrapulmonary cryptococcosis including meningitis.
- Disseminated endemic mycosis (extrapulmonary histoplasmosis, coccidiomycosis or penicilliosis).
- Chronic cryptosporidiosis(with diarrhoea).
- Chronic isosporiasis.
- Disseminated non-tuberculous mycobacterial infection.
- Cerebral or B cell non Hodgkin lymphoma.
- PML.
- Symptomatic HIV nephropathy or cardiomyopathy.

Pneumocystis carinii pneumonia (PCP)

PCP is an important cause of ARI in children, and the leading cause of ARI among children aged 2–6mths. Treatment of ARI in the latter group should always include PCP treatment; treat older children for PCP when suspected clinically.

- *Co-trimoxazole:* 15–20mg/kg TMP plus 75–100mg/kg SMX IV or oral daily in 3 or 4 divided doses for 21d. Treatment can be switched to oral therapy once acute pneumonitis subsides, provided no diarrhoea or malabsorbtion.
- *Alternative therapies include:*
  - *pentamidine*—4mg/kg IV od 7–10d then atovaquone for 14d
  - *atovaquone*—30–40mg/kg/d oral in 2 divided doses (max 750mg bd)
  - *dapsone*/TMP—2mg/kg/d of dapsone and 5mg/kg tds of TMP (dose as above)
  - *clindamycin/primaquine*—clindamycin 10mg/kg/dose 6-hourly and primaquine base 0.3mg/kg/d.
- *Prednisolone:* 2mg/kg for 5d, 1mg/kg for 5d then 0.5mg/kg for 5d, should be added if hypoxic (PaO2 <70mmHg (<9.3kPa) in room air).

Continue 2° prophylaxis until 5yrs of age if CD4 count of >500cells/mm^3 or >15% in children 1–5yrs and >15% or 200cells/mm^3 in children >6yrs.

Toxoplasmosis

- *Congenital:* treat for 6mths with pyrimethamine (2mg/kg od for 2d then 1mg/kg od for 2–6mths, then 1mg/kg 3× weekly), plus folinic acid 10mg with each dose, plus sulphadiazine 50mg/kg bd.
- *Acquired:* treat for 6wks with pyrimethamine (2mg/kg [max 50 mg] od for 3d then 1mg/kg [max 25mg] od) plus sulphadiazine 25–50mg/kg qds, plus folinic acid 10–25mg od.
- *Clindamycin:* 5–7.5mg/kg (max. 600mg/dose) oral/IV qds can be substituted for sulfadiazine.
- *Corticosteroids:* recommended for children with CNS disease with highly elevated CSF protein (>1000mg/dL) and with focal lesions that may cause a mass effect.
- Consider discontinuing 2° prophylaxis once the child has been on stable ART for >6mths, has demonstrated sustained immune reconstitution (as for PCP) and is asymptomatic.

Cryptosporidiosis No consistently effective therapy exists and the best treatment is ART.

Microsporidiosis The best treatment is ART although albendazole 7.5mg/kg (max 400mg) bd is effective against all forms except *Enterocytozoon bieneusi.*

Tuberculosis

- *Pulmonary TB and lymph node disease:* standard triple therapy, rifampicin, isoniazid, pyrazinamide, (RHZ) for 2mths (intensive phase) followed by RH (continuation phase) for 4mths. In children who are clinically unstable with severe TB, and HIV+ or malnourished, consideration should be given for treating with 4 drugs in the intensive phase, using ethambutol as the 4th drug.
- Extrapulmonary disease: as above except for bone and joint TB where duration should be 12mths.
- TB meningitis: ethambutol is recommended by WHO, however ethionamide (Eth) can also be used as the 4th drug, as it penetrates CSF better than ethambutol. Treat for 12mths in total: 2mths RHZEth (intensive phase) and 10mths continuation phase (RH). Some experts suggest 4 drugs (RHZEth) for 6mths at high dose for treatment of TB meningitis and miliary TB.
- If there is a poor response to TB treatment the child requires repeat investigation for MDR TB, other mycobacterial infections, e.g. MAC or other pathologies (e.g. lymphoma).
- See 🕮 Combining ART with TB treatment in children: special considerations, p. 141 for notes on prescribing anti-TB medication with ART.
- Adjunctive treatment with corticosteroids is often added for CNS TB, pericardial TB and intrathoracic TB lymph nodes with airway obstruction.

BCG immunization in children

- Immunization with BCG is recommended despite HIV exposure in countries with high TB prevalence (🕮 Immunization, p. 904).

Mycobacterium avium complex

- *Minimum of two drugs given:* clarithromycin 7.5-15mg/kg (max. 500mg) bd plus ethambutol 15–25mg/kg (max. 1g) od.
- In severe disease rifabutin 10–20mg/kg (max. 300mg/d) can be added and azithromycin 10–12mg/kg (max. 500mg) od can be substituted for

clarithromycin. Azithromycin has fewer interactions than clarithromycin with PIs and NNRTIs and may be considered in children on ART.

Candidiasis

- *Oropharyngeal options:*
  - fluconazole 3–6mg/kg (max 400mg) oral od for 7–14d
  - itraconazole 2.5mg/kg oral bd (max 200mg daily). Nystatin suspension 4–6mL oral qid
  - clotrimazole troches 10mg troche oral qds.
- *Oesophageal:* fluconazole and itraconazole as for oropharyngeal candidiasis, but extend treatment for 21d.
- *Invasive:* amphotericin 0.5–1.5mg/kg IV od. Continue for at least 2–3wks after last +ve blood culture. If amphotericin is unavailable, fluconazole can be used at 5–6mg/kg bd (max 800mg/d).

Coccidioidomycosis

- *Diffuse pulmonary or disseminated:* amphotericin 0.5–1.0mg/kg IV od for several weeks, followed by chronic suppressive therapy with an azole.
- *Meningeal infection:* fluconazole 5–6mg/kg bd (max 800mg/day) for several weeks followed by 2° prophylaxis.

Cytomegalovirus

- *Congenital:* ganciclovir 6mg/kg IV bd for 6wks; trials are investigating extended use of valganciclovir in congenital CMV (HIV+ and HIV–).
- *Retinitis and visceral disease:* ganciclovir 5mg/kg IV bd for 14–21d followed by 5mg/kg IV od 5–7d/wk as suppressive therapy. *Alternative:* foscarnet 60mg/kg IV tds for 10–21d then 90–120mg/kg od for chronic suppression.
- *CNS disease*: ganciclovir 5mg/kg IV bd *plus* foscarnet 60mg/kg IV tds continued until symptoms improved, followed by chronic suppressive therapy.

Cryptococcosis

- *Amphotericin:* 0.7–1mg/kg IV od for at least 2wks (induction therapy) plus flucytosine 25mg/kg oral qds or fluconazole 12mg/kg/day for 2 weeks. (May ↑ amphotericin dose to 1.5mg/kg/day if flucytosine is not tolerated.). Follow with consolidation and continuation therapy as below.
- *If amphotericin unavailable:* fluconazole 12mg/kg (max 800mg/day) on day 1, then 6–12mg/kg/d plus flucytosine 25mg/kg/dose qds.

Induction therapy must be followed by consolidation and continuation therapy:

- Fluconazole 12mg/kg/d on day 1 then 6–12mg/kg/d for at least 8wks.
- Continuation therapy must then be followed by chronic suppressive therapy with fluconazole.

Discontinue maintenance therapy

- Viral load monitoring available: virally suppressed, on maintenance for at least 1 year and CD4 count > 100 cells/mm^3.
- No viral load monitoring: maintenance therapy for at least a year and CD4 greater than 200 cells/mm^3.
- HIV-infected children aged between two and 5 years, with successfully treated cryptococcal disease if child is stable and adherent to ART, anti-fungal maintenance treatment for at least one year and CD4 cell count percentage greater than 25% or absolute count greater than 750 cells/mm^3.
- Maintenance therapy for cryptococcal disease should NOT be discontinued in children less than two years.

- Maintenance therapy should be restarted if CD4 count drops to 100 cells/mm^3 or below in HIV-infected adults and adolescents (or CD4 cell count less than or equal to 25% or 750 cells/mm^3 in children aged between two and five years), or if a WHO stage 4 clinical event occurs, irrespective of patient age.

Histoplasmosis

- *Mild:* itraconazole 2–5mg/kg/dose tds (max 600mg daily) oral for 3d (induction), followed by 2–5mg/kg (max 200mg) bd for 12mths (consolidation).
- *Severe and disseminated:* amphotericin 1mg/kg IV od for 2–3wks followed by consolidation therapy as above.
- Lifelong 2° prophylaxis with itraconazole is recommended.

HSV

- *Neonatal:* aciclovir 20mg/kg IV tds for 21d if CNS and disseminated disease and 14d if limited to skin, eyes, and oral lesions.
- *CNS:* outside neonatal period aciclovir 10mg/kg IV tds run over 1h for 21d.
- *Gingivostomatitis, orolabial lesions:* aciclovir 20mg/kg/dose oral tds. If moderate or severe ideally treat with aciclovir 5–10mg/kg IV tds then switch to oral therapy.
  - closely evaluate hydration status in children with gingivostomatitis as oral intake may be impaired
  - add analgesia as necessary.
- *Genital herpes:* aciclovir 20mg/kg (max 400mg) oral tds for 7–10d. Foscarnet can be given for aciclovir-resistant disease.
- *Aciclovir analogues:* valaciclovir, famciclovir, penciclovir are not fully evaluated in children.

VZV

- *Chickenpox:* aciclovir 10mg/kg IV tds for 7–10d or until no new lesions in severely immunosuppressed children (CDC immune category 3). Oral aciclovir (20mg/kg qds) can be used for children with mild chickenpox or children in CDC immunologic category 1 and 2.
- *Zoster:* aciclovir 20mg/kg oral qds for 7–10d.
- If trigeminal nerve involvement or extensive multidermatomal zoster: IV aciclovir 10mg/kg tds; switch to oral therapy when lesions resolving.

HBV

- *Treat if:* detectable HBV RNA (with or without HBeAg +ve) for >6mths, persistent (>6mths) elevation of transaminases >2 × upper limit normal, signs chronic hepatitis on liver biopsy.
- *If needs HBV treatment:*
  - *if not on ART*—interferon-alfa (6mths) or adefovir (12mths).
  - *if on ART*— 3TC and TDF have activity against HBV and should be used in combination in the ART regimen to avoid resistance.
- *If does not need HBV treatment:* select an ART regimen not containing either 3TC or TDF to avoid → resistant HBV.

NB. TDF is not approved for use in children <18yrs, although careful use may be warranted in older children (over 15yrs and >40kg in weight).

HCV

- Treat with interferon-α-2b plus ribavirin. Treat for 48wks regardless of HCV genotype.
- Treatment is expensive and not usually available in resource-poor settings.

Antiretroviral therapy in children

Effective prevention of MTCT is the best way to reduce paediatric HIV. Transmission rates of <5% can be achieved by giving ART to the mother and giving the baby prophylaxis, e.g. daily nevirapine. However 430 000 new infections occurred in 2008 in children <15yrs, the majority in resource-poor regions, 90% as a result of MTCT. Untreated, 50% of children with HIV will die by their 2nd birthday. ART in children needs to be started as soon as possible if the child meets criteria for ART.

When to start ART

WHO recommends all children <5yrs, regardless of clinical or immunological criteria, start ART. Priority needs to be give to initiating infants <1yr on ART.

Other indications are:

- WHO Stage III or IV disease, irrespective of CD4 count.
- >5yrs: WHO stage 3 or 4 Or CD4 ≤500 cells/mm^3 (CD4 ≤350 cells/mm^3 as a priority). WHO Stage I or II disease with CD4 count < threshold for severe immunodeficiency (see Tables 3.14 and 3.15). Do not treat if CD4 count is not available. Total lymphocyte count should not be used in decisions to initiate ART in children.

General principles

- Use one formulation or a fixed drug combination (FDC) if possible.
- Use syringes to accurately dose liquid formulations.
- Avoid large volumes of liquid drugs; switch to solids when possible.
- If solid paediatric formulations unavailable, adapt adult forms. Many tablets can be divided in half or capsules may be opened and contents mixed with water or sprinkled on a small amount of food.
- Some adult FDC (e.g. those containing NVP) may under-dose during induction and should be avoided during this phase.
- Do not use d4T and AZT together.
- Avoid differing a.m. and p.m. regimens where possible.
- If a dose is forgotten, reassure the family it can be given within 3h of the usual time.
- Weigh the child at each visit and adjust doses accordingly.
- If capsules or tablets are broken into food, ensure all food is eaten.
- If the child vomits within 30min of taking ART, repeat dose.

Recommended first line ART regimens

In children < 3 years of age

In young children, nevirapine is inferior to ritonavir boosted lopinavir (LPV) regardless of previous NNRTI exposure in terms of virological suppression and mortality and thus should only be used if LPV/r not available.

Children < 3yrs ABC/AZT + 3TC+LOP/r
or if LOP/r not available, ABC/AZT +3TC+ NVP

Children > 3yrs ABC + 3TC+ EFV
(NVP can replace EFV, AZT can replace ABC)

Caution with using TDF in children due to bone mineral density and renal complications.

Although triple NRTI may simplify drug interaction and toxicity, this is not a widely recommended regimen as virological suppression may be inadequate with the possibility of resistance, and should be avoided.

Paediatric ART dosing

Weight-banded dosing charts are available in the WHO 2010 updated guidelines, which provide simple dosage guidance for ART in children (Table 3.16). (http://whqlibdoc.who.int/publications/2010/9789241599801_eng.pdf)

Where body surface area (BSA) has been used this is calculated by the formula:

$$\text{BSA} = \sqrt{[[\text{weight (kg)} \times \text{height (cm)}]/3600]}$$

Table 3.14 Recommendations for initiating ART in HIV+ infants (WHO, 2010)

WHO paediatric stage	CD4 available?	Age specific treatment recommendation	
		>5yrs	**<5yrs**
Stage 4	N/A	Treat all irrespective of availability of CD4 and age	
Stage 3	Yes No	Treat all	Treat all
Stage 2	Yes	CD4 guided	
Stage 1	Yes	CD4 guided	

Table 3.15 Immunological criteria for initiating ART (WHO, 2013)

Marker	<5yrs	≥5yrs
CD4 count	N/A	$<500/mm^3$

Table 3.16 Paediatric ART dosing: WHO guidelines[1]

3TC	*Target dose:* 4 mg/kg (max 150mg) bd, 2mg/kg bd if <30d old
d4T	*Target dose:* 1mg/kg bd (<30kg), 30 mg/dose bd
AZT	*Target dose:* for infants >6wks: 180–240mg/m² (max 300mg) bd *Prevention of MTCT in infants:* 4mg/kg oral bd; start <12h after birth and continue up to 6wks. IV alternative (until oral administration possible): 1.5mg/kg qds, infused over 30min.
ABCv	*Target dose:* 8mg/kg (max 300mg) bd
ddI	*<3mths:* 50mg/m² bd *3mths–12yrs:* 90–120mg/m² bd *Max dose, >12yrs or >60kg:* 200mg/dose bd or 400mg od
TDF	Little data on use in children, but consider in children >15yrs and >40kg; dose 300mg oral daily
EFV	*>40kg:* 600mg od *<40kg:* 19.5mg/kg od (syrup) or 15mg/kg od (capsule/tablet) Not recommended children <3yrs or weight <10kg
NVP	*Target maintenance dose:* 160–200mg/m² bd (max 200mg bd) *Induction dose:* for first 14d omit evening dose of NVP (A mild rash may be observed during induction—defer escalation if necessary. A serious rash requires discontinuation.) NVP for PMTCT (preferred method currently) *Birth to 6wks:* • weight <2.5kg 10mg/d • weight >2.5kg 15mg/d
Etravirine (ETR)	Age 6wks to 6mths 20mg/d Age 6–9mths 30mg/d Age 9mths to end of breastfeeding 40mg/d 5.2mg/kg bd from 6yrs to a max adult dose of 200mg bd
Saquinavir (SQV)	33mg/kg tds (not licensed for use in children <16yrs or <25kg)
LPV ritonavir co-formulation	*Lopinavir:* target doses (children ≥6wks): 230–350mg/m² bd *Ritonavir:* used to boost other PI's and should not be used alone. Dose equivalent to 75mg/m²
	Max dose: 400mg LPV+ 100 mg ritonavir bd, 10–20mg/kg/dose bd. Boost with ritonavir (≥6yrs)
Darunavir Atazanavir	*Treatment-naïve daily dose:* • weight 15kg to <25kg: 150mg AZT/80mg ritonavir (RTV) • weight 25kg to <32kg: 200mg ATV/100mg RTV • weight 32kg to <39kg: 250mg ATV/100mg RTV *Treatment-experienced* • weight 25kg to <32kg: 200mg ATV/100mg RTV • weight 32kg to <39kg: 250mg ATV/100mg RTV

¹ ww.who.int/hiv/pub/guidelines/paediatric020907.pdf

ART toxicity in children

Overall the spectrum of adverse events is similar to adults (see Antiretroviral therapy side-effects, pp. 120–3).

- Hypersensitivity and hepatitis due to NVP are less frequent.
- Severe toxicities and potential drugs to switch to are listed in Table 3.17 (source WHO).
- In general acute serious adverse reactions require discontinuation of all ART until the symptoms resolve.
- More chronic or subacute toxicities may be managed by withdrawing and then substituting the most likely offending drug (e.g. AZT-induced bone marrow suppression).
- Note that children who demonstrate ABC hypersensitivity should not be re-challenged with the drug as re-challenge may be fatal.
- Lipoatrophy or metabolic syndromes are the most common side-effect in children treated with ddI, d4T, and to a lesser extent AZT. These drugs should be switched to ABC or TDF (in older children) early if the child demonstrates recent virological suppression as the switch is aimed at halting progression, rather than reversing lipoatrophy. Children who are still receiving d4T should be switched to ABC/AZT/TDF as these drugs are associated with less long term toxicity than d4T.

Table 3.17 Severe toxicities and potential drugs to switch to

Drug	Toxicity	Suggested substitution
ABC	Hypersensitivity	AZT/d4T
AZT	Haematological toxicity	d4T or ABC
	Lactic acidosis	ABC
	Severe gastrointestinal intolerance	d4T or ABC
d4T	Lactic acidosis	ABC
	Peripheral neuropathy	AZT or ABC
	Pancreatitis	AZT or ABC
Lop/r	Lipoatrophy/metabolic syndrome	ABC or AZT
	Lipoatrophy/metabolic syndrome	Switch to NNRTI
EFZ	CNS toxicity	NVP or PI
	Potential teratogenicity	
NVP	Acute hepatitis	EFZ
	Hypersensitivity	PI or 3rd NRTI (less potent)
	Stevens–Johnson syndrome	PI or 3rd NRTI (less potent)

Switching to second line therapy due to treatment failure

Treatment failure can be defined as:

- *Clinical:* a new and recurrent WHO stage 3 or 4 condition whilst on ART may indicate disease progression.
- *Immunological:* failure indicated by returning to the following in a child adherent to ART for >24wks:
    - 2 to <5yrs—CD4 count of <200cells/mm^3 or <10%
    - >5yrs—CD4 count <200cells/mm^3.
- *Virological:* child adherent to ART with a viral load >1000copies/mL.

Poor adherence or drug absorption and viral drug resistance can contribute to treatment failure. Prior to switching therapy ensure that:

- ≥24wks of treatment have been completed.
- Adherence has been optimized.
- CD4 count has been measured at least twice if viral load monitoring is not available.
- As far as possible exclude IRIS (p. 128) as a cause of clinical deterioration.
- The clinician must be aware that although it is recommended that children >3yrs of age on a LPV/r-based regimen change to EFV/NVP, these drugs have a low genetic threshold for resistance and unless adherence has been corrected, this change may be unsuccessful with continued virological failure.

It is best to switch early if a child is on an NNRTI-based regimen to prevent the accumulation of further resistance mutations. PI resistance is less likely and children can remain on these regimens without the accumulation of resistance. See Table 3.18 for WHO 2013 recommended 2nd line regimens.

Table 3.18 Second line ART regimens for children. Adapted from WHO guidelines 2013

Second line ART			**Preferred regimens**	**Alternative regimens**
Children	If NNRTI-based first-line regimen was used		ABC+3TC +LPV/r[a]	ABC+3TC +LPV/r[a] TDF+3TC (or FTC) + LPV/r[a]
	If a PI-based first-line regimen was used	<3yrs	No change from first line regimen in use[b]	AZT (or ABC) +3TC+NVP
		3 yrs to <10yrs	AZT (or ABC) +3TC + EFV	ABC (or TDF) +3TC+NVP

[a] ATV/r can be used as an alternative to LPV/r for children older than 6yrs

[b] Unless failure caused by lack of adherence due to poor palatability of LPV/r.

Combining ART with TB treatment in children: special considerations

HIV/TB is a complex area.

- TB is an indication for ART.
- The development of TB during ART may be a sign of ART failure.
- Alternatively TB may become manifest ('umasking IRIS') or worsen ('paradoxical IRIS') during ART.
- Rifampicin-based therapy for TB complicates the choice of ART.

When to start ART in HIV/TB

For WHO stage 4 disease and for stage 3 disease, where no CD4 is available ART should be commenced 2wks after starting TB therapy. TB and HIV co-infection → significant morbidity and mortality and ART should be started as soon as possible after 2wks of TB treatment.

Optimum drug regimens in HIV/TB

Background regimen of 2 NRTIs plus:

In children <3yrs

- NVP.
- Lop/r (4:1).

Dose needs to be super-boosted with additional ritonavir to create a 1:1 ratio of lopinavir to ritonavir or lop/r dose can be doubled.

- *Another NRTI:* not widely recommended as ↓ rates of virological suppression but is included in WHO 2013 guidelines.

In children >3yrs 2 NRTIs plus

- EFZ.
- Lop/r as above if on second line therapy.
- *Another NRTI:* not widely recommended as ↓ rates of virological suppression.

TB IRIS

An alternative explanation for clinical deterioration of TB, or rapid appearance of TB during ART, is TB IRIS. This syndrome is poorly characterized in children, but typically occurs within weeks of starting ART. A pronounced inflammatory component is characteristic, and history of previously good response to TB treatment. Wherever possible ART should be continued and IRIS treated symptomatically. Steroid therapy may be considered in children with severe and life-threatening forms of IRIS involving vital structures or the CNS (prednisolone 1–2mg/kg/d).

HIV prevention strategies

In the absence of a vaccine, prevention is the only method of controlling the AIDS pandemic. Strategies to control HIV infection should be aimed at sexual, parenteral, and mother to child transmission.

Sexual transmission

Changing high-risk sexual behaviour through health education could have a major effect on sexual HIV transmission. It would also → ↓ STI transmission. Creative educational approaches that respect cultural traditions are necessary to make the population aware of the dangers of HIV/AIDS and to encourage protective measures. These programmes have to be accompanied by approaches that influence the social determinants of risk, such as gender inequality, to enable those vulnerable to infection to protect themselves. Key interventions are the promotion of condom use and prevention and treatment of STIs.

Antiretroviral therapy

Suppression of HIV viral load in infected partner with ART in HIV discordant sexual couples dramatically ↓ risk of transmission. Earlier ART at a population level likely ↓ HIV incidence, the magnitude of this effect needs to be tested in prospective studies to assess policy implications. Post-exposure prophylaxis (PEP) should be prescribed to all victims of sexual assault and to anyone who has had an unprotected sexual encounter where there is a risk of HIV exposure (see below).

Clinical trials have also demonstrated the efficacy of pre-exposure prophylaxis with antiretroviral drugs given to people involved in high risk sexual practices (e.g. commercial sex workers) and the efficacy of tenofovir-based microbicide gel for HIV prevention in women living in a high HIV prevalence setting.

Male medical circumcision

Three clinical trials have demonstrated similar beneficial effects of male medical circumcision: reducing HIV acquisition by the circumcised male by ~60%. Circumcision must be accompanied by adequate counselling about using other preventive measures as the procedure is only partially protective against HIV infection.

Blood transfusion

Screening of blood donations for HIV antibody is highly effective at ↓ risk of blood transfusions. Drawbacks are cost, logistics, and the lack of detectable HIV antibodies in the window period (3–6wks after infection). Efforts to identify and exclude high-risk donors are difficult, but they can ↓ risk of infected persons donating blood in the window period.

Injections

Prevention of infection through contaminated needles is feasible with the use of universal precautions. Health workers should be trained to give as few injections as possible. Wherever possible disposable needles and syringes should be used. Where these are absolutely not available, adequate sterilization of all equipment is imperative.

The risk of transmission after a needlestick injury may be ↓ by PEP (see 📖 Post-exposure prophylaxis following needlestick injuries, p. 146). Injecting drug use transmission can be ↓ through programmes that promote harm reduction, clean needles and opiate maintenance.

Mother-to-child transmission

Most importantly, this involves the prevention of HIV infection in women of childbearing age and advice on contraception to HIV+ women to prevent unwanted pregnancies.

Prevention of mother to child transmission

The cumulative risk of MTCT is 30–40% in the absence of preventive interventions. All pregnant women should be tested for HIV as early as possible during pregnancy to enable preventive interventions to be offered if HIV+. HIV testing should ideally be repeated in 3rd trimester.
Interventions include:

- ART.
- Consideration of mode of delivery.
- Appropriate breast feeding advice.
- WHO recommends that where causes of infant deaths are infectious disease and malnutrition, pregnant women (including those known to be HIV+) should breastfeed for the first 6mths, introduce complementary feeds thereafter and continue breastfeeding for 12mths.
- Where this is not the case, HIV+ women are advised not to breastfeed, and to use a safe formula feeding alternative for their babies. However, if exclusive formula feeding cannot be guaranteed, then exclusive breastfeeding is advisable as it ↓ risk of MTCT compared with mixing breast and formula feeding.
- Risk of transmission to breastfed infants can be substantially ↓ if the mother is on virally suppressive ART (usually 3 ART drugs), while breastfeeding. Initiation criteria of ART for pregnant women for their own health are the same as non-pregnant women (see Table 3.8). However, WHO now also recommends 'Option B+' where ART is maintained after delivery and cessation of breastfeeding, regardless of WHO clinical stage or cell count.

HIV+ pregnant women in need of treatment for their own health should:

- Start ART irrespective of gestational age and continue it through pregnancy, delivery, breastfeeding, and thereafter.
- Maternal ART should be coupled with daily NVP or bd AZT to infants from birth until 4–6wks of age, irrespective of mode of feeding.

HIV+ pregnant women who do not need ART for their own health are recommended either:

Option B

For the mother

Triple ART using FDC of EFV/3TC/TDF starting from 14wks until end of pregnancy and breastfeeding regardless of whether the mother needs ART for her own health or whether she will only take ART as part of PMTCT during pregnancy, delivery, and breastfeeding. See note above that some programmes may continue ART, irrespective of WHO clinical stage or CD4 count, termed 'Option B+'.

For all infants regardless of breastfeeding

NVP or AZT for 4-6 wks.

The use of single-dose nevirapine at delivery alone is also used to ↓ transmission (to 8% at delivery, excluding breastfeeding risk), but is less effective in preventing MTCT than option A (risk of transmission ~2%) or B (risk of transmission ~1%). It also carries the risk of causing NNRTI resistance in the mother and infected infant, and compromising future ART options. Covering the nevirapine 'tail' with 7d of AZT/3TC to the mother will ↓ this risk.

Triple drug ART is the optimal form of MTCT prevention, and with increased availability of FDC this option has become possible even in resource limited settings. If there is a contraindication to FDC or it is not available then option A can be implemented.

Option A: no longer recommended in WHO 2013 guidelines.

For the mother

- AZT from 14wks pregnancy *plus*
- Single-dose nevirapine (sdNVP) during labour and delivery *plus*
- Consider AZT + 3TC bd for 7d post-partum.

If maternal AZT >4wks, omission of sdNVP and AZT + 3TC tail can be considered.

For breastfeeding infants

NVP from birth to 1wk after breastmilk exposure ends (min. 4–6wks).

For non-breastfeeding infants

NVP or single dose NVP + AZT for 4–6wks.

Elective caesarean section

↓ Risk of MTCT, particularly in women with high viral loads, but is not practical as a routine procedure in most resource-poor settings.

Antiretroviral drugs for treating pregnant women and preventing HIV infection in infants are given in detail at: http://www.who.int/hiv/pub/guidelines/arv2013/en/

Post-exposure prophylaxis following needlestick injuries

Prevention of injuries

Occupational exposures are almost entirely preventable. A culture of 'standard precautions' should be promoted continuously in all health care settings. All blood and body fluid samples should be handled as potentially infectious. Sharps containers should be immediately available whenever needles are used.

Health care workers (HCWs) are at risk of HIV infection if they sustain a needlestick injury with a needle that has been used in someone who is HIV+. The risk of infection is ~0.3% per needlestick event.

Injuries are regarded as high risk if:

- Needle was in a blood vessel.
- Injury was deep.
- There was visible blood on the needle or in an attached syringe.
- It was a hollow-bore needle.
- The source patient has a high viral load.

Splash injuries with HIV-infected blood onto non-intact skin (e.g. dermatitis or open wound) or mucous membranes, including conjunctivae, may also result in HIV infection (risk of transmission ~0.1%). Other fluids, such as CSF and serous effusions are also potentially infectious. Following a significant exposure, the risk of transmission can be substantially ↓ by taking PEP for 28d.

Other infections that can be potentially transmitted in such circumstances are HBV, HCV, and syphilis.

Action that should be taken following a needlestick or splash injury:

- *Local measures:* prolonged washing with soap.
- ART PEP should start as soon as possible (within 1h if possible). This should be taken before the source patient's status is known. If the patient is found to be HIV-uninfected, the PEP can be stopped. See Table 3.19 for recommended regimens.
- Obtain consent from the source patient for HIV testing if status is unknown. Also test for hepatitis B and C and syphilis (do the same tests for HCW—if the HCW is HIV+, then PEP should NOT be prescribed).
- Counsel the HCW.
- Psychological support is necessary.
- Document details of event and all investigations and management. This is critical for compensation of HCWs who seroconvert.
- If patient is HIV-seronegative, stop PEP unless it is suspected that the patient has an HIV seroconversion illness.
- If the patient is HIV+ or the status is unknown, continue PEP for 28d.
- In HCW on PEP regimens containing AZT, the Hb and neutrophil count should be checked at baseline and 2wks.
- The HCW should have an HIV ELISA test performed at 6wks, 3mths, and 6mths (PEP may delay seroconversion).

- The HCW should be advised to use condoms or abstain from sexual intercourse until seronegativity is documented.
- If the HCW is not HBV immunized and the source patient is HBV infected, then HBV immunoglobulin and vaccination should be administered. HCWs who have been immunized but have inadequate antibody titres (<10mLU/mL) may require booster vaccination.
- If source patient is on ART and suspected to have drug resistance, then standard PEP should be instituted as soon as possible, but modification in the regimen, based on likely resistance patterns, should be discussed with an expert.

Side-effects such as nausea are common with AZT and anti-emetics may be required. Drugs used for PEP are potentially toxic. Thus, PEP should not be administered if the risk of infection is negligible.

- Guidelines are similar for splash injuries to non-intact skin or mucous membranes, but generally 2 drugs are used unless there is a large volume of blood from a high-risk patient. No PEP is required for a blood or body fluid splash to intact skin.
- Every health institution must maintain at least a 'starter' supply of PEP, which is available to be provided rapidly (within 1h) even after hours.
- PEP should also be prescribed to victims of sexual assault and to those who had unprotected sex with a risk of HIV exposure.

Table 3.19 Recommended HIV PEP for percutaneous injuries

Exposure type[1]	**HIV-infected source**	**HIV-infected source—high risk[2]**	**Source of unknown HIV status[3]**	**HIV –ve**
Less severe	2 drugs	3 drugs	? PEP*	No PEP
More severe	3 drugs	3 drugs	? PEP*	No PEP

2 drugs = AZT + 3TC (or TDF + 3TC or TDF +FTC or d4T + 3TC) for 28d.

3 drugs = Above combination + lopinavir 200mg/ritonavir 50mg (Kaletra®) 2 tablets bd or an alternative PI.

[1] *Less severe*—solid needle, superficial injury; *more severe*—large-bore hollow needle, deep wound, visible blood on needle, needle in patient's vessel.

[2] *High-risk source patient*—patient with AIDS or acute seroconversion illness or who is known to have high viral load.

[3] *Unknown source*—e.g. needle from sharps container.

*In these settings, if source patient has risk factors for HIV infection or exposure to HIV-infected blood is likely, then 2 drug PEP should be considered. In areas with high HIV prevalence rates it is advisable to prescribe PEP in all needlestick injuries where HIV status of source is unknown.

Running an antiretroviral therapy clinic

The following are key components of a successful ART service:

- *Staffing:* medical, nursing, counselling, pharmacy, and clerical staff all form an important part of the service. Some clinical services are run by doctors, others by nurses with the doctor seeing complicated cases only. Enabling nurses to manage patients on ART will ↓ ART waiting times by enabling more patients to be seen.
- *Adequate counselling services:* often lay people who have been trained to be HIV and ART adherence counsellors play a very important part in the preparation of patients for ART. Coming from the patients' community, speaking their language, and having time specifically for counselling, they can ensure the patient has a thorough knowledge of HIV and its treatment, and address any concerns.
- *Team work:* all members of the clinical team are important. The decision whether a patient is ready to commence ART is best made collectively, with all members of the team contributing their insights as to the patient's medical and psychosocial readiness.
- *A reliable drug supply is essential:* the health service must not let patients down. The pharmacist should play a role in educating patients how to take their medication and what side-effects they might expect.
- *Data collection and management:* clerical staff play an important role in ensuring accurate data are collected and stored. Often those funding ART programmes will require outcome data, and audit of clinic practice is important for quality of care assurance.
- Psychological, social worker, and nutritional input are also important.

Palliative care

Pain

- Pain in late-stage HIV+ patients is often multi-factorial, and treatment plans should recognize this.
- Common problems include painful peripheral neuropathies, post-zoster pain, disseminated KS involving a limb, HIV cholangiopathy, oral and perineal aphthous ulceration, and bedsores.
- Start by attempting to address the cause, e.g. treating bacterial pneumonia can control the chest pain associated with it.
- More commonly, the cause cannot be remedied, and attention should be given to appropriate analgesia.
- Neuropathic pain may respond to amitriptyline 10–25mg nocte.
- Musculoskeletal pain may respond to ibuprofen 400mg tds.
- In patients with poorly characterized pain, or where side-effects may be an issue, start with paracetamol 1g qds (max in 24h).
- When control is inadequate with simple analgesics, codeine or tramadol can be added. Frequently, it is appropriate to move on to the use of oral morphine (📖 Fever without localizing features p. 732, for regimen). Give laxatives to prevent and treat opiate-induced constipation.

Chronic diarrhoea

Simple attention to nursing basics (gloves for attendants, disposable nappies for patients) may make a considerable impact. ART often relieves chronic diarrhoea. Consider use of antidiarrhoeals such as loperamide.

Dyspnoea

Patients with terminal pulmonary malignancy (e.g. KS) are often very dyspnoeic. Tapping a large effusion may cause some relief, as may supplementary O_2 via face mask or nasal prongs. Most severely ill patients with profound dyspnoea will, however, require careful sedation with morphine.

Family support

Family support for late-stage HIV+ individuals can be very helpful, but requires considerable counselling input. If breadwinners (e.g. a spouse) need to temporarily become care-givers, then short-term assistance with social grants can help. Time and effort spent on empowering and encouraging families can ↓ hospital admissions.

Palliative care

Pain

Chapter 4

Tuberculosis*

Invited author **Robert J. Wilkinson**

* This chapter is intended for use in conjunction with the relevant national TB programme manual.

Current global situation and trends

TB has been curable for >50yrs, yet the global burden of morbidity and mortality due to TB remains great, especially in sub-Saharan Africa. Nearly 9 million develop active TB and ~2 million people die of TB each year. ~95% of cases occur in low-income countries and 75% of patients are aged 15–50yrs. Both globally and within countries, there is a strong link between poverty and TB.

TB treatment regimens of 6–8mths are highly effective in curing patients and preventing transmission.

Several important developments have occurred:

- TB incidence ↑ dramatically in communities highly endemic for HIV, especially in Africa.
- ↑ Drug resistance → ↓ cure rates and complicates TB control.
- Expansion of directly observed therapy, short-course 'DOTS' TB control programmes in resource-poor regions, → stabilizing or ↓ incidence except in sub-Saharan Africa (Box 4.1).

Box 4.1 Elements of the WHO 'DOTS' (directly observed therapy, short course) TB control strategy

Sustained political commitment

- *Microscopy:* case detection using sputum smear microscopy among symptomatic patients presenting to the health services.
- *SCC/DOT:* standardized short-course chemotherapy (SCC) using regimens of 6–8mths at least for all confirmed smear+ cases. Good case management includes directly observed therapy (DOT) during the intensive phase for all new smear+ cases, during the continuation phase when rifampicin is used, and throughout a re-treatment regimen.
- *Drug supply:* establishment and maintenance of a system to supply all essential anti-TB drugs and to ensure no interruption in their availability.
- *Recording and reporting:* establishment and maintenance of a standardized recording and reporting system, allowing assessment of treatment results.

Lessons learned in TB treatment and control

- TB treatment and control is a core public health activity, since identifying and curing infectious patients is the principal means by which we can ↓ transmission and prevent new infections in the community.
- In stable political situations, the public sector has primary responsibility for ensuring the proper functioning of TB treatment and control, usually through the establishment of a National Tuberculosis Programme.
- TB treatment should be provided free of charge to patients.
- TB treatment and control must be integrated with the general health services of the community, since that is where TB cases present.

Public health note: TB and public health

Impact

Globally, *M. tuberculosis* is the 2nd commonest cause of death among all infectious agents (after HIV).

TB control

- Identification and cure of smear+ pulmonary cases.
- BCG in infants.
- ↓ Poverty; HIV prevention and treatment.
- Prevention of TB transmission in healthcare settings.

Key lessons of TB control

- Application of the DOTS principles.
- Treatment must be free to the patient.
- The public healthcare sector must play a strong role.

Threats and obstacles to TB control

- Failure of the programme to provide a sustainable diagnostic service, TB drugs, supervision of therapy, and outcome monitoring.
- Drug resistance.
- HIV and poverty.

Disease and pathogenesis

Microbiology

Mycobacteria are slender aerobic bacilli which are 'acid-fast' on ZN staining. Members of the genus *Mycobacterium* which are of particular interest in the tropics include *M. leprae* and *M. ulcerans*, the causes of leprosy, and Buruli ulcer (see 🕮 Ocular leprosy, p. 584 and 🕮 Ulcers, p. 592). The *M. tuberculosis* complex comprises *M. tuberculosis, M. africanum*, and *M. bovis*: *M. africanum*, seen mainly in Africa, behaves clinically and epidemiologically like *M. tuberculosis. M. bovis* is a pathogen of cattle and other species of domestic and wild animals, which can cause TB-like disease in humans.

M. tuberculosis multiplies slowly so that up to 6wks are required for growth in culture. Correspondingly, disease due to *M. tuberculosis* tends to progress relatively slowly, and responds slowly to treatment.

Transmission

Individuals with active pulmonary TB produce airborne droplet nuclei containing infectious *M. tuberculosis* in the course of speaking, sneezing, and particularly coughing. Infection occurs when these are inhaled by a susceptible person. Crowding, poor ventilation, and duration of exposure ↑ risk of transmission. *M. bovis* can also be transmitted by the airborne route, but human infection may occur through ingestion of unpasteurized milk from infected cows. Other sources of *M. tuberculosis* infection, except for handling TB cultures in the laboratory, are extremely rare.

TB infection

Aerosolized particles containing *M. tuberculosis* reach the alveoli where they initiate a non-specific response. The bacilli are ingested by phagocytic cells and transported to regional lymph nodes. They may either be contained there or spread via the lymphatics or bloodstream to other organs. With the development of specific cell-mediated immunity, cytokines secreted by lymphocytes recruit and activate macrophages, which organize into the granulomas characteristic of TB, effectively 'walling in' the bacteria.

In immunocompetent hosts, the most common outcome of infection with *M. tuberculosis* is containment of the infection without the development of clinical illness. A granuloma can sometimes be seen on CXR; more commonly, the lesion is not detectable radiographically and a +ve TST or Interferon gamma release assay (IGRA) is the only evidence of infection. *M. tuberculosis* has the ability to persist intra-cellularly in a quiescent state, within macrophages, retaining the ability to reactivate at a later time. This is referred to as 'latent tuberculous infection'.

Active TB disease

On average 10% of immunocompetent adults infected with *M. tuberculosis* ultimately develop active TB. About half of this risk is concentrated in the first 1–2yrs after infection, the other half is distributed over the remainder of the individual's lifetime. A number of factors greatly ↑ the risk of disease reactivation (see Box 4.2).

In a minority of cases, infants or those with depressed cell-mediated immunity being at particular risk, 1° infection is not contained and symptomatic disease develops directly from 1° infection (progressive 1° TB).

Post-1° TB occurs as a reactivation of latent infection, sometimes years after the 1° infection; sometimes, but not always, due to an identifiable immunosuppressive condition.

Patients, especially HIV+ individuals, can be re-infected with a new strain of *M. tuberculosis* after successful treatment of TB. The proportion of TB cases attributable to reinfection varies by location, proportion of cases HIV co-infected, and by incidence.

Box 4.2 Risk factors for development of active TB disease in individuals infected with *M. tuberculosis*

- HIV is the most powerful known factor.
- Recent infection—the risk per year of developing active TB is much greater in the first 1–2yrs after infection.
- Age: weakened immunity at the extremes of age.
- Malnutrition, including vitamin D deficiency.
- Diabetes mellitus.
- Silicosis or other types of lung fibrosis.
- Intercurrent infections (e.g. measles, visceral leishmaniasis).
- Toxic factors (e.g. alcohol and smoking).
- Poverty: probably many biological mechanisms involved.
- Immune suppression (e.g. corticosteroid therapy, malignancy).

Clinical features

The diagnostic resources available vary widely in different settings where TB is treated. This section mentions technologies such as TB culture and histology of biopsies, which may be required for the diagnosis of extra-pulmonary TB. However, most TB cases, especially those with the poorest prognosis and those most infectious to others, can be diagnosed with basic resources, particularly smear microscopy.

TB in adults

One or more non-specific systemic symptoms are present in the majority of patients: weight loss, anorexia, fever, night sweats, or malaise.

Pulmonary TB (PTB) is the most common presentation. It is also the most important epidemiologically since it is the form which is infectious to others. However, TB may affect any organ → a variety of clinical presentations.

Pulmonary TB

Involves the lung parenchyma. Many patients have a cough, which is often productive. A cough for >3wks should always raise the suspicion of TB. Haemoptysis, chest pain, or breathlessness are present in some patients.

Physical examination is often normal or the findings non-specific. Some patients may look ill and wasted with a fever and tachycardia, others can appear surprisingly well. Chest examination may reveal localized crackles or findings of a pleural effusion. Finger clubbing suggests a diagnosis other than TB, such as lung cancer, bronchiectasis, or empyema, but occasionally bronchiectasis may be 2° to lung damage from chronic or previous PTB.

~65% of PTB cases are sputum smear +ve. Smear +ve patients are most infectious (more likely to transmit TB than patients who are smear –ve, even if culture +ve) and also sickest (without treatment, their average mortality is considerably higher than that of smear –ve patients). HIV+ individuals with TB are less likely than HIV- individuals to be smear +ve because they are less likely to have cavities. A +ve smear for acid-fast bacilli in a high TB prevalence area strongly suggests TB since *M. tuberculosis* occurs much more frequently than non-tuberculous mycobacteria in these settings.

Smear –ve PTB is relatively common, but the diagnosis involves a degree of uncertainty unless confirmed by culture. Many of these patients will become smear +ve later if not treated. While under-diagnosis of smear –ve PTB is clearly undesirable, over-diagnosis also creates problems, by misusing the scarce resources of the TB programme, overlooking other treatable diagnoses, and undermining the programme's credibility in the community by ↓ success rate of treatment.

Complications of pulmonary TB

Acute complications include haemoptysis which is occasionally life-threatening, and pneumothorax. Chronic complications include post-TB bronchiectasis, extensive lung fibrosis, and aspergillomas (fungus balls) in residual cavities.

Pleural TB

An effusion can often be detected on examination and confirmed by X-ray and/or diagnostic aspiration. TB effusions are exudates (fluid protein >50% serum protein concentration) and contain ↑ lymphocytes, but seldom smear +ve. ~30–70% will be culture +ve. In TB endemic areas, in the absence of obvious alternative explanations such as heart failure, acute pneumonia, or malignancy, TB will be the most common cause of a 'straw-coloured' effusion. Some patients with pleural TB also have involvement of the pulmonary parenchyma. Hence, sputum smear and culture should be performed. Culture of pleural biopsy tissue may also be helpful and histology of a pleural biopsy usually shows granulomas.

TB lymphadenitis

Can involve any site, but cervical lymph nodes (LNs) are most common, especially low down on the right side of the neck (TB bacilli ascend from the paratracheal chain into the neck LNs). The LNs have typically been present for weeks or months, and are seldom acutely inflamed, distinguishing them from most lymphadenopathy due to acute viral or bacterial infections. LNs may initially feel rubbery and non-tender, becoming matted or fluctuant, and sometimes discharging spontaneously through the skin to produce chronic sinuses with scar formation. By the time a TB LN has enlarged to >3cm diameter, it should contain necrotic areas—when needled, a little pus should be obtained. Thus if a large LN is entirely solid, suspect another diagnosis. Paradoxically, TB LNs sometimes enlarge during anti-TB therapy. These characteristics, and the asymmetrical involvement, help to distinguish most cases of TB adenitis from the persistent generalized lymphadenopathy of HIV.

A needle aspiration can be smear +ve in HIV+ individuals, less frequently among HIV– individuals. If the smear is –ve, diagnosis can be confirmed by excision biopsy of a node, usually a minor procedure in adults, with histologic examination and/or culture.

Osteomyelitis

Most commonly affects the spine (Pott's disease). Any level can be involved, commonly 2 or more adjacent vertebrae are infected and in ~30% there is more than one level of spinal involvement. Vertebral collapse may ultimately produce a characteristic angular deformity. Paravertebral cold abscesses or psoas abscesses may accompany Pott's disease, but do not generally require surgical drainage. The presence of a characteristic angular kyphosis or 'gibbus' in a TB-endemic area is highly suggestive of spinal TB. In the absence of this striking clinical finding, X-ray changes with intervertebral disc and adjacent bone involvement +/– paravertebral soft tissue densities suggest an infectious aetiology, but cannot reliably distinguish between TB and other infections (e.g. brucellosis, staphylococcal). Where available, MRI scanning is extremely valuable in aiding diagnosis; CT scanning is 2nd choice; plain radiographs often of little help. If present, a cold abscess can be aspirated for ZN staining +/– culture; most abscesses will be smear–ve, but culture +ve. Imaging-guided biopsy of the infected disc or adjacent bone can provide a histologic or microbiologic diagnosis, but requires sophisticated resources. Spinal TB generally responds well to drug treatment. Some patients may present with rapidly progressive spinal cord or cauda equina compression and these patients may require urgent surgery to decompress the spinal cord and stabilize the spine. If surgery is not available, strict bed rest and steroids should be used until the neurological features improve after several weeks of treatment. Occasional patients with severe deformities (adults with >60° angulation or children with >30° angulation on X-ray) or chronic neurological compromise benefit from neurosurgery or orthopaedic surgery if available. With these exceptions, medical therapy alone will result in neurologic improvement or complete recovery in most patients. Spinal deformity will persist. TB of other joints such as hip and knee generally requires synovial biopsy to distinguish TB from other chronic infections.

Miliary TB

Is an aggressive form of haematogenously disseminated TB; more common in infants and the immune suppressed. Typically, there is a rather non-specific, but progressive history of fever (sometimes with rigors, which are rare in other forms of TB), malaise, and weight loss without other identifiable cause. Clinical suspicion is raised by a history of known or likely recent contact with infectious TB. Physical findings are commonly non-specific, but can include hepatomegaly, mild splenomegaly (which is not a feature of other forms of TB), tachypnoea, and wasting.

A CXR (or, preferably, CT scan) demonstrating diffuse, tiny, nodular opacities is the clue to miliary TB and warrants initiation of TB treatment if the clinical picture is compatible. Sputum smear examination and TST are often negative. If available, biopsy of liver, bone marrow, lymph nodes, or lung parenchyma often yield granulomas and/or acid-fast bacilli. Without prompt treatment, the patient with military TB will inevitably deteriorate and die, often when respiratory distress or TB meningitis occur. Steroids are often added for extremely ill patients with cachexia, tachycardia, and respiratory distress—initially prednisolone 1mg/kg/d, tapering over ~6wks as the clinical situation improves.

TB meningitis (TBM)

More common in children and the immune suppressed as the patient experiences a progressive febrile illness which may be accompanied by headache, irritability, vomiting, and ↓ consciousness, ultimately → coma. The pace of illness is characteristically slower than in acute bacterial meningitis. Neck stiffness is variable, especially early in the course. Cranial nerve palsies (particularly III, IV, VI, and VIII) are common, as these nerves run through inflammatory exudate at the base of the brain. Other focal neurological signs may develop, indicating vasculitis, tuberculomas, or hydrocephalus. Seizures can also occur. Diagnosis of TBM rests on CSF examination. Typically, the CSF white blood count is ↑ with a lymphocytic predominance, the protein is ↑ and glucose ↓, although all 3 abnormalities are not present in every case. CSF should also be examined to exclude cryptococcus in HIV+ individuals. CSF is rarely smear +ve for acid-fast bacilli; culture is +ve in ~80%, especially if a large volume of CSF is taken and concentrated by centrifugation.

A decision to start TB treatment must be made on the basis of clinical features, suggestive CSF abnormalities, and the absence of a likely alternative diagnosis, since delay in TBM treatment → poor outcome. In some mild cases where the diagnosis is unclear, the patient can be observed and the CSF examination repeated after a few days. The diagnosis is likely if the clinical illness and CSF abnormalities persist (vs. the rapid improvement anticipated with alternative diagnoses such as viral or bacterial infection). There is evidence for using adjunctive steroids in TBM: adults (>14yrs) should start treatment with oral or IV dexamethasone 0.4mg/kg/24h with a ↓ course over 6–8wks. Children should be given prednisolone 4mg/kg/24h (or dexamethasone: 0.6mg/kg/24h) for 4wks, followed by ↓ course over 4wks.

Intracranial tuberculomas (presenting as epilepsy or focal neurological deficit, and seen on brain scans) may accompany TBM, or may develop in isolation or as part of disseminated (miliary) TB. Tuberculomas may also develop or enlarge 'paradoxically' during treatment of these forms of TB, and require prolonged courses of steroids along with TB treatment.

Abdominal TB

The patient with abdominal TB characteristically experiences fever and night sweats with abdominal pain, ↓ weight, ↑ abdominal girth, diarrhoea or partial bowel obstruction. TB can affect any site in the GI tract, most commonly, the terminal ileum and peritoneum.

Diagnosis is usually made from specimens taken at surgery or endoscopy; the histology resembles that of Crohn's disease. Often peritoneal tuberculosis supervenes after some time, increasing abdominal distension being the first sign. Peritoneal TB may be suspected on the basis of ascites without another obvious cause such as liver disease. The ascitic fluid resembles TB pleural fluid (see above). The peritoneum appears covered in white nodules and fibrinous exudate at surgery or laparoscopy; culture and histology of a peritoneal biopsy, preferably taken at laparoscopy, are diagnostic. Ultrasound or CT scans may show thickened terminal ileum, mesenteric lymph nodes, thickened contrast-enhancing peritoneum, and ascites.

Pericardial TB

This is often first suspected on the basis of globular enlargement of the cardiac silhouette on CXR in patients investigated for systemic and cardiorespiratory symptoms. It is more common in HIV+ individuals. Clinical features of tamponade (↑ jugular venous pressure, pulsus paradoxus, hypotension, muffled heart sounds, +/−oedema, hepatomegaly) may be present and a pericardial rub is occasionally audible. Ultrasound readily confirms an effusion. Some cases of pericardial TB are purely effusive; others have features of pericardial constriction. Therapeutic pericardial aspiration for tamponade requires ultrasound or at least ECG control; pericardial fluid is similar to pleural fluid in TB (see above), although often bloodstained. In practice, the diagnosis is often made by a pericardial effusion in the absence of other likely causes. The risk of tamponade and later constriction ↓ by adding corticosteroids—the recommended adult dose is prednisolone 60mg/d tapered during the first 6–12wks of TB treatment.

Genitourinary TB

Can involve any part of the male or female genitourinary tract. Renal TB may present with dysuria, haematuria, and pain or a mass in the flank. The urinalysis typically shows pus cells, but routine culture is –ve ('sterile pyuria'). Diagnosis usually requires TB culture of urine. TB of the uterus or adnexae presents as infertility, pelvic pain or mass, or bleeding. Epididymal swelling is the most common presentation of genital TB in males. Biopsy is usually required to distinguish TB from other possible causes; though imaging (CT scan) may be suggestive of TB.

TB in children

Infants and young children are more likely than adults to progress to disease following *M. tuberculosis* exposure. Infants who develop TB have a high fatality rate without prompt treatment. By contrast, children aged 7–12yrs have the lowest risk, of any age group, of developing active TB.

Even where culture, X-ray, and other facilities are available, diagnosis of childhood TB is often very difficult. TB may be suspected clinically in the presence of persistent fever, malaise, and cough. A history of close contact with a smear +ve pulmonary TB patient makes TB more likely. A +ve TST (or +ve interferon gamma release assay, IGRA) indicates infection at some time by *M. tuberculosis* and, hence, is supportive, but not diagnostic of TB in a child with an unexplained illness. Children are less likely to develop pulmonary cavities and may be unable to expectorate sputum, and for these reasons children with PTB are often sputum smear –ve. A CXR may show enlarged intra thoracic lymph nodes +/– lung consolidation. Culture of specimens obtained by gastric lavage, sputum induction, or nasopharyngeal aspirate can ↑ the rate of confirmed diagnosis. Several scoring systems have been developed to rationalize the diagnosis of childhood TB; none has been validated and they often disagree, but they can guide the puzzled clinician. An example is given in Box 4.3.

Box 4.3 Example of a scheme to aid diagnosis of TB in children*

1. Score chart for child with suspected TB

Score	0	1	3
Length of illness	<2wks	2–4wks	>4wks
Weight for age	>80%	60–80%	<60%
Family TB (past or present)	None	Reported by family	Known sputum +ve

2. Score for other features if present

Feature	Score
Positive TST	3
Large painless lymph nodes—firm, soft, and/or sinus in neck, axilla, and groin	3
Unexplained fever, night sweats, no response to malaria treatment	2
Malnutrition, not improving after 4wks	3

3. If the TOTAL score is 7 or more—treat for TB

Treat children with a score less than 7 if:

- CXR is characteristic of TB infection.
- The child does not respond to two 7d courses of two different antibiotics.

* Dr Keith Edwards, University of Papua New Guinea, published in Crofton J, *et al.* (1997) *Clinical tuberculosis*, Oxford: MacMillan.

Diagnosis

Sputum smears

Access to reliable, quality controlled sputum smear microscopy is a prerequisite for a TB treatment programme. At least 2 sputum samples should be examined microscopically in any patient who has been coughing for 2–3wks. When patients must travel some distance to the clinic, the 'spot-morning-spot' protocol can be used: the 1st specimen is collected and submitted at presentation, the 2nd is an early-morning sputum produced at home the next morning and submitted at a clinic visit that day, and the 3rd is produced and submitted during that clinic visit (see Box 4.4).

Nucleic acid amplification tests

Until recently, molecular diagnostics were only useful in a research setting. The GeneXpert multi-drug resistant (MDR)/rifampicin (RIF) test is a fully automated nucleic acid amplification test (NAAT), which is a practical alternative to microscopy and culture; other systems are likely to follow. WHO has called for the GeneXpert MDR/RIF test to be rolled out under clearly defined conditions and as part of national plans for TB and MDR-TB care and control. It has been adopted as a 1st-line test to diagnose active TB throughout South Africa, and is becoming rapidly adopted elsewhere. This self-contained system automates sample processing on sputum, providing a result in <2h. The test also detects the presence of rifampicin resistance, which generally indicates MDR-TB. The GeneXpert does not require a sophisticated laboratory set-up or a highly trained laboratory technician—nurses or other staff can be trained to perform the test. In addition to the equipment cost, the reagent cost is ~$16 per test. The test is positive on a single sputum sample in all smear +ve and ~75% smear –ve cases; a second test increases sensitivity by ~10%, a third test, by another ~5%. The sensitivity in extra-pulmonary samples is lower than in sputum.

Chest X-ray

CXR is not necessary for the diagnosis of TB. It is most useful in patients with undiagnosed chest symptoms who are repeatedly smear –ve and in identifying other findings such as pleural effusions or nodules. A normal CXR does not exclude TB especially in HIV+ individuals. The interpretation of a CXR varies with the skill of the reader and even between skilled readers. However, a CXR cannot distinguish reliably between TB and other diseases or between changes of active and past, inactive TB. The presence of cavities usually predicts a smear +ve patient who is infectious, but sputum smear is the most reliable predictor of infectiousness.

Box 4.4 Diagnosis of sputum smear-negative TB

Reassessment and repeat sputum examinations after 2–3wks, following a therapeutic trial of a broad-spectrum antibiotic, may clarify the diagnosis. CXR, interpreted with caution, may help to estimate the likelihood of TB in suspects who remain smear –ve. Culture and sputum induction can ↑ sensitivity of diagnosis. Before diagnosing smear –ve PTB, consider alternative diagnoses such as:

- Pneumonia.
- Asthma.
- Chronic bronchitis.
- Non-TB respiratory complications of HIV.
- Bronchiectasis.
- Lung abscess.
- Lung cancer.

NAATs (currently GeneXpert, with others to follow) can provide a positive diagnosis in around 75% of smear –ve, culture +ve pulmonary TB cases.

In some TB programmes, a decision to start treatment for smear –ve PTB can only be made by a doctor or individual with particular expertise in TB.

Tuberculin skin testing

This is a test immune sensitization by *Mycobacterium tuberculosis* (MTB); it is insufficient to diagnose active TB. It relies on the fact that cell-mediated hypersensitivity develops after infection with MTB. Following intradermal injection of tuberculin (purified protein derivative), the transverse diameter of skin induration (swelling, not redness) is measured at 48–72h. Training and experience in interpreting skin test responses is critical to achieving accurate results. In most situations, 10mm of induration to a standard tuberculin dose is the cut-off between negative and positive; 5mm is considered positive in HIV+ individuals. Both false –ve and false +ve TST results are relatively common (see Box 4.5). The larger the area of induration, the less likely it is to be a false +ve. IGRA using blood samples are more specific than the TST, but are costly and their prognostic significance is still being determined.

Uses of the TST

- *Epidemiologic:* determining prevalence or incidence of *M. tuberculosis* infection in a population or specific group, e.g. healthcare workers.
- *Diagnostic:* to aid in assessing the likelihood of TB as the cause of a clinical illness. In high-prevalence countries, it is used mainly in children because the 'background' prevalence of TST positivity in the general population ↑ with age.
- Identification of candidates for treatment of latent TB infection (e.g. paediatric contacts of pulmonary TB patients, HIV+ individuals).

Box 4.5 False TST results

A false positive TST can be caused by

- *BCG:* TST response following BCG is variable; BCG in infancy is unlikely to account for a strongly +ve TST (>15mm induration) in adulthood.
- Exposure to environmental mycobacteria.
- Incorrect interpretation.

A false negative TST can be caused by

- Normal variation.
- Long interval since infection.
- Reduced cell-mediated immune response (HIV, old age, corticosteroid therapy, measles, malnutrition).
- Severe illness, including overwhelming TB.
- Incorrect TST technique or interpretation.

Tuberculosis treatment

Aims of treatment

- To cure the patient and prevent disability.
- To prevent transmission.
- To prevent development of resistant TB.

Principles of anti-TB therapy

- Treatment must always include a minimum of 2 drugs to which the organism is sensitive.
- *The correct duration:* generally 6–8mths for drug-sensitive TB.
- *Assured adherence:* the TB programme must ensure that each patient completes the full course of therapy.

Treatment supervision

DOT was initially intended to mean observed swallowing of each dose by a healthcare worker. Because this is not always feasible, a range of alternatives have been tried, some successfully. Treatment supervisors can include teachers, employers, community-chosen volunteers, ex-TB patients, and family members. If these strategies for treatment supervision are used, there must be adequate provision for selection, training, and regular monitoring of the treatment supervisor, a reliable mechanism for delivery of drugs, proper record keeping, and rigorous monitoring of treatment outcomes.

Drug dosage and standard regimens (see Table 4.1)

Standard TB treatment and duration appears to be effective regardless of disease site, although some recommend prolonging the consolidation phase for TB meningitis and bone disease (up to 12mths total). Preferably, TB drugs should be provided in the form of fixed-dose combination (FDC) tablets which make monotherapy impossible and provide an extra defence against the development of drug resistance.

Most national TB programmes have a standard regimen and a re-treatment regimen—the latter for patients who have defaulted, failed treatment, or relapsed after initially successful treatment.

Table 4.1 Drug dosage and standard regimen

	Recommended dose (mg/kg)	
Anti-TB drug	**Once daily regimen**	**3×/wk regimen**
Isoniazid (H)	5	10
Rifampicin (R)	10	10
Pyrazinamide (Z)	25	35
Streptomycin (S)	15	15
Ethambutol (E)	15	30

Anti-TB drugs

- Isoniazid *(INH; 'H')*: potent anti-TB activity. Main serious adverse effect is liver toxicity; can cause peripheral neuropathy.
- Rifampicin *(rifampin in North America; 'R')*: essential to the success of short course (<12mths) TB therapy. Important interactions with warfarin, anticonvulsants, oral contraceptives, opiates incl. methadone, nevirapine, efavirenz, and protease inhibitors.
- Pyrazinamide *('Z')*: 'sterilizing' activity allows treatment courses of 6mths. Contribution to 1st-line regimens limited largely to the first 2mths of therapy. May cause hyperuricaemia and arthralgias; most hepatotoxic 1st-line TB drug.
- Ethambutol *('E')*: weak anti-TB agent; main role is prevention of resistance to other drugs. Main serious adverse effect is ocular toxicity, which is uncommon at recommended doses.
- Streptomycin *('S')*: now limited to 2nd-line or re-treatment regimens because of the desire to avoid unnecessary injections in the HIV era. Ototoxicity (vertigo>hearing loss) and renal toxicity are the main adverse effects. The drug should be avoided or dosage adjusted carefully in renal dysfunction. Contraindicated in pregnancy.

Special groups

- Isoniazid causes peripheral neuropathy more commonly in diabetic, malnourished, alcoholic, and pregnant patients, and in those with pre-existing neuropathy including HIV+ individuals. Give pyridoxine 10–15mg/d to protect against peripheral neuropathy.
- *Women on oral or injectable (hormonal) contraceptives:* must use another form of contraception (e.g. an intra-uterine contraceptive device (IUD)) during rifampicin therapy and for 4–8wks after stopping rifampicin.
- *Pregnancy:* TB drugs, except for streptomycin, may be used in pregnancy. Any theoretical risks to the fetus are much less than the risks from untreated TB.

1st-line regimen (WHO) 2HRZE 4HR or 2HRZE 4H_3R_3

- Isoniazid, rifampicin, pyrazinamide, and ethambutol od for 2mths.
- Followed by a 'continuation phase' of isoniazid and rifampicin either od (4HR) or 3×/wk (4H_3R_3) for 4mths.

'Re-treatment regimen' (defaulters, treatment failure, relapse) 2HRZES 1HRZE 5$H_3R_3E_3$

- Isoniazid, rifampicin, pyrazinamide, ethambutol, and streptomycin od for 2mths.
- Followed by isoniazid, rifampicin, pyrazinamide, ethambutol od for 1mth.
- Then isoniazid, rifampicin, ethambutol 3×/wk for 5mths.

It is increasingly recognized that this regimen is suboptimal in patients who have failed fully supervised 1st-line therapy, but at the moment, no satisfactory alternative exists for low-income settings. If possible, culture and drug sensitivity testing should be obtained in these patients and treatment guided by the results.

Monitoring treatment

Smear +ve patients should be monitored by sputum smear examination after 2mths of treatment and at least one other time prior to treatment completion. All other patients should be monitored clinically.

Education

Regarding adverse drug reactions is essential. Of particular importance, every patient should be advised to present to a clinic or hospital immediately if jaundice is noted. The symptoms of hepatitis should be emphasized: nausea, vomiting, anorexia, dark urine before the daily dose of rifampicin.

Treatment adherence

Good adherence is the most important determinant of successful treatment. As patients feel better ~2mths after starting treatment, their motivation to continue therapy wanes. It is a responsibility of the treating healthcare worker to ensure that patients complete TB therapy. The patient and community must be well informed of the risks of drug resistance. The relationship between the patient and clinic staff is a major factor promoting adherence. Practical measures, e.g. clinic hours convenient for working patients are very important. Individualized approaches to the patients at risk of defaulting include help with transportation, nutritional support, addiction treatment, home visits, etc. Early identification and tracing of defaulters is essential. See Box 4.6.

Box 4.6 A 'therapeutic trial' of treatment

A therapeutic trial is used in many settings to diagnose TB. This strategy has not been validated, is not recommended by WHO, and risks creating confusion in a TB programme. If a 'therapeutic trial' is to be used:

- All efforts to make a diagnosis should have been exhausted. WHO has provided guidelines for this purpose.*
- An objective indicator of success (e.g. fever) and the planned trial duration (fever resolves within 14d of starting treatment in most cases) should be established before starting the trial.
- Preferably, the drugs used for the trial should have anti-mycobacterial activity (isoniazid, ethambutol, and pyrazinamide), but not be effective against other infections (rifampicin and streptomycin).
- The trial patient should be clearly distinguished from other patients in the TB programme records.

* WHO. Improving the diagnosis and treatment of smear-negative pulmonary and extra-pulmonary tuberculosis among adults and adolescents. Recommendations for HIV-prevalent and resource-constrained settings. Geneva, WHO 2006.

TB and HIV

TB incidence has ↑ up to 6-fold in communities severely affected by the HIV pandemic. 80% of TB patients in some settings are HIV +ve. Among HIV+ individuals, TB is the most common cause of death. The mechanism underlying the powerful interaction between these two diseases is the suppression, by HIV, of the cell-mediated immune response to TB (CD4+ helper T-cells and macrophages).

Preventive therapy of latent TB infection

Preventive therapy with isoniazid for 6–9mths ↓ by 60% the risk of developing active TB among HIV+ individuals who are TST+. This benefit ↓ over time, especially if the patient lives in a community where the risk of TB re-infection is high. It is difficult to implement this intervention on a large scale in poor countries. Anti retrovirals are very effective in ↓ the risk of TB in HIV+ individuals by ↑ immune function.

HIV testing of TB patients All TB patients should be encouraged to undergo HIV testing. TB programmes should offer HIV testing and coordinate follow-up and support with the HIV programme.

TB testing of HIV patients All HIV+ individuals should be screened at programme entry for systemic or pulmonary symptoms of active TB and monitored subsequently. If a program for treatment of latent TB is available, then all HIV+ individuals should be offered tuberculin skin testing.

Management of TB in HIV+ individuals

Many patients presenting with HIV-related TB do not know their HIV status. Some will have clinical features of HIV infection such as oral candidiasis, chronic diarrhoea, skin and hair changes, peripheral neuropathy, herpes zoster scars. However, since TB can occur early during the course of HIV disease, these clinical features of HIV are often absent.

Extra-pulmonary TB is common in HIV+ individuals, particularly lymphadenopathy, pleural and pericardial effusions, miliary TB, and meningitis. However, PTB, which may co-exist with other sites of disease, remains the most common form of disease. The radiographic appearance of PTB in HIV+ individuals is often atypical, depending on the degree of immune suppression. HIV+ individuals less commonly have upper lobe disease and cavities and, more commonly, have intrathoracic adenopathy, effusions, and miliary shadowing.

Diagnosis

Sputum smear microscopy remains the primary investigation, but is less sensitive in HIV+ individuals. If the smear is –ve, the differential diagnosis of lung disease in HIV+ individual includes:

- *Bacterial* (most often pneumococcal) pneumonia: a short history and a response to antibiotic therapy are suggestive.
- *Pneumocystis jiroveci* pneumonia (PJP, also called PCP): characteristic features include severe dyspnoea and hypoxia, diffuse changes on X-ray, absence of effusions, and response to high-dose co-trimoxazole.
- *Pulmonary KS*: most patients have cutaneous or oral lesions.

Treatment regimens

TB drug treatment regimens are the same in HIV+ and HIV- individuals although some studies suggest a benefit of prolonging therapy in HIV+ individuals. Cure rates are similar provided rifampicin-containing regimens are used. Recurrence rates are higher in HIV+ individuals, partly due to ↑ rate of reinfection. Mortality during and after treatment is ↑↑ among HIV+ individuals, mainly due to HIV-related causes other than TB, in the absence of ART.

The widespread provision of ART in resource-poor countries has greatly expanded. Treatment with ART and TB drugs at the same time creates the potential for a variety of complex and challenging problems:

- Adverse effects which could be due to either TB drugs or ART and which could → treatment interruption.
- Complex, clinically important drug interactions, particularly involving rifampicin and protease inhibitors.
- Immune reconstitution reactions (📖 Immune reconstitution inflammatory syndrome, p. 128).

Knowledge in this area is evolving rapidly. Participation of someone with current knowledge and expertise in HIV/TB management highly desirable.

IRIS most likely to occur in a patient with a very low initial CD4 cell count or clinical evidence of profound immune suppression. May occur days to 3mths (median 14d) after starting ART. IRIS involves an inflammatory reaction to a pre-existing opportunistic organism (especially *M. tuberculosis*) as cell-mediated immunity ↑ in response to ART. Reaction is usually characterized by fever and localized appearance or worsening of opportunistic disease process, e.g. enlarging lymph nodes or worsening pulmonary infiltrate. Treatment failure, drug resistance in the case of TB, or a 2nd complicating infectious process must be excluded as far as possible, before arriving at a diagnosis of IRIS.[1] Prednisolone 1.5mg/day for 2–4wks, sometimes longer, is effective in ↓ duration of symptoms. ART should be continued during IRIS.

Patients taking ART prior to diagnosis of TB should continue when TB treatment is started, but may require modifications in the ART regimen to ensure compatibility with rifampicin (R). In patients not taking ART at the time of TB diagnosis, starting TB treatment is the first priority. ART should be provided to TB patients with CD4 counts <350cells/mm^3 or with clinical features of advanced HIV disease. Try to initiate ART ~2wks after TB treatment has been established, provided the patient is tolerating anti-TB medications.

Regimen consisting of efavirenz + 2 nucleosides analogues (e.g. zidovudine/lamivudine or emtricitabine/tenofovir), if otherwise appropriate, is currently best established regimen for patients receiving simultaneous ART and TB therapy. Alternatives are limited: nevirapine levels are ↓ by

1 TB and HIV drug interactions website: http://www.cdc.gov/tb/publications/guidelines/TB_HIV_Drugs/PDF/tbhiv.pdf

R and thus viral suppression may be ↓. An established strategy for using a PI is to replace R with rifabutin, a costly drug not widely available. Most patients are prescribed PI with low dose ritonavir (100mg or 200mg oral daily) to take advantage of ritonavir's CYP3A4 enzyme-inhibiting properties. Ritonavir boosts the concentration of the other PI allowing easier dosing. The use of 3 or 4 nucleoside antiretroviral regimens largely eliminates concerns about drug interactions, but these regimens appear less efficacious than standard antiretroviral combinations.

HIV+ TB (Box 4.7) patients may also need prophylaxis with co-trimoxazole. HIV+ individuals with MDR TB have a very high mortality rate without ART; there is very little published information to guide the concomitant use of ARVs and MDR treatment.

Box 4.7 HIV and TB

In HIV+ individuals, by comparison with HIV–individuals:

- ↑↑ incidence of TB .
- The clinical and radiographic presentation may be different.
- TB treatment is the same and cure rates are similar.
- ↑ Recurrence and ↑ mortality.
- Concomitant ART may complicate TB treatment, but should be started < 2wks if possible.

Paediatric note: paediatric TB

- Probably under-recognized.
- High case fatality, particularly in infants.
- Diagnosis commonly difficult and uncertain.
- *Diagnostic clues:* clinical.
- History of close contact with smear +ve TB.
- Unexplained fever, unresponsive to other therapy.
- Unexplained, unresponsive weight loss.
- Persistent lymphadenopathy.
- *Diagnostic clues:* laboratory and imaging.
- +ve TST.
- Intrathoracic adenopathy +/– infiltrate on CXR.
- Smear (culture more sensitive) of gastric aspirate or induced sputum or lymph node sample.

Multi-drug resistant and extensively drug resistant TB

Development of acquired drug resistance in a TB patient requires 2 steps:

- A random mutation in the TB bacillus conferring resistance to that drug, followed by
- Selection 'pressure' from the use of that drug.

The resistant organisms will then replicate more rapidly than drug-sensitive organisms, unless suppressed by the use of one or more other effective TB drugs. Once an organism has acquired resistance, the resistant strain can be transmitted to another individual who will then have transmitted drug resistance, even if they have never taken TB drugs. The original cause of drug resistance is inadequate treatment; it is a responsibility of the TB programme to prevent this from occurring. TB drug resistance is preventable by a TB programme which assures adequate adherence to effective therapy.

The definition of MDR TB is resistance to isoniazid and rifampicin +/– other drugs. ~5% of TB patients worldwide have MDR disease, highest in settings where TB programmes have been weak. Recently, some programmes have implemented treatment of MDR TB. Treatment of MDR TB is much longer (>18mths), much more toxic, much more costly, and considerably less effective than treatment of drug-sensitive TB, averaging ~60% cure rates in low income settings. Thus, the most important response to the MDR TB problem is to strengthen prevention of acquired resistance and of healthcare associated transmission. MDR treatment should only be introduced in settings where a DOTS programme is established and demonstrating good outcomes. MDR TB treatment ('DOTS Plus') requires supervision of treatment for 18+mths, specialized medical expertise, a well-structured programme and guidelines, appropriate laboratory and culture resources, and an assured supply of 3rd line drugs. Expert advice and drugs at ↓ cost can be obtained through the WHO 'Green Light Committee' by programmes which meet its standards. Typical regimes for the treatment of MDR TB include an injectable (e.g. amikacin), a fluoroquinolone (e.g. moxifloxacin) plus other 2nd and 1st line drugs as determined by local policy. The treatment of extensively drug resistant (XDR)-TB requires the addition of drugs such as prothionamide, capreomycin, cycloserine, and linezolid. The therapeutic margin of these drugs is narrow and expert advice is recommended (Box 4.8).

Box 4.8 Extensively drug resistant (XDR) tuberculosis

A large outbreak of XDR TB amongst HIV+ individuals occurred in South Africa that brought this problem dramatically to attention. XDR is defined as resistance to at least rifampicin and isoniazid plus resistance to any quinolone plus resistance to at least one injectable 2nd line agent (capreomycin, amikacin, kanamycin). For some years, such strains have been known to exist in Asia, the Americas, and Europe. Of 17 000 TB isolates collected from around the world between 2000–2004, 2% of MDR strains were also XDR, being most frequently found in eastern Europe, western Asia, and South Korea. Population-based data from the USA, Latvia, and South Korea revealed that 4%, 19%, and 15% of MDR strains, respectively, were XDR. A substantial proportion of MDR and XDR TB represent transmitted resistance both in community and healthcare settings.

TB control programmes

TB control programmes require a structure, usually extending up to the national level, that coordinates programme regimens and protocols, training, drug supply, laboratory quality assurance, and monitoring of programme outcomes.

Smear +ve PTB patients are the main source of TB transmission. Detecting and curing infectious cases is the most effective means to ↓ new infections.

The 1st priority of a TB programme is to achieve a high rate of treatment success, since treating cases badly can → drug resistance. Once a TB programme is achieving good treatment outcomes (>85% treatment success), the next priority is to ↑ case finding. This activity must be integrated with the 1° healthcare service since it depends upon recognition and appropriate investigation (mainly sputum smear examination) of symptomatic TB suspects presenting to 1° healthcare workers.

Bacille Calmette–Guérin (BCG) is a live attenuated vaccine derived from *M. bovis*. Protective efficacy ranges from 0 to 80% for reasons which remain controversial. BCG provides some protection against miliary TB and TB meningitis in children, and should be given at birth to all children in high TB prevalence countries (except HIV+ children, see 🕮 Immunization of HIV-infected persons, p. 902). BCG appears to have little or no impact on the overall incidence or transmission of TB in a community.

Household and close contacts of TB cases

Symptomatic contacts of smear +ve PTB cases should be sought out and investigated for active TB. This is a particularly efficient form of case finding. Treatment of latent TB infection should be given to household contacts aged <5yrs of smear +ve PTB patients, after an assessment to rule out active TB.

In high HIV-prevalence countries, both HIV prevention and ART are likely to ↓ TB incidence. Ultimately, poverty reduction with improved housing and nutrition may be the most definitive TB control measures.

Chapter 5

Chest medicine

Invited author **Stephen Gordon**

Symptoms of respiratory disease

Cough

Acute cough without serious systemic symptoms usually requires no investigation or treatment. Persistent cough (>2–3wks) associated with phlegm, fever, dyspnoea, or chest pain warrants further investigation. Nocturnal coughing is a feature of asthma (spirometry helpful), LVF, tropical pulmonary eosinophilia (TPE), and gastro-oesophageal reflux disease (GORD). Most causes of cough can be diagnosed by a careful history, physical examination, a blood count, and a CXR.

Common causes of cough

Acute

- Viral ARIs.
- Pneumonia.
- Inhaled foreign body (especially in children).
- Acute sinusitis.

Chronic

- Asthma (can be without wheezing).
- TB, including mediastinal lymph node.
- Gastro-oesophageal reflux disease (GORD)—usually non-productive.
- Chronic bronchitis including chronic obstructive pulmonary disease (COPD).
- Bronchiectasis.
- Chronic sinusitis, with a post nasal drip.
- Drugs—(ACE inhibitors and beta blockers).

Uncommon causes of cough

- Larva migrans (Ascaris, Strongyloides).
- TPE.
- Pleural effusion.

Haemoptysis

Severe haemoptysis is an emergency—maintain a clear airway, as patients die of asphyxiation (clot in trachea) or aspiration rather than exsanguination. Careful history needed to differentiate haemoptysis from haematemesis, oropharyngeal bleeding or posterior epistaxis; sometimes needs to be witnessed. Patients should be placed under close observation and investigated. Patients with haemoptysis will continue to expectorate blood for 24h after the acute event.

Common causes of haemoptysis

- *Infections:* TB, acute LRTI, acute bronchitis.
- *Neoplastic:* carcinoma of bronchus.
- *Cardiovascular:* mitral stenosis, pulmonary embolism (PE) (with infarction).
- *Pulmonary disease:* bronchiectasis.

Other causes of haemoptysis

- *Infections:* lung abscess, parasitic disease (e.g. paragonimiasis), fungal disease (e.g. aspergillosis), pleuro-pulmonary amoebiasis.
- *Trauma:* lung contusions, foreign body aspiration, post endotracheal intubation or following aggressive endotracheal suctioning.
- *Diffuse pulmonary parenchymal disease:* Goodpasture's syndrome, Wegener's granulomatosis, systemic vasculitides.
- *Cardiovascular:* pulmonary oedema , pulmonary hypertension, aortic aneurysm.
- *Bleeding tendency:* sepsis, DIC, snake bite, haemorrhagic fevers.

Dyspnoea/breathlessness

Breathlessness can be due to respiratory, cardiac, or haematological causes (or combinations). Look for anaemia, wheezing (may have both pulmonary and cardiac causes), signs of LVF and note the pattern of breathing. Acidosis → sighing breathing (Kussmaul) and the breath may smell (ketones). In most instances, clinical examination, CXR, ECG, and blood count will guide appropriate treatment. In patients with COPD, type 2 respiratory failure may → CO_2 retention—do blood gas measurements for optimal management (📖 COPD, pp. 220–1).

Diagnosis

- ***Pulmonary***: often associated with wheezing or chest pain. Consider pneumothorax, pulmonary embolism, pneumonia and pleural effusions, as well as asthma, COPD, interstitial lung disease, pulmonary fibrosis, and pulmonary hypertension.
- ***Cardiac***: often with paroxysmal nocturnal dyspnoea, orthopnoea or ankle oedema—inability to lie flat is a crucial observation. Examination for ↑ JVP and swelling of ankles is important. Cor pulmonale is common, along with LVF due to valvular or ischaemic heart disease or myocardial disease due to myocarditis or cardiomyopathy.
- ***Diseases of the chest wall (rare)***: severe kyphoscoliosis, GBS, neurotoxic snake envenoming, myasthenia gravis, ankylosing spondylitis.
- ***Anaemia:*** if acute, or chronic and severe.

Wheeze

Wheezes are (generally expiratory) musical sounds coming from the lower airways. Wheezes may vary in pitch and intensity and can be heard at the mouth in some patients. Localized wheeze may be due to partial endobronchial obstruction.

Causes of wheeze

- Lower airways obstruction, especially asthma and COPD.
- Infection, especially *Mycoplasma pneumoniae* and rarely, parasitic disease—Katayama fever in schistosomiasis, ruptured hydatid cyst.
- LVF → peribronchial oedema → bronchospasm.
- Inhalation of toxic chemicals or smoke.
- Endobronchial obstruction from a tumour or foreign body (localized wheeze).

Multiple causes of a wheeze may exist in a single patient.

In children consider causes above, but also:

- Bronchiolitis (usually <2yrs, commonest <1yr).
- Viral induced wheeze (related to concurrent URTI).

Stridor

Stridor is less common, especially in adults. It is a harsh sound heard in inspiration, due to obstruction of the trachea or larynx. If severe, it is also heard in expiration.

Stridor is more common in children, due to the susceptibility of the upper airways to obstruction from inflammation.

Acute

- Foreign body.
- Infections: viral croup (📖 Acute laryngotracheobronchitis: croup p. 194), bacterial tracheitis (📖 Bacterial tracheitis, p. 196), diphtheria (📖 Diphtheria, p. 198), epiglottitis (📖 p. 192), and retropharyngeal abscess.

Chronic

- Tumour.
- Retrosternal goitre.
- Laryngomalacia (in infancy: usually resolves with time).

Pneumonia

Pneumonia kills ~2 million children/yr in resource-poor regions. It affects adults especially the elderly and HIV+ individuals. Most serious cases are bacterial, although it can occur as part of a severe systemic viral infection (especially measles or influenza).

Epidemiology

The incidence, aetiology, and clinical severity of pneumonia depends on the patient's age (see Table 5.1), and presence of other co-morbidity. *Streptococcus pneumoniae* (pneumococcus) is the most common cause of bacterial pneumonia at all ages, hence the worldwide drive for pneumococcal vaccination (📖 p. 906). It causes 25–50% of ARIs in children admitted to hospital and >1 million deaths/yr in children. It is commonest in crowded communities with poor living conditions.

In order to determine the likely cause of pneumonia and severity (see Table 5.2), consider age, immunization status and:

Was infection acquired in the community or hospital?

- In a previously healthy person with community-acquired pneumonia (CAP):
  - *S. pneumoniae* is most likely
  - Atypical organisms are implicated less often
  - TB is a possibility, especially if response to antibiotics is poor.
- In hospital acquired (nosocomial) pneumonia—Gram –ve infections and antibiotic resistance are common, so treat with broader spectrum antibiotics (see 📖 Management of pneumonia: adults, p. 186).

Are risk factors for disease present?

- Malnutrition.
- HIV+.
- Asplenia/hyposplenism (e.g. due to sickle cell disease).
- Chronic lung disease.
- Diabetes.
- Cerebral palsy.
- Immune deficiency (e.g. hypogammaglobinaemia).
- Alcoholism or IV drug use.
- Poor dental/gingival hygiene.

Some risk factors are associated with particular organisms:

- Chronic lung disease → colonization, e.g. with *H. influenzae*.
- Alcoholism or IV drug use → Gram –ve bacterial infection, ↑ risk TB, pneumococcal infection, and aspiration pneumonia.
- ↓ Consciousness (e.g. head injuries or epilepsy) and children with cerebral palsy are at ↑ risk of aspiration pneumonia.
- Poor dental hygiene → anaerobic infection from oral or gum flora → pneumonia which often → lung abscess (see 📖 Lung abscess, p. 204).

Table 5.1 Organisms common in particular age groups

Age	Organism*
Neonates	Gram +ve organisms (Group B *Strep.*, Group A *Strep.*, *Strep. pneumoniae, Staph. aureus.)*
	Gram –ve organisms (*E. coli, Salmonella* sp., *Klebsiella*)
	Less common: *Chlamydia, Listeria, Bordetella pertussis*
<5yrs	*Streptococcus pneumoniae*
	Haemophilus influenzae
	Group A Streptococcus
	Staphylococcus aureus (severe), especially post measles infection
	Bordetella pertussis
	Viral: RSV, human metapneumovirus, measles, influenza, adenovirus, parainfluenza
School age	*Streptococcus pneumoniae*
	Mycoplasma, Chlamydia
	Viral pneumonias as above
Adults	*Streptococcus pneumoniae*
	'Atypical' organisms (*Mycoplasma, Chlamydia, Legionella*)
	H. influenzae
	Viral pneumonias: influenza, adenovirus, *Varicella zoster*

*Aetiology studies in resource-poor settings are very limited. The pneumonia etiology research for child health study (PERCH) a multi-site international study is ongoing and seeks to address this question. http://www.jhsph.edu/ivac/projects/perch/

Clinical features: adults

- Systemically unwell with malaise, fever, anorexia, body aches, and headache, may have delirium if severe.
- ↑ Respiratory rate and respiratory signs including cough, sputum production, dyspnoea, pleural pain, and, rarely, haemoptysis.
- Chest movements might be ↓ on the affected side; ↓ percussion note, inspiratory crackles, and pleural rub may be present on auscultation. After a few days, an effusion often occurs. Sputum is often initially scanty or absent, becoming purulent or blood-streaked later.
- Lower lobe pneumonia with diaphragmatic pleurisy may mimic an acute abdomen—abdominal pain, ileus, rigidity.
- In the elderly, or debilitated, there may be fewer signs. Look for ↑ respiratory rate and perform a careful chest examination.

Table 5.2 Markers of severity

Clinical features	**Investigations**
Confusion/sepsis	Blood urea >7mmol/L
Respiratory rate >30/min	WCC <4 × 10^9/L or >30 × 10^9/L
Diastolic BP <60mmHg	Arterial PO_2 <8kPA
New atrial fibrillation	Serum albumin <25g/L
	Multilobe involvement

A poor prognosis is associated with

- Bacteraemia (e.g. the fatality rate ↑ from 5% in isolated *S. pneumoniae* pneumonia to 25–35% if bacteraemic).
- Infections with *S. aureus, H. influenzae* type B, and Gram –ve bacteria.
- Previous illness, either chronic (e.g. COPD, cardiac disease, HIV+, malnutrition) or acute (influenza, measles).

Common pathogens in community acquired pneumonia have particular clinical features which may be helpful.

Streptococcus pneumoniae

URTI → sudden onset fever, rigors, malaise, headache, myalgia. At extremes of age, onset is often less clear, children show ↑ RR in addition to fever and cough, elderly may have little fever and present with confusion. Chest pain (pleuritic, sometimes referred to shoulder if diaphragm is involved) and cough (initially painful and dry → blood-tinged → purulent) commonly follow. Lower lobe involvement can result in abdominal pain and guarding. WCC is often ↑.

Haemophilus influenzae Type B

Occurs in children <5yrs old, with lobar pneumonia, pleural involvement, and effusion. Also in adults as a 1° infection or in previously damaged lungs. Onset may be slow and accompanied by infection elsewhere (e.g. meninges, epiglottis). Hib vaccine has ↓ incidence dramatically.

Staphylococcus aureus

Affects patients with pre-existing lung disease, especially following viral infections, such as influenza. Influenza infection may be subclinical. Alternatively, haematogenous spread from a distant site (e.g. skin, bones and joints, or heart) may produce pneumonia in a previously healthy lung and *S. aureus* may be isolated from blood. It is always a serious condition with high fever and cyanosis; common complications include pulmonary abscess formation, cavitation, empyema.

Clinical features: children

- *Symptoms:* systemically unwell, fever, cough, difficulty breathing.
- Non-specific symptoms such as abdominal pain, vomiting, and refusal of feeds may be the only symptoms.
- *Signs of respiratory distress:* ↑ RR (note: age-dependent—see Box 5.1 and Table 5.3), nasal flaring, lower chest wall in drawing, tracheal tug, head-nodding, grunting, or nasal flaring.
- Signs such as bronchial breathing, crackles, pleural rub are less common. Absence of sputum is common.

WHO classifies pneumonia in children (as pneumonia, or severe pneumonia (SP), see Box 5.1) according to the presence of specific signs and symptoms. A poor prognosis is associated with:

- Presence of bacteraemia or clinical signs of shock or sepsis.
- Hypoxia and other signs of SP.
- HIV infection and/or severe malnutrition.

Table 5.3 Respiratory rates in children of different ages: count RR for 1min in calm circumstances—crying gives a falsely ↑ RR

Age	Normal RR/min	Severe respiratory distress
<2mths	40–30	>60
2–11mths	40–30	>50
12mths–5yrs	30–25	>40
>5yrs	25–20	>30

Box 5.1 WHO classification of pneumonia in children

Severe pneumonia

Cough or difficulty in breathing, plus at least one of the following: central cyanosis or O_2 sats <90%, severe respiratory distress (e.g. grunting, very severe chest indrawing), presence of a general danger sign (inability to breastfeed or drink), lethargy/unconsciousness/convulsions or clinical signs such as bronchial breath sounds and/or signs of pleural effusion/empyema. Other signs of pneumonia, as below, may also be present.

Pneumonia

Cough or difficult breathing with at least one of fast breathing (as per Table 5.3) or lower chest wall indrawing. They may also have signs of pneumonia on auscultation such as crackles, or pleural rub.

Atypical pneumonia

'Atypical' organisms cause <10% of all pneumonias in resource-poor countries; consider TB in cases of non-resolving infection. In HIV+ individuals, mixed infections, PCP, and KS are common (see 🕮 Respiratory disease, pp. 90–1).

- Atypical pneumonias include; *Mycoplasma pneumonia, Chlamydia pneumoniae, C. trachomatis,* and *C. psittaci, Coxiella burnetti, Legionella pneumophila* (see 🕮 Legionnaires´ disease, p. 184), and viruses, e.g. influenza and adenovirus.
- Organisms are difficult to culture and diagnosis is clinical, supported by CXR, blood picture, serology, or nasopharyngeal aspirate (if available).
- Atypical pneumonia affects previously healthy individuals of all ages.
- Symptoms are dyspnoea, dry cough, fever, and malaise.
- Chest signs are uncommon.
- CXR often shows bilateral, fluffy infiltrates, and appears worse than the clinical signs suggest.
- Treatment with doxycycline or macrolide; if severe → ICU admission.

Legionnaires' disease

The importance of *Legionella pneumophila* in the tropics is unknown. It is transmitted by inhalation of aerosolized water droplets from air conditioning, water tanks, showerheads, and medical equipment, e.g. nebulizers.

Clinical features

Vary from subclinical or mild infections to severe pneumonia. In severe infection, after 2–10d, there is abrupt high fever, rigors, myalgia, and headache → the dry cough, dyspnoea, and crackles. Patient appears toxic, sometimes with delirium or diarrhoea. Complications include respiratory failure, pericarditis, myocarditis, and acute renal failure.

Diagnosis

Gram –ve slender rods of variable length in biopsy or sputum samples; bacterial antigen in urine for first 1–3wks.

Management

Erythromycin 0.5–1g/6h IV or oral (+/– rifampicin 600mg bd, moxifloxacin 400mg od, or ciprofloxacin 500mg bd) for 2–3wks. Exclude TB if rifampicin or quinolones used, as these have potent anti-TB activity.

Prevention

Maintenance of stored water and tanks to prevent bacterial colonization and spread.

Recurrent pneumonia

>2 episodes of pneumonia may be caused by:

- Respiratory disease: COPD, bronchiectasis, bronchial obstruction (foreign body, bronchial carcinoma, lymphadenopathy, bronchial stenosis), intrapulmonary sequestration.
- Non-respiratory, e.g. recurrent aspiration, immunosuppression, HIV.

Nosocomial pneumonia

Definition Pneumonia >48h after admission to hospital. This is a ↑ problem in sub-Saharan Africa, with a high case fatality rate in children admitted to hospital.

Aetiology Aspiration of nasopharyngeal secretions, inhalation of bacteria from contaminated instruments, haematogenous spread (e.g. from abdominal infection, infected cannulae, or catheters left in for too long).

Risk factors Malnutrition, low birth weight, elderly, smoking, long pre-operative stay, prolonged anaesthesia, intubation, abdominal/thoracic operations, plus risk factors for aspiration pneumonia (see 📖 Aspiration pneumonia p. 185).

Clinical features Development of fever, cough.

Diagnosis ↑ WCC, purulent sputum, lung infiltrate on CXR.

Management Chest physiotherapy post-op may help ↓ nosocomial pneumonia. IV antibiotics (see 📖 Management of pneumonia: adults, p. 186).

Prevention Infection control measures in hospitals including hand washing. Prevent smoking pre-operatively, good respiratory equipment hygiene.

Aspiration pneumonia

Risk factors

↓ Consciousness (e.g. epilepsy, excess alcohol), dysphagia, immobility, neuromuscular diseases, inability to clear bronchial secretions or cough after surgery. In children, also consider GORD, especially if underlying neurological/neuromuscular disorders.

Aetiology

- *In the community:* anaerobes from oropharynx and teeth crevices (normally penicillin-sensitive).
- *In hospital:* aerobic bacteria become more important, especially Gram –ve enterobacteria and *P. aeruginosa*.

It may be possible to diagnose anaerobic infection from a history of poor dental hygiene, aspiration, or ↓ consciousness. As the infection proceeds, tissue necrosis → foul-smelling purulent discharge.

Management of pneumonia: adults

Treatment

Follow local antimicrobial guidelines if available - or use empiric treatment (see Table 5.4).

Supportive care

- *Oxygen:* if ↑ RR measure O_2 sats provide O_2 (usually by concentrator at 4l/min). In extreme hypoxia, two concentrators can be used (one by nasal cannulae, the other by mask. If concentrators are scarce, the supply can be split to two patients.
- *Analgesia.*
- *Fluids (IV if necessary):* treat dehydration and maintain adequate urine output (>1mL/kg/h). Losses ↑ if the patient is febrile. Syndrome of Inappropriate Antidiuretic Hormone (ADH) secretion (SIADH) is common in severe pneumonia.
- *Rest:* the patient should sit up, rather than lie flat.
- Physiotherapy not recommended in acute pneumonia; useful when pleuritic pain has subsided.

Antimicrobial use: general points

- Obtain culture specimens if microbiological facilities available, then immediately begin empirical antibiotics. Give IV therapy if the patient is very ill, cannot swallow/vomits, or if GI tract is not functioning.
- Give antibiotics for 3–7d in mild pneumonia. For severe pneumonia, continue treatment according to the clinical response. In the presence of cavitation and abscess, treat for 3–4wks.
- *Streptococcus pneumoniae* has progressively become less sensitive to penicillin: >50% of pneumococcal isolates in some countries have ↓ laboratory sensitivity to penicillin, but this is of limited significance except in meningitis. Treat with high dose penicillin unless local guidelines indicate otherwise.
- Nosocomial infections include Gram –ve organisms and require broad-spectrum antibiotics.
- Aspiration pneumonia includes anaerobes, so cephalosporin and metronidazole, or penicillin, aminoglycoside and metronidazole are used.

Chest X-rays in pneumonia

The value of CXR for each patient should be carefully considered:

- Is the diagnosis already clear from the clinical features? Typical pneumococcal pneumonia need not be X-rayed.
- Cavitation on CXR shifts the diagnosis to include TB, *Staph. aureus, Klebsiella*, meliodosis, or rarely paragonamiasis.

Note: CXR changes in pneumonia may take 3mths to resolve following successful treatment and clinical improvement by the patient.

Table 5.4 Empiric treatment of pneumonia

Clinical picture	Likely organisms	Antibiotic route Oral	 IV
Community acquired pneumonia			
Mild to moderate	*S. pneumonia*	Ax	A or Ax
If 'atypical'		Add E	
2° pneumonia			
Previous lung disease (e.g. COPD)	*S. pneumoniae* *H. influenzae*	Co or C	Co or C
If following flu, measles or URTI	*S. aureus*	Add F to above regimen	
Aspiration	*S. pneumoniae*, *Klebsiella* spp., anaerobes, Gram −ve organisms	Co	P + M + G
Immunosuppression (e.g. leukaemia)	*Pseudomonas* spp.		Cz + G
Nosocomial (especially if 2° disease)	Gram −ve		Ct + G
Sepsis elsewhere	Treat as for sepsis		F + G + M
Severe pneumonia	Widest possible range		Ct + E + G
Cavitation	TB, *Klebsiella* (South Africa), Meliodosis (Southeast Asia), *S. aureus*		

Key to antimicrobials (dose indicated is for adults)

A Ampicillin 500mg qds IV

Ax Amoxicillin 500mg tds oral or IV

C Cefuroxime 750mg tds IV or 500mg bd oral

Co Co-amoxiclav 1 tablet (500mg/125 mg) tds oral or 1.2g (1000mg/200mg) tds IV

Ct Ceftriaxone 1–2g IV or cefotaxime 1g tds IV

Cz Ceftazidime 2g tds IV

E Erythromycin 500mg qds oral or 500mg qds slowly IV

F Flucloxacillin 500mg qds oral or 250–1000mg qds slowly IV

G Gentamicin 3–5mg/kg od IV

M Metronidazole 500mg po tds (for up to 7d)

P Benzylpenicillin 1.2–1.8g qds IV (dose may be increased)

A, Ax, and oral Co doses can be doubled in severe infections; the IV Co dose can be increased in frequency to qds.

Complications

Pneumococcal pneumonia often → complications if poorly treated. A reactive effusion may be present → complicated parapneumonic effusion → empyema (see 📖 Empyema, p. 203). Haematogenous spread can → infection of meninges, joints, eyes, or abscess formation in distant organs. Rare complications include: septicaemia in patients with underlying conditions, such as asplenia; endocarditis; peritonitis in patients with ascites.

Prevention

Protein-conjugate vaccines prevent disease from pneumococcus and Haemophilus (📖 *Haemophilus influenzae* type b (Hib) vaccine, p. 905) in children and HIV+ individuals. Pneumonia should prompt a HIV test. A common preventable cause of pneumonia is smoking.

Viral pneumonia (SARS and H1N1)

In 2002–2003 an unusual coronavirus was responsible for a large number of cases of a severe acute respiratory syndrome (SARS) which had a high morbidity and mortality and spread rapidly across continents from its origin in China and Hong Kong. In 2009–2010, an influenza A (H1N1) outbreak in Mexico initially had a high mortality in young adults and became a global pandemic. In other regions the severity was similar to seasonal 'flu, but with a younger age distribution. Zoonotic viral outbreaks will continue to be important globally. Influenza, parainfluenza, RSV, human metapneumovirus and adenovirus can all cause viral pneumonia in children and adults, especially those with chronic disease.

Clinical features

Fever, cough, malaise, diarrhoea, myalgias, and headache occur after an incubation period of 2–7d. In many patients CXR shows infiltrates and patchy consolidation especially in the lower zones. As the illness progresses CXR shadowing worsens → development of ARDS and multi-organ dysfunction. Recovery may be slow and some patients develop pulmonary fibrosis. Diagnosis is based on the clinical sequence of events during an outbreak. Cultures of viruses are not possible in routine laboratories and an RT-PCR diagnostic test in a surveillance laboratory (where available) should be requested on initial cases using blood, urine, and nasopharyngeal samples.

Management

Specific antiviral therapy is of value if started early in the course of the illness. Steroids have been tried in SARS, but no benefit has been found; their role in influenza is unclear. Supportive treatment in intensive care unit (ICU) may be required. 2° bacterial infection contributed to mortality in the H1N1 pandemic (2009–2010), and staphylococcal pneumonia also ↑ in incidence following influenza infection.

Management of pneumonia: children

Treatment

- Use local guidelines if available, otherwise use empiric treatment (see Table 5.5). WHO guidelines are given in Table 5.5 (for pneumonia and severe pneumonia (SP)). Parenteral antibiotics should be given for at least 5 days in SP.
- HIV+ and/or severely malnourished children should always be treated as SP. Treatment of HIV+ children should include high dose co-trimoxazole for PCP according to risk (see 🕮 Special aspects of paediatric HIV/AIDS, p. 130).

Supportive care

- O_2—use paediatric SaO_2 probes for children.
- Analgesia.
- Ensure adequate fluids, but avoid overhydration.
- Use IV antibiotics sooner in very young children, and in all neonates, as they become unwell very rapidly (see 🕮 Multi-system diseases, p. 729).

Review treatment after 48h. Clinical deterioration or failure to improve → CXR to check for lung abscess, empyema, cavities, or TB and change to 2nd line antibiotics or treat as indicated by the CXR.

Table 5.5 Empiric treatment of childhood pneumonia (adapted from WHO guidelines)

Clinical picture	**Parenteral**	**Oral (may follow IV in SP)**
SP 1st line	A + G	Ax
	Or Ct*	
SP 2nd line if staphylococcal pneumonia is suspected	Clox + G	Clox
Pneumonia		Ax

*Ct is an alternative, but it best to reserve Ct for treatment failures.

Key to antimicrobials dosing for children (>1mth)

A Ampicillin 50mg/kg IM or IV qds

Ax Amoxicillin 40mg/kg per oral dose bd

Clox Cloxacillin 50mg/kg qds IV/IM, 25mg/kg qds oral

Ct Ceftriaxone 80mg/kg IM/IV od

G Gentamicin 7.5mg IM or IV od

Further reading

British Paediatric Formulary available online (free to many low resource countries through HINARI and UK users): Available at: http://www.bnf.org/bnf/index.htm

WHO guidelines available at: http://www.who.int/maternal_child_adolescent/documents/9241546700/en/index.html.

Paediatric acute respiratory infections: epiglottitis

Epiglottitis is an acute bacterial infection of the epiglottis and arytenoids, the surrounding tissue and cartilages, mainly affecting children aged 2–7yrs and mainly caused by *Haemophilus influenzae* type b (Hib).

Direct or haematogenous infection of the upper airway → rapid swelling and risk of airway obstruction. Hib conjugate vaccine substantially ↓ incidence of life-threatening infections. Severe disease occurs where immunization coverage is low. In older individuals, *Streptococcus pneumoniae*, *Haemophilus parainfluenzae*, group A Streptococcus, and *Staphylococcus aureus* can cause a similar illness.

Clinical features

Typically starts suddenly and progresses rapidly. The affected child presents with sudden onset of high fever, sore throat, and muffled voice → stridor, respiratory distress, and drooling of saliva. The child appears toxic, refuses to eat or drink and prefers to sit upright, leaning forward in an effort to maintain patency of the airway; may have loss of voice (aphonia) and dysphagia.

Diagnosis

Consider epiglottitis in any young child with compatible clinical presentation, especially if not immunized against Hib. Intubation is dangerous and should be undertaken only if expert. Visualization of a large, swollen, cherry-red epiglottis by laryngoscopy at the time of intubation confirms the diagnosis.

Management

Epiglottitis is a medical emergency. The goals of management are prevention of airway obstruction and eradication of infection. Before a definitive airway is established, **make all attempts to minimize distress to the child, as this will compromise the airway.**

- Give humidified O_2.
- Make urgent arrangements for inserting an artificial airway (preferably nasotracheal); even if there is no current respiratory distress.
- Be prepared to perform a tracheostomy if endotracheal intubation fails.
- Until the airway has been inserted *do not:*
  - examine the throat (reflex laryngeal spasm may cause complete airway obstruction)
  - attempt venepuncture (associated anxiety and pain may precipitate acute laryngeal spasm)
  - send the child for CXR (immediate intervention will be necessary if airway obstruction occurs).
- Once definitive airway inserted take samples for FBC and cultures of blood and epiglottic surface.
- *Give antibiotics when the airway is safe:* IV ceftriaxone.

Note Adrenaline and corticosteroids are NOT effective in epiglottitis. Once the airway is inserted, most children improve rapidly. The epiglottitis resolves after a few days of antibiotics, and the patient can be weaned from the endotracheal or NGT.

Differential diagnosis of acute upper airways obstruction in children

- Croup (most common).
- Bacterial tracheitis.
- Epiglottitis.
- Diphtheria.
- Severe tonsillitis.
- Infectious mononucleosis.
- Laryngeal foreign body.
- Smoke or steam inhalation.
- Trauma.
- Laryngomalacia.

Acute laryngotracheobronchitis: croup

Laryngotracheobronchitis (LTB; croup) is the commonest form of upper airway obstruction in childhood, usually occurring between 3mths–5yrs of age. LTB initially affects the mucosa of the nose and nasopharynx, → larynx, and bronchial tree. In young children inflammation → submucosal oedema and narrowing of the airway. Human parainfluenza viruses cause ~75% cases; other causes include adenoviruses, RSV, influenza, and measles.

Clinical features

LTB begins as a mild URTI with mild barking cough, low grade fever, and intermittent stridor. Over the ensuing few days, progressive compromise of the airway → ↑ coughing, stridor becomes continuous (+/– wheeze), and signs of respiratory distress develop, including nasal flaring, suprasternal, intercostal and subcostal recession (lower chest wall in drawing), associated with a prolonged, laboured expiratory phase of respiration. Symptoms are characteristically worse at night. Crying and agitation ↑ symptoms and the child prefers to sit up in bed or be held upright. Examination reveals reduced breath sounds, wheezes, and crackles. Most children improve spontaneously within 48–72h, but some → severe airway compromise and require further intervention to avert respiratory failure. The *croup score* is useful for assessment and evaluating response to treatment (see Table 5.6).

Diagnosis Clinical.

Management

Indications for admission are listed in Box 5.2.

- Give dexamethasone 150micrograms/kg IV/IM/oral, or prednisolone 1–2mg/kg oral, or nebulized budesonide 2mg stat; repeat at 12h if necessary.
- Give humidified O_2.
- Give IV fluids to children with moderate to severe respiratory distress.
- Ensure minimal disturbance as symptoms worsen on agitation.
- Observe closely for signs of ↑ airway obstruction.
- If severe airway obstruction develops (cyanosis, air hunger, restlessness) consider nebulized adrenaline (give 400micrograms/kg up to max 5mg, of 1 in 1000 (1mg/mL) solution, repeated after 30min if required), +/– tracheostomy or nasotracheal intubation.

Note

- Sedation is contraindicated in croup because it masks restlessness, which is a major indicator of the severity of airway obstruction and the need for tracheostomy or nasotracheal intubation.
- Expectorants, bronchodilators, and antihistamines are not helpful in croup.

Table 5.6 Croup score

Clinical parameter	Score 1	2	3
Colour	normal	cyanosed in room air	cyanosed on 40% O_2
Stridor	absent	inspiratory	expiratory
Cough	nil	mild, barking	severe
Respiratory distress	absent	nasal flaring	intercostal recession, in drawing
Air entry	normal	slightly reduced	greatly reduced

A croup score of ≥ 6 is an indication for ICU care

Box 5.2 Indications for admission in a child with croup:

- ↑ Stridor or respiratory distress.
- Severe stridor at rest.
- Hypoxia or cyanosis.
- Restlessness, lethargy, or unconsciousness.

Managing milder episodes at home

- Children with mild croup can be managed at home, but must be watched closely for signs of worsening respiratory obstruction.
- Management is supportive.

Bacterial tracheitis

Presentation similar to croup, but patient is systemically more unwell. It may affect any age group and does not respond to croup treatment. Unlike epiglottitis, bacterial tracheitis rarely causes airway obstruction. Causes include *S. aureus*, Group A streptococci, *H. influenzae*, *Moraxella catarrhalis*, *Klebsiella* species, other Gram –ves, and anaerobes. There is diffuse inflammation of the larynx, trachea, and bronchi with formation of an adherent or semi-adherent mucopurulent membrane in the trachea.

Clinical features

Include:
- Fever.
- Bark-like/brassy cough.
- Hoarseness.
- Respiratory distress.
- Sepsis.

Other differential diagnoses include:
- Diphtheria.
- Epiglottitis.
- Peritonsillar or retropharyngeal abscess.

Diagnosis

Is clinical supported by ↑ WBC, CXR may show narrowing of trachea, and blood culture. Direct visualization and culture of purulent tracheal secretions by laryngotracheobronchoscopy provides definitive diagnosis.

Treatment

Involves airway management and administration of broad-spectrum antibiotics. Affected children may decompensate acutely with worsening respiratory distress and sepsis.

Bronchiolitis

Bronchiolitis is common among children aged <2yrs (peak 3–6mths). In >50% of cases it is caused by RSV. Other causes include human metapneumovirus, adenovirus, parainfluenza virus. Source of infection is usually an older child or adult with a minor respiratory illness. Risk factors for severe bronchiolitis include low birth weight, age <6wks, and co-morbidity such as lung disease, congenital heart disease, and immune deficiency.

Clinical features

Characteristically begins as a URTI; the infant appears slightly unwell, with low grade fever, a blocked nose, serous nasal discharge, cough, and feeding difficulty. Within 24–48h, the signs of airway obstruction appear with paroxysmal wheezy cough, dyspnoea, and irritability. Breast and bottle-feeding become difficult as ↑ RR does not give enough time for sucking and swallowing. Clinical features tend to be most severe days 4–6 of illness. Examination reveals tachypnoea, nasal flaring, intercostal, and subcostal recession. Chest is hyper-resonant with obliteration of the cardiac dullness due to hyperinflation. Wheeze and fine crepitations are heard on auscultation. The liver and spleen may be palpable due to hyperinflation.

Diagnosis

Is primarily clinical, CXR may show hyperinflation (flattening of the diaphragm) +/– increased perihilar infiltrates.

Management

Markers of severity requiring admission:

- Apnoea.
- Hypoxia (O_2 sats <92%).
- Reduced feeding <50%.
- Respiratory rate (RR) >70.
- Moderate or severe recessions.
- Nasal flaring.
- Grunting.

Consider admission in the absence of markers of severity in the presence of risk factors or if early in the course of illness; ~50% of infants are asymptomatic by 2wks.

- Give humidified O_2 via a nasal catheter, CPAP if more severe and available. Need for intubation is very rare.
- Ensure adequate fluid intake, feed via nasogastric tube (NGT) or give IV fluids for severe respiratory distress.
- Keep propped up in bed (30–40° above horizontal).

Note

- Antibiotics are indicated if any associated pneumonia.
- Corticosteroids are of no benefit.

Whooping cough

Bordetella pertussis commonly affects infants and young children, with the highest mortality <3mths. Mild infections in adolescence and adults are likely under-diagnosed and are the source of infection for infants. *B. parapertussis* causes a similar illness to *B. pertussis*.

Clinical features

Incubation is 6–20d.

- Initially has URTI symptoms and lasts 1–2wks. Fever not usually prominent.
- Paroxysms of severe coughing with a 'whoop' are the classical feature. The 'whoop' is caused by forced inspiration against a partly-closed glottis and can → cyanosis and hypoxic syncope.
- Child commonly drools and vomits after coughing, and may become exhausted.
- Wheezing does not occur.
- After 1–3wks of whooping, a more tolerable chronic cough may persist for several weeks; adults and older children may have a chronic cough throughout.
- Infants <6mths do not whoop, but may become apnoeic and have non-specific signs of respiratory distress (difficult to differentiate from bronchiolitis see 📖 Bronchiolitis, p. 197 caused by respiratory viruses).
- Many cases, especially older children are uncomplicated and self-limiting; however, illness can persist for weeks to months and → bronchiectasis and malnutrition.
- Prolonged coughing may → petechiae, conjunctival haemorrhages, and rectal prolapse.
- Death is usually in older age groups, may be due to 2° pneumonia, or encephalopathy (↓ consciousness not due to hypoxia, seizures, or brain damage).

Diagnosis

Normally made clinically. The WCC usually shows a lymphocytosis. Culture is difficult—a per-nasal swab or a nasopharyngeal aspirate sample can be taken (PCR if available).

Management Essentially supportive. Erythromycin is recommended, and ↓ transmission, but has little effect in modifying whooping cough.

Prevention Routine immunization.

Lymphocytic interstitial pneumonitis

LIP accounts for 22–75% of pulmonary disease in paediatric HIV+ patients, but is uncommon in adults. LIP also occasionally occurs in EBV, human T lymphotrophic virus (HTLV), lymphoproliferative disorders, and autoimmune disease. Pathologically, there is a pleomorphic lung infiltrate of activated lymphocytes, plasma cells and immunoblasts.

Clinical features

May be asymptomatic in the early stages. Symptoms usually progressive:
- Chronic cough.
- Dyspnoea.
- Parotid enlargement.
- Generalized lymphadenopathy.
- Hepatosplenomegaly.
- Digital clubbing.
- Wheezing.

+/– other features of underlying HIV.

Diagnosis Is clinical.
- CXR findings include bibasal interstitial or small nodular infiltrates which coalesce into alveolar consolidation; widened mediastinum; and peri hilar adenopathy.
- Serum LDH is often ↑ to 300–500IU/L.
- Look for underlying immunosuppressive disease, especially HIV.

Differential diagnoses include varicella pneumonia, miliary TB, and metastatic carcinoma. Definitive diagnosis requires open lung biopsy, which is rarely performed in view of its attendant complications.

Treatment

Asymptomatic children require no treatment, but follow up for clinical and/or radiological signs of deterioration. For symptomatic children:
- O_2.
- Prednisolone 2mg/kg oral daily; treat for 4wks then gradually ↓ dose.
- Long-term steroid therapy may be required if symptoms recur.
- Bronchodilators may be used to treat children with wheeze.
- Treat the underlying cause: ART for HIV+ patients.

Diphtheria

Corynebacterium diphtheriae causes infection of the nasopharynx and occasionally skin and mucous membranes. Its endotoxin has potentially fatal effects on the heart, kidney, and peripheral nerves. Death occurs in ~50% without treatment, and in 5–10% despite treatment. Children <5yrs and adults >40yrs have a worse prognosis. Although incidence is ↓ worldwide, it remains a significant problem in some developing countries without vaccination programmes.

Transmission By droplets or secretions from infected humans. Incubation is 2–5d. Patients are infectious for ~1mth; however, some become carriers.

Clinical features

Incubation is ~2–5d (7d cutaneous diphtheria).

There may be non-specific symptoms:

- Fever.
- Chills.
- Malaise.
- Nausea.
- Vomiting.
- Headache.

Local

Mucosae are initially red and oedematous; → necrosis of epithelium. An inflammatory grey-white pseudo-membrane forms at the site of infection (commonly the tonsils and oropharynx); it is adherent and separates with bleeding. There is sore throat (may cause dysphagia), cervical lymphadenopathy, and halitosis (see Box 5.3). Neck is often swollen with oedema and enlarged lymph nodes. Palatal paralysis by toxin produces a 'nasal' quality to the speech.

Tracheolaryngeal

- Hoarseness.
- Dry cough.
- Rarely, airway obstruction.

Cutaneous Pustules and ulcers with a grey membrane (rare).

Systemic effects of toxin

- Myocarditis (10%).
- Heart block (often >1wk after acute infection; can cause death up to 8wks after).
- Murmurs.
- Heart failure.
- Demyelination → peripheral neuritis (often ~6wks after initial illness).
- → Paralysis (soft palate, ocular, and intercostals muscles).

There may be renal failure (tubular necrosis) and pneumonia.

Malignant diphtheria Indicates rapid spread of membranes, neck oedema, adenitis, stridor, and shock.

Diagnosis

Treat on suspicion—do not wait for confirmation. Arrange for throat swabs of membrane, ECG (look for ectopics, ST and T wave changes, right bundle branch block (RBBB), complete heart block (CHB)), U&Es, FBC.

Treatment

Give antitoxin urgently. A test dose of diluted diphtheria antitoxin should 1st be given intradermally to exclude hypersensitivity; then give 10 000–40 000 units by IV infusion for mild-moderate disease, and 40 000–100 000 for severe disease by IV infusion. Antitoxin is made from horse serum, so beware anaphylaxis which is rare, but potentially fatal. Have adrenaline drawn up. Tracheostomy may be lifesaving; do not delay if there are signs of respiratory distress. Give high-dose antibiotics IV (penicillin, erythromycin, cephalosporin, tetracycline are all effective).

Prevention Routine childhood vaccination prevents disease. Recovering patients should also receive vaccine as a booster dose, as well as close contacts.

Box 5.3 Causes of sore throat and tonsillar exudates

- *Streptococcus pyogenes* (sequelae are rheumatic heart disease and glomerulonephritis).
- *Mild viral infections* (less common to have exudates).
- *Corynebacterium* diphtheria.
- *EBV:* infectious mononucleosis.
- *Neisseria gonorrhoeae.*
- 2° syphilis.
- Herpes simplex virus—especially if HIV+.
- Lassa virus.
- *Fusobacterium necrophorum* (part of Lemierre's syndrome).

Pleural effusion

Pleural effusion is the presence of fluid in the pleural cavity, this is generally unilateral, but may be bilateral. See Box 5.4 for causes.

- Exudates are inflammatory fluid collections caused by an underlying infective/inflammatory disease. They are generally straw coloured, unilateral, cellular pleocytosis is common and fluid LDH levels are generally high. Protein is >50% of serum protein or >30g/L.
- *Transudates:* low protein content, are generally bilateral, and cellular pleocytosis is minimal. All oedema-causing conditions—congestive cardiac failure (CCF), nephrotic syndrome, liver cell failure, anaemia, and hypoproteinaemia may cause transudative pleural effusions.
- *Chylothorax:* fluid looks milky with a high lipid content, caused by leakage from the thoracic duct due to damage by filariasis or a tumour.
- *Empyema:* is infected effusion. Cells are neutrophils, and in some cases, frank pus; pH <7.2 (Box 5.5).
- *Haemothorax:* pure blood or heavily bloodstained fluid.

Box 5.4 Causes of pleural effusion

Exudates

- TB.
- Lung cancer.
- Pneumonia.
- Mesothelioma.
- Collagen diseases.
- Sub diaphragmatic infections/ abscesses.
- Metastatic carcinoma.
- Pulmonary embolism.
- Pancreatitis.

Haemothorax

- Trauma.
- Mesothelioma.
- Metastatic carcinoma.
- Vascular pleural adhesions.

Transudates

- LVF.
- Liver disease especially with ascites.
- Nephrotic syndrome.
- Anaemia and hypoproteinaemia.
- Pericardial disease.

Chylothorax

- Filariasis.
- Lymphoma.
- Trauma to the thoracic duct.
- Metastatic carcinoma.

Clinical features of pleural effusion

Pleuritic pain may be present if acute—less common in TB (chronic inflammation). Patients are tachypnoeic and may be dyspnoeic. Chest wall expansion is ↓ on affected side and there is stony dullness to percussion with ↓ tactile fremitus and ↓ or absent breath sounds. Signs are commonly detected at the bases posteriorly, and in the mid-axillary line.

Box 5.5 Empyema

- Pus in the pleural space.
- A complication of a bacterial pneumonia, aspiration pneumonia, or rupture of a liver or lung abscess and less commonly TB.
- Suspect in any patient with persistent (often high spiking) fever, with signs of fluid in the pleural space.
- Diagnosis by aspiration of pleural fluid for Gram stain and culture.
- Putrid odour indicates anaerobic bacterial infection.
- High protein, high cell count, pH <7.1 or high LDH level (>60% of serum LDH or >1000) suggests an empyema is developing, and needs to be drained.
- Give broad spectrum antibiotics (co-amoxiclav; ceftriaxone; cefotaxime: plus metronidazole). Cultures are often –ve in which case empirical therapy must continue.
- Intercostal tube drainage to dryness (<20mL fluid in 24h) and 6wks antibiotics will cure in most cases.
- Decortication may be required if a prolonged course of IV antibiotics combined with repeated ultrasound guided aspiration fails.
- Recurrent empyema presents a particular problem if HIV+. Culture often shows mixed growth, response to therapy poor and surgical risk too high for decortication. In these cases, palliation with antibiotics and fistula or short drain into ileostomy bag can be effective.

Diagnosis

The presence of fluid is confirmed by CXR or US. Aspiration of 50–100mL is generally done for diagnosis, but in patients with respiratory distress 700–1000mL is aspirated to relieve symptoms. Fluid is best withdrawn posteriorly with the patient leaning forward and the needle inserted above the rib one or two intercostal spaces below the upper level of dullness. Fluid should be sent for protein, pH, cytology, Gram and AFB staining, adenosine deaminase (ADA) and lactate dehydrogenase (LDH) levels and appropriate cultures (see Box 5.6).

Management Treat cause of effusion. Where fluid → dyspnoea, repeated aspirations or chest tube insertion may be beneficial. Where recurrence is a problem, pleurodesis may be performed.

Box 5.6 Diagnostic features of pleural effusions

- *Exudates:* protein >30g/L (+ normal serum proteins) or fluid protein >0.5 X serum albumin, LDH >200IU fluid: serum LDH ratio >0.6.
- *Transudates:* protein <30g/L, LDH <200, LDH ratio <0.6.
- *Neutrophilia:* bacterial pneumonias, empyemas.
- *Lymphocytosis:* TB, lymphomas, viral infections.
- *Abnormal cytology:* carcinomas, mesotheliomas.
- *Low pleural fluid sugar:* rheumatoid arthritis (RA), infections, malignancies.
- pH <7.2 indicates need for tube drainage.
- Gram stain indicates empyema.

Lung abscess

This is a suppurative cavitating infection of the lung parenchyma, commonly caused by aspiration of mouth anaerobes, and less often by blood-borne infection. Meliodosis is a particularly severe cause of abscess in Southeast Asia, Indian subcontinent, North Australia (see Box 5.7 for causes).

Clinical features

Patients present with a cough, fever with chills, chest pain, and haemoptysis. Gingivitis with poor dentition, the usual source of the bacteria, is often found. When the abscess communicates with a bronchus, copious quantities of purulent sputum often blood streaked are expectorated. Clubbing develops rapidly and if the abscess ruptures into the pleural space an empyema will result. Chronic abscesses with waxing and waning symptoms may result from inadequate antibiotic therapy.

Diagnosis

Characteristically the CXR shows a rounded opacity with an air-fluid level. Multiple abscesses suggest a blood-borne infection, e.g. infected pulmonary emboli or tricuspid endocarditis. Leukocytosis with ↑ ESR and CRP are typical. If abscess does not resolve with antibiotics, bronchoscopy may be performed to seek an endobronchial obstruction (foreign body, malignancy, bronchial adenoma).

Management

IV antibiotics are mandatory until fever and leukocytosis settles—this may take weeks. Co-amoxiclav, ceftriaxone or cefuroxime are good initial choices plus metronidazole and may be modified according to cultures. Consider an antistaphylococcal antibiotic, e.g. flucloxacillin or clindamycin in influenza outbreaks or when cultures indicate.

Box 5.7 Causes of lung abscesses

Pulmonary aspiration

Most occur in the right lung; aspiration while supine results in abscesses in apical segment of the lower lobe or posterior segment of the upper lobe. Often caused by anaerobes of gingival origin.

Bronchial obstruction

Due to lung CA or inhaled foreign body. Caused by mixed anaerobes.

Bacteraemia/septicaemia

Often multiple abscesses from sites such as right-sided endocarditis, infected IV cannulae, IV drug abuse. Common causes are *S. aureus*, *Streptococcus milleri*.

Primary infection with cavitation

TB or as a complication of severe pneumonia with *S. aureus*, *Klebsiella pneumonia*, or *Nocardia asteroides* (especially in immunosuppression).

Spread from subphrenic or hepatic abscess

Produces 2° abscess, often in the right lower lobe. Due to *Entamoeba histolytica*, coliforms, *Streptococcus faecalis*.

Cavitating lesions seen on CXR, mimicking abscesses

May be caused by :

- TB.
- Paragonimiasis.
- Fungal infection.
- Cavitating squamous cell CA.
- Pulmonary infarction.
- Wegener's granulomatosis.

Fungal pulmonary infections

Fungal spores are found airborne and in soil; often growing in large numbers in bird and bat faeces. Human–human transmission does not appear to be a problem. The infections depend on the immune status of the individual and the level of exposure. Many cases are asymptomatic, illness may present as:

- Self-resolving pneumonitis (acute pulmonary form): cough, chest pain, fever, joint pains, malaise, occasionally erythema nodosum, or multiforme. Specific therapy may be required in more severe cases.
- Localized cavitation, nodules, or calcification may be asymptomatic and found on CXR for other reasons. No treatment is required. However, since they can be similar to lung tumours, they may be diagnosed only at surgery.
- Persisting or spreading cavitation → chest pain, cough, and sometimes haemoptysis (which can be heavy). Surgery and antifungal therapy may be required. Resembles pulmonary TB.
- Acute or chronic systemic spread. Patients present with fever, often marked ↓ weight, skin lesions. If acute, there may be signs of lung disease and purpura due to thrombocytopenia and hepatosplenomegaly. Disseminated disease is fatal in the absence of systemic antifungal therapy.

Severe fungal pneumonia is rare. Diabetes, elderly, pregnant women, and children (especially neonates) predispose to spreading and cavitation. Immunosuppression or neoplasia predispose to acute disseminated disease.

Aspergillosis

Aspergillus is ubiquitous and clinical infection is rare. Most infections are caused by *Aspergillus fumigatus*, *A. flavus*, or *A. niger* in predisposed hosts, especially patients with asthma or post-TB cavitation.

Clinical forms and management

- *Allergic bronchopulmonary aspergillosis (APBA):* persistent endobronchial infection → severe asthma and, with time, a chronic cough (producing mucoid plugs) and dyspnoea. CXR may show shadowing in the peripheral fields. Eosinophilia is a feature. Manage with steroids and itraconazole if possible. May → proximal bronchiectasis.
- *Aspergilloma:* a fungal ball that often develops in a pre-existing cavity (commonly due to TB). Intermittent cough is often the only sign, but haemoptysis may develop. If possible, the aspergilloma should be surgically excised. CT scan appearances are distinctive, showing a mass attached to the interior of the cavity, and overlying pleura usually thickened.
- *Invasive aspergillosis:* occurs in brain; kidney, liver, and skin of the severely immunocompromised (e.g. bone marrow transplant recipients). Attempt to ↓ immunosuppression, if possible. Amphotericin B (0.5–1.0mg/kg IV od, to a total dose of 2–2.5g) has been standard therapy (it is a toxic drug), but for confirmed invasive aspergillosis voriconazole may be more effective.

Diagnosis of Aspergillus infection

This is often difficult.

- Microscopic analysis of skin lesion scrapings, sputum, or pus for evidence of fungal infection.
- Serology (*Aspergillus* precipitins), specific fungal cultures.
- Skin prick tests to *Aspergillus* and *Aspergillus* RAST test are useful in ABPA.
- In invasive aspergillosis, the CXR or CT appearances may give a clue, being typically more severe than expected from clinical examination.
- Isolated chronic lung lesions (mycetomas) may only be distinguished from lung tumours at surgery.
- Galactomannan levels (cell wall component of *Aspergillus*) are being used in some high-risk patients in high-resource settings, but require careful interpretation.

Histoplasmosis

This occurs in two forms, and commonly causes disseminated disease in HIV infected patients:

- *Small-form histoplasmosis:* (caused by *Histoplasma capsulatum* var. *capsulatum*) occurs in the Americas plus Asia and eastern Africa. This → acute or chronic pulmonary infections, pericarditis, or progressive disseminated histoplasmosis in immunocompromised individuals. Disseminated small-form histoplasmosis affects bone marrow, spleen, liver, lymph nodes, and skin (papules, ulcers). A chronic form in immunocompetent patients presents with persistent painful oral ulceration and/or hypoadrenalism. Complications include laryngeal ulceration, endocarditis, and meningitis.
- *Large-form or African histoplasmosis:* (*H. capsulatum* var. *duboisii*.) occurs in central and west Africa. African histoplasmosis is either a focal disease affecting bone, skin, and lymph nodes or a progressive disseminated disease affecting mucosal surfaces, especially the GI tract and lungs.

Blastomycosis

A systemic infection caused by *Blastomyces dermatitidis* that occurs in northern America, Africa, India, and Middle East. It causes chronic pulmonary or disseminated disease (involving both lung and skin). Skin lesions are commonly an initial single nodule, then crusted plaques, ulcers, and abscesses. Complications include lytic bone lesions (especially axial skeleton), and GI tract disease (especially epididymitis).

Coccidioidomycosis

A disease of semi-arid regions of the Americas caused by the fungus *Coccidioides immitis*. It is inhaled into alveoli, where it rounds up and divides to form a large spherule with thick outer wall. The clinical features are typically varied with dissemination occurring particularly to meninges, joints, and skin. It commonly disseminates in patients with advanced HIV.

Paracoccidioidomycosis

A granulomatous disease caused by the fungus *Paracoccidioides brasiliensis*. It occurs sporadically in south and central America where it is the most common systemic mycosis. An acute form of the disease occurs in children and adults <30yrs, while a chronic form is more common in 30–50-yr-olds, especially agricultural workers living in endemic areas. The M:F ratio is ~10:1.

Acute form

Presents with generalized lymphadenopathy, moderate hepatosplenomegaly, fever, and ↓ weight over several months. The nodes may become fluctuant. Involvement of mesenteric and hepatic perihilar nodes → an appendicitis-like picture or obstructive jaundice. Complications include lytic bone lesions, small bowel disease, multiple mucocutaneous lesions (lymphatic/haematogenous spread). Pulmonary involvement is uncommon. Immunosuppression can → severe superinfection (e.g. TB, cryptococcus, pneumonia).

Chronic disease

Normally presents with lung disease—dyspnoea, cough, (rarely haemoptysis and fever), with extensive involvement on CXR. Mucocutaneous lesions are common on skin (face, limbs); painful lesions in the mouth, pharynx, or oesophagus inhibit eating, → marked ↓ weight. Other features—ulcerated tongue, hypoadrenalism. Chronic inflammation and fibrosis may → tracheal/laryngeal fibrosis, pulmonary fibrosis, and bowel obstruction due to enlarged lymph nodes.

Management of systemic fungal infections

- Follow local guidelines.
- Amphotericin B (↑ daily dose (after test dose) from 0.25mg/kg/day IV to 1.0mg/kg/day, if renal function permits) to a cumulative total of >15mg/kg.
- (Alternative: fluconazole 200–400mg oral od for 6–18mths depending on specific fungus.)
- Meningitis due to coccidioidomycosis requires fluconazole 400–800mg oral od for 9–12mths.
- Patients with histoplasmosis may be switched to oral itraconazole (200mg oral tds for 3d, then 200mg oral bd for total treatment duration of 12 wks) after improvement on amphotericin B.

Surgery may be required for management of chronic sequelae in paracoccidioidomycosis.

Paragonimiasis (lung flukes)

A persistent lung disease, occurring widely around the globe, but especially in East Asia, which is caused by >15 different species of *Paragonimus* trematodes; ~22 million people are infected world-wide (Fig. 5.1).

Transmission

Humans are infected by eating undercooked freshwater crabs and crayfish infected with the metacercariae. The immature flukes burrow out of the human intestine into the peritoneum, where they mature and tunnel their way into the lungs (see Fig. 5.1). Here, they cause inflammation, haemorrhage, and necrosis of the lung parenchyma. Adult flukes (stout, bean-shaped, ~1cm long) live in cavities in proximity to airways. Ova are expelled either in expectorated sputum or in the faeces after being swallowed. Flukes that miss the lungs produce extra-pulmonary symptoms (due to cysts, granulomas, and abscesses) in muscles, abdominal viscera, brain, genitalia.

Clinical features of paragonimiasis

Days or weeks after eating infected food, migration of the flukes within the peritoneum and pleura → causes signs of inflammation and fever, rashes, urticaria, abdominal, and chest pain, wheeze, cough, or discomfort.

The classic feature of chronic pulmonary disease is a persistent cough with production of thick brownish-red sputum (due to the presence of ova and flukes). The CXR resembles TB, except that cavities are often basal. CXR changes may also include areas of consolidation, and pleural effusions. Physical examination of the chest often reveals little and the patients appear quite well.

Aberrant migration of the flukes may produce signs of a cerebral SOL (epilepsy, ↑ ICP, psychiatric syndromes, meningeal irritation) or spinal SOL, necrosis of abdominal viscera, transitory subcutaneous swellings. Extra-pulmonary disease may occur in the absence of pulmonary signs, but this is uncommon.

Diagnosis

Presence of large characteristic ova or adult flukes in the sputum, faeces, or effusion; serology.

Management

Praziquantel 25mg/kg oral tds for 2–3d → rapid symptomatic improvement, although radiological changes may take some months to improve. Treatment of cerebral infection may result in neurological deterioration, in some cases → seizures and coma. Beware of ↑ ICP due to dying parasites. Treat cautiously and consider dexamethasone 4mg IV qds as cover.

Prevention Improve health education to decrease consumption of undercooked crustaceans; mass treatment of persons in endemic areas.

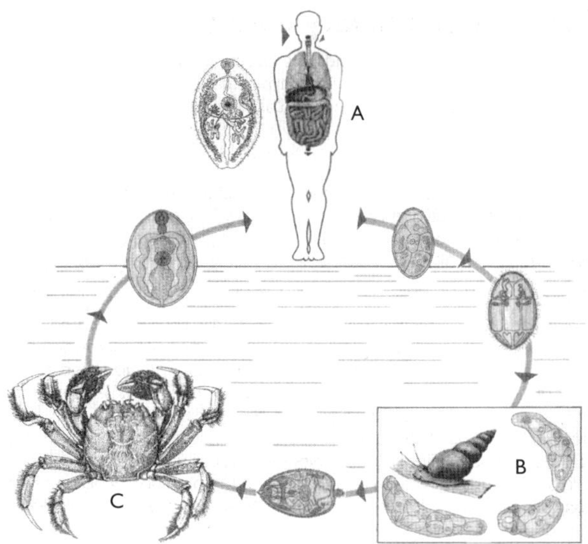

Fig. 5.1 Life cycle of *Paragonimus* lung flukes.

(A) Man is the definitive host, along with a range of domestic canines and felines. The adult fluke lives in cavities in the lung; ova are either coughed or defecated into fresh water. Miracidia emerge, and infect aquatic snails (B), in which development into cercaria takes place. These encyst as metacercariae on the muscles of freshwater crabs and crayfish (C), which are eaten uncooked. The metacercariae contain immature flukes which bore through the intestinal wall, migrate through the diaphragm into the lungs. The mature flukes are hermaphrodite, and without mating produce ova 2–3mths after infection, completing the life cycle.

Tropical pulmonary eosinophilia

This acute or chronic lung syndrome occurs in areas where lymphatic filariasis is endemic. TPE results from hypersensitivity to microfilarial antigens. In most instances the diagnosis is based on a therapeutic response to diethylcarbamazine (DEC).

Pathology

Culex mosquitoes carry the larvae that mature into adult worms of *Wuchereria bancrofti* and *Brugia malayi* within lymphatics. Female worms discharge millions of microfilaria many of which are trapped and destroyed within the lungs eliciting an eosinophilic hypersensitivity reaction.

Clinical features

Young adults are generally affected. Nocturnal cough associated with wheezing may occur, due to the nocturnal periodicity of microfilaraemia. Low grade fever, malaise, and ↓ weight may occur. Wheezes and crackles are heard in severe or advanced cases, but in many patients respiratory examination is normal. Significant eosinophilia is typical with total eosinophil counts 3000–50 000mm^3. Symptoms do not correlate with the degree of eosinophilia. Filarial serology is +ve, but is unhelpful in endemic areas. CXRs may be normal or show a reticulonodular appearance. In long-standing cases features of pulmonary fibrosis are seen. Pulmonary function tests (PFTs) show a mixed restrictive and obstructive pattern with diffusion abnormalities prominent in longstanding cases.

Management

Diethylcarbamazine 5mg/kg daily in three divided doses × 3wks. Patients who respond poorly should have a 2nd course of DEC for a longer duration. Doxycycline kills the endosymbiont bacteria *Wolbachia* in filarial worms, but this is not of proven efficacy in TPE.

Asthma

Asthma is a syndrome of reversible bronchial obstruction → episodic wheezing and shortness of breath (SOB). There is genetic susceptibility and triggers include

- Protein allergens, e.g. dust, food, pets in atopic individuals.
- Low molecular weight allergens, e.g. isocyanate in industry.
- Infections, especially viral in children, e.g. RSV.
- Environmental or occupational pollutants, e.g. smoke, automobile exhausts, and industrial dusts → irritation and can ↑ existing asthma.

Epidemiology of asthma

~10% young adults in resource-poor countries are atopic, with ↑ prevalence in Ghana and similar areas. This is likely multifactorial and theories include the immunological effect of ↓ parasite exposure, altered diet, and obesity and ↑ house dust allergen exposure.

Pathology

Constant exposure to environmental triggers → constant mucosal inflammation. Acute symptoms may be caused by exposure to any exacerbating factor and may ↑ by beta blocker therapy or aspirin or NSAIDS; exercise commonly → wheezing.

Diurnal variation is common, due to the circadian variation in endogenous cortisol. Symptoms are generally worse on waking and in severe cases may cause nocturnal awakening with cough, chest tightness, and dyspnoea.

Exacerbating factors (e.g. cold dry air, pollen, fumes) → bronchial hyperresponsiveness, inflammatory bronchial wall oedema, and intra-luminal mucus accumulation → airway narrowing, airflow obstruction and distal air trapping.

Acute severe asthma either occurs for no reason or with infection or exposure to allergen/irritant.

Clinical features

- Breathlessness.
- Cough.
- *Expiratory wheezing:* best heard towards full expiration.
- Chest tightness.

Diagnosis of asthma

- Based on characteristic clinical features and history.
- Measurement of variability in peak expiratory flow rate (PEFR) measurements is useful.
- Typical spirometry shows ↓ PEFR with >15% reduction in response to stimulus challenge, e.g. 6–10min of strenuous exercise. PEFR is <60% predicted or varies by >30%; or PEFR improves by >20% with bronchodilators or steroids.

Management

- Identify and avoid triggers (limited evidence of efficacy).
- Relieve acute symptoms with β-agonist inhalers and suppression of chronic inflammatory airways hyper-reactivity with inhaled or oral steroids (good efficacy) or leukotriene antagonists (very expensive) (see Fig. 5.2).
- Once asthma is controlled, therapy should be stepped-down. Regular review of patients is important during this process. Patients should be maintained on the lowest possible dose of inhaled steriod. See http://www.brit-thoracic.org.uk/Portals/0/Guidelines/AsthmaGuidelines/sign101%20Jan%202012.pdf for further information.

Aims of treatment

- Freedom from symptoms, especially nocturnal asthma.
- Lung function in the normal range varying by <20% during 24h.
- Normal quality of life with self-management of condition.

Paediatric note

- Ask about eczema and hay fever (in child and in family) as these suggest atopy, and are associated with asthma.
- In children <2yrs, a formal diagnosis of asthma is not usually given. Children <2yrs who wheeze and may need treatment, (often caused by a viral trigger), may or may not later develop asthma and these episodes are termed 'viral induced wheeze'.
- Management of asthma in children is based on age and response to treatment. In those aged 2–5yrs, start with occasional relief bronchodilators, then add regular preventer therapy if needed. This may be an inhaled steroid (or a leukotriene receptor antagonist if inhaled steroid cannot be used). A step-up from this would be to use both of these agents. If control is not achieved, specialist advice should be sought if possible.

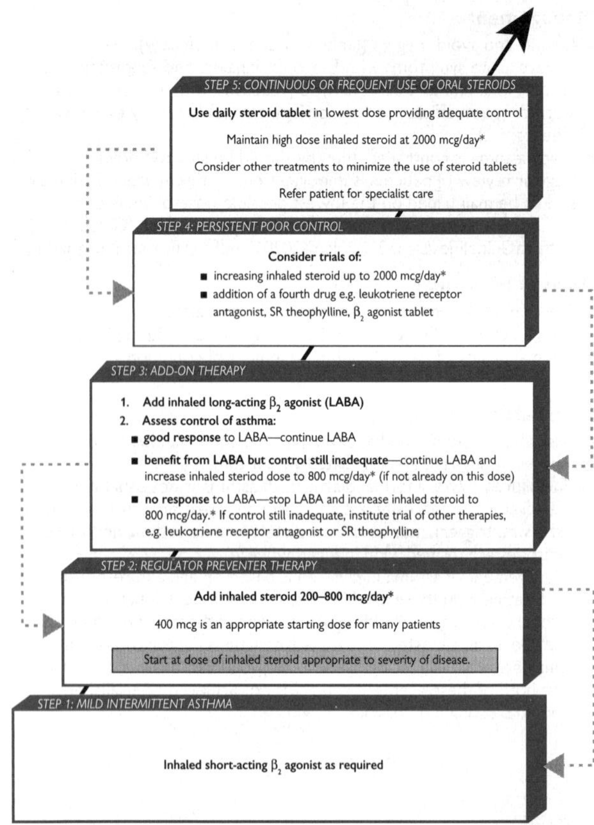

STEP 5: CONTINUOUS OR FREQUENT USE OF ORAL STEROIDS
Use daily steroid tablet in lowest dose providing adequate control
Maintain high dose inhaled steroid at 2000 mcg/day*
Consider other treatments to minimize the use of steroid tablets
Refer patient for specialist care
STEP 4: PERSISTENT POOR CONTROL
Consider trials of:
■ increasing inhaled steroid up to 2000 mcg/day*
■ addition of a fourth drug e.g. leukotriene receptor antagonist, SR theophylline, β_2 agonist tablet
STEP 3: ADD-ON THERAPY
1. Add inhaled long-acting β_2 agonist (LABA)
2. Assess control of asthma:
■ good response to LABA—continue LABA
■ benefit from LABA but control still inadequate—continue LABA and increase inhaled steriod dose to 800 mcg/day* (if not already on this dose)
■ no response to LABA—stop LABA and increase inhaled steroid to 800 mcg/day.* If control still inadequate, institute trial of other therapies, e.g. leukotriene receptor antagonist or SR theophylline
STEP 2: REGULATOR PREVENTER THERAPY
Add inhaled steroid 200–800 mcg/day*
400 mcg is an appropriate starting dose for many patients
Start at dose of inhaled steroid appropriate to severity of disease.
STEP 1: MILD INTERMITTENT ASTHMA
Inhaled short-acting β_2 agonist as required
* BDP or equivalent

Fig. 5.2 Summary of stepwise management in adults. BDP = beclometasone dipropionate; LABA = long acting beta agonist. Reproduced with kind permission from the British Thoracic Society, BMJ Group.

Acute severe asthma

Ascertain the recent best or predicted PEFR, the current medication, especially that recently taken for relief of this attack and when was the last severe attack.

Features of severe asthma

- Cannot speak in whole sentences.
- Respiration >25breaths/min.
- Pulse >110beats/min.
- PEFR <50% of best or predicted.

Life-threatening asthma

- Silent chest, cyanosis, or feeble respiratory effort.
- Bradycardia, dysrhythmia, or hypotension.
- Exhaustion, confusion, or coma.
- O_2 saturations <92%, pO_2 <8kPa(60mmHg), pCO_2 normal or ↑, pH ↓.
- PEFR <33% of best or predicted.
- *Rule out airway obstruction:* foreign body, epiglottitis, mediastinal mass.

Immediate management

- Sit the patient up and give high flow O_2.
- Give salbutamol 5mg or terbutaline 10mg by O_2-driven nebulizer. (Alternately give 10 puffs of salbutamol 100mcg via a spacer and repeat every 10–20min as necessary.)
- Give hydrocortisone 100mg IV or prednisolone 40–60mg oral.
- Do oximetry, CXR, PEFR.

If there is no improvement or there are signs of life-threatening asthma

- Add ipratropium 0.5mg to the nebulized salbutamol.
- Give aminophylline 5mg/kg by IV infusion over 20min, but avoid or use with great caution in patients already taking oral aminophylline.
- Contact an anaesthetist about possible emergency intubation if patient continues to deteriorate.

If the patient is improving continue with

- Oxygen (high flow) guided by O_2 saturations which should be >92%.
- Prednisolone 40–60mg oral od or hydrocortisone 100mg IV qds.
- Salbutamol 5mg nebulized 4–6-hourly and as required.

If the patient is not improving

- Continue with O_2 and steroids.
- Nebulized salbutamol 5mg up to every 15–30min until bronchospasm is relieved.
- Ipratropium 0.5mg qds.
- IV magnesium 1.2–2g single dose over 20min if bronchodilator not working.
- Intubation if exhausted.

Monitoring response to therapy

- PEFR 15–30min after treatment and at least 6-hourly.
- Maintain SaO_2 >92% with supplemental oxygen.
- Recheck ABG to monitor potential respiratory failure.

On discharge from hospital

The patient should have been:

- Stable on discharge medication for 24h and have had their inhaler technique checked and recorded.
- PEFR >75% of best or predicted and PEFR diurnal variability <25% (no nocturnal dipping).
- Treatment initiated with high dose inhaled steroids to cover tapering oral steroid therapy.
- Follow up in 1wk and provide emergency plan.

Paediatric note

Acute severe asthma in children >2yrs includes those with:
O_2 saturation <92%, PEFR 33–50% of best or predicted, too breathless to talk, using accessory muscles and:

- *Pulse:*
  - >140 in children 2–5yrs
  - >125 in children >5yrs.
- *Respiration:*
  - >40breaths/min aged 2–5yrs
  - >30breaths/min aged >5yrs.

Life-threatening features include: O_2 saturation <92%, silent chest, cyanosis, poor respiratory effort, hypotension, exhaustion, agitation, and confusion. PEFR <33% predicted.

Management is initially with O_2, bronchodilators (salbutamol 1st line) and steroids.

- Nebulizers repeated in acute severe asthma every 20–30min.
- Ipratropium bromide 250micrograms/dose (nebulised) can be effective in acute severe asthma, given frequently in the first few hours of admission (can be mixed with salbutamol). It should then be weaned to 4–6-hourly.
- Give prednisolone early in acute asthma attacks (20mg oral prednisolone 2–5yrs, 30–40mg >5yrs). Course usually 3d. Repeat dose if the child vomits, or give IV hydrocortisone if necessary.
- Seek help for further management and parenteral therapy (IV salbutamol or aminophylline may be used).

For further information: http://www.brit- thoracic.org.uk/Portals/0/Guidelines/AsthmaGuidelines/sign101%20Jan%202012.pdf

Chronic obstructive pulmonary disease

This is a chronic progressive disease of the airways and alveoli, which occurs in smokers, ex-smokers, and non-smokers exposed to smoke or high levels of indoor air pollution.

Pathology

Inhalation of smoke → neutrophil inflammatory response in the airways which overcomes the protective effects of pulmonary protease inhibitors and → chronic bronchial inflammation and airway damage. Lung defences are ↓ by smoke → recurrent respiratory infections and bacterial colonization of the proximal airways. Bronchial mucosal gland, hyperplasia, and hypertrophy → excessive mucus secretion and airway thickening and narrowing → chronic productive cough, often seasonal and worse in winters. Alveoli are particularly damaged in emphysema → loss of lung units and over-distension of the remaining alveoli → compression of the terminal bronchioles → further airway obstruction.

Clinical features

Patients with chronic obstructive pulmonary disease (COPD) experience chronic productive cough, recurrent respiratory infections, and/or exertional dyspnoea. PFTs deteriorate after respiratory infections, and may take weeks to recover. Minor respiratory infections may → respiratory failure and necessitate hospitalization. Patients are often wheezy, tachypnoeic, and use accessory muscles during exacerbations. In advanced cases patients may be plethoric, cyanosed, and have cor pulmonale. Type I (hypoxic, normocapnic) or Type II (hypercapnic) respiratory failure is common. Confusion, drowsiness, and flapping tremor indicates CO_2 retention.

Management

Stopping smoking is essential (see Box 5.8 for advice to smokers). Long-acting bronchodilators provide relief. Inhaled corticosteroids ↓ exacerbations and ↓ the rate of lung function deterioration. Combination inhalers are effective and should be given with a spacer device to improve delivery. Tiotropium once daily provides further symptomatic relief if available. Chest physiotherapy and mucolytics may help in clearing mucus and ↑ respiratory muscle strength.

In exacerbation

Oral steroids and antibiotics are helpful, but the risk of steroid side-effects (proximal muscle weakness, obesity, osteoporosis, skin bruising etc.) is high. In acute exacerbation, non-invasive ventilation can be life-saving and full ventilation often has difficulty weaning.

O_2 therapy should be closely monitored; high concentrations of O_2 may → CO_2 retention and narcosis. Home and portable O_2 therapy helps many patients—long-term oxygen therapy (LTOT; Box 5.9) is life-prolonging in chronically hypoxic patients, but not often available in developing countries.

Box 5.8 Advice to smokers regarding smoking cessation

- *Preparation:* make a positive decision and list reasons for quitting. Get the support of family/friends. Set a target date. Recognize the difficulty. Know that most relapses occur in the 1st week after quitting.
- *Switch brands:* to one that is distasteful and low in tar/nicotine.
- *Cut down the number of cigarettes:* smoke only half of each cigarette. Postpone the first cigarette of each day by 1h. Smoke only during odd or even hours of the day. Remember that cutting down is not a substitute for quitting.
- Do not smoke automatically, do not empty ashtrays.
- *Make smoking inconvenient:* buy one packet/cigarette at a time.
- *Make smoking unpleasant:* only smoke alone
- *Prepare for the target day:* practice going without cigarettes.
- *On the day of quitting:* throw away all cigarettes and matches; hide ashtrays and lighters. Make a list of things you want to buy, price them in terms of cigarettes, and put the money aside to buy them. Keep busy on the target day. Remind family/friends about the day.
- *Immediately after quitting:* develop a clean, fresh, non-smoking environment. Go to places where smoking is not allowed.
- *Avoid temptation:* avoid situations you associate with smoking; socialize only where smoking is not allowed.

Reproduced from Dilworth JP, Baldwin DR *Respiratory Medicine: A Specialist Handbook*, with permission from Informa Healthcare 2001.

Box 5.9 Oxygen therapy

- If the patient has a PaO_2 <8kPa on air, give a trial of O_2 at 2L/min via a mask. Recheck ABG after 1h.
- If there is no ↑ in $PaCO_2$, ↑ the O_2 to 4L/min and recheck ABGs after another hour. If you do not have blood gases, observe carefully for confusion, cyanosis, or flap.
- If the patient is not CO_2 retaining, they may have O_2 therapy without risk.
- If CO_2 does ↑, ↓ O_2 delivery to the level before which CO_2 was retained. Balance the risks of hypoxia and acidosis.
- At this point, if available, it is worth considering non-invasive ventilation via mask (e.g. BiPAP) to improve hypoxia and acidosis.

Bronchiectasis

Long-standing damage and dilatation of bronchi and bronchioles → inflammation and accumulation of infected mucus. Persistent infection within the bronchiectatic airways with *H. influenza*, *S. pneumoniae*, *M. catarrhalis*, or *P. aeruginosa* causes the clinical symptoms.

Aetiology

Most cases are 2° to inadequately treated pneumonia, pulmonary TB, TB lymph node disease, necrotizing pneumonias, whooping cough, foreign body inhalation, allergic bronchopulmonary aspergillosis (proximal bronchiectasis). In developed countries congenital conditions (e.g. cystic fibrosis, Kartagener's syndrome, or hypogammaglobulinaemia) are common, but these are almost unknown in Africa.

Clinical features of bronchiectasis

Depending on the severity, patients may produce large volumes (several cupfuls) of mucoid or purulent sputum daily. In milder disease, patients may be asymptomatic between acute exacerbations. Fever, haemoptysis, and chest pain are features of exacerbation, especially when infection spreads to the lung parenchyma → bronchopneumonia. Chronic sinusitis and otitis media may be associated. Clubbing is prominent, expiratory crackles with occasional wheezes are heard in the lungs.

Complications Recurrent episodes of pneumonia, hypoxia, and respiratory failure, massive haemoptysis, 2° amyloidosis, brain abscesses, and arthropathy.

Diagnosis

Largely based on the history and clinical features. Bronchiectatic cysts with fluid levels and 'tram lining' may be seen on CXRs, but CT scans are far more accurate. Airways obstruction and reversibility can be measured by PFTs to determine the usefulness of bronchodilators. Sputum should be cultured frequently if possible to choose appropriate antimicrobial therapy.

Management

- Physiotherapy is useful especially during acute exacerbations. Patients should be taught postural drainage and deep breathing/coughing exercises.
- Underlying conditions will require separate and continuous treatment. Focal disease with severe recurrent symptoms may be suitable for surgical resection, but CT often shows bronchiectasis is widespread and bilateral, which rules out surgery.
- Severe haemoptysis can be life-threatening → angiographic embolization or surgical resection in specialist centres.
- Airways obstruction requires bronchodilators and hydration.
- Broad-spectrum antibiotics, e.g. co-amoxiclav are indicated as soon as the patient is symptomatic with purulent sputum. Continue for 1–2wks.
- *Pseudomonas* colonization requires use of fluoroquinolones or IV ceftazidime or aminoglycosides—depending on sensitivities.
- If patients are requiring frequent repeated treatment with antibiotics, then use three or four oral antibiotics (amoxicillin, erythromycin, chloramphenicol, doxycycline) in rotation.

Prevention Hib, pneumococcal, and influenza vaccination. Early identification and treatment of TB and whooping cough.

Lung cancer

>95% of cases occur in smokers and is related to the quantity and duration of exposure to cigarette smoke ('pack-years'). Most patients are incurable, hence, prevention is essential.

Clinical features of lung cancer

Patients may be asymptomatic until late, then have:

- *Pulmonary features:* persistent cough or alteration in the previous chronic cough; haemoptysis; chest pain; dyspnoea. Distal pneumonia, pleural effusions, localized wheezing or stridor.
- Local/mediastinal invasion → vocal cord paralysis, Horner's syndrome, SVC obstruction, chest wall invasion, bony pains, brachial plexus involvement, dysphagia, and pericardial effusion.
- Metastatic spread → symptoms and signs affecting brain, liver, adrenal, skin, and bones (especially ribs, spine, and femoral). Lymph node involvement is common especially mediastinal and supraclavicular.
- Systemic symptoms → fatigue, lassitude, anorexia, marked ↓ weight. Fever may occur without infection.
- Endocrinopathies → SIADH, hypercalcaemia (from secretion of PTH-like substances or from bony metastases). Ectopic ACTH production, gynaecomastia and testicular atrophy can also occur.
- *Others:* clubbing is common, occasionally severe, with hypertrophic pulmonary osteoarthropathy. Neuromuscular syndromes (e.g. Lambert-Eaton syndrome) are rare.

Diagnosis

Based on CXR or CT imaging, which shows a mass, collapse/consolidation or invasive disease; CT is also useful in staging the disease. Histology is obtained from a biopsy/cytology obtained via a bronchoscopy/bronchoalveolar lavage (BAL), fine needle aspirate cytology (FNAC), CT-guided or open biopsy. The yield from sputum cytology is low; pleural fluid cytology is useful in patients with disseminated lung cancer and mesotheliomas. In many developing countries, bronchoscopy is possible, but histology is difficult to obtain. In this case it is important to consider treatable alternative diagnoses, e.g. TB.

Management

Surgery is often impossible because of spread or coexistent COPD. <20% of patients with localized non-small cell disease may be cured by surgery. Palliative chemotherapy and radiotherapy both prolong life and improve complications such as haemoptysis, SVC obstruction and recurrent pleural effusions. Patients with small cell cancer generally have disseminated disease and palliative chemotherapy and radiotherapy can extend and improve quality of life and manage complications.

Prevention Anti-smoking campaigns benefit patients and those exposed to passive smoke. ↓ chemicals and dust in the work environment.

Lung cancer: tumour types

- *Squamous cell carcinoma:* tumours with a medium rate of growth that often present with obstruction. Metastatic spread is common (80% at presentation).
- *Small-cell (oat-cell) carcinoma:* fast-growing tumours that often present with disseminated disease. They may secrete hormones.
- *Adenocarcinoma:* includes bronchoalveolar cell carcinoma; the most common peripheral tumour, it may produce mucin and can surround associated bronchi, stenosing the lumen. May not be smoking related.
- *Large-cell carcinoma:* large, necrotic, pleomorphic, mucin-producing tumours; frequently peripheral and locally invasive. Metastatic spread is common, survival rates post-surgery are good.
- *Carcinoid tumours:* unrelated to smoking and occur in a younger age group. May be benign adenomas or malignant. Most occur in proximal airways.
- *Metastases:* often from primaries in the breast, colon, kidney, prostate, and lung. Less often choriocarcinoma, testicular cancer, sarcomas, melanoma.
- *Mesotheliomas:* malignancies of the pleural space caused by exposure, often remote, to asbestos. Spread is local, but rarely may metastasize.

Interstitial lung disease

Painless progressive shortness of breath may indicate interstitial lung disease. Fortunately this is very much less common than infection as it is rarely treatable.

Clinical features

Careful history taking may define a risk factor for pulmonary fibrosis, e.g. mining or asbestos exposure. Clubbing is common; fine inspiratory crackles may be heard at both bases in the absence of signs of heart failure, or there may be no signs at all.

Investigation with CXR may show fine interstitial shadowing bilaterally or very little change in early disease. HRCT if available will detect early disease, and PFTs will show ↓ gas transfer. In advanced disease, clinical signs will be obvious, CXR abnormality will be marked and the patient will become hypoxic on minimal exertion.

Differential diagnosis

The classification of interstitial lung disease is based on CT appearance and histology, both of which have limited availability. Occupational lung diseases are diagnosed by the history, but most cases will not have an obvious cause. Sarcoidosis may be underdiagnosed.

Management

In resource-poor settings, palliation of symptoms is very difficult and treatment is impossible. Exacerbations due to infection can be treated, as can congestive cardiac failure (CCF). Steroids have limited benefit, and opiates are useful to control breathlessness.

Prevention

Control of industrial exposures is rudimentary in resource-poor countries, and exposures are often high in the absence of protective equipment. Prevention of occupational lung disease is best achieved with education and provision of better equipment.

Acute respiratory distress syndrome

Any severe infection or illness can be complicated by non-cardiogenic pulmonary oedema.

Aetiology

Burns, infection, surgery, trauma, pancreatitis, or poisoning can all → extensive pulmonary inflammation. Inflamed lung parenchyma then becomes leaky and fluid exudates, fills the alveolar space.

Clinical features

Severely ill patients become markedly hypoxic over a short period of time despite adequate circulation and Hb. Examination shows bilateral poor air entry, fine crackles, or large airway noise. CXR shows marked bilateral shadowing 'white out'.

Management

ARDS is very hard to manage, even in ICUs. Mechanical ventilation is essential. Treatment of the underlying diagnosis offers a chance of recovery, with organ support as can best be managed in the interim. Steroids are not usually helpful.

Pulmonary embolism

Risk factors for venous thrombosis are ↑ coagulability, stasis and damage to the vascular endothelium. Most PEs occur as a result of migration of soft thrombi of recent onset from the deep veins of the leg or pelvis to the pulmonary venous vasculature. Embolism from mural intracardiac thrombi and right sided endocarditis may also occur. Septic thrombophlebitis due to infected central lines or IV drug abuse is ↑ common.

- Oral contraceptives and pregnancy ↑ coagulability.
- Young patients with no underlying risk factors may present with severe thrombotic disease due to congenital or acquired thrombogenic states (protein C, S, antithrombin III deficiency, antiphospholipid antibody syndrome, etc.).
- Pregnancy or recent surgery and protracted immobility after injury/travel ↓ venous return.
- In resource-poor countries, severe dehydration (e.g. diabetic ketoacidosis), trauma, and obstetric emergencies often → PE owing to lack of prophylactic heparin.

Clinical features

Most patients will have minor and subacute symptoms with tachypnoea, mild dyspnoea, a cough and occasionally low grade fever. Some report a sudden onset of pleuritic chest pain and shortness of breath. In a few patients, haemoptysis indicates pulmonary infarction. If the diagnosis is missed, repeated emboli will occur. In patients with showers of low grade emboli over many years, pulmonary hypertension and cor pulmonale may ensue and patients may present with CCF and marked exertional dyspnoea. In cases of massive PE the patient has circulatory collapse and may die acutely.

On examination, respiratory findings are sparse, but hypoxia with a normal CXR suggests the possibility of a PE. A DVT may be present. Investigations: CXR, ECG (any abnormality particularly tachycardia, R axis deviation, or RBBB; classical S3Q3T3 is rare), V/Q scan, CT pulmonary angiogram, Doppler ultrasound of the legs and D-dimer levels. These tests are useful in both the confirmation and exclusion of DVTs and PEs.

Management

Anticoagulate with IV heparin or with twice daily low molecular weight heparin (expensive). The diagnosis of PE is not easy to make and so the Wells score (see Box 5.10) is used to define high, medium and low risk of recurrent PE. Using this score, a clinical decision can be made to institute oral anticoagulation with warfarin. Once a target INR of 2.5–3.0 is maintained for 48–72h then heparin can be safely discontinued. It is problematic, however, to manage warfarin anticoagulation where INR cannot be measured and the risk of haemorrhage is significant. In acute massive PE, thrombolysis with streptokinase may be useful if the diagnosis can be made confidently.

Box 5.10 The Wells score

- Clinically suspected DVT: 3.0 points
- Alternative diagnosis less likely than PE: 3.0 points
- Tachycardia: 1.5 points
- Immobilization/surgery in previous 4wks: 1.5 points
- History of DVT/PE: 1.5 points
- Haemoptysis: 1.0 points
- Malignancy (treatment for <6mths, palliative): 1.0 points

Traditional interpretation

Score >6.0	High (probability 59% based on pooled data)
Score 2.0 to 6.0	Moderate (probability 29% based on pooled data)
Score <2.0	Low (probability 15% based on pooled data)

Alternate interpretation

Score > 4	PE likely. Consider diagnostic imaging.
Score 4 or less	PE unlikely. Consider D-dimer to rule out PE.

Pneumothorax

Air leak into the pleural space → collapse and sometimes compression of the underlying lung. If a rapid ongoing accumulation of air occurs with each bout of coughing → tension pneumothorax; relief of the tension pneumothorax is an emergency. A small or moderate pneumothorax may be sufficient to cause respiratory failure in a patient with pre-existing lung disease. Pneumothorax may be asymptomatic in an otherwise healthy patient.

Causes

Spontaneous/1° pneumothorax

Common in tall and thin men with no pre-existing lung disease. 20% recur after 1st episode and 65% after a 2nd episode.

2° Pneumothorax

Occurs in patients with scars of previous TB or in patients with active TB, often cavitary. Also common in patients with COPD, and can complicate severe necrotizing lung infections such as staphylococcal pneumonia, aspiration pneumonias and in some cases of PCP.

Traumatic pneumothorax Occurs from penetrating injuries, e.g. stabbing or road traffic accident.

Iatrogenic pneumothorax May be a complication of central line insertion, transbronchial lung biopsy, or high pressure mechanical ventilation.

Clinical features

Most patients will complain of sudden onset of pleuritic chest pain and dyspnoea. Hyper-resonance to percussion is accompanied by ↓ movement and ↓ or absent breath sounds on the affected side. Breathing is generally shallow on account of splinting due to pain. A tension pneumothorax causes mediastinal displacement away from the pneumothorax, with severe tachypnoea, dyspnoea often with hypoxia and shock.

Management

- *Small pneumothoraces* (CXR shows pneumothorax occupies <15% of hemithorax) in asymptomatic, otherwise healthy, individuals need no treatment other than observation. Follow up X-rays should demonstrate gradual absorption of the pneumothorax (1% of lung area per day).
- *Symptomatic pneumothoraces* require needle aspiration. A plastic venous cannula is placed into the pleural space (above a rib in mid-axillary line) and a 3-way tap attached. A large syringe is used to draw air out of the chest and expelled through tubing held under water. Count the volume of air withdrawn and stop when resistance is felt on the cannula. Needle aspiration is suitable for iatrogenic pneumothoraces, because these are unlikely to recur.
- If aspiration fails or if > 2L of air is freely withdrawn it is likely that a bronchopleural fistula exists and an intercostal chest drain should be placed. Use the 5/6th intercostals space in the mid-axillary line. In developed countries, the method is to place pigtail drains by Seldinger technique under ultrasound guidance. This may not be practicable in

which case use traditional blunt dissection to place a drain with an underwater seal. Clamp the drain when the drain has stopped bubbling for 24h. Ideally repeat CXR, but if not possible, remove drain after 24h clamped if no recurrent symptoms.

- *Pleurodesis* may be required if pneumothorax fails to resolve despite 1–2wks of intercostal drainage and suction (Box 5.11).
- *Tension pneumothorax* is a medical emergency and requires the immediate placement of a wide bore needle into the 2nd intercostal space on the affected side. Air usually bubbles out in a rush and the relief is immediate. Intercostal tube drainage should follow.

Box 5.11 Pleurodesis

This procedure aims to cause sterile inflammation of the pleura and obliterate the pleural space by adhesions and fibrosis. It is painful and needs adequate analgesia: 20mL of 1% lidocaine is diluted with saline to 100mL and this is inserted into the chest tube which is then clamped. The patient is placed on his back, side and chest to disperse the lidocaine and after this is drained off, 1–1.5g of tetracycline dissolved in 30–50mL normal saline, or 20mL of povidone-iodine 10% in 80mL normal saline, is inserted into the chest drain and the procedure repeated. The solution is kept in the chest for 3–4h and then drained off. The chest drain is maintained in situ until air ceases to bubble through it.

Chapter 6
Diarrhoeal diseases

Invited authors **Mary E. Penny**
Fulton P. Rivera

Introduction

Diarrhoea is the passage of abnormally loose or fluid stools more frequently than normal. Normal bowel habit varies, but recent onset >3 liquid/loose stools per day is considered abnormal (see Box 6.1 for classification).

Infective diarrhoea is the 3rd highest cause of death due to infection in the world, with ~1–2 million deaths each year; 80% of deaths are in children <2yrs, most of these during and shortly after the introduction of complementary foods between 6–12mths. Micronutrient deficiencies, especially zinc deficiency, ↑ incidence of infective diarrhoea. Breastfeeding, especially exclusive breastfeeding, confers significant protection. Repeated attacks of diarrhoea initiate a vicious cycle of malnutrition, reduced immunity, and more intestinal infections. Diarrhoea is a common symptom of HIV/AIDS.

An accurate history will give clues to the aetiology and severity of diarrhoea. Ask about previous episodes and current medication.

The treatment of most diarrhoeal episodes depends on managing and preventing dehydration regardless of the aetiology. Antimicrobials are only recommended for dysentery and cholera, and for severe episodes with laboratory diagnosis in certain vulnerable groups (see Box 6.2).

Anti-diarrhoeal agents should be avoided in young children.

Some key questions to be asked

- How long has the diarrhoea been present?
- Is there (or was there) fever or other systemic symptoms?
- Is there blood (bright red or dark) and/or mucus?
- How frequent are the motions?
- What is the stool volume?
- Is there abdominal pain—if so, where?
- Is there tenesmus (a sense of incomplete emptying following defecation)?
- Has the patient vomited—if so, how much, when, what?
- Has the patient lost weight?
- Have any household or close contacts had diarrhoea?
- What did they eat and drink in the 72h before getting diarrhoea—anything unusual?
- If the diarrhoea is recurrent/remittent, is it related to any particular food or drink?
- Is anyone else in the family ill?
- Is there a history of recent travel? If so, where?
- Has the patient been exposed to malaria?
- Is the patient at risk of HIV infection?

In examining the patient, one should look for signs of dehydration and malnutrition, as well as for clues to the aetiology (Box 6.3).

Box 6.1 Classification of diarrhoea

- Subdivide diarrhoeal diseases according to presence or not of blood in the stool, since the causes are generally different. Be aware that both shigellosis and *Campylobacter* infections may present as acute watery or bloody diarrhoea.
- Divide the diseases into acute diarrhoea with blood (dysentery) and acute diarrhoea without blood (enteritis).
- Persistent diarrhoea lasts >14d. Additional diseases need to be considered—see other topics in this chapter and always consider HIV.

Box 6.2 Antimicrobial drugs

Antimicrobials are only indicated in:

- *Bloody diarrhoea (dysentery) that does not improve after 3 days of rehydration therapy:* if a specific cause is found, it should be treated appropriately (see 🕮 Acute diarrhoea with blood, p. 238). If no cause can be found, an antimicrobial effective against *Shigella* (e.g. ciprofloxacin) should be given. Local antibiotic resistance should be taken into account.
- *Cholera with severe dehydration*: any suspected case of cholera should be treated with an effective antimicrobial (e.g. azithromycin) and control agencies notified.
- *Laboratory-proven symptomatic cases of* Giardia intestinalis *infection that* do not improve after 3d of ORS therapy should be treated with an antimicrobial (e.g. tinidazole).
- *Laboratory-proven enteropathogenic* E. coli *infections:* respond to antibiotics (e.g. ciprofloxacin) and should be used in vulnerable individuals.
- *Travellers' diarrhoea:* duration ↓ when treated with an antibiotic (e.g. ciprofloxacin).

The direct faecal smear

See Fig. 6.1.

1. Write the patient's name on a clean slide. Place a drop of sterile saline in the centre of the left-hand side of the slide and place a drop of iodine in the centre of the right-hand side of the slide.
2. With a match or applicator, pick up a small portion of faeces (~2mg—or about the size of a match head) and add it to the drop of saline. Repeat and add to the iodine. Mix the faeces with the drops to form suspensions.
3. Cover each drop with a coverslip.
4. Examine each drop with the x10 objective or, for identification, with the higher-power objectives, searching in a systematic manner. When organisms are seen, switch to higher power for more detail.

Box 6.3 Investigations

- Most uncomplicated cases of diarrhoea can be managed without laboratory tests. In a hospital setting, or if diarrhoea continues beyond 2–3d, do FBC, U&E, and glucose.
- Stool culture and microscopy are often requested, but few centres can offer diagnostic tests for all enteropathogens (see Fig. 6.2):
  - mixed infections are common; single-stool cultures are insufficient for some pathogens (e.g. *Giardia*, amoebae, *Shigella*)
  - results often come back too late to influence management.
- Faecal lactoferrin appears more sensitive than faecal leukocyte smear, and accurately rules out inflammatory diarrhoea. Presence of faecal lactoferrin supports use of immediate empiric therapy in the very young, elderly and immunocompromised individuals.
- Apart from investigation of outbreaks, surveillance, and research purposes, stool culture in uncomplicated cases should be limited to exclusion of pathogens for which antibiotic treatment is indicated (e.g. parasites, *Shigella* species, and *Vibrio cholerae*).
- If appropriate, do a blood film for malaria.

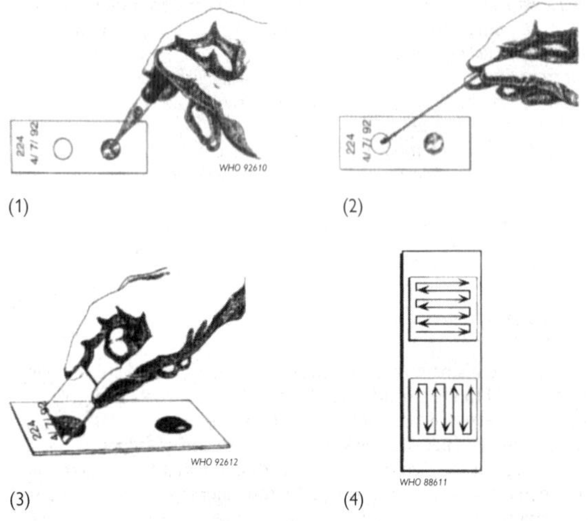

Fig. 6.1 How to make a direct faecal smear.

Reproduced with permission, from *Bench Aids for the Diagnosis of Malaria*, 2nd edition, Geneva: WHO.

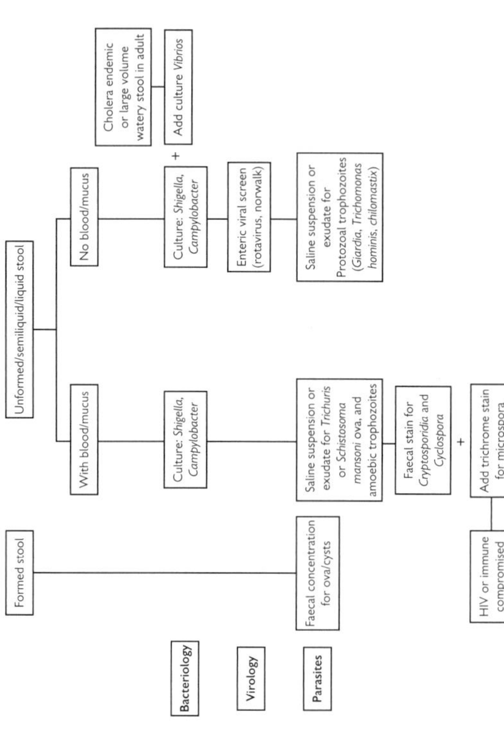

Fig. 6.2 Recommended diagnostic tests for enteropathogens depending on stool characteristics.

Acute diarrhoea with blood

Presence of blood in diarrhoea is called *dysentery* and usually signifies ulceration of large bowel. The most common bacterial agents causing dysentery are *Shigella* (bacillary dysentery), *Campylobacter* and *Entamoeba histolytica* (amoebic dysentery). Dysentery should be treated on clinical diagnosis with antibiotics that cover *Shigella* (e.g. ciprofloxacin). If no improvement after 48h, antibiotics should be changed taking into account stool culture findings. If culture results are –ve or unavailable, still change the antibiotic (e.g. from co-trimoxazole to ciprofloxacin, or from ciprofloxacin to azithromycin) on the basis of a lack of clinical response to initial therapy.

Shigellosis (bacillary dysentry)

Shigella dysenteriae, S. flexneri, S. boydii, and *S. sonneii* cause bacillary dysentery (Box 6.4), with the former two species responsible for most morbidity and mortality (which may reach 20% in untreated cases). The disease may occur both endemically and epidemically, with children most frequently affected. Humans are the only natural host. The incubation period is 1–5d following direct person to person contact (often with asymptomatic excreters) or ingestion of contaminated water and food.

Clinical features

Range from mild disease in which there is intermittent watery diarrhoea, to severe systemic complications. In severe cases, onset is usually rapid, with tenesmus, fever, and passage of frequent (up to 100/d or ~every 15min) bloody mucoid stools.

Intestinal complications Include toxic megacolon, perforation, and protein-losing enteropathy.

Systemic complications Include dehydration, hypoglycaemia, and electrolyte imbalance (particularly hyponatraemia), haemolytic-uraemic syndrome (Box 6.5), convulsions (particularly in children, often before the onset of diarrhoea), Reiter's syndrome, thrombotic thrombocytopenic purpura, and pneumonia. Invasive disease may give 'rose spots'—crops of 2–4mm papules, which fade on pressure, usually appearing on the upper abdomen and lower chest.

Diagnosis

The clinical distinction between bacillary and amoebic dysentery is difficult. Stool microscopy often shows leukocytes (pus cells) in shigellosis vs. haematophagus trophozoites in amoebic dysentery. Confirmation is made by stool culture, serological and biochemical tests.

Management

Oral rehydration is sufficient for mild disease. In severe disease, ampicillin or trimethoprim (or co-trimoxazole) should be given, although resistance is common; quinolones (e.g. ciprofloxacin) are an alternative. Antimicrobial therapy should be tailored to the local sensitivity pattern if individual sensitivity of isolates is not possible.

Prevention

Food and hand hygiene; specific vaccines are under development, but are not yet widely available.

Reiter's syndrome

Classic Reiter's syndrome is a triad of urethritis, conjunctivitis, and a seronegative, large joint, mono- or oligoarthritis; it can follow dysentery.

Associated features Iritis, enthesopathy, keratoderma blenorrhagica, and circinate balanitis.

Box 6.4 Infective causes of acute diarrhoea with blood (dysentery)

- Bacillary dysentery (shigellosis).
- Enterohaemorrhagic *E. coli.*
- *Campylobacter* enterocolitis.
- *Salmonella* enterocolitis.
- *Clostridium difficile* associated (pseudomembranous) colitis.
- *Yersinia* enterocolitis.
- Amoebic dysentery.
- *Balantidium coli* enterocolitis.
- Massive *Trichuris* infection.
- *S. mansoni* or *S. japonicum.*
- CMV in immunosuppressed (📖 HIV/AIDS, p. 69).

All may also cause diarrhoea without blood. Non-infectious causes include IBD, colorectal cancer or polyps, ischaemic colitis.

Enterohaemorrhagic *E. coli*

These bacteria produce vero cell cytotoxins similar to the toxin produced by *Shigella dysenteriae*, known as Shiga-like toxin. The most common EHEC is *E. coli* 0157. However, many other serogroups (non-0157) of these bacteria can cause disease, including *E. coli* serogroups 026, 0111, 0103. These bacteria have been associated with a number of outbreaks of inflammatory, haemorrhagic colitis, and HUS. Infections occur most frequently in the summer months. Contaminated food is the most common cause, particularly ground beef in hamburgers or milk. Fruit, vegetables, and cider may be contaminated by animal faeces. Cross-contamination of meat products has been responsible for outbreaks.

Clinical features

Illness usually starts with watery diarrhoea, blood appearing after 2–3d. Vomiting and abdominal tenderness are common (can mimic appendicitis, intussusception, or IBD). HUS (see Box 6.5) may complicate EHEC infection.

Diagnosis

In patients who present with an acute onset of bloody diarrhoea (especially without fever) or HUS, faecal testing for Shiga toxin should be performed, along with cultures for *E. coli* 0157:H7. The presence of an outbreak and exposure risk is often found in the history.

Management

- Oral rehydration and supportive care.
- Antibiotics are not indicated: they have been associated with ↑ duration and may ↑ risk of HUS.
- Antimotility drugs should be *avoided.*

Prevention

Improve animal husbandry and slaughterhouse management to prevent contamination of meat with intestinal content; pasteurize dairy products; cook beef adequately; wash hands frequently with soap including after contact with farm animals or meat.

Box 6.5 Haemolytic uraemic syndrome

- HUS complicates 6–9% of EHEC infections and ~15% of EHEC infections in children <10yrs. However, 30% of cases, 80% of whom were adults followed an outbreak of 0104:H4 infection in Germany.
- As a whole, the non-0157 serogroups are less likely to cause severe illness than *E. coli* 0157; but occasionally, non-0157 serogroups can cause the most severe manifestations.
- HUS is characterized by a microangiopathic haemolytic anaemia, thrombocytopenia, renal failure, and CNS involvement. Clinical features overlap with those of thrombotic thrombocytopenic purpura (TTP) in which CNS involvement is much more common.

Campylobacter enterocolitis

C. jejuni (also *C. coli* and *C. lari*) cause epidemics in nurseries or paediatric wards and are common in the community in resource-poor regions. Bacteria may be excreted in the faeces up to 3wks after cessation of diarrhoea. *Campylobacter* spp. infect most mammals and birds and transmission may be by contact with animal or poultry excreta or contaminated food or water.

Clinical features

Episodes typically start with fever, abdominal pain, and watery diarrhoea. This may be followed by bloody diarrhoea, indistinguishable from *Shigella* and *Salmonella* infections. Abdominal pain may be prominent even after diarrhoea settles. The disease normally settles in 5–7d. Severe, disseminated infection can occur in presence of malnutrition, liver disease, malignancy, diabetes, renal failure, and immunosuppression. Complications include bacteraemia, meningitis, deep abscesses, cholecystitis, reactive arthritis/Reiter's syndrome, and GBS.

Diagnosis

Gram stain or dark-field microscopy of faecal smears shows curved Gram –ve rods with 'gull wing' and 'S-shapes'; confirmed on culture. In severe disease, colonoscopy/biopsy may be needed.

Prevention
Campylobacter infection is an almost ubiquitous zoonosis. Prevention depends on breaking the chain of food and water contamination. No vaccine is currently available.

Yersinia enterocolitis

Yersinia enterocolitica is a rare cause of diarrhoea in the tropics. There may be low-grade fever, bloody diarrhoea, and abdominal pain affecting mainly children <5yrs, plus nausea, vomiting, headache, or pharyngitis. Infection may spread to cause

- Septicaemia.
- Peritonitis.
- Hepatic, renal, and splenic abscesses.
- Pyomyositis.
- Osteomyelitis.

These complications are more common in immunocompromised patients or those who are iron overloaded (e.g. haemochromatosis).

Diagnosis Culture from stool or other sites of infection.

Management of *Campylobacter and Yersinia* enterocolitis

Rehydration and supportive care are usually sufficient for *Campylobacter* and *Yersinia* infections. Severe disease may require antibiotics.

Campylobacter Use erythromycin; resistant strains (especially *C. coli*) may need trimethoprim (or co-trimoxazole), ciprofloxacin, or azithromycin.

Yersinia In complicated disease, use one of the following: gentamicin, cefotaxime, ciprofloxacin, or doxycycline.

Salmonella enterocolitis

Salmonella typhimurium and *S. enteritidis* enterocolitis are an important public health problem in resource-poor regions. Transmission is usually by ingestion of contaminated food (they survive freezing at –20°C). The organisms are common among wild and domestic animals. Reptiles kept as pets may also be a source of *Salmonella* infection. The incubation period is 24–48h (up to 72h); bacteria are then excreted in the faeces for up to 8wks following infection. More common in HIV+ individuals.

Clinical features
Range in severity according to the serotype involved. Two (often overlapping) clinical syndromes are seen:

- *Acute enterocolitis:* nausea and vomiting, headache, fever, and malaise, rapidly progressing to diarrhoea with cramping abdominal pains. Initially voluminous and watery, the stool changes to bloody with mucus as the disease progresses. There may be left iliac fossa (LIF) pain and rebound tenderness. Infrequently, ileal involvement is dominant with symptoms mimicking appendicitis. Toxic megacolon may complicate severe colitis.

- *Invasive salmonellosis:* bacteraemia rates of 8% have been recorded, with ↑ rates for certain serotypes. Predisposing factors are:
  - extremes of age
  - immunosuppression, especially HIV
  - malignancy
  - gastric hypoacidity (e.g. antacid use)
  - severe comorbidity
  - malarial anaemia
  - sickle cell disease.
- Invasive salmonellosis is characterized by swinging fevers, rigors, and toxaemia accompanying diarrhoea, or a typhoid-like illness characterized by sustained fever, splenomegaly, rose spots, and minimal diarrhoea.
- There may be spread to CSF (children <2yrs), bones and joints, lungs, heart valves and arteries, liver, spleen, ovaries, or kidneys, and a reactive arthritis can occur.
- Patients with chronic schistosomiasis are prone to 2° *Salmonella* bacteraemia, since the bacteria live within the worm and are protected from antibiotics.

Diagnosis

Requires isolation of the bacteria from faecal or blood cultures. Sigmoidoscopy may be necessary in severely ill patients. *Salmonella typhi* and *S. paratyphi* (📖 Typhoid and paratyphoid fevers, p. 748) do not usually present with diarrhoea and should not be confused with enterocolitis due to non-typhi *Salmonellae*.

Management

- Rehydration and supportive care are usually sufficient.
- Most antibiotics do not ↓ duration and may ↑ bacterial carriage.
- Treat patients with severe colitis and/or invasive disease, or in whom the risk of developing severe disease is high (e.g. neonates, immunosuppressed, and elderly).
- Ciprofloxacin 500mg oral bd for 5d is commonly used in adults. There are very limited data on quinolone use in neonates, although it is increasing. Possible risks should be balanced against substantial risk of invasive disease and availability of alternative therapies.
- Chloramphenicol, amoxicillin, trimethoprim, or co-trimoxazole may be effective in systemic disease, but there is ↑ resistance.
- Cefotaxime/ceftriaxone still highly effective, where available.

Amoebic dysentery

~ 48 million people worldwide are infected by the protozoan *Entamoeba histolytica* and, although only ~10% are symptomatic, it is an important parasitic cause of death with an annual mortality of ~70 000. Severe infection occurs in pregnant women, very young children, the malnourished, and people on steroids. Most of those previously thought to have asymptomatic *E. histolytica* infection are actually infected with the related amoeba *E. dispar*, which is morphologically indistinguishable but non-pathogenic to humans.

Transmission

Usually via food and drink contaminated with human faeces; prevalence is highest where human faeces are used as fertilizer. Faeco-oral sexual transmission also occurs. Cysts are ingested and pass into the small and large intestine, dividing to form metacysts and trophozoites. As trophozoites pass through the colon they desiccate to form 'precysts' and then cysts. Mature cysts are evacuated in the stool, and remain viable and infective for up to 2mths in cool, damp conditions. *E. histolytica* has the capacity to destroy almost any tissue in the body, with amoebic liver abscess being the most common extra-intestinal manifestation.

Clinical features

- Related to degree and location of tissue damage by trophozoites and range from an asymptomatic carrier state to fulminant colitis and invasive extra-intestinal disease (see Box 6.6).
- Intestinal amoebiasis usually has an insidious onset with abdominal discomfort and diarrhoea becoming increasingly bloody and mucoid as severity increases.
- Rectosigmoid involvement is frequently associated with tenesmus.
- On palpation, there may be tenderness over the caecum, transverse, and sigmoid colon; if there is a liver abscess (which rarely accompanies dysentery), the liver may be enlarged and tender.
- Colonoscopy may reveal hyperaemic, necrotic ulcers covered with a yellowish exudate, particularly in the region of the flexures.

Complications

Include toxic megacolon and bowel perforation. Following repeated infection, an amoebic granuloma (amoeboma) may develop (most frequently at the caecum) where it may be palpable and mistaken for a malignant mass.

Diagnosis

Often difficult and relies on identification of *E. histolytica* cysts or trophozoites in the stool. Demonstration of cysts does not prove amoebiasis as cause of symptoms—*E. histolytica* cysts are microscopically identical to common, non-pathogenic *E. dispar* cysts.

- Examine at least three stool samples for cysts, using concentration and permanent stain techniques, preferably before administration of medications or contrast media, since these interfere with amoebae recovery.
- A 'hot stool' (examined <30min) is required to look for trophozoites. Examine a wet mount preparation for motile amoebae. The presence of *E. histolytica* trophozoites containing ingested erythrocytes is diagnostic of amoebiasis.
- Techlab Entamoeba 11® is a faecal ELISA that will differentiate invasive *E. histolytica* cysts or trophozoites from those of *E. dispar*.
- *E. histolytica* serology useful in non-endemic areas.

Management

- Metronidazole is effective against the trophozoites, but because it has little effect on the cysts, treatment should be followed by a luminal amoebicide, such as diloxanide or paromomycin.

- Give metronidazole 800mg oral tds for 5d, *followed by* diloxanide furoate 500mg oral tds for 10d (alternative to metronidazole: tinidazole 2g daily × 3d; alternative to diloxanide: paromomycin 25-35mg/kg/d in three divided doses × 7d).
- If there are signs of peritonism, add a broad-spectrum antibiotic.

Prevention

Ensure safe disposal of human faeces; prevent faecal contamination of water supplies. Filtering water with sand or diatomaceous earth is effective. Address personal hygiene, including hand washing.

Box 6.6 Extra-intestinal amoebiasis

- Following colonic invasion, trophozoites may travel to the liver via the portal circulation; further direct or haematogenous spread may occur to almost any tissue of the body.
- The most common form of extra-intestinal disease is amoebic liver abscess (ALA; 📖 Amoebic liver abscess, p. 316). ~10% ALA patients have diarrhoea; ~20% have a history of previous dysentery.
- Digestion of hepatocytes by trophozoites leads to foci of liver necrosis, which coalesce to form abscesses containing reddish-brown 'anchovy sauce' fluid. This fluid is digested liver, not pus (WBC not seen on microscopy) and has no odour; it seldom contains visible amoebae.
- Rupture into the pericardium (especially of left lobe abscesses) causes *pericardial amoebiasis*, often → cardiac tamponade and death; adequate pericardial drainage usually requires thoracotomy.
- ALA rupture through the diaphragm to form a bronchohepatic fistula and cause pleuro-pulmonary amoebiasis, with cough, dyspnoea, and expectoration of 'anchovy sauce' material.
- *Peritoneal amoebiasis* occurs due to colonic or ALA rupture, *cutaneous amoebiasis* due to percutaneous rupture, and *cerebral amoebiasis* due to haematogenous spread.
- All may occur without diarrhoea.

Diagnosis

Usually clinical +/– demonstration of trophozoites (which may be scarce) in the affected tissue and/or in the stool. Amoebic serology is sensitive.

Management

- Medical management as for amoebic dysentery.
- Liver abscess often aspirated to differentiate from bacterial liver abscess (fluid is pus, usually yellow or blood-streaked, often foul-smelling).
- In bacterial liver abscess, drainage or aspiration is important for cure.
- In ALA, drainage or aspiration of abscess is indicated if poor response to medical therapy or high risk of rupture (especially for abscess in left lobe of liver).

Balantidium enterocolitis

Balantidium coli is a rare protozoal pathogen of humans, existing in cyst and trophozoite forms; cysts are responsible for faeco-oral transmission. Trophozoites invade intestinal mucosa producing inflammation and ulceration. Clinical features resemble amoebic colitis and include:

- Asymptomatic carrier state (80%).
- Acute dysentery that may be associated with nausea, abdominal pain, and weight loss. This is potentially fatal.
- Chronic diarrhoea, frequently without blood.

Diagnosis Rests upon identification of the trophozoite in the faeces.

Management

- Symptomatic plus rehydration.
- Give tetracycline 500mg oral qds for 10d in severe disease.
- *Alternatives:* ampicillin, metronidazole.

Trichuriasis (whipworm)

Thought to infect ~25% of world's population, *Trichuris trichiura* are 3–4cm long. Colonize colon and rectum after ingestion of faecally contaminated soil.

Life cycle

- Ingested eggs hatch in the small intestine releasing larvae which mature in the villi for ~1wk before colonizing the caecum and colorectum.
- Released eggs pass out in the stool and can resist low temperatures, but not desiccation.
- The time from ingestion to appearance of eggs in the faeces is 60–70d (See Fig. 6.3). Heavy infection is most common in children.

Clinical features

Often absent in mild infections, but co-infection with *Ascaris lumbricoides* or hookworms common and may result in abdominal distension, flatulence, RIF pain, vomiting, and weight loss. Heavy worm burden can → GI haemorrhage, mucopurulent stool, dysentery +/– rectal prolapse (worms usually seen attached to prolapsed mucosa), and growth retardation. Massive worm burdens may cause protein-losing enteropathy, severe anaemia, and finger clubbing. Severe infection with *E. histolytica* or *B. coli* can aggravate mucosal ulceration and exacerbate dysentery.

Diagnosis

By detection of eggs in stool (>30000/g stool = heavy infection (several hundred adult worms)). There may be anaemia, hypoalbuminaemia, and eosinophilia. Proctoscopy may reveal worms attached to reddened, ulcerated rectal mucosa. AXR can show changes similar to those seen in Crohn's disease.

Management

Mebendazole 500mg or albendazole 400mg, both oral once, are equally effective, although there may be regional differences in albendazole sensitivity. 3-d courses may be used for heavy infections.

Prevention Control is as for other soil-transmitted helminths.

Clostridium difficile associated diarrhoea and colitis

Condition (also known as antibiotic-associated colitis and pseudomembranous colitis) caused by infection with *C. difficile* following disruption of normal bowel flora by antibiotic therapy. An important cause of hospital-acquired diarrhoea.

Clinical features

Due to production of toxins and vary from asymptomatic to severe colitis with toxic megacolon. Disease severity probably depends on combination of patient co-morbidity, and degree of exposure to both antibiotics and *C. difficile* spores. In elderly hospitalized patients or those with significant co-morbidity, carries a high mortality. Sigmoidoscopy shows characteristic yellow mucosal plaques (pseudomembranes).

Management

- Metronidazole 800mg po stat, then 400mg oral tds for 10 days.
- Oral vancomycin (125mg qds for 7–10d) is an expensive alternative.

Prevention

Avoid indiscriminate or unnecessarily prolonged use of antibiotics. Hand washing, barrier nursing, and environmental cleaning to eradicate spores are fundamental to preventing transmission in hospitals.

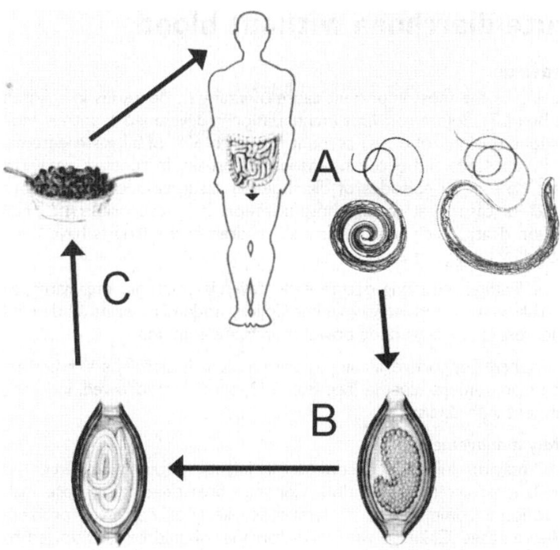

Fig. 6.3 Life cycle of *Trichuris trichiura*. The adult worms (A) are 75cm long (male, shown on the left, is more tightly curled) and live mainly in the large bowel. The eggs (B) are shed in large numbers and become embryonated (infectious form, C) after ~2wks to ~6mths in the environment. They are then ingested, e.g. on food or on fingertips, to become new adult worms.

Acute diarrhoea without blood

Rotavirus

Rotavirus is the most important cause of viral gastroenteritis in children (see Box 6.7). Before rotavirus immunization in developed countries, viral infections (mainly rotavirus) account for up to 60% of all gastroenteritis in children <5yrs and occur in seasonal outbreaks. In contrast, rotavirus causes <5% of all episodes of diarrhoea in resource-poor regions, but 40–50% of cases that require hospitalization. It is responsible for ~half a million deaths each year. Nearly all children in the tropics have been infected by the age of 2yrs.

Clinical features Vomiting occurs early; fever is common; the diarrhoea is usually watery and large volume. Colicky abdominal pains, ill-defined tenderness, and exaggerated bowel sounds are common.

Management Supportive, aiming to prevent dehydration. The WHO diarrhoea management scheme (see Box 6.13) should be followed, including treatment with zinc salts.

Dietary management

Since rotavirus infection is common in infants, dietary management is important to avoid malnutrition. Continue breastfeeding. Lactose malabsorption is common, but intolerance is usually only a clinical problem in severe cases. Children with mild diarrhoea should be encouraged to continue eating a normal diet in order to limit weight loss. If diarrhoea continues or is severe, lactose can be reduced by mixing milk with cereals or changing to a lactose-free diet, but calorie intake should be maintained. As with all diarrhoeal episodes, once the child improves or is hungry, extra food should be given to make up for weight loss. Beware confusion with surgical causes of diarrhoea in the neonate, such as necrotizing enterocolitis, intussusception, and Hirschsprung's disease.

Prevention

Rotavirus infection is highly contagious, difficult to prevent, and causes outbreaks in hospitals. Two rotavirus vaccines are available which prevent severe illness and hospitalizations (📖 Immunization, p. 893).

Other viral causes of diarrhoea

Astroviruses

Are single-stranded RNA viruses that occur worldwide and cause diarrhoea, mainly in children and the elderly. The diarrhoea is similar to rotavirus, although generally milder.

Diagnosis PCR; ELISA may be useful for diagnosis of outbreaks.

Enteric adenovirus

Serotypes 40 and 41 cause diarrhoea, possibly more in developed countries. Clinical features similar to other viral diarrhoeas.

Diagnosis Electron microscopy or ELISA.

Noroviruses (small, round structured viruses e.g. Norwalk virus)
Human enteric caliciviruses are the most important viral cause of water- and food-borne diarrhoeal outbreaks in both developing and developed countries. Shellfish have been implicated in some outbreaks. They are the most common viral cause of epidemic diarrhoea and vomiting in adults ('winter vomiting disease').

Transmission Faeco-oral +/– airborne; nosocomial transmission common.

Clinical features Vomiting common at onset—may be severe; watery diarrhoea rarely severe, usually lasts 12–24h.

Diagnosis Immunoassays or PCR may be used in an epidemic.

Sapoviruses and caliciviruses These infections are associated with sporadic gastroenteritis in young children.

Diagnosis Electron microscopy or PCR.

Management of viral diarrhoea Rehydration. Follow WHO diarrhoea treatment guidelines for management of diarrhoea in children (see 🕮 Chapter 1).

Box 6.7 Causes of acute diarrhoea without blood

Systemic infections
- Malaria, especially *P. falciparum*.
- Sepsis.

Viruses
- Rotavirus.
- Astrovirus.
- Enteric adenovirus.
- Noroviruses.
- Sapoviruses.

Bacteria
- Early or mild shigellosis; *Salmonella* or *Campylobacter* infections.
- Enterotoxigenic *E. coli* (ETEC) (e.g. traveller's diarrhoea).
- Enteropathogenic *E. coli* (EPEC).
- Enteroaggregative *E. coli* (EAEC).
- Enterotoxin-producing strains of *Staphylococcus aureus*.
- *Cholera*.
- *Clostridia* spp.

Protozoa
- Giardiasis.
- Cryptosporidiosis.
- *Cyclospora cayetanensis*.

Strongyloidiasis

Food toxins

Causes of bloody diarrhoea may also cause diarrhoea without blood (🕮 Acute diarrhoea with blood, p. 238, Box 6.4).

Enterotoxigenic *E. coli*

Enterotoxigenic *E. coli* (ETEC) accounts for 20% of diarrhoeal cases, second only to rotavirus as a cause of in-patient gastroenteritis in developing countries. Transmission is by the faeco-oral route mainly via contaminated food, less commonly water. It accounts for ~80% of travellers' diarrhoea.

Clinical features

After an incubation period of 1–2d ETEC produces diarrhoea through heat-labile enterotoxin (LT) and/or heat-stable enterotoxin (ST) toxin. These toxins stimulate Cl^-, Na^+, and water efflux into the intestinal lumen, resulting in voluminous, watery diarrhoea. Vomiting and abdominal cramps are frequently a feature and up to 10 motions per day may be passed.

Diagnosis

Depends on identification of the LT and/or ST toxins from *E. coli* cultured from faeces, but these tests are usually only available in specialized laboratories. Immunoassays or PCR may be used in an epidemic. Simple culture of *E. coli* in stools is not helpful.

Management:

Supportive. Children should be managed according to WHO guidelines. See 📖 Travellers' diarrhoea, p. 290.

Prevention:

General methods to prevent food contamination. Specific ETEC vaccines are under development but are not yet widely available.

Enteropathogenic *E. coli* (EPEC)

EPEC are a major cause of infantile diarrhoea that can be devastating. Transmission is by the faeco-oral route. Epidemics of hospital-acquired infection occur and recent hospitalization is a risk factor for infection. It is also a cause of travellers' diarrhoea.

Clinical features

Range from acute watery to severe, prolonged, or relapsing diarrhoea, usually with mucus, but no blood. Initially, there may be vomiting and fever. Epidemics can occur affecting mainly infants, with an untreated fatality reaching 50%.

Diagnosis

Depends on either serotyping of *E. coli* in stools, adherence pattern to HEp-2 cells in culture, DNA probes for the virulence plasmid or PCR. Serotyping is not very reliable or specific, and cell culture techniques and molecular methods are usually only available in specialist centres.

Management

Rehydration. Give antibiotics to vulnerable individuals, such as infants (e.g. co-trimoxazole 15mg/kg qds for 5d for infants >1mth), depending on local resistance patterns.

Prevention

Avoid routinely placing newborns in nurseries (encourage mothers and babies to stay together; avoid shared equipment). Enforce strict hand-washing in neonatal nurseries and special care units.

Enteroinvasive *E. coli*

Enteroinvasive *E. coli* (EIEC) are endemic in developing countries and cause 1–5% of episodes of diarrhoea presenting to health services. Like *Shigella*, EIEC can invade and multiply in epithelial cells. Clinically resembles shigellosis, but dysentery is less common. Specific diagnosis is only available in reference laboratories. Management is supportive; treat as for *Shigella*.

Enteroaggregative *E. coli* and diffuse-adherent *E. coli*

They are an important cause of diarrhoea—enteroaggregative *E. coli* (EAEC) mainly in infants and travellers' diarrhoea and diffuse-adherent *E. coli* (DAEC) in preschool children. EAEC have also been associated with persistent diarrhoea in adults with (especially advanced) HIV. Clinical features vary from asymptomatic infection to watery diarrhoea, often persistent. Definitive diagnosis by HEp-2 cell assay or PCR is only available in specialist centres. Management is supportive. Antibiotics may be indicated for severe episodes; ciprofloxacin is most effective.

Cholera

Vibrio cholerae is the main cause of dehydrating diarrhoea in adults. Clinical episodes range from asymptomatic infection to acute fulminant watery diarrhoea which, if untreated, may be fatal.

Microbiology

Vibrios are Gram –ve, aerobic, comma-shaped bacteria. Several serovars of *V. cholerae* are recognized. Serovar 01 is responsible for most cholera epidemics (see Box 6.8). Killed by heating at 55°C for 15min and by most disinfectants, yet it can survive in seawater for up to 2wks. In most cases, bacteria survive for only limited periods on foodstuffs, with notable exception of prawns, crayfish, etc., upon which they may survive for 14d if refrigerated.

Transmission

V. cholerae is found in brackish water, estuaries, and seawater in association with copepods and other zooplankton but the most important reservoir is thought to be humans. Infection via contaminated food or water usually requires a large infective dose. The incubation period ranges from a few hours to 5 d. Only a minority of infected people develop symptoms. There are 740 asymptomatic carriers of the El Tor biotype for every symptomatic case (75:1 for classical biotype). This is true both in endemic areas and during outbreaks, hence the need for meticulous hygiene of even asymptomatic individuals.

Clinical features:

If symptomatic, varies from mild, self-limiting diarrhoea to severe, watery 'rice water' diarrhoea of up to 30L/d. Diarrhoea → electrolyte imbalances, metabolic acidosis, prostration, and can cause death from dehydration within hours. Vomiting starts shortly after the onset of diarrhoea in 80% of cases. Shock typically follows ~12h later, with ↓ consciousness due to hypovolaemia and hypoglycaemia. Particularly serious in children who may have a mild fever (adults are afebrile). Renal failure, ileus, and cardiac arrhythmias may precede death; the elderly or those with ↓ gastric acid, such as alcoholics, are especially vulnerable. Muscular and abdominal cramps are common due to loss of Ca^{2+} and Cl^- ions.

Diagnosis
In epidemics, the diagnosis of cholera may be made clinically. In non-epidemic situations, acute watery diarrhoea → severe dehydration or the death of a patient >5yrs suggests cholera. Dark-field microscopy of faecal material shows comma-shaped bacteria darting about; this is quickly halted upon addition of diluted 01 antisera. Transportation of samples should be in alkaline peptone water; samples should be kept cool. Culture requires selective media such as thiosulfate-citrate-bile salts-sucrose agar (TCBS) agar. If possible, specimens should be sent to a reference laboratory for bio- and serotyping.

Management
Treatment consists mainly of prompt and sufficient rehydration, usually with oral fluids. This will reduce mortality to <1% (see 📖 General management of dehydration, p. 272 for rehydration regimens). Most common error is underestimation of volume of ORS or IV fluid required. In emergencies where ORS is not available, sucrose and rice-water-based solutions can be given with success.

Antibiotics should be given to severe cases, where they ↓ volume and ↓ duration of diarrhoea.

Adults
Azithromycin 1g oral, given as single dose, is drug of choice. Doxycycline 300mg oral, given as single dose, is an alternative (except in pregnant women). If resistance reported, alternative antibiotic regimes are furazolidone 100mg oral qds, erythromycin 250mg oral qds, or co-trimoxazole 960mg oral bd, all for 3d; or ciprofloxacin 1g as a single oral dose.

Children
Give azithromycin 20mg/kg (max 1g) oral stat; or erythromycin 12.5mg/kg oral qds, furazolidone 1.25mg/kg oral qds, or co-trimoxazole 5–25mg/kg oral bd, all for 3d.

In pregnancy Use erythromycin 250mg oral qds for 3d; furazolidone 100mg oral qds for 3d is an alternative.

Prevention
Public health measures aimed at improving food and water hygiene, and sanitation are most important. Currently, two oral cholera vaccines are available (📖 Immunization, p. 910) and are recommended for travellers to areas known to have a cholera epidemic. The use of vaccines in epidemics has not been fully evaluated and should not deflect resources from treatment facilities and prevention of spread.

Box 6.8 Epidemiology of *V. cholera*

- *V. cholerae* serovar 01 is the causative agent of cholera.
- There are two biotypes of the 01 serovar: *classical* and *El Tor*, each of which is further divided into three serotypes: Ogawa, Inaba, and Hikojima.
- The classical biotype caused the first six cholera pandemics in South Asia during the 19th and early 20th centuries.
- The El Tor biotype was first recognized in 1906, but until 1963 was restricted to Sulawesi in Indonesia.
- During the 1960s, the 7th pandemic started with the spread of El Tor biotype, Inaba serotype, out of Indonesia into South Asia, Africa, and, since 1991, Latin America. This biotype has now replaced the classical biotype throughout much of the world, except Bangladesh.
- The 0139 *V. cholerae* serovar first appeared in southern India in 1992. It causes cholera similar to 01. In Bangladesh, it is reported to affect mainly adults. Previous exposure to the 01 serovar does not confer protection.
- Recent cholera epidemics include the 2008–9 epidemic in Zimbabwe and the 2010 epidemic following the earthquake in Haiti. The *V. cholerae* strain responsible for the Haiti epidemic is almost identical to the El Tor 01 strains predominant in Southeast Asia, suggesting introduction of the strain from Asia. This strain was subsequently identified in cholera cases in the Dominican Republic and Florida.
- New cholera strains have been identified in Bangladesh, East Africa, and Asia and appear to be very virulent.

Health education

Is essential in preventing outbreaks and limiting the spread of infection during an outbreak. Advice should include food and water hygiene, as well as other measures to ↓ transmission such as disinfecting patients' clothing by boiling for 5min, drying out bedding in the sun, burying stools, etc. In larger health centres, patient excreta may be mixed with disinfectant (e.g. cresol) or acid before disposal in pit latrines. Semi-solid waste should be incinerated. Funerals have been a source of spread and preventative measures should be instigated to minimize the risk of mourners arriving from uninfected areas, and potential contamination from ritual washing of the dead and funeral feasts.

Cholera outbreaks

It is obligatory to notify the WHO of all cholera cases. Suspected cases should be reported immediately by health authorities and laboratory confirmation sent as soon as it is obtained. This should be followed by weekly reports containing the number of new cases and deaths since the last report, the cumulative totals for the year, and, if possible, the age distribution and number of patients admitted to hospital, recorded by region or other geographical division. This data should be sent to WHO headquarters, as well as to the appropriate regional office.

Usually, there is a national coordinating committee to implement and regulate control and prevention measures, although often it is up to the front-line doctors to initiate the process and maintain close collaboration. Mobile control teams may be needed in inaccessible areas or in countries with no national coordination, and these are responsible for establishing and operating temporary treatment centres, training local staff, educating the public, carrying out epidemiological studies, collecting stool, food, and water samples for laboratory analysis, and providing emergency logistical support to health posts and laboratories. Emergency treatment centres may be needed if appropriate facilities do not exist or are swamped with patients. Strict isolation or quarantine measures are not needed. The most crucial factor affecting survival is access to treatment centres with trained staff and intravenous and oral rehydration capability.

Public health note: estimated minimum supplies needed to treat 100 patients during a cholera outbreak[1]

- 50 packets of ORS solution (1L).
- 20 bags of 1L Ringer's lactate solution,[2] with giving sets.
- 10 scalp vein sets.
- 3 adult NGTs, 5.3mm outside diameter (16 French), 50cm long.
- 3 paediatric NGTs, 2.7mm diameter (8 French), 38cm long.

For adults with severe diarrhoea

- 60 doxycycline 100mg capsules (3 capsules per patient) *or*
- 40 azithromycin 500mg tablets (2 tablets per patient).

For children 120 erythromycin 250mg tablets (6 tablets per patient broken into half).

For pregnant women 240 furazolidone 100mg tablets (12 tablets per person).

If selective chemoprophylaxis is planned

The additional requirements for 4 close contacts per severely dehydrated patient (~80 people) are 240 capsules of doxycycline 100mg (3 capsules per person).

Other necessary supplies

- 2 large water dispensers with tap for bulk ORS preparation.
- 20 1-L bottles, 20 500-mL bottles for ORS dispensing.
- 40 200-mL cups.
- 20 teaspoons.
- 5kg cotton wool to sterilize skin (e.g. with 70% alcohol) for IV access prior to insertion of cannulae.
- 3 reels of adhesive tape to secure IV cannulae and NG tubes.

[1]The supplies listed are sufficient for IV fluid followed by oral rehydration salts for 20 severely dehydrated patients and for ORS alone for 80 patients.

[2]If Ringer's lactate solution or equivalent unavailable, physiological saline may be substituted.

Giardiasis

Giardia intestinalis (also known as *G. lamblia* and *G. duodenalis*) is the most common human protozoan GI pathogen, having a worldwide distribution. Its prevalence can reach ~30% in the tropics, with infection highest in infants and children especially among children <5yrs. It causes ~3% of travellers' diarrhoea.

Transmission

Cysts can survive for long periods outside the host in suitable environments (e.g. surface water). *Giardia* cysts are NOT killed by chlorination. Infection follows ingestion of cysts in faecally contaminated water (from humans or animal hosts) or through direct person to person contact. Partial immunity may be acquired through repeated infections.

Clinical features

In endemic areas, asymptomatic carriers are common. Symptoms usually begin within 3–20d of infection; most patients recover within 2–4wks, although in 25% of travellers, symptoms persist for up to 7wks. Diarrhoea is the major symptom; it is watery initially, becoming steatorrhoeic and often associated with nausea, abdominal discomfort, bloating, weight loss, and sometimes sulfurous, offensive burps. Giardiasis can be the cause of abdominal pain without diarrhoea in children. Some patients develop a chronic diarrhoea associated with weight loss of up to 20% of body weight, fat malabsorption, deficiencies (particularly of vitamins A and B12), and, in some cases, 2° hypolactasia.

Complications

In endemic settings, infections are common and usually asymptomatic but some studies have documented ↓ growth and development in severely affected infants and children, in whom malabsorption exacerbates malnutrition. Chronic giardiasis is associated with allergic and inflammatory conditions such as lymphoid nodular hyperplasia. Protein-losing enteropathy, lactose intolerance, and irritable bowel syndrome can also occur.

Diagnosis

Detection of cysts (and occasionally trophozoites) in faecal samples by light microscopy. Examine three separate samples, since cysts are excreted intermittently and diagnostic sensitivity is low. Trophozoites may be detected in biopsies of small intestine mucosa. ELISA tests can detect faecal *Giardia* antigens. Since mixed enteric infections and asymptomatic carriage of *Giardia* are common, identification of the parasite does not guarantee it is the cause of diarrhoea. Serology is not useful because of cross-reactivity in non-infected individuals in endemic areas. Research tools include serology, culture, and PCR techniques.

Management

- Rehydration and symptomatic relief are usually sufficient.
- If symptoms persist, an anti-giardial drug will ↓ severity and duration of symptoms.
  - There is ↑ drug failure due to resistance.
  - Recommended drugs include metronidazole 2g od oral for 3d, or tinidazole 2g as a single oral dose.

- In pregnancy, possible treatment is paromomycin 25–35mg/kg/d oral in four divided doses for 10d, although efficacy is only 60–70%.
- In the 2nd and 3rd trimesters, lower dose metronidazole is an alternative, 250mg tds oral for 5–7d.

Prevention Attention to personal hygiene, appropriate treatment of water supplies, encouraging breastfeeding (shown to partially protect against infection).

Cryptosporidiosis

The protozoan *Cryptosporidium parvum* is a common opportunistic infection in HIV+ individuals. It is also a common cause of childhood diarrhoea in the immunocompetent. Transmission is mainly through contaminated water. It accounts for 2–20% of childhood diarrhoea in resource-poor regions, and infections contribute to growth faltering during the 1st year of life. Although usually mild, severe, or persistent diarrhoea may occur.

Clinical features

Acute diarrhoea is indistinguishable from diarrhoea due to other causes. Abdominal cramping pain is often a feature. *Cryptosporidium* should be sought in persistent (chronic) diarrhoea; in HIV+ individuals it may be severe, mimicking cholera, and/or be very prolonged.

Diagnosis

Faecal detection of the oocysts (4–6μm diameter red spheres on modified ZN stain). Oocysts may also be present in duodenal aspirates, bile secretions, biopsy specimens from affected GI tissue, or respiratory secretions on occasions. ELISA detection kits are available.

Management

Rehydration with symptomatic relief; as yet, no drug has been shown to be effective against this organism. Wider use of HAART in people with AIDS has reduced the prevalence of severe cryptosporidiosis.

Cyclospora

Cyclospora cayetanensis is a protozoan coccidian parasite now recognized to be a frequent cause of diarrhoea in developing and developed countries. Cyclospora can occur as a locally-acquired infection, among travellers or in patients with HIV/AIDS. Transmission is via contaminated water or food; raspberries, basil, and lettuce have been incriminated.

Diagnosis

Is by finding typical oocysts in faeces which are 7–10μm diameter and contain a 'morula' of 8 spherical bodies. The oocysts are also irregularly acid-fast when stained with modified ZN stain. It is important to distinguish the *Cyclospora* oocysts from those of *Cryptosporidium*, which are also acid-fast, but smaller (5μm in diameter). Fluorescence microscopy can also be used for detection of oocysts, which are autofluorescent.

Clinical features Watery diarrhoea which is most severe in non-immune travellers. Mild fever, fatigue, anorexia, and weight loss may occur. The illness can last for weeks.

Management Co-trimoxazole 960mg oral bd for 7–10 d.

Strongyloidiasis

The nematode *Strongyloides stercoralis* commonly infects humans worldwide, particularly in parts of South America and Southeast Asia. It is a serious condition in the immunosuppressed and may cause acute, relapsing, or persistent diarrhoea. There are two adult forms of the worm and two larval forms, one of which is infective.

Life cycle

Complex (see Fig. 6.4), since reproduction can take place in either of two cycles: an external cycle involving free-living worms or an internal cycle. Contamination of skin or buccal mucosa with damp soil or mud containing larve → penetration of larvae. The larvae travel to the lungs and enter the bronchi, eventually passing into the small intestine, where they mature into adults. Eggs produced by the female pass out in the faeces and continue the external cycle.

Autoinfection occurs by either bronchial larvae producing progeny or filariform larvae not passing out in the stool but reinvading bowel or perianal skin. This can produce indefinite (>40yrs) multiplication within the host, not requiring further infection. The pre-patent period from infection to the appearance of larvae in the stools is ~1mth.

Clinical features

- Immune response limits the infection to the small bowel and also the number of adult worms. Infection is usually asymptomatic.
- Larval penetration causes petechial haemorrhages and pruritis at the site of entry (e.g. peri anal skin).
- Characteristic linear, urticarial eruption (larva currens) as larvae migrate under skin (see Colour plate 5). This is normally transient, but may be followed by congestion and oedema. A creeping urticarial rash may occur in pre-sensitized individuals following re-infection.
- Symptoms similar to bronchopneumonia with consolidation may result from larval invasion of the lungs; accompanied by eosinophilia and resembles TPE.
- Watery diarrhoea with mucus is a frequent symptom; its intensity depends on worm burden, often alternating with constipation.
- In severe cases, chronic diarrhoea with malabsorption may ensue.

In immunosuppressed, those co-infected with HTLV-1, malnourished, or debilitated, massive tissue invasion may occur with severe diarrhoea, ileus, hepatomegaly, and multi-system disease due to blood/lymphatic spread ('hyperinfection syndrome'). Granulomas and/or abscesses occur in liver, kidneys, and lungs, and there may be serous effusions; CNS involvement → pyogenic meningitis and encephalopathy. Eosinophilia usually absent in hyperinfection. Death usually results from Gram –ve septicaemia.

Diagnosis

Adult or rhabditiform larvae may be detected in stool, although simple stool microscopy is insensitive. Other methods include modified Baermann technique, agar plate culture, stool ELISA, serology, and stool culture using charcoal. Look for infection in those who are, or are about to be, immunosuppressed (e.g. on steroids).

Management

- Treat all infected patients, not just the symptomatic.
- Give ivermectin 200micrograms/kg oral od for 2d.
- *Less effective alternatives:* albendazole 400mg oral bd for 7d; thiabendazole 25mg/kg oral bd for 2d, or 5d in disseminated infection.

Prevention Requires improving hygiene, encouraging footwear, and education on a community level, as well as monitoring and evaluation.

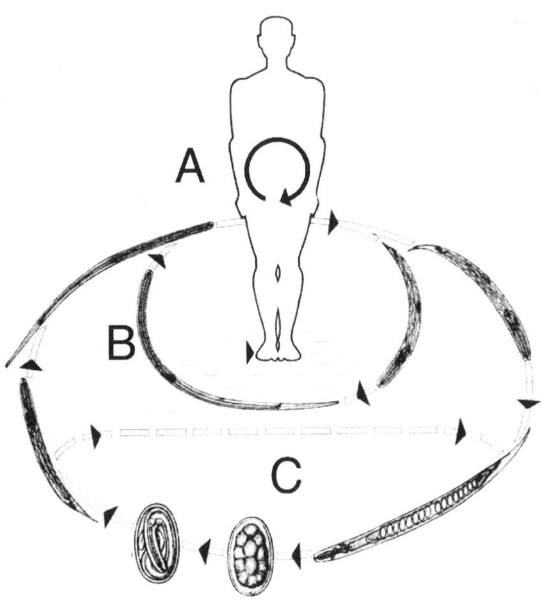

Fig. 6.4 Life cycle of *Strongyloides stercoralis*: The female worms are ~2mm in length and live in the small intestine; produce eggs parthenogenetically. In auto-infectious life cycle (A), these hatch within bowel and larvae penetrate intestinal wall to produce more adult worms. Alternatively (B), larvae may be passed in faeces into environmental surface water, and infect new hosts through intact skin (when walking barefoot in puddles). In a third life cycle (C), free-living adult worms give rise to eggs, then larvae, which infect new hosts. Infective larvae are called 'filariform', and those freshly passed in stool are 'rhabtidiform' larvae.

Food poisoning

Food poisoning is a general term referring to gastrointestinal symptoms occurring within a few hours of ingesting the food containing a toxin. Microbial infections usually have a longer incubation period as the pathogen proliferates in the intestine (see Table 6.1).

Clostridium perfringens

Clostridium perfringens produces two forms of GI disease: simple food poisoning (caused by type A, see Table 6.1) and necrotizing enterocolitis (type C).

Necrotizing enterocolitis (pigbel)

This high fatality illness has become less common following vaccination, but still occurs, particularly in the highlands of Papua New Guinea and also in Uganda, Southeast Asia, and China. It occurs when *C. perfringens* type C is eaten, normally in meat that has been cooked some time previously. It has been associated with malnutrition, infestation with *Ascaris lumbricoides*, and a diet rich in sweet potatoes. The latter two are associated with high levels of heat-stable trypsin inhibitors that inhibit the luminal proteases, preventing them inactivating the type C toxin.

Clinical features

Symptoms usually begin 48h following ingestion but may start up to one week later. It is classified into four types:

- *Type I (acute toxic):* presents with fulminant toxaemia and shock. Usually occurs in young children; 85% mortality.
- *Type II (acute surgical):* presents as mechanical or paralytic ileus, acute strangulation, perforation, or peritonitis; 40% mortality.
- *Type III (subacute surgical):* presents later, with features similar to type II; 40% mortality.
- *Type IV:* of mild diarrhoea only, although it may → type III. In types II and III, a thickened segment of bowel is sometimes palpable. Blood and pus are passed with the stool in severe disease.

Diagnosis Isolation of *C. perfringens* from stool or peritoneal fluid culture. Serological diagnosis is also possible.

Management

Type I and II disease require urgent surgery after appropriate resuscitation. Surgery may also be required for type III. Give IV chloramphenicol or benzylpenicillin and *C. perfringens* type C antiserum, where available. Milder cases may require glucose and electrolyte infusions, with IV broad-spectrum antibiotics if signs of extra-intestinal spread. Give an antihelminthic effective against *Ascaris*. Oral food intake should begin after 24h.

Prevention Immunization with type C toxoid.

Table 6.1 Food poisoning from bacteria or their toxins

Organism/toxin	Principal foods	Time after food	Clinical features
Staph. aureus	Meat, poultry, dairy produce, prepared foods	1–6h	D, V, AP
Bacillus cereus	Fried rice, sauces, vegetables	1–5h	V
		6–16h	D, AP
Red bean toxin		1–6h	D, V
Scombrotoxin (bacteria produce histamine)	Fish (especially dark fleshed)	1–6h	D, flushing, sweating, mouth pain
Mushroom toxin		1–6h	D, V, AP
Ciguatera	Fish	1–6h	Fits, coma, renal/ liver failure
Salmonella spp.	Meat, poultry, eggs, dairy produce	8–72h (mean 12–36h)	D, V, AP, fever
Campylobacter spp.	Poultry, raw milk, eggs	1–10d (mean 2–5d)	D, AP
Clostridium perfringens	Cooked meat	8–24h (mean 8–15h)	D, AP, V
Vibrio parahaemolyticus	Seafood	4–96h (mean 12h)	D, V, AP, cramp, headache
Shigella spp.	Faecal contamination	1–7d (mean 1–3d)	D(bloody), V, fever
Clostridium botulinum	Poorly canned food, smoked meats	2h–8d (mean 12–36h)	Diplopia, paralysis
Listeria monocytogenes	Dairy produce, meat, vegetables, seafood	1–7wks	Septicaemia, septic abortion
E. coli	Dirty water	8–44h	D, V, cramps
Y. enterocolitica	Pork and beef	24–36h	Fever, AP, D

V = vomiting, D = diarrhoea, AP = abdominal pain

Public health note: prevention of food poisoning from bacteria or their toxins

Five rules for safe food:

- Keep food clean.
- Cook thoroughly.
- Separate raw and cooked food.
- Keep food at safe temperatures.
- Use safe water and raw materials.

Food handlers should be particularly careful about personal hygiene, especially hand washing after defecation and before touching food. Especial attention should be taken to prevent *S. aureus* contamination from skin, nose, and eye infections of food handlers, who are the most common source of contamination of food (~25% people are carriers). The toxin is not destroyed at boiling temperatures.

Persistent diarrhoea and malabsorption

Persistent diarrhoea (PD) refers to diarrhoea episodes that start acutely and continue >2wks. Several mechanisms may be implicated (see Box 6.9). In areas where sanitation and clean water are lacking, and ↑ diarrhoea incidence, most PD seems to be caused by frequent new infections combined with delayed recovery, often due to nutrient deficiencies. PD is accompanied by malnutrition and ↑ mortality in children. Rehydration and dietary management with continued feeding, correction of micronutrient deficiencies, and treatment of concomitant infections and dysentery is effective in 80% of children.

Malabsorption

May be due to a range of causes (see Box 6.9). The key features are:

- Chronic diarrhoea +/– steatorrhoea (see Fig. 6.5): stool typically loose, bulky, offensive, greasy, light-coloured, and difficult to flush away.
- Abdominal discomfort, distension, flatulence.
- *Signs of nutritional deficiency:* e.g. glossitis, pallor, muscle pain, bruising.
- *General ill health:* anorexia, ↓ weight, lethargy, dyspnoea, fatigue.
- Features related to underlying cause: surgical scars, systemic disease.

Investigations

FBC, U&Es, erythrocyte sedimentation rate (ESR), LFTs, stool microscopy, and culture. Other tests include faecal fat, INR (deficiency of fat-soluble vitamins), carbohydrate absorption (after glucose or xylose), Schilling test (measure of ileal function), small bowel biopsy via endoscopy, or Crosby capsule.

Hypolactasia and lactose intolerance

- 1° hypolactasia occurs normally because most humans, like most mammals, lose the digestive enzyme lactase as they mature and no longer depend on milk (a genetic variant in some ethnic groups preserves the enzyme).
- 2° hypolactasia occurs after injury to the intestinal mucosa and is common after GI infections.

In both types the limited capacity to hydrolyse lactose leads to malabsorption (Box 6.10). *Lactose intolerance* occurs when incompletely hydrolysed lactose reaches the colon and causes osmotic diarrhoea, abdominal pain, distension, and flatulence. Symptoms depend on the amount of lactose reaching the small intestine at a given time.

Diagnosis History of worsening symptoms with increased lactose intake (lactose tolerance test), acid stools with +ve reducing substances, the hydrogen breath test, or a lactase assay in jejunal biopsy.

Management

Symptoms can often be controlled by allowing only small amounts of lactose at a time; slowing gastric emptying, e.g. by adding chocolate to milk or mixing milk with cereals; ↓ lactose by fermentation, as in yogurt; or

Box 6.9 Causes of persistent or chronic diarrhoea

Secondary events

- Lactose intolerance due to 1° or 2° hypolactasia.
- Tropical sprue.
- Cow's milk protein intolerance.

Continuing infection

- Strongyloidiasis.
- Cryptosporidiosis.
- Microsporidiosis.
- Enteropathogenic *E. coli.*
- Giardiasis.
- Intestinal flukes.
- Chronic intestinal schistosomiasis.

Delayed recovery

- Malnutrition.
- Zinc deficiency including acrodermatitis enteropathica.
- Sequential new infections.

Other causes

- HIV enteropathy (see 🕮 Gastrointestinal disease in HIV, p. 92).
- Chronic calcific pancreatitis.
- Short bowel disease (e.g. recovered pigbel disease).
- Ileocaecal TB.
- *Lymphoma:* Burkitt's and Mediterranean.
- Acute and chronic liver disease.
- IBD and coeliac disease.
- Irritable bowel syndrome.

taking lactase supplements with milk drinks. Total exclusion of milk to avoid lactose is rarely necessary and should be avoided whenever possible in infants, because it is often difficult to provide alternative sources of the many nutrients in milk. Care should be taken to maintain energy and nutrient intakes. If, in severe cases, it is necessary to eliminate lactose-containing products, these may be introduced slowly after 6wks depending on symptom recurrence.

HIV and diarrhoea Diarrhoea is common in HIV+ individuals; up to 80% will present diarrhoea (see 🕮 Gastrointestinal disease in HIV, p. 92).

Post-infective malabsorption; tropical enteropathy; tropical malabsorption, tropical sprue

This syndrome of malabsorption, haematological abnormality, ↓ weight and diarrhoea can occur in residents and long-term visitors (>3mths) to the tropics, especially Central America, northern South America, parts of Africa, the Mediterranean coast, Middle East, and Asia. It is by definition a

Box 6.10 Causes of malabsorption

- *Infective:* acute enteritis; intestinal TB; helminths *Strongyloides stercoralis, Capillaria philippinensis*; protozoa *Giardia intestinalis, Isospora belli, Cryptosporidium parvum, Enterocytozoon bieneusi, Encephalitozoon intestinalis, Cyclospora cayetanensis, Leishmania donovani*; bacteria *Mycobacterium tuberculosis*; viruses HIV; Whipple's disease, and other causes of travellers' diarrhoea.
- *Anatomical/motility:* blind loops, diverticuli, intestinal resection, strictures, fistulae, small bowel lymphoma, systemic sclerosis, diabetes mellitus, pseudo-obstruction, radiotherapy, amyloidosis, lymphatic obstruction (2° to TB).
- *Defective digestion:* chronic pancreatitis,tropical pancreatitis, cystic fibrosis, food sensitivity (lactose, gluten), malnutrition, gastric/intestinal surgery, Zollinger–Ellison syndrome, pancreatectomy, biliary obstruction, terminal ileal disease/resection (short bowel syndrome), parenchymal liver disease, bacterial overgrowth, tropical sprue.
- *Inflammatory and/or immune related:* coeliac disease, Crohn's disease, 1° immunodeficiency.
- *Malignancy:* immunoproliferative small-intestinal disease, small intestinal lymphomas.
- *Drugs:* antibiotics, colestyramine, metformin, methyldopa, alcohol, antacids, purgative misuse, para-aminosalicylic acid.

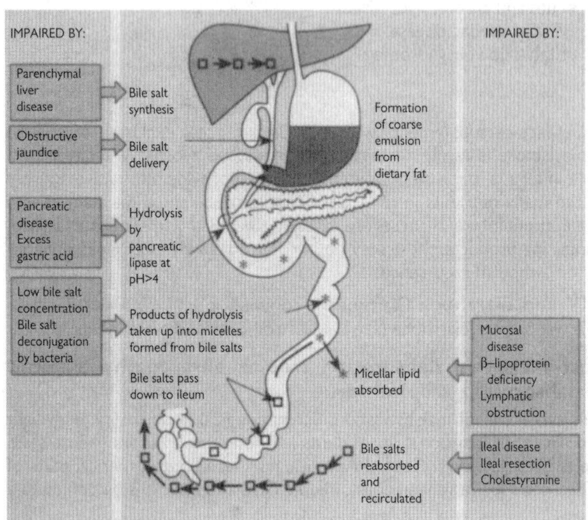

Fig. 6.5 Mechanisms of steatorrhoea.

chronic condition; ≥2mths of symptoms are needed to make the diagnosis. Malabsorption significantly ↓ energy and nutrient intake quickly → malnutrition, especially in children, and to anaemia. For reasons that are not clear, post-infective malabsorption (PIM) seems to be becoming less common.

Aetiology

It is not clear whether PIM is a distinct entity that occurs with persistence of malabsorption after acute infective diarrhoea, or a severe form of tropical enteropathy (tropical sprue; see Fig. 6.6). Both tropical enteropathy and PIM show abnormal jejunal morphology with partial villous atrophy. There is crypt hyperplasia, with T cell infiltration. Changes in gut hormones, disturbed gut motility, and colonic function have been described. Bacterial overgrowth of the small intestine is found, but no single organism can be held responsible. An association with certain HLA antigens has been reported suggesting a genetic predisposition.

Clinical features

- Chronic diarrhoea with or without steatorrhoea +/– flatulence of >2mths duration. Other features include ↓ weight, glossitis, macrocytic anaemia, fluid retention, depression, lethargy, amenorrhoea, and infertility. Serum folate and vitamin B12 may ↓ to very low levels. Hypoalbuminaemia and oedema are late signs.
- Foreign travel or recent GI infection can unmask other chronic GI disorders, such as coeliac disease, inflammatory bowel disease, and GI malignancy.
- Irritable bowel syndrome is reported in 3–10% of people following travellers' diarrhoea episodes.

Investigations

- 1h Blood xylose concentration following a 5 or 25g loading dose.
- 72h Faecal fat estimation.
- Schilling test.
- Serum B12.
- Red blood cell (RBC) folate.
- Serum albumin.
- Exclude faecal parasites.
- Barium meal and follow-through will show dilated loops of jejunum with clumping of barium.
- Endoscopy and jejunal biopsy may show a ridged or convoluted mucosa, depending on the duration of the disease, with T lymphocyte infiltration.

Management

- Eliminate bacterial overgrowth with tetracycline 250mg oral qds for >2wks.
- Aid mucosal recovery by providing folate supplements.
- Provide a suitable diet to promote weight gain.
- Give symptomatic relief in the acute stages: codeine phosphate 30mg oral tds or loperamide 4mg oral initially, then 2mg after each loose stool. Usual dose 6–8mg od; maximum dose 16mg od.

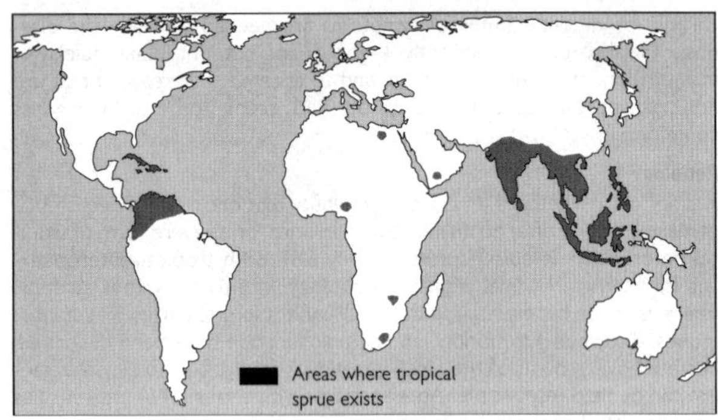

Fig. 6.6 Distribution of post-infective malabsorption (tropical sprue).

Tropical enteropathy and subclinical malabsorption

Individuals living in highly contaminated environments, commonly found in the tropics, fight a constant battle against repeated low-grade viral, bacterial, and parasitic GI infections. This is associated with chronic changes in the jejunal mucosa with blunted villi and nutrient malabsorption, which recover when subject leaves the environment. Tests of nutrient absorption, e.g. B12 and xylose absorption tests, usually abnormal. Tropical enteropathy probably contributes to child growth retardation in resource-poor regions, together with energy and micronutrient deficiencies and frequent infectious diseases. Improvement of the condition occurs spontaneously when travellers return to a clean environment, or it may be treated as for PIM (see 📖 Post-infective malabsorption, p. 265). In resident infants, mucosal changes improve with age, but persist into adulthood.

Chronic calcific pancreatitis

A syndrome of pancreatic calcification associated with both exocrine and endocrine impairment, commonly encountered in the tropics, especially equatorial Africa, southern India, and Indonesia. Aetiology unknown, but genes that ↓ activity of PIs in pancreas, which prevents premature activation of trysinogen to trypsin in acinar cells (SPINK1) have been found to be risk factors.

Clinical features Chronic malabsorption with ↓ weight, often associated with diabetes mellitus (DM; 10% of diabetes in East and West Africa) and (sometimes severe) pain. Association with pancreatic malignancy.

Management Diabetic control, low-fat diet, and enzyme supplementation (e.g. pancreatin BP 6g oral with food; dose tailored to individual patient).

Intestinal lymphoma

Wide variety of lymphomas may affect the GI tract, originating in either intestinal lymph nodes (e.g. Hodgkin's lymphoma) or mucosa-associated lymphoid tissue (MALT lymphomas). Small bowel lymphoma is recognized complication of HIV. Weight loss a common feature and nodal disease may be confused with intestinal TB, as X-ray changes appear similar. Diagnosis requires biopsy.

Whipple's disease

Rare condition caused by actinomycete bacterium, *Tropheryma whipplei*. Classically, there is ↓ weight, diarrhoea, and malabsorption, but clinical features are protean and often non-specific. Other features include fever, lymphadenopathy, arthralgia (may be transient or migratory), uveitis, culture –ve endocarditis, coronary arteritis, myocarditis, and encephalopathy. A histopathological diagnosis is often made incidentally on examination of intestinal biopsy material showing granulomatous inflammation and periodic acid-Schiff (PAS) staining deposits. PCR for the presence of *T. whipplei* in affected tissues confirms the diagnosis.

Treatment 2wks ceftriaxone 1g bd IV, then oral co-trimoxazole (alternatives: tetracycline or minocycline) for 1yr.

Other causes of malabsorption

Lymphangiectasia Lacteal dilatation (either 1° or 2° to abdominal malignancy) causes a protein-losing enteropathy, hypoproteinaemia, and oedema. Diagnosis requires small bowel biopsy.

Treatment Low-fat diet.

Abetalipoproteinaemia Rare autosomal recessive disorder, usually presenting in childhood due to defective triglyceride transport from the liver and gut. Eventually, neurological dysfunction (peripheral neuropathy, cerebellar ataxia) may follow.

Diagnosis By small bowel biopsy. Symptomatic treatment with low-fat diet and vitamin supplementation.

Intestinal parasites Many GI parasites (e.g. *Giardia, Cryptosporidium, Trichuris, Strongyloides*) can cause diarrhoea. Others (e.g. schistosomiasis, trichinellosis, cysticercosis, clonorchiasis, opisthorchiasis, ecchinococcus) → hepatic or pancreatic dysfunction. Pancreatic duct obstruction may be caused by ascariasis.

Intestinal flukes

Common throughout Asia (particularly Southeast Asia), where prevalence may reach 30% in certain populations. Children more heavily infected and prone to symptoms.

- *Fasciolopsiasis:* caused by *Fasciolopsis buski*; infection follows ingestion of metacercaria attached to the seed pods of water plants contaminated by human and pig faeces (see Fig. 6.7 for life cycle).

- *Echinostomiasis:* at least 15 *Echinostoma* species infect humans via the consumption of raw or undercooked freshwater snails, clams, fish, and tadpoles. In Northeast Thailand, commonly associated with *Opisthorchis* infection.
- *Heterophyasis:* numerous species of small (2.5mm) *Heterophyes* flukes infect humans following consumption of raw aquatic foods and/or insect larvae.

Clinical features

- Attachment of parasites to intestinal mucosa results in inflammation and ulcer formation.
- Infections frequently asymptomatic; when symptoms do occur, they are usually mild and non-specific—diarrhoea, flatulence, mild abdominal pains, vomiting, fever, and anorexia.
- Fasciolopsiasis may produce severe disease with anaemia, malabsorption, oedema, and ascites.
- Eggs (and sometimes adult worms) of *Heterophyes* spp. may enter lymphatics after mucosal penetration and be transported to other sites (notably heart, spinal cord, brain, lungs, liver, and spleen) where they cause granulomatous reactions. Myocarditis and neurological deficits may result.

Diagnosis

Faecal examination for eggs (Fig. 6.8), after concentration. Differentiation between *F. hepatica*, *F. buski*, and echinostomes is often difficult. Similarly, heterophydiae eggs closely resemble those of *Clonorchis* and *Opisthorchis*. Recovery of adult worms from post-treatment faeces allows definitive diagnosis, although in case of heterophyids, this is difficult owing to small size. Extra-intestinal cases of heterophyiasis are also difficult to diagnose—often only revealed during surgery or autopsy.

Management

- Praziquantel is drug of choice, 25mg/kg oral tds for 1d.
- Mebendazole or albendazole may be used for echinostomiasis, although praziquantel is recommended in areas where other trematodes are present, due to its broad efficacy.

Prevention

Concentrate on breaking the faeco-oral cycle (e.g. stopping the use of human and pig excreta as fertilizer) possibly combined with community-based praziquantel treatment and education regarding the consumption of raw/undercooked foodstuffs.

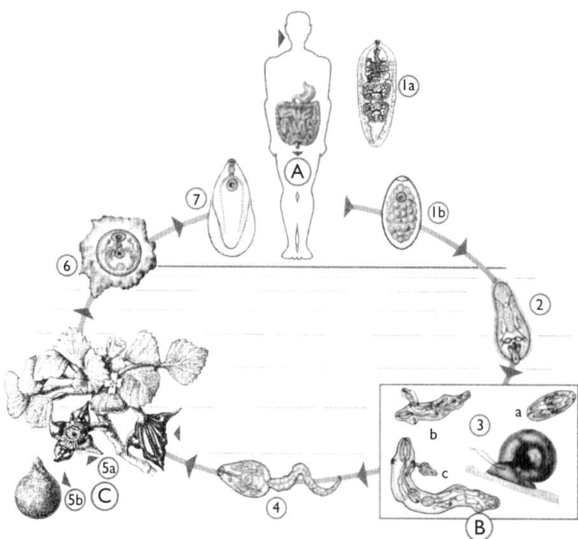

Fig 6.7 Life cycle of *Fasciolopsis buski*. Adult fluke (1a) lives attached to the intestinal wall. Eggs (1b) are passed in faeces into fresh water, where they release miracidia (2). These invade a suitable snail (B) in which the parasites undergo several developmental stages (3a–c). The cercariae (4) are released into water and encyst as metacercariae on aquatic plants (C). The human or pig hosts become infected by ingesting metacercariae (6), which excyst in the duodenum and attach to the intestinal wall. There they develop into adult flukes (20–75mm × 8–20mm) in ~3mths; adult flukes live ~1yr.

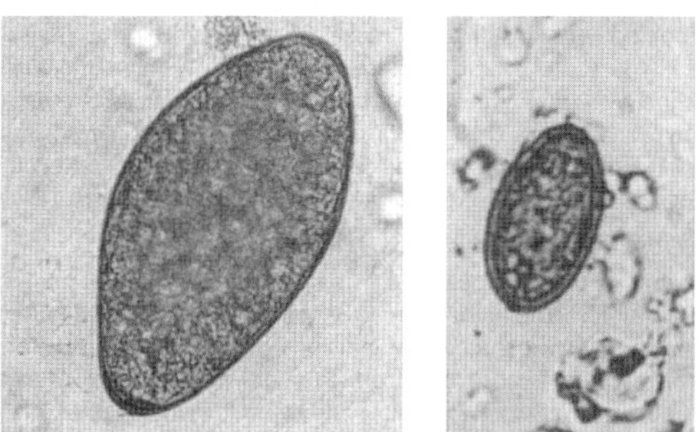

Fig. 6.8 Eggs of *Fasciolopsis buski* (left, 140 × 85μm) and *Heterophyes heterophyes* (right, 25 × 15μm).

General management of dehydration

Dehydration due to diarrhoea is a major cause of childhood death. Volume of fluid lost in stool can vary from 5mL/kg to >200mL/kg in 24h. Electrolyte loss also varies. Total body Na+ deficit in young children with severe dehydration owing to secretory diarrhoea is usually about 70–110mmol/L water lost. Degree of dehydration is assessed clinically. In early stages of dehydration, there are no signs or symptoms. As dehydration ↑, thirst, restlessness or irritable behaviour develop. Examination reveals ↓ skin turgor, dry mucous membranes, sunken eyes, sunken fontanelle (in infants), and absence of tears when crying. In severe dehydration, effects become more pronounced and the patient may develop signs of hypovolaemic shock, including ↓ consciousness, anuria, cool moist extremities, rapid and feeble pulse, low BP, delayed capillary filling, and peripheral cyanosis. Death may follow swiftly without prompt rehydration. In adults with dehydration, dry mucous membranes, sunken eyes and ↓ skin turgor are very inaccurate signs. Look for cool peripheries, a rapid, thready pulse, hypotension and especially postural hypotension (Box 6.11).

Types of dehydration

Isotonic dehydration

Occurs most frequently and is due to net losses of water and Na^+ in similar proportion to that in the extracellular fluid (ECF). The serum Na+ concentration (130–150mmol/L) and serum osmolality (275–295mOsmol/L) are normal. Hypovolaemia occurs due to excess ECF losses. Clinical features are those of hypovolaemic shock (thirst, ↓ skin turgor, dry mucous membranes, sunken eyes, oliguria, and a sunken fontanelle in infants). This → anuria, hypotension, a weak pulse, cool extremities, and eventually → coma and death.

Hypertonic (hypernatraemic) dehydration

Reflects a net loss of water in excess of Na^+ and tends to occur in infants only. It usually results from attempted treatment of diarrhoea with fluids that are hypertonic (e.g. sweetened fruit juices/soft drinks, glucose solution) combined with insufficient intake of water and other hypotonic solutes. Hypertonic solutions cause water to flow from the ECF into the intestine, → ↓ ECF volume and hypernatraemia. There is a deficit of water, hypernatraemia (Na^+ >150mmol/L), and ↑ serum osmolality (>295Osmol/l). Clinical features include severe thirst, irritability and convulsions (especially if Na^+ is >165mmol/l).

Hypotonic (hyponatraemic) dehydration

Occurs in patients with diarrhoea who drink large amounts of water or other hypotonic fluids containing very low quantities of salt and other solutes and in patients who receive IV infusions of 5% glucose in water. It occurs because water is absorbed from the gut while the loss of salt continues, producing a net excess of water and hyponatraemia. Serum Na^+ and osmolality are low (Na^+ <130mmol/L, Osm <275mOsmol/L). Clinical features include lethargy and, rarely, convulsions.

All three types of dehydration can be managed with same oral rehydration fluid and intravenous regimes described on the following pages.

Box 6.11 Assessment of dehydration in children with diarrhoea

1. Look at			
Condition	Well, alert	Restless, irritable	Lethargic[1] or unconscious
Eyes[2]	Normal	Sunken	Sunken
Thirst	None	Drinks eagerly, very thirsty	Drinks poorly, unable to drink
2. Pinch the skin to assess skin turgor[3]			
	Goes back immediately	Goes back slowly	Goes back very slowly
3. Decide			
	No dehydration	Some dehydration	Severe dehydration
4. Treat			
	Plan A (see p. 276)	Plan B (see p. 278)	Plan C (see p. 280)
	Plans B and C require at least two of the four signs to be +ve		

Notes

[1]A lethargic patient is not simply asleep; patient's mental state is dull and patient cannot be fully awakened. Patient may appear to be drifting into unconsciousness.

[2]In some infants, eyes normally appear a little sunken, so ask mother if child's eyes appear normal to her.

[3]Pinch abdominal skin in a longitudinal manner with thumb and bent forefinger. 'Goes back slowly' means that it is visible for more than 2s (see Fig. 6.9).

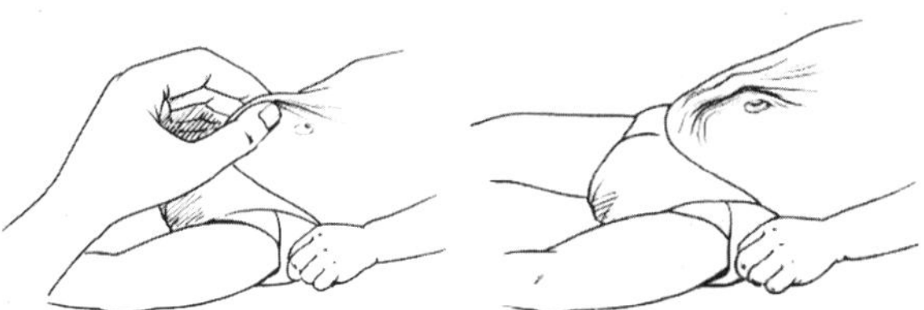

Fig. 6.9 Skin pinch to assess skin turgor. Pinch skin midway between umbilicus and flank, then release skin to observe how quickly it goes back. Skin pinch returns very slowly (≥2 seconds) in severe dehydration due to reduced skin turgor.

Reproduced from *Management of the Child with a Serious Infection or Severe Malnutrition* with permission from WHO.

Undress and observe the child for signs of severe malunutrition—no fat plus muscle wasting = marasmus, pitting oedema = kwashiorkor.

Check for fever and signs of pneumonia.

Estimation of fluid deficit

A child's fluid deficit may be estimated by following Table 6.2.

Children with dehydration should be weighed without clothing to estimate fluid requirements. If weighing is not possible, use the child's age to estimate weight. Treatment should never be delayed because scales are not available.

Suitable fluids

Recommended home fluids should be used in the prevention of dehydration only (i.e. treatment plan A). These should include at least one fluid that normally contains salt (e.g. ORS; salted drinks such as salted rice water or salted yoghurt; vegetable or chicken soup with salt). Other fluids recommended are those that are frequently given to children in the area, and mothers consider acceptable for children with diarrhoea, and that may be likely given in ↑ amounts if advised to do so. Such fluids should be safe and easy to prepare.

If there are signs of dehydration (Box 6.12), ORS should be used as per treatment plans B and C.

- Teaching mother to add salt (about 3g = level teaspoon/L) to unsalted drinks or soups during diarrhoea is beneficial, but requires education and (initially) supervision. Teach the mother to *always* taste fluid herself before giving it to child. It should not taste saltier than tears.
- A home-made solution containing 3g/L salt and 18g/L of sugar (sucrose) is effective, but recipe is often forgotten, made up incorrectly, and/or the ingredients hard to obtain.

Unsuitable fluids

A few fluids are potentially dangerous and should be avoided during episodes of diarrhoea. Avoid drinks sweetened with sugar that can cause osmotic diarrhoea and hypernatraemia (e.g. soft drinks, cola, sports drinks, energizing drinks, sweetened fruit drinks, sweetened tea).

Oral rehydration solution

The formula for ORS recommended by WHO and UNICEF in 2004 is given in Box 6.13. This formula contains less Na^+ than the original ORS, and is safer and more effective. Where bulk preparation is required, multiply the amounts shown by the number of litres required. WHO-ORS is also available in pre-prepared packets for dissolution in water. ORS should be used within 24h of preparation. When given correctly, ORS provides sufficient water and electrolytes to correct the deficits associated with acute diarrhoea.

Table 6.2 Estimation of child's fluid deficit

Assessment	Fluid deficit as % body weight	Fluid deficit mL/kg
No signs of dehydration	<5%	<50mL/kg
Some dehydration	5–10%	50–100mL/kg
Severe dehydration	>10%	>100mL/kg

Box 6.12 Dehydration in children with malnutrition

Signs of dehydration are more difficult to assess in children with severe malnutrition, and can be difficult to distinguish from signs of sepsis. As a result, the degree of dehydration may be over- or underestimated.

- Eyes appear sunken because of the absence of orbital fat. Ask the mother if there has been a change.
- Skin turgor more difficult to assess by skin pinch because of oedema in kwashiorkor and redundant skin in marasmus, but characteristic dough-like feel of severe dehydration may still be useful.
- Thirst is a useful sign if present. Check by offering water or ORS rather than by asking. Inability to drink also occurs in sepsis.
- Lethargy and coma may be due to sepsis.
- ReSoMal should be used for rehydration, 📖 p. 696.
- Reserve IV fluids for dehydration with shock. See 📖 Management of the sick child, Management of shock in children with severe malnutrition, p. 12 for further information.

Box 6.13 WHO and UNICEF recommended reduced osmolarity ORS recipe: to make 1L from bulk ingredients

1. Sodium chloride	2.6g	Na+	75mmol/L
2. Glucose (anhydrous)	13.5g	Chloride	65mmol/L
3. Trisodium citrate, dihydrate	2.9g	Glucose	75mol/L
4. Potassium chloride	1.5g	K^+	20mmol/L
If glucose and trisodium citrate are not available, use:		Citrate	10mmol/L
Sucrose	18g	Total osmolarity	245
Sodium bicarbonate	2.5g		

- Completely dissolve the sugar and salts in 1L clean water—boiled or chlorinated water is best.
- ORS solution should be used within 24h, after which time it should be discarded and fresh solution prepared.
- To make 1L of rice-based ORS, boil 50g of rice powder in 1.1L of water. Mix in sugar and salt in the quantities stated above. Use within 12h.

Treatment plan A: treat diarrhoea without signs of dehydration at home

Use this plan to teach the mother to:
- Continue to treat her child's current episode of diarrhoea at home.
- Give early treatment for future episodes of diarrhoea.
- Prevent dehydration.

Counsel the mother on the four rules of home treatment:

Give extra fluid (as much as the child will take).
- Breastfeed frequently and for longer at each feed.
- If not exclusively breastfed, give one or more of the following:
  - ORS solution
  - food-based fluids (such as soup, rice water, and yoghurt drinks)
  - clean water.

It is especially important to give ORS at home when:
- The child has been treated with Plan B or Plan C during this visit.
- The child cannot return to a clinic if the diarrhoea gets worse.

▶ Teach the mother how to mix and give ORS. Give the mother 2 packets of ORS to use at home.

▶ Show the mother how much fluid to give in addition to the usual fluid intake (see Table 6.3).

Tell mother to:
- Give a teaspoon every 1–2min for a child <2yrs.
- Give frequent small sips from a cup for older children.
- Wait 10min if child vomits, then continue, but more slowly.
- Continue giving extra fluid until the diarrhoea stops.

Give zinc supplements

▶ Tell the mother how much zinc to give:
- <6mths → half a 20mg tablet (10mg total) per day for 14d.
- ≥6mths → one 20mg tablet (20mg total) per day for 14d.

▶ Show the mother how to give zinc supplements:
- Infants → dissolve the tablet in a small amount of expressed breastmilk, ORS, or clean water, in a small cup or spoon.
- Older children → tablets can be chewed or dissolved in a small amount of clean water in a cup or spoon.

▶ Remind the mother to give the zinc supplements for the full 14d.

Continue feeding
- Give the child plenty of food to prevent malnutrition.
- Continue to breastfeed frequently. If the child is not breastfed, give the usual milk, in small quantities spread throughout the day.
- If the child is >6mths, or already taking solid foods, also give cereal or another starchy food mixed, if possible, with pulses, vegetables, milk, meat, or fish. Give fresh fruit juice or mashed banana to provide K^+. Give freshly prepared foods. Cook and mash/grind food well.

- Encourage the child to eat; offer food >5× per day taking advantage of any time the child will accept food.
- Fever is often accompanied by anorexia, offer food again when fever subsides.
- Give same foods after diarrhoea stops and give an extra meal each day for 2wks.

When to return

Take the child to a health worker if the diarrhoea does not improve within 3d or the child develops any of the following:

- Many watery stools.
- Fever.
- Repeated vomiting.
- Eating/drinking poorly.
- Unable to breastfeed.
- Marked thirst.
- Blood in the stool.

Table 6.3 Amount of ORS to give according to child's age

Age	After each loose stool	At home
<2yrs	50–100mL	500mL/day
2–10yrs	100–200mL	1L/day
>10yrs	As much as tolerated	2L/day

What to do if patient does not improve with ORT

In ~5% of patients the signs of dehydration do not improve or worsen after starting treatment with ORS. The usual causes are:

- Continuing rapid stool loss (>15–20mL/kg/h), e.g. cholera.
- Insufficient ORS intake due to fatigue, lethargy, or lack of supervision.
- Frequent severe vomiting.

Admit such patients to hospital and give ORS by NGT or Ringer's lactate solution 75mL/kg IV over 4h. Consider possibility of cholera. Close monitoring of patient's progress, hourly at first, is essential.

When not to give ORS

Rarely, ORS should not be given. This is true for children with:

- Abdominal distension due to paralytic ileus (often owing to opiates, e.g. codeine, or loperamide, or to hypokalaemia).
- Glucose malabsorption, indicated by a marked ↑ in stool output when ORS is given. There is no improvement and the stool contains large amounts of glucose.

In these situations, rehydration should be given IV until diarrhoea subsides.

Table 6.4 Amount of ORS to give during the first 4h

Age*	<4mths	4–11mths	12–23mths	2–4yrs	5–14yrs	>14yrs
Weight	<5kg	5–7.9kg	8–10.9kg	11–15.9kg	16–29.9kg	≥30kg
Volume	200–400mL	400–600mL	600–800mL	800–1200mL	1.2–2.2L	2.2–4.0L

*Use the child's age only when you do not know the weight. Approximate amount of ORS required (in mL) can be calculated by multiplying the child's weight (in kg) × 75.

Treatment plan B: treat some dehydration with ORS

In clinic, give the recommended amount of ORS over a 4h period:

▶ Determine the amount of ORS to give during first 4h (see Table 6.4).
- If the child wants more ORS than shown, give more.

▶ Show the mother how to give ORS solution:
- Give a teaspoon every 1–2min for a child <2yrs.
- Give frequent small sips from a cup for an older child.
- If the child vomits, wait 10min; then continue, but more slowly.
- Continue breastfeeding whenever the child wants.

▶ After 4h, reassess the patient using the chart on Box 6.11 and continue plan A, B, or C as appropriate:
- If there are no signs of dehydration, shift to plan A. When dehydration has been corrected, urine will start to be passed, and child may become less irritable and fall asleep.
- If signs indicating some dehydration are still present, repeat plan B, but start to offer food, milk, and juice as in plan A.
- If there are signs indicating severe dehydration, treat using plan C (Fig. 6.10).

▶ If the mother must leave before completing treatment:
- Show her how to prepare ORS solution at home.
- Show her how much ORS to give to finish 4-h treatment at home.
- Give her enough ORS packets to complete rehydration. Also give her 2 packets as recommended in plan A.
- Make sure that children receive breastmilk, or if >6mths, are given some food before being sent home. Emphasize to mother importance of continuing feeding throughout the diarrhoeal episode.

Explain the four rules of home treatment:
- Give extra fluid (see plan A for recommended fluids).
- Give zinc supplements.
- Continue feeding.
- When to return.

Monitoring signs during oral rehydration therapy

Check the patient from time to time during rehydration to ensure that ORS is being taken satisfactorily and signs of dehydration are not worsening. If, at any time, patient develops severe dehydration, switch to treatment plan C. After 4h, reassess patient following guidelines in Box 6.11. Decide what treatment to give next:

- If signs of severe dehydration have appeared, IV therapy should be started immediately, following plan C. This is very unusual, however, and tends to occur in children who drink ORS poorly and continue to pass large volumes of watery stool during the rehydration period.
- If patient still has signs of mild dehydration, continue oral rehydration therapy, following plan B. At same time start to offer food, milk, and other fluids as described in treatment plan A. Reassess the patient frequently.
- If no signs of dehydration, patient should be considered fully rehydrated. If this is the case, the skin pinch will be normal; thirst will have subsided; urine passed normally; and child will no longer be irritable and may fall asleep.

Teach the mother to treat child at home using ORS following plan A. Give her enough ORS sachets for 3d and teach her signs that indicate she must bring her child back to health post.

Meeting normal fluid needs

While treatment to replace existing water and electrolyte deficit is in progress, child's normal daily fluid requirements must also be met. This may be done as follows:

- *Breastfed infants:* continue to breastfeed as often and as long as infant wants, even during oral rehydration therapy.
- *Non-breastfed infants <6mths of age:* during rehydration with ORS, give 100–200mL of plain water by mouth. After completing rehydration, resume full-strength milk or formula feeds. Give water and other fluids normally taken by infant.
- *Older children and adults:* throughout rehydration treatment, in addition to ORS, offer as much plain water, milk, or other fluids that do not contain large amounts of sugar as is accepted. Avoid processed juices and sodas.

Treatment plan C: treat severe dehydration quickly

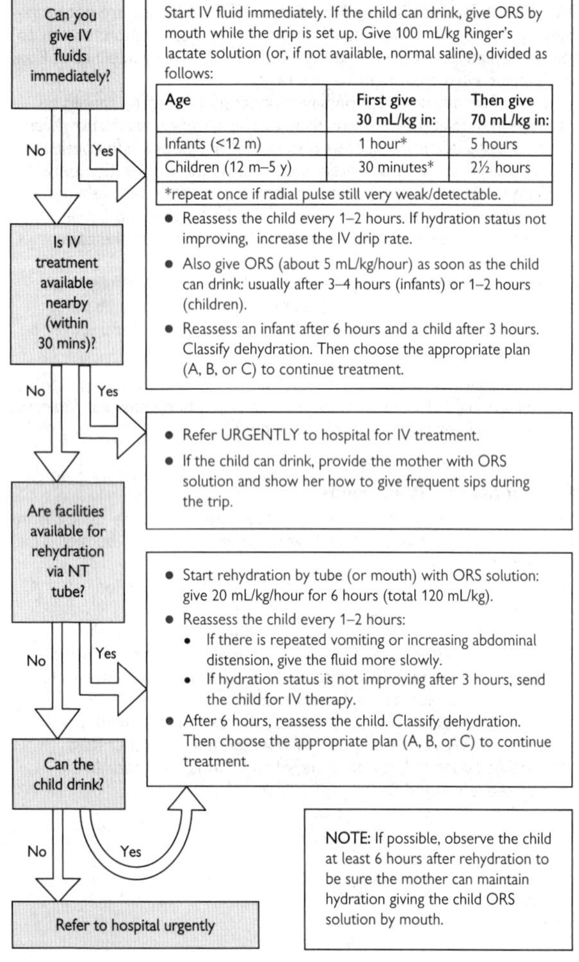

Fig. 6.10 Treatment plan C.

Reproduced from *Diarrhoea Treatment Guidelines for Clinic-based Healthcare* Workers, 2005, with permission of WHO.

Monitoring IV rehydration therapy

Patients should be reassessed every 15–20min until a strong radial pulse is present. Thereafter, assess hourly to confirm that hydration is improving. If it is not, IV fluid may be run at a faster rate.

When the planned amount of IV fluid has been given (6h for infants, 3h for older patients), patient's state of hydration should be reassessed using the chart in Box 6.11.

- If the child's eyelids become puffy, liver enlarges, or tachycardia and tachypnoea appear, these may be signs of fluid overload and cardiac failure, especially in malnourished children. ↓ Rate of IV infusion and monitor closely.
- If there are still signs of severe dehydration, repeat plan C (see Fig. 6.10). Unusual, but may occur in cases of cholera and in children who pass frequent, watery stools during rehydration period.
- If the patient shows signs of mild dehydration, discontinue IV fluid replacement and commence oral rehydration with ORS for 4h according to plan B.
- If no signs of dehydration, discontinue IV therapy and commence ORS treatment according to plan A.

Observe the patient for >6h before discharging. For children, ensure that mother is able to continue giving ORS at home and is aware of signs that indicate she must bring the child back.

Alternative solutions for IV rehydration

Preferred

- *Ringer's lactate solution with 5% glucose (also called Hartmann's solution):* provides glucose to help prevent hypoglycaemia. If available, it is preferred to Ringer's lactate solution without glucose.

Acceptable

- *Physiological saline (0.9% NaCl, also called normal saline):* widely available; an acceptable alternative to Ringer's lactate solution, but contains neither a base to correct acidosis nor potassium to correct K^+ losses. KCl (5–15mmol/L) may be added.

Unsuitable

- *Plain glucose (dextrose) solution should* ***not*** *be used:* does not contain Na^+, base, or K^+; does not correct hypovolaemia effectively.

Some difficulties encountered in home therapy for diarrhoea

Mother is disappointed because child is not prescribed an antibiotic or given an injection

Explain that diarrhoea will usually stop by itself after a few days. Zinc supplements will help the child get better quicker and will increase the child's appetite. In most cases, antibiotics do not help and sometimes can make the diarrhoea go on longer. It is better to see how child progresses and, if necessary, check to see what is causing diarrhoea so that, if antibiotics are needed, doctor can give the right one. Fluid replacement and continued feeding will help shorten illness, and maintain child's strength and growth.

Mother believes that food should not be given during diarrhoea

Ask her to explain her beliefs about how diarrhoea should be treated. Discuss with her importance of feeding in order to keep her child strong and growing, even during diarrhoea. There are almost always some foods that are acceptable—find out and encourage these alternatives.

Mother does not know what fluids to give her child at home

Ask her what fluids she can prepare at home and reach an agreement on appropriate fluids for her child.

Mother does not have ingredients to make a recommended fluid

Ask her if she can obtain necessary ingredients easily. If she cannot, suggest another home fluid.

Child vomits after drinking ORS or other fluids

Explain that more fluid is usually kept down than is vomited. Tell her to wait 10min, then start giving fluid again, but more slowly, just sips at a time from a spoon or cup.

Child refuses to drink

A child who has lost fluid and is dehydrated will usually be thirsty and want to drink, even when there are no signs of dehydration. If child is not familiar with taste of ORS, some persuasion and patience may be needed at first. When child drinks well to begin with, but then loses interest, it usually means that sufficient fluid has been given. If child is not dehydrated, it is not necessary to insist on ORS; other clear fluids can be given as suggested in Table 6.2.

Mother is given some ORS packets for use at home, but is afraid they will be used up before diarrhoea stops

Explain that after the ORS has been used up she should give a recommended home fluid (e.g. rice water), or water, or she should return to health facility for more packets of ORS. In any event, she should continue to give extra fluid until diarrhoea stops.

Paediatric note: summary of important points in management of diarrhoea in children

- Infectious diarrhoea very common, especially ages 6mths–2yrs.
- Always examine child and follow WHO guidelines for assessing dehydration (Box 6.11).
- Keep in mind possibility of non-infectious causes, such as intussusception, appendicitis.
- Exclusively breastfed babies may have frequent explosive loose stools, but appear well, are not dehydrated, do not lose weight, and usually follow a similar daily pattern of stooling.
- Treat dysentery (visible blood in stools) with antibiotics.
- Avoid antibiotics in non-dysenteric diarrhoea unless severe diarrhoea in a high-risk group (neonates, immune compromised).
- Avoid antimotility drugs (loperamide) in children <2yrs.
- Give oral zinc supplements: 20mg elemental zinc daily for 10–14d (10mg daily in children <6mths).
- Continue breastfeeding.
- Continue normal diet, fractioning* diet, and ↑ frequency of servings. ↓ Lactose if necessary by mixing milk with other foods. Do not dilute formula with water.
- *Advise carer of signs of alarm in small children:*
  - undue sleepiness
  - abdominal distension
  - worsening of diarrhoea
  - fever
  - drinking poorly/unable or unwilling to breastfeed
  - visible blood in stools.
- Use opportunities of contact with carers of young children to advise preventative measures:
  - exclusive breastfeeding to 6mths
  - introduce complementary foods from 6mths
  - continue breastfeeding together with other foods to 2yrs
  - give locally appropriate nutritional advice to ensure sufficient calories and micronutrients
  - wash hands frequently with soap
  - dispose of infant stools safely, use potties, avoid faecal contamination of play areas
  - make up infants' food fresh for each meal
  - avoid storing prepared food and bottles at room temperature
  - boil water for children if clean water source is not guaranteed.

*Fractioning diet: divide diet into small frequent amounts. Especially useful for lactose intolerance—reduces amount reaching duodenum and having to be hydrolysed at any one time.

Management of persistent diarrhoea

Diarrhoea, with or without blood, that begins acutely and lasts >14d. Clinically, these episodes cannot be differentiated from sequential episodes of acute diarrhoea over a prolonged period, and management is the same. Usually associated with ↓ weight and, often, with serious non-intestinal infections. Many children with persistent diarrhoea are malnourished before diarrhoea starts. Persistent diarrhoea seldom occurs in infants who are exclusively breastfed. Take a careful history and examine the patient well.

The object of treatment is to restore weight gain and normal intestinal function. In most cases, patient will need to be admitted to hospital for diagnostic tests, treatment, and observation.

Treatment of persistent diarrhoea

- *Appropriate fluids:* to prevent/treat dehydration (see 🕮 General management of dehydration, p. 272; 🕮 Some difficulties encountered in home therapy for diarrhoea, p. 282).
- *Appropriate antimicrobial therapy:* to treat infections, in particular non-intestinal infections (e.g. pneumonia, otitis media, UTI). Send stool to look for *Giardia*, *Shigella*, or *Entamoeba* infection.
- *A nutritious diet:* that does not cause worsening of the diarrhoea. Children will require a >110cal/kg/d, which may need to be given via a NGT if the child is too weak or refuses to eat. For infants <6mths, encourage exclusive breastfeeding, but check baby is gaining weight. If possible, help mothers who are not breastfeeding to re-establish lactation (see 🕮 Nutrition, p. 683).
- Where possible, replace animal milk with yoghurt, a lactose-free formula, or a local diet with ↓ lactose (<3.5g lactose/kg body weight/d). For older infants and young children, use standard diets made from local ingredients. Two diets are given in Table 6.5: the first contains ↓ lactose, the second is lactose-free for the 30% children who do not improve with the first diet.
- *Supplementary vitamins and minerals:* all children with persistent diarrhoea should receive supplementary multivitamins and minerals each day for 2wks. Aim to provide >2 RDAs of folate, vitamin A, Fe, Zn, Mg, and Cu. As a guide, RDAs for a 1-yr-old child are:
- Folate 150micrograms.
- Zinc 10mg.
- Iron 10mg.
- Vitamin A 400micrograms.
- Copper 1mg.
- Magnesium 80mg.

Table 6.5 Low lactose and lactose free diets

Diet 1 (low lactose)	Diet 2 (lactose-free)
83cal/100g	75cal/100g
11% of calories as protein	15% of calories as protein
2.7g lactose in 130mL/kg body weight/day	
Ingredients	
Full-fat dried milk 11g (or 85mL whole milk)	Whole egg (without shell) 36g
Uncooked rice 15g	Uncooked rice 10g
Vegetable oil 3.5g	Vegetable oil 5g
Cane sugar 3g	Glucose 5g
Water to make up to 200mL final volume	Water to make up to 200mL final volume
130mL/kg provides 110cal/kg	*145mL/kg provides 110cal/kg*
Boil rice to a slurry with some of the water, add other ingredients and rest of water to make up to 200mL final volume.	Boil rice to a slurry with some of the water, add the whole beaten egg and continue to cook for another minute, stirring well. Add the rest of the ingredients and the water to make up to 200mL final volume.

Malnutrition and diarrhoea

Diarrhoea is as much a nutritional disease as one of fluid and electrolyte loss. Children who die from diarrhoea, despite good management, are usually malnourished—often severely so.

During diarrhoea, ↓ food intake, ↓ nutrient absorption, and ↑ nutrient requirements often combine → ↓ weight and failure to grow. The child's nutritional status declines and any pre-existing malnutrition is made worse. Malnutrition itself makes diarrhoea worse, prolonging it and making it more frequent. This vicious cycle may be broken by continuing to give nutrient-rich foods during diarrhoea and giving a nutritious diet, appropriate for the child's age, when the child is well.

When these steps are followed, malnutrition can be either prevented or corrected, and the risk of death from a future episode of diarrhoea is much reduced.

Other complications of diarrhoea

Electrolyte disturbances

Knowing serum electrolyte concentrations rarely changes management of patients dehydrated due to diarrhoea. In most cases, hypernatraemia, hyponatraemia, and hypokalaemia are all adequately treated by oral rehydration with ORS or IV rehydration with Ringer's lactate. In severe dehydration, however, plasma Na^+ concentrations may reach extremes and hypokalaemia may produce muscular weakness, cardiac arrhythmias, and paralytic ileus.

Fever

Fever in a patient with diarrhoea may be due to the organism causing the diarrhoea or, particularly in children, another infection (e.g. pneumonia, otitis media, malaria). Presence of fever should suggest infection, particularly if it persists after patient is fully hydrated. In malaria-endemic areas, children with fever should be urgently tested for malaria. High fevers (>39°C) in children should be treated with an antipyretic, such as paracetamol to ↓ irritability and prevent febrile convulsions.

Convulsions

In a child with diarrhoea and convulsions during illness, the following diagnoses should be considered:

- *Febrile convulsions:* usually occur in children aged 6mths to 6yrs (Box 1.12).
- *Meningitis:* needs to be considered in any child or adult following a convulsion. Look for neck rigidity and Kernig's sign (classical signs less common in young children). Do a lumbar puncture after checking the retinae for papilloedema (↑ ICP) and looking for focal neurological signs.
- *Hypoglycaemia:* occasionally occurs in children with severe malnutrition, due to their small hepatic glycogen reserves and insufficient gluconeogenesis. If suspected, give 2–5mL/kg of 10% glucose solution (or 2.5mL/kg of a 20% glucose solution) IV over 5min. If hypoglycaemia is the cause, recovery will usually be rapid. In such cases, Ringer's lactate with dextrose should be given to the child for IV rehydration. Feed child as soon as possible to restore liver glycogen.
- *Shigellosis: Shigella* infections can sometimes cause convulsions—do stool culture.

Vitamin A deficiency

Diarrhoea ↓ absorption of, and ↑ the need for, vitamin A. In areas where vitamin A deficiency is already prevalent, young children with diarrhoea have an ↑ risk of developing eye problems. Treat if vitamin A deficiency common locally or suspected clinically.

Doses

50 000IU vitamin A for children <6mths; 100 000IU for children 6–12mths; 200 000IU for children >12mths. Give dose on day 1, day 2, and 14 days later or at discharge.

Metabolic acidosis

During episodes of diarrhoea, a large amount of bicarbonate may be lost from the stool. If renal function is normal, this will be replaced. However, renal impairment due to hypovolaemia may → rapid development of acidosis. Poor tissue perfusion → excess lactate production. Features of metabolic acidosis are: respiratory compensation (look for deep 'Kussmaul' breathing +/– tachypnoea); vomiting; low serum bicarbonate (<10mmol/L); acidaemia (pH <7.3).

Antidiarrhoeal drugs

These agents, though commonly used, have no practical benefit and are never indicated for the treatment of acute diarrhoea in children. Some of them are dangerous.

- *Adsorbents:* e.g. kaolin, attapulgite, smectite, activated charcoal, colestyramine, are of no proven value.
- *Antimotility drugs:* e.g. loperamide, diphenoxylate with atropine, tincture of opium, paregoric, codeine, ↓ frequency of stools in adults, but are less effective in children. Moreover, they may → severe paralytic ileus and prolong infection by delaying the elimination of the causative organism or toxin. Loperamide is useful in travellers' diarrhoea in adults; it should never be used in infants.

Other drugs

- Antiemetics: e.g. prochlorperazine, chlorpromazine, metaclopramide, should not be given since they often cause sedation and may interfere with ORS treatment. Vomiting will cease as the patient becomes hydrated.
- Cardiac stimulants (inotropes): should never be used to overcome shock and hypotension, which may occur in severe dehydration with hypovolaemia. Cardiac output will be restored by fluid resuscitation.
- *Blood or plasma:* is only indicated if there is proven shock.
- *Steroids and purgatives:* are of no benefit and should not be used.

Prevention of diarrhoea

Correct treatment of diarrhoeal diseases is highly effective in preventing death, but has no impact on the incidence of such diseases. Teach family members to adopt preventative measures. Do not overload the mother with technical advice, but emphasize the most important points for each particular mother and child.

Measures that interrupt the transmission of pathogens

The infectious agents that cause diarrhoea are usually transmitted by the faeco-oral route. Focus on:

- Giving only breastmilk for the first 6mths of life.
- Avoiding the use of infant feeding bottles and dummies.
- Improving the preparation and storage of weaning foods (to minimize microbial contamination).
- Using only clean water for drinking.
- Washing hands with soap after defecation and disposal of faeces, and before preparing food.
- Disposing of all faeces in a safe manner.

Measures that strengthen host defences

- Continuing to breastfeed for the first 2yrs of life.
- Improving a child's nutritional status by giving more nutritious food, including foods of animal origin that contain essential minerals such as zinc and other micronutrients. Giving complementary foods more often, from 3 × per day when first introduced at 6mths to 5 × per day at 12mths.
- Immunizing against measles.
- Immunizing against rotavirus.

How doctors can help to prevent diarrhoea

- Ensure appropriate in-service training of health facility staff.
- Make sure that staff are giving consistent messages on diarrhoea prevention and infant feeding.
- Display promotional material on how to treat and prevent diarrhoea.
- Be a good role model (breastfeeding, hand washing, water hygiene, latrine hygiene).
- Take part in community-based activities to promote health.
- Coordinate efforts for disease prevention with those of relevant government programmes.
- Prescribe zinc supplements rather than antibiotics.

Public health note: household strategies for safe drinking water

Provision of safe drinking water requires a safe water source and a safe storage system. Clean water alone is not enough; food hygiene and hand washing are also essential measures to ↓ diarrhoea.

- *Boiling:* bring water to rolling boil for 1min and allow to cool. Most effective sterilization method: kills most microbes even at high altitude. But is slow, expensive, requires ~1kg firewood/L, contributes to deforestation, danger of scalding, and recontamination is possible.
- *Chlorination:* add 0.5–1.0mg/L sodium hypochlorite solution (e.g. liquid laundry bleach, but check no other ingredients), mix well, and leave for 30min to kill all bacteria, viruses, and most protozoa; longer exposure in tightly closed container kills *E. hystolytica* and *Giardia* spp. and reduces chlorine taste; not effective against cryptosporidia. Works less well (requires more time) when water is turbid: works best if turbid water filtered or sediment left to settle first. Taste may reduce acceptability. During disinfection, use two containers: while one is in use, the water in the other remains exposed to the chlorine increasing the effectiveness against viruses and protozoa and also reducing the chlorine taste.
- *Iodination:* 8mg/L iodine sterilizes most microbes within 10–30min at 20°C; longer periods for colder water; and up to 8h to ensure complete sterilization. Taste may reduce acceptability.
- *Sand filtration (0.15–0.3mm particles ≥0.5m deep, either in a settling tank or a specially designed receptacle):* removes particulate matter and ~50% bacteria, 20% viruses, and 50% protozoa (not cryptosporidia oocysts). Cotton cloth filters remove ~50% bacteria, but less effective for viruses and oocysts. Both methods remove the copepod vector of dracunculiasis. Helpful as preliminary stage before boiling or chlorination.
- *Ceramic filters:* require 1μm pore size; use a coarser filter first if water turbid to prevent clogging. Relatively expensive. Ideally, boil water first.
- *Sunlight UV-irradiation:* put 0.5–1L water in clean transparent container (e.g. plastic Cola bottle), shake vigorously, and expose to sunlight (e.g. on roof of hut) for 6 h. UV light kills many bacteria and protozoa, but some viruses resistant; more effective if water gets hot. Usually only suitable for small volumes; needs plenty of sunlight.
- *Flocculation/coagulation:* not usually used domestically. Reduces turbidity, removes ~30% microbes, enhances action of chlorination or sunlight.
- *Safe carriage and storage of water:* water is often contaminated by dirt, dust, animals, or bird droppings during collection and storage, e.g. by dipping hands or containers into the water store. To minimize contamination use vessels of sufficient size, with smallest possible opening to prevent hand entry or dipping of utensils, preferably with a cap or lid, and a spout or tap, which prevents hand contact. Disinfectant such as sodium hypochlorite may be added to the water container (as above).

Travellers' diarrhoea

Travellers' diarrhoea affects ~20–50% of the ~12 million travellers to the tropics/subtropics annually, especially those from resource-rich regions; small children and young adults (perhaps because of higher risk behaviour); backpackers; campers; adventure tourists; and those staying in low-cost accommodation or cruise ships. In addition to upset business or holiday plans, longer-term consequences include chronic or persistent diarrhoea (1–3%), irritable bowel syndrome (3–10%), and Guillain–Barré syndrome (rare). The most common causes are:

- Enterotoxigenic *E. coli:* 30–80%
- *Campylobacter jejuni:* ~20%
- *Shigella* spp.: 5–15%
- *Salmonella* spp: 3–15%
- *Giardia intestinalis:* 0–3%

Management (see Fig. 6.11)

- Most episodes are self-limiting.
- ↑ Fluid intake. Eating, e.g. broth with noodles or salty crackers with sweetened drinks, will provide a balance of carbohydrate and salt.
- ORS is preferable if diarrhoea frequent or severe, or if there are signs of dehydration, weakness, or muscle cramps, as it more effectively restores both salts and water deficits.
- Drinks designed for rehydration during sports activities do *not* contain the correct balance of salts for diarrhoea treatment. Sodas and fruit juices are often hyper-osmolar or have high sugar content and can make diarrhoea worse.
- Prompt antibiotic treatment reduces symptom duration (e.g. ciprofloxacin 500mg bd oral for 3d).
- Loperamide (4mg oral once followed by 2mg after each loose stool) shortens the episode in older children and adults with frequent small volume stools. (Do not use loperamide in infants, nor if blood in stools, fever, tenesmus, or other signs of dysentery.)

Prevention

Avoid unpeeled fruit and uncooked vegetables, sauces that are not freshly prepared, and food prepared and handled in unhygienic conditions, e.g. by street vendors. Where there is no reliable source of chlorinated water, sterilize water by boiling or with chlorine tablets, or drink bottled water from a reputable source. Avoid bottled water where the bottles are immersed in water or ice to keep them cool. Beware of ice or ice cream, which may be made using contaminated water. When trekking or in isolated places, it is advisable to carry packets of ORS and a course of treatment. Hand sanitizers are useful when handwashing is impossible.

Prophylaxis

Short-term travellers may take prophylactic bismuth subsalicylate (525mg qds oral) or antibiotics such as norfloxacin 400mg od oral or ciprofloxacin 500mg od oral, but both are associated with some side-effects including risk of *Clostridium difficile* associated diarrhoea; early treatment of episodes is therefore preferable.

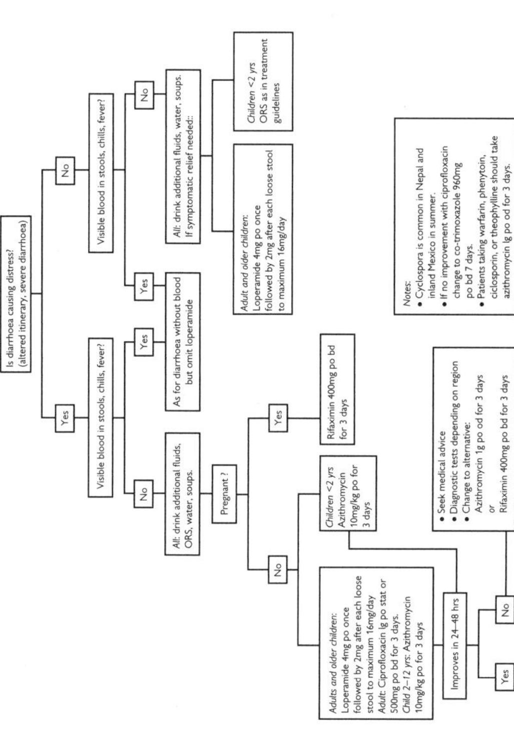

Is diarrhoea causing distress?
(altered itinerary, severe diarrhoea)
Yes
No
Visible blood in stools, chills, fever?
Visible blood in stools, chills, fever?
No
Yes
Yes
No
All: drink additional fluids, ORS, water, soups.
As for diarrhoea without blood but omit loperamide
All: drink additional fluids, water, soups. If symptomatic relief needed::
Pregnant ?
No
Yes
Adults and older children: Loperamide 4mg po once followed by 2mg after each loose stool to maximum 16mg/day
Adult: Ciprofloxacin lg po stat or 500mg po bd for 3 days.
Child 2–12 yrs: Azithromycin 10mg/kg po for 3 days
Children <2 yrs Azithromycin 10mg/kg po for 3 days
Rifaximin 400mg po bd for 3 days
Adult and older children: Loperamide 4mg po once followed by 2mg after each loose stool to maximum 16mg/day
Children <2 yrs ORS as in treatment guidelines
Improves in 24–48 hrs
Yes
No
• Seek medical advice
• Diagnostic tests depending on region
• Change to alternative:
Azithromycin 1g po od for 3 days
or
Rifaximin 400mg po bd for 3 days
Notes:
• Cyclospora is common in Nepal and inland Mexico in summer.
• If no improvement with ciprofloxacin change to co-trimoxazole 960mg po bd 7 days.
• Patients taking warfarin, phenytoin, ciclosporin, or theophylline should take azithromycin lg po od for 3 days.

Fig. 6.11 Empirical treatment of travellers' diarrhoea.

Chapter 7
Gastroenterology

Invited author **Marc Mendelson**

Disorders of the mouth and pharynx

A common feature of tropical infections, particularly in HIV+ malnourished individuals.

Gingivostomatitis and mouth ulcers

Gingivostomatitis (inflammation of the gums/oral mucosa) may be caused by HSV, EBV, or enteroviruses. Treat HSV gingivostomatitis with aciclovir (📖 Common cutaneous viral infections, p. 615).

Aphthous ulcers may be idiopathic or due to HIV, Behçet's, Crohn's, coeliac, or Stevens–Johnson syndrome.

Treatment

Topical steroid (e.g. hydrocortisone 2.5mg oromucosal tablet), or inhaled beclametasone applied directly to ulcers. Consider oral prednisolone or thalidomide for major aphthous ulceration in HIV. Consider biopsy of persistent ulcer(s) to exclude malignancy.

Oral candidiasis

Small, white mucosal flecks with surrounding erythema, common in HIV. Treat with nystatin liquid 1mL (infants) or 5mL (adults) kept in mouth for as long as possible then swallowed. Continue until symptoms gone for 48h. Severe disease may require oral fluconazole, particularly if oesophageal involvement is suspected (200mg od × 2wks).

Oral hairy leukoplakia (OHL)

Poorly demarcated, painless, raised, corrugated white patches on the side of the tongue or buccal mucosa. Cannot be scraped off. Caused by EBV, qualifying as a WHO stage III HIV diagnosis. No specific treatment, but usually regresses on ART (see 📖 HIV/AIDS, p. 69).

Gingivitis

Causes include anaerobic infection (Vincent's angina), drugs (phenytoin, ciclosporin, or nifedipine), acute myeloid leukaemia (AML), pregnancy and vitamin C deficiency (scurvy). Prevent periodontal disease by encouraging better oral hygiene.

Glossitis

Glossitis is a feature of iron deficiency, vitamin B deficiency, and tropical sprue. Overgrowth of papillae and *Aspergillus niger* result in a black, hairy tongue.

Acute necrotizing ulcerative gingivostomatitis

Painful ulceration of the mouth with halitosis and gingivorrhoea. Predisposing factors include malnutrition, HIV, poor oral hygiene, and smoking. Treat with warm saline mouth washes and metronidazole 200mg oral tds plus penicillin 500mg oral qds for 5–7d.

Pharyngitis

Typically due to Streptococci, viruses, or diphtheria, rarely in Lassa fever, rabies, or following ingestion of *Fasciola hepatica*. In high incidence acute rheumatic fever settings, treat children (especially >3yrs) with sore throat with single dose benzathine benzylpenicillin 1.2MU IM (↓ risk of acute rheumatic fever from 2.8 to 0.2%). Severe pharyngitis with spread to neck, thrombosis of internal jugular vein, +/– embolization of infected thrombus typifies necrobacillosis (Lemierre's disease). Treat with IV penicillin and metronidazole.

Malignant lesions of the mouth and pharynx

Buccal squamous cell carcinoma (associated with tobacco, chewing betel nut, +/– alcohol) and Burkitt's lymphoma (due to EBV infection) are common, especially in India, Southeast Asia, and tropical Africa. Nasopharyngeal carcinoma (due to EBV infection, see 🕮 EBV Ch 18, p. 798) is common in the Far East and S. China. Malignant change may be preceded by leukoplakia and epithelial atrophy. Optimum management and outcome rely on early diagnosis. Consider malignancy in chronic (>3wks), solitary lesions: examine for cervical lymphadenopathy and biopsy lesion +/– lymph nodes. KS causes purple lesions, often on the hard palate. It is usually associated with HIV; treatment is ART therapy (see 🕮 HIV/AIDS, p. 69, and 🕮 Dermatology, p. 587).

Other lesions of the mouth

- *Salivary gland hypertrophy:* common in malnourished children. Other causes include *Ascaris lumbricoides* and diffuse inflammatory lymphocytosis syndrome (DILS) in HIV.
- *Angular stomatitis:* common in iron-deficiency anaemia, HIV, and riboflavin deficiency.

Paediatric note: *Cancrum oris* (Noma)

A serious and often fatal condition in which gangrenous stomatitis rapidly spreads to involve the palate and face following anaerobic infection. Occurs mainly in young, malnourished African children. Management requires wound debridement and antisepsis, antibiotics (IV penicillin plus metronidazole), and nutritional rehabilitation (+/– surgical reconstruction).

Upper gastrointestinal tract symptoms

Dysphagia and odynophagia

Dysphagia = difficulty in swallowing; odynophagia = painful swallowing. Dysphagia that has progressed from solids to liquids implies severe narrowing of the oesophagus. Endoscopy +/– biopsy is the investigation of choice where available; barium swallow is an alternative. In HIV, a trial of empirical fluconazole 200mg od oral for 2wks for oesophageal candidiasis reduces the need for endoscopy.

Dyspepsia

Epigastric or retrosternal discomfort associated with eating. Clues lie in the history (see Box 7.1).

Causes

Peptic ulcer disease (PUD), gastro-oesophageal reflux, dysmotility, drugs, and GI tract parasites (including hookworm, *Taenia*, *Ascaris*, *Giardia*, and *Entamoeba histolytica*). Suspect malignancy if age >45yrs, weight loss, dysphagia, vomiting, haematemesis, or anaemia (see Boxes 7.2 and 7.3).

Management

- Review any drugs that may cause dyspepsia.
- Trial of antacids, unless malignancy suspected.
- Endoscopy (or barium meal) if malignancy or PUD suspected.
- Stool microscopy if GI parasites suspected. *Note*: presence of parasites does not exclude other causes of dyspepsia.
- Stop smoking and avoid alcohol.

Box 7.1 Dysphagia: key questions in the history

- Can fluid be drunk normally?
  - *Yes*—suspect stricture (benign or malignant).
  - *No*—possible motility disorder.
- Is the dysphagia constant and painful?
  - *Yes*—suspect malignant stricture.
- Is it difficult to initiate swallowing?
  - *Yes*—suspect bulbar palsy, especially if swallowing causes cough.
- Does the neck bulge or gurgle upon swallowing?
  - *Yes*—suspect pharyngeal pouch.
- Is the patient HIV-infected?
  - *Yes*—suspect oesophageal candidiasis.
- Are there signs of systemic infection or illness?
  - *Yes*—may be manifestation of systemic disease.

Box 7.2 Causes of dysphagia

- *Malignancy:* carcinoma of the oesophagus, stomach, or pharynx.
- *Extrinsic compression*: mediastinal lymphadenopathy, lung carcinoma, retrosternal goitre, left atrial enlargement.
- *HIV-associated:* candidiasis, CMV, HSV, severe aphthous ulceration. TB less common.
- *Motility disorders:* achalasia, Chagas disease, bulbar/pseudobulbar palsy (including bulbar poliomyelitis), diffuse oesophageal spasm, myasthenia gravis, syringobulbia, systemic sclerosis.
- *Benign strictures:* peptic stricture, ingestion of caustics, oesophageal web, iron deficiency anaemia (Plummer–Vinson syndrome).
- *Pharyngeal pouch.*
- *Others:* trauma, foreign body (e.g. bezoar, swallowed fish or animal bone), anxiety (globus hystericus).

Box 7.3 Causes of dyspepsia and their typical clinical features*

- *Peptic ulcer disease:* epigastric pain, night waking, and relief by eating food, drinking milk, or taking antacids.
- *Gastro-oesophageal reflux:* retrosternal discomfort, heartburn, and regurgitation/acid brash. Worse lying flat or after large meals.
- *Dysmotility:* early satiety, bloating, and nausea.
- *Drugs:* e.g. non-steroidal anti-inflammatory drugs (NSAIDs), calcium antagonists, nitrates, pyrazinamide.

*Note that, although history often gives a clue to cause of dyspepsia, it does not replace further investigation of specific causes where indicated.

Helicobacter pylori **and peptic ulcer**

Helicobactor pylori are motile, Gram –ve rods that live in the mucus layer of the stomach. In resource-poor countries *H. pylori* colonization is almost universal by 20yrs. Clinical associations include:

- *PUD:* up to 90% patients with duodenal ulcer (DU) and >50% patients with gastric ulcer (GU) are colonized with *H. pylori.*
- *Gastric cancer: H. pylori* causes intestinal metaplasia and atrophic gastritis, which are risk factors for adenocarcinoma of the stomach.
- *MALT lymphoma:* generally, a benign monoclonal proliferation of lymphocytes; tumour histology and clinical features improve with *H. pylori* eradication.
- *Non-ulcer dyspepsia:* the role of *H. pylori* remains uncertain; trials of *H. pylori* eradication have shown little benefit.

Diagnosis

Options include endoscopy + biopsy, serology, urea breath test, and stool antigen test, depending on resources.

Eradication therapy

Proton pump inhibitor or bismuth-based regimens with two antibiotics, e.g. omeprazole 20mg od oral (or bismuth subsalicylate 2 tabs qds oral) + amoxicillin 1g bd oral (or tetracycline 500mg bd oral) + metronidazole 400mg bd oral (or clarithromycin 500mg bd oral) for 7d.

Disorders of the oesophagus

Gastro-oesophageal reflux disease

Heartburn and regurgitation with a bitter, acid taste (acid brash), particularly when lying flat, are the hallmarks. Gastro-oesophageal reflux disease (GORD) may also cause a chronic nonproductive cough or wheezing.

Diagnosis

Usually clinical; barium swallow may identify a hiatus hernia.

Management

Stop smoking, lose weight if obese, and raise the head of the bed. Antacids after meals and at bedtime. Severe cases require H_2 receptor antagonists (e.g. ranitidine 150mg bid or 300mg nocte oral) or proton pump inhibitors (e.g. omeprazole 20–40mg nocte oral) +/– metoclopramide.

Hiatus hernia

Herniation of the stomach through the oesophageal hiatus of the diaphragm. Often asymptomatic; may predispose to GORD or present with acute chest and/or epigastric pain. A fluid level behind the heart on erect CXR, or on Ba meal, is diagnostic. Management is as for GORD.

Columnar-lined (Barrett's) oesophagus

Columnar-lined oesophagus (CLO) represents the severe end of the spectrum of GORD in which there is columnar metaplasia of a segment of the oesophagus. Its importance derives from the risk of progression to oesophageal adenocarcinoma.

Management

Treat GORD. Repeated endoscopy + biopsy for early detection of malignancy advised.

Paediatric note: gastro-oesophageal reflux disease

Gastro-oesophageal reflux (GOR) commonly occurs in infants, normally ↓ by 12–18mths. Symptomatic reflux is termed gastro-oesophageal reflux disease (GORD).

Clinical features

Infants

Most commonly vomiting and ↑ crying (may see back-arching). May also present with abdominal pain, feeding difficulties, failure to thrive, cough, wheeze, and apnoea. Children with neurodevelopmental problems are particularly prone to GORD; it is more likely to persist and to be more severe.

Older children

May present with dysphagia and heartburn, similar to adults.

Management

Infants

In milder cases (well babies with ↑ regurgitation and/or crying) give smaller feeds more often; this may ↓ symptoms sufficiently. Feed thickeners or sodium alginate preparations (such as Gaviscon® Infant) may also be trialled. H_2 antagonists (e.g. ranitidine) are usually then used (may be appropriate earlier if breastfed and sterile water a problem for Gaviscon®/thickeners). PPIs (e.g. omeprazole) may benefit if not improved with ranitidine. In the most severe, Nissen fundiplication may be required, usually after failure of medical treatment. In some cases, cow's milk protein intolerance may cause symptoms of GORD.

Older children Advice and treatment similar to adults.

Oesophageal cancer

Commonest in adults (males: females 73:1) aged >30yrs. Highest incidence Central/East Africa, Iran, Southeast Asia, and northern China. Pre-malignant associations include CLO (for adenocarcinoma), and Plummer–Vinson syndrome or achalasia (squamous cell carcinoma). Other risk factors include smoking, alcohol, and malnutrition.

Clinical features

Dysphagia, ↓ weight, retrosternal pain (lymphadenopathy). Coughing due to aspiration or development of oesophago-tracheal fistula, aspiration pneumonia, Horner's syndrome, recurrent laryngeal nerve palsy (hoarse voice).

Management and prognosis

Usually rapidly progressive; late presentation common, so <5% 5-yr survival; chemo/radiotherapy slightly ↑ survival in adenocarcinoma. Palliative treatment includes nutrition (+/– oesophageal stenting), pain relief, and treatment of complications including aspiration pneumonia.

Gastric cancer

Incidence varies; common in Costa Rica and Northeast Brazil.

Risk factors Chronic gastritis, bile reflux, *H. pylori*, pernicious anaemia, ingestion of corrosives, and diet—↑ salt intake, lack of fresh fruit, and ingestion of toxic nitrosamines from fish.

Clinical features

Dyspepsia, ↓ weight, malaena, anaemia, and abdominal mass. In metastatic disease there may be hepatomegaly, deranged LFTs, lymphadenopathy (left supraclavicular lymphadenopathy = Virchow's node), umbilical deposits (Sister Mary Joseph's nodule), or peritonism.

Diagnosis Biopsy for histology and staging.

Management Surgical resection offers the only hope of cure. Palliation aims to relieve pain and obstruction and control haemorrhage.

Upper GI bleeding

Assessment

Haematemesis and/or malaena due to a number of causes (see Box 7.4) indicate upper GI bleeding. Ask about previous GI bleeds, history of PUD, liver disease, varices, dysphagia, vomiting or ↑ weight, co-morbidity, alcohol, and drugs. Look for signs of liver disease and portal hypertension; rectal examination for malaena.

- *Mild to moderate bleed:* pulse/BP normal, <60yrs, insignificant co-morbidity, and Hb >10g/dL (unless chronic anaemia present).
- *Severe bleed:* age >60yrs, pulse >100bpm, systolic BP <100mmHg, Hb <10g/dL, significant co-morbidity.

Immediate management

- IV access (two large bore venous cannulae; central venous access to assist fluid resuscitation if severe).
- Blood for FBC, U&E, LFT, clotting, group and save/cross-match.
- Resuscitate with normal saline or colloid while waiting for blood (if blood required); in dire emergency, use O Rhesus –ve blood.
- Correct clotting abnormalities (vitamin K, FFP, platelets).
- Catheterize if severe bleed. Monitor urine output to ensure >0.5mL/kg/h.
- Monitor vital signs closely.
- Consider urgent endoscopy, and notify surgeons of all serious bleeds on admission; keep patient nil by mouth until stable.

Further management

Depends on severity, response to initial treatment, and diagnosis.

- High-dose IV proton pump inhibitor therapy ↓ re-bleeding (but has little effect on mortality).
- Endoscopy to define cause, assess risk of re-bleeding, and plan treatment; repeat endoscopy may be required for re-bleeding.
- Endoscopic therapy may be possible for some lesions (e.g. adrenaline injection, sclerotherapy, variceal banding).
- If stable 4–6h post-endoscopy, allow to eat and drink.
- Treat peptic ulcers and *H. pylori*. Avoid NSAIDs if possible.
- Repeat endoscopy at 6wks for gastric ulcers to ensure response to proton pump inhibitors and exclude gastric cancer.

Oesophageal varices

In portal hypertension, portal-systemic shunts develop in the lower oesophagus causing dilated oesophageal veins. Variceal bleeding occurs in 20–50% cirrhotic patients, usually <2yrs of diagnosis. Mortality from 1st bleed is 75% and is related to severity of liver disease.

Common causes Liver cirrhosis, schistosomiasis, portal vein thrombosis, and Budd–Chiari syndrome (hepatic vein thrombosis).

Management of acute variceal bleed

- Assess and resuscitate as for any upper GI bleed (see 📖 Upper gastrointestinal symptoms, p. 296).
- *Protect airway:* may need intubation and ventilation if uncontrolled bleeding, encephalopathy, hypoxia, or aspiration pneumonia.
- *Control bleeding:* endoscopic variceal band ligation or sclerotherapy. Balloon tamponade with a Sengstaken–Blakemore tube may be used for emergency short-term control of bleeding; ideally, patient should be intubated and ventilated to reduce aspiration and aid passage.
- Give octreotide (50micrograms/h IV) for 2–5d.
- Correct clotting abnormalities (FFP, vitamin K, platelets).
- Prophylactic antibiotics, e.g. ciprofloxacin 500mg bd oral for 1wk.

Primary and secondary prevention of variceal bleeding

- Endoscopic variceal band ligation is effective if available; sclerotherapy also works.
- ↓ Portal vein pressure with propranolol 40–80mg bd oral (and/or isosorbide mononitrate 20mg bd oral).
- Manage underlying cause, especially schistosomiasis—periportal fibrosis regresses after treatment. Advise to abstain from alcohol.

Box 7.4 Causes of upper GI bleeding

Most common causes	Rarer causes
• Peptic ulcer disease. • Gastritis/gastric erosions. • Mallory–Weiss tear. • Oesophageal varices. • Oesophagitis. • Duodenitis. • Malignancy. • Drugs (NSAIDs, anticoagulants, steroids).	• Portal hypertensive gastropathy. • Angiodysplasia. • Dieulafoy lesion. • Bleeding disorders. • Aortoenteric fistula. • Haemobilia (bleeding from biliary tree).

Acute abdomen

An acutely ill person whose symptoms and signs are chiefly related to the abdomen. Thorough history and examination are essential—abdominal pain may be misinterpreted as body aches and treatment given for malaria, only for peritonitis to be found later. Prompt laparotomy can be essential: *repeated examination is the key to making the decision.* Most common causes of an acute abdomen are given in Fig. 7.1.

Clinical syndromes that usually require laparotomy

- *Organ rupture (e.g. spleen, aorta, ectopic pregnancy):* there may be shock and abdominal swelling. Note history of trauma (especially if pre-existing splenomegaly, but splenic rupture may occur weeks after trauma, and in the absence of trauma).
- *Peritonitis due to perforated viscus:* the patient lies still and has signs of shock, abdominal tenderness, board-like abdominal rigidity, and absent bowel sounds. Acute pancreatitis may present similarly, but does not require laparotomy, so check serum amylase.

Syndromes for which laparotomy may not be indicated

Local peritonitis

For example, cholecystitis, salpingitis, appendicitis (the latter *will* need surgery). If abscess formation suspected (swelling, swinging fever, ↑ WCC) look for sentinel loop on plain AXR; abdominal ultrasound scan (USS) or CT if available. Drainage of a collection may be percutaneous (USS- or CT-guided) or by laparotomy.

Colic

Is pain that regularly waxes and wanes due to muscular spasm of a hollow viscus (e.g. gut, ureter, uterus, or gallbladder), causing restlessness, unlike peritonitis.

Bowel obstruction

Causes colic, distension, vomiting, and (often absolute) constipation, with active 'tinkling' bowel sounds (c.f. ↓ bowel sounds in functional ileus). Causes include adhesions (previous surgery), herniae (internal or external), sigmoid/caecal volvulus, tumours, intussusception, TB, and ascariasis. AXR shows dilated loops of bowel. Fluid levels help to distinguish small and large bowel obstruction.

Immediate management

- Resuscitate with normal saline, colloid, or blood as appropriate. Anaesthesia ↓ BP, so resuscitate properly before taking to theatre — unless losing blood faster than it can be replaced (e.g. ruptured ectopic pregnancy, leaking abdominal aortic aneurysm).
- FBC, U&E, LFT, Ca^{2+}, clotting, amylase, culture, cross-match.
- Insert NGT and keep patient nil by mouth; give IV maintenance fluids.
- Consider erect CXR, AXR, +/– ECG.
- Broad-spectrum empiric antibiotics if infection suspected; rationalize therapy later in light of investigations and progress.

Non-surgical causes of an acute abdomen

Several non-surgical conditions may present with an acute abdomen. The most common causes are listed in Box 7.5.

Box 7.5 Medical causes of acute abdominal symptoms

- Gastroenteritis.
- Typhoid.
- Malaria.
- Myocardial infarction.
- Cholera.
- Porphyria.
- Heroin addiction.
- Pneumonia.
- UTI.
- Sickle cell crisis.
- Polyarteritis nodosa.
- Herpes zoster.
- Thyroid storm.
- Lead colic.
- Diabetic ketoacidosis.
- Abdomino-peritoneal TB.
- *Yersinia enterocolitica.*
- Fitz-Hugh-Curtis syndrome (*Chlamydia*).
- Pneumococcal peritonitis.
- Henoch–Schölein purpura.
- Irritable bowel syndrome.

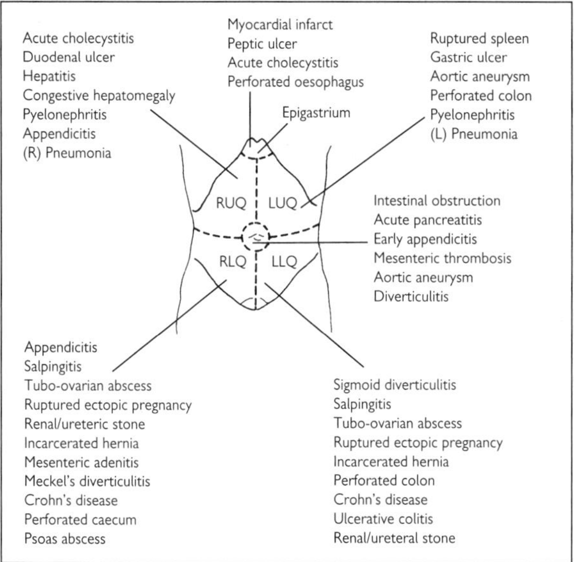

Fig. 7.1 Causes of acute abdominal pain.

Appendicitis

Appendicectomy is the commonest emergency abdominal operation. Without surgery, appendicitis may → gangrene, perforation, peritonitis, and death. Mortality is highest at the extremes of age, but also in young adults in malaria-endemic areas, where non-specific symptoms may be misinterpreted.

Aetiology

Obstruction due to lymphoid hyperplasia or faecolith; super-infection is usually bacterial (rarely, amoebae, *S. mansoni, S. stercoralis, T. trichiura, A. lumbricoides*, or *Taenia* spp. implicated).

Clinical features

Increasing central abdominal colic, usually shifting to the RIF, depending on the anatomical position of the appendix. Anorexia common; vomiting or diarrhoea may occur. Flushing with mild fever, tachycardia, RIF tenderness, guarding, rebound tenderness, and Rovsing's sign (left iliac fossa (LIF) palpation causes pain in RIF) are common. Appendix mass or abscess may be palpable, due to encasement of appendix or pus in omentum and bowel loops.

Diagnosis

Clinical Examine the patient repeatedly, since the severity may change. Do a per rectum (pr) (painful on right side), and a per vagina (pv) in women to exclude salpingitis.

Differential diagnosis

See Table 7.1. USS may differentiate between an appendix mass and an abscess.

Management

- Prompt appendicectomy to prevent perforation, unless appendix mass present or surgery contraindicated. Metronidazole 500mg IV or 1g pr plus cefuroxime 1.5g IV prior to surgery.
- If appendix mass present, manage conservatively initially. Metronidazole 1g pr tds plus either gentamicin 3–5mg/kg IV daily or chloramphenicol 12.5mg/kg IV qds. Monitor vital signs and size of appendix mass closely. Surgery indicated if patient's condition worsens. Any abscess should be drained. Elective appendicectomy is carried out at ~3mths, once inflammatory adhesions have subsided.

Paediatric note: mesenteric adenitis

A viral inflammation of the mesenteric lymph nodes affecting children. Suspect it if there is high fever, vomiting, a history of URTI, and cervical lymphadenopathy. Abdominal signs are usually less severe than in appendicitis and usually subside within 48h.

Table 7.1 Differential diagnosis of RIF pain

Inflammation	Clinical features
Mesenteric adenitis (children)	High fever, vomiting, cervical nodes; improvement with observation
Meckel's diverticulitis	Usually discovered at appendicectomy; rarely bleeds or causes obstruction
Caecal diverticulum	May be inflamed, perforate, or bleed; blood pr cannot be attributed to other causes
Inflammatory masses	?Abdominal mass, weight loss
TB	Other systemic signs of TB; ascites common, lymphadenopathy
Crohn's disease/UC	Systemic, eye, joint, and/or anorectal manifestations
Worm infection	Worms or ova in stool. Chronic history; weight loss; pruritus ani
Amoebic colitis	Diarrhoea with blood and mucus; trophozoites in hot stool; patient may be critically ill
Malignancy	
Lymphoma	Weight loss; lymphoma elsewhere
Caecal cancer	Anaemia, ↓ weight, intermittent pain
Large bowel tumour	Diarrhoea; blood pr; eventually obstruction with caecal distension
Genital tract pathology	
Salpingitis	Vaginal discharge; pelvic pain; tender on pv
Ectopic pregnancy	Amenorrhoea, vaginal bleeding, abdominal distension; may be in shock; +ve pregnancy test
Pelvic abscess	Previous salpingitis; ? history of illegal abortion.
Ovarian torsion or bleeding	Severe pain, minimal signs; requires USS. Ovarian cyst/fibroid
Testicular torsion	Testis is swollen and very tender +/– referred pain
Intra-abdominal testis	Torsion or malignancy (teratoma/seminoma)

Peritonitis

In the tropics, most commonly due to appendicitis, perforated DU, salpingitis, typhoid perforation, or amoebic colitis. If less acute, consider TB peritonitis, especially in HIV+ individuals.

Clinical features

Abdominal pain, immobile and anxious +/– fever, sweating, tachycardia, and tachypnoea. Sepsis → hyperdynamic circulation initially (warm peripheries, bounding pulse), but shock (cold peripheries, thready pulse) may develop. Abdomen may be distended, rigid, moves poorly with respiration; rebound tenderness, guarding, and absent bowel sounds. In chemical peritonitis: (bile, gastric acid, or pancreatic enzymes) pain is intense; the abdomen may be so rigid that distension is minimized. Signs of peritonism may be less in the very young or critically ill (e.g. post-operatively). Abdominal signs usually mild in cirrhotic patients with spontaneous bacterial peritonitis.

Diagnosis

Is clinical; +/– gas under the diaphragm on CXR (see Fig. 7.2 for causes); AXR may show fluid between thickened loops of bowel or distended bowel and fluid levels. USS may show intraperitoneal fluid or collections/abscesses. Aspirate free fluid in the abdomen and send for microscopy (pus cells suggest bacterial peritonitis, lymphocytes suggest TB) and protein (to confirm fluid is an exudate). FBC, CRP, U&E, serum amylase, blood cultures are helpful. Diagnostic laparotomy may be required in severe cases.

Treatment

- Resuscitate as for acute abdomen (📖 Acute abdomen, p. 306).
- Insert NGT and keep patient nil by mouth.
- Broad-spectrum antibiotics (e.g. IV cefuroxime 750mg tds or IV ceftriaxone 1g od, plus IV metronidazole 500mg tds).
- Monitor vital signs and urine output closely.
- Drain any intra-abdominal collections under USS guidance. If USS not available, or deteriorates, drain by laparotomy.
- If no contraindications, laparotomy is usually indicated for severe, generalized peritonitis.

Female genital tract sepsis

Salpingitis usually causes local pelvic peritonitis. Many cases may be managed with antibiotics alone—but if patient's condition deteriorates, pelvic mass expands, or perforated uterus suspected (e.g. septic abortion), urgent laparotomy +/– hysterectomy is indicated. Rupture of tubo-ovarian abscesses carries a high mortality.

Amoebic colitis

Failure to respond to metronidazole (see 📖 Acute diarrhoea with blood, Amoebic dysentery, p. 238) within 48h suggests transmural disease and ischaemic necrosis for which laparotomy indicated.

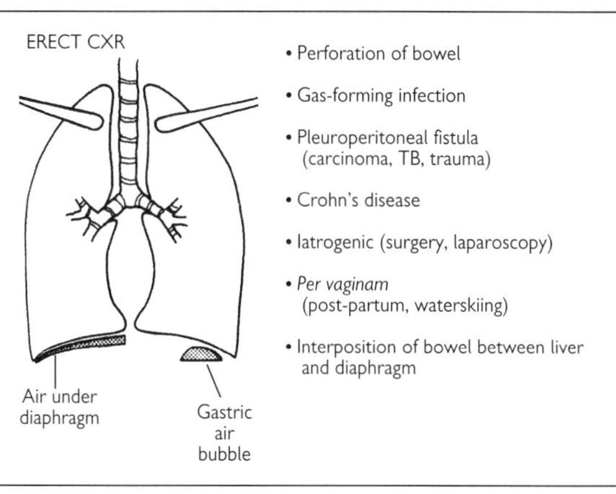

Fig. 7.2 Causes of gas under the diaphragm.

Right upper quadrant pain

Right upper quadrant (RUQ) pain is usually due to liver or gallbladder pathology; other causes shown in Box 7.6. Important tropical causes include amoebic liver abscess, AIDS cholangiopathy, complicated hydatid cysts.

Box 7.6 Causes of RUQ pain

Gastrointestinal/hepatobiliary

- Acute hepatitis
- Amoebic liver abscess
- Hydatid liver disease (if complicated)
- Liver tumours
- AIDS cholangiopathy
- Gallstones (biliary colic)
- Cholecystitis
- Cholangitis
- Liver flukes

Other

- RLL pneumonia
- Right heart failure
- Pyelonephritis
- Duodenal ulcer
- Trichuriasis (whipworm)

Acute pancreatitis

Rare in most tropical countries. Progression to haemorrhagic, necrotizing disease may be rapid with high mortality.

Causes

Gallstones (50%), alcohol abuse (20–25%), other causes of duct obstruction (e.g. *Ascaris*, tumour, hydatid cysts in common bile duct), drugs (e.g. stavudine, sodium stibogluconate and meglumine antimoniate, thiazides, steroids, tetracycline), viruses (mumps, coxsackie, EBV, hepatitis A virus (HAV), HBV), hypercalcaemia, hyperlipidaemia, trauma, scorpion venom, autoimmune diseases (e.g. polyarteritis nodosa (PAN)), hypothermia.

Clinical features

Abdominal pain and vomiting (90% cases) + raised amylase/lipase are typical. Peritonism may develop, but as the pancreas is retroperitoneal, abdominal signs are often mild. Jaundice may occur due to oedema around the common bile duct. Severe disease may cause peri-umbilical (Cullen's sign) or flank (Grey Turner's sign) discoloration.

Investigation

Serum amylase/lipase (levels peak early and ↓ over 3–4d), U&Es, Ca^{2+}, glucose, fasting lipids, ABG. Exclude other causes of acute abdomen (📖 Acute abdomen, p. 306). USS for gallstones. If patient deteriorating with severe pancreatitis, CT may show pancreatic necrosis requiring surgery.

Treatment

- Resuscitate as for acute abdomen (📖 Acute abdomen, p. 306).
- *Severe pain:* strong analgesia (e.g. morphine 10mg q4h plus prochlorperazine 12.5mg tds IM).
- Broad-spectrum antibiotic prophylaxis.
- Consider surgery (necrosectomy) in very severe cases.
- Following recovery, consider cholecystectomy if gallstones.

Complications

- *Early:*
  - organ failure
  - acute respiratory distress syndrome
  - acute renal failure
  - DIC
  - hypocalcaemia (may require albumin replacement or 10mL of 10% calcium gluconate IV slowly)
  - transient hyperglycaemia.
- *Late (>1wk):* pancreatic pseudocyst (may resolve spontaneously or require surgical drainage; if it becomes infected, it requires drainage). A few patients develop persisting DM.

Chronic pancreatitis

Destruction of pancreas with atrophy results in some permanent loss of exocrine and endocrine function → pain, DM, and malabsorption (steatorrhoea).

Biliary disease

Gallstones

Gallstone impaction in the gallbladder outlet. In tropical regions, pigmented gallstones may be more common than in non-tropical regions, due to ↑ haemolysis (e.g. from malaria).

- *Clinical:* severe, constant pain lasting up to several hours, radiating to the interscapular region, and associated with nausea and vomiting. Complications include acute cholecystitis and ascending cholangitis.
- *Management:* strong analgesia and antispasmodics (e.g. hyoscine butylbromide 20mg IV/IM, repeated after 30min if necessary).

Acute cholecystitis Acute inflammation of the gallbladder (90% caused by gallstones but also consider biliary parasites).

- *Clinical:* fever and local peritonism, tender, palpable gallbladder especially on inspiration (+ve Murphy's sign), and/or jaundice.
- *Management:* treat with broad-spectrum antibiotics e.g. cefuroxime 750mg IV tds + metronidazole 500mg IV (or 1g pr) tds as inflammation may be associated with infection; usually followed by cholecystectomy when the patient's condition allows.

Ascending cholangitis Bacterial infection of the biliary tract, usually a result of bile stasis due to chronic obstruction from gallstones or biliary parasites.

- *Clinical:* RUQ pain, fever, and jaundice (Charcot's triad).
- *Management:* broad-spectrum antibiotics, e.g. cefuroxime 750mg IV tds + metronidazole 500mg IV (or 1g pr) tds. Biliary drainage may be needed, followed by cholecystectomy when patient's condition allows.

Bilary parasites

Biliary parasites are an important concern in tropical regions. They include biliary ascariasis (📖 p. 348), and liver flukes: fascioliasis (📖 p. 342), clonorchiasis (📖 p. 340) and opisthorchiasis (📖 p. 340).

AIDS cholangiopathy

Biliary obstruction resulting from infection-related strictures of the biliary tract, usually seen with low CD4 count. RUQ pain (>90%) and cholestasis +/– low-grade fever. May present with asymptomatic cholestatic jaundice. Cryptosporidium, CMV, and microsporidiosis are common causes, but often no organism is identified. ART markedly improves prognosis.

Cholangiocarcinoma

Bile duct cancer. Liver flukes are endemic in the Far East and can cause chronic irritation resulting in far higher risk of cholangiocarcinoma in endemic regions (📖 Liver flukes, p. 338).

- *Clinical:* usually become symptomatic with blockage of biliary drainage, causing painless jaundice. May also see weight loss and abdominal pain.
- *Management:* staging, surgery. Prognosis is generally very poor.

Amoebic liver abscess

Amoebic liver abscess (ALA) is the most common form of extra-intestinal amoebiasis (📖 Acute diarrhoea with blood, p. 238). It may complicate acute amoebic dysentery (10%) or present months after exposure. 70% recall no history of diarrhoea.

Clinical presentation

- *Usually acute (over 2–7d):*
  - fever, rigors, sweats, and RUQ +/– right shoulder tip pain, +/– vomiting
  - left lobe abscesses often → LUQ pain.
- May also present subacutely with dull RUQ ache, weight loss, fatigue, low-grade pyrexia, and anaemia.
- Use of empiric antimalarials may make onset less acute.
- Clinical signs include hepatomegaly (often tender); 'punch tenderness' may be elicited if abscess concealed beneath the ribs.
- Extreme tenderness or oedema of the abdominal wall or intercostal space suggests imminent rupture.
- There is seldom jaundice or ascites.
- Right-sided pleural effusion/empyema/lung collapse may occur due to rupture into the pleura.
- Rupture of a left lobe abscess into pericardium usually rapidly fatal.

Diagnosis

- Neutrophilia, ↑ESR, +/– ↑ ALT/alkaline phosphatase (ALP).
- CXR may show raised hemi-diaphragm +/– pleural reaction and/or basal atelectasis.
- *USS:* large (usually unilocular) necrotic lesion with some internal debris. During the early 'amoebic hepatitis' stage of the disease, USS may miss the lesion: repeat USS after 24–48h may be required.
- *E. histolytica* serology is +ve in >95% patients after the first week.
- Stool microscopy is +ve for amoebic cysts in 50%.
- Indications for aspiration are shown in Box 7.7. Abscess fluid is odourless and reddish-brown (resembles 'anchovy sauce') vs. yellow pus of bacterial abscesses. Microscopy shows debris (c.f. pus cells in bacterial liver abscess) and Gram stain does not show organisms; rarely *E. histolytica* trophozoites may be seen.
- Beware misdiagnosing acute ALA as acute cholecystitis or appendicitis.

Management

- Drug therapy is sufficient to cause healing without scarring in most cases. Metronidazole 800mg tds (or tinidazole 2g od) oral 5d, followed by diloxanide furoate 500mg tds (or paromomycin 500mg tds) oral 10d for intraluminal *E. histolytica* cyst eradication.
- Indications for percutaneous drainage are given in Box 7.8. Drains may be removed when drainage is minimal (usually after 2–3d).
- Follow up ALA clinically. (Note: USS may show large liver defects even after successful cure.)

Box 7.7 Percutaneous aspiration-injection-reaspiration (PAIR)

- Puncture cyst under USS or CT guidance.
- Aspirate >30% of cyst fluid volume.
- Inject* an equal volume of a scolicidal agent, such as hypertonic saline (30% saline = 300g NaCl/L) or 95% ethanol into the cyst.
- Reaspirate complete cyst contents after 30min.

**Note*: Injection of a scolicidal agent is contraindicated if cyst fluid is bile stained suggesting communication with the biliary tree.

Box 7.8 Indications for drainage of amoebic liver abscess

- Left lobe abscess (risk of rupture into pericardium).
- Severely ill patients in whom rupture is considered imminent either clinically or on USS.
- *Diagnostic uncertainty*: diagnostic aspirate for Gram stain/culture.*
- Lack of response to drug therapy after 3–4d.

* Adequate drainage is usually indicated for pyogenic liver abscess.

Hydatid disease

Echinococcus granulosus (cystic hydatid disease) and *E. multilocularis* (alveolar hydatid disease) are responsible.

Cystic hydatid disease

E. granulosus is a small (3–6mm) cestode (tapeworm) that lives in the small intestine of dogs (also jackals, foxes). Eggs passed in canine faeces are infective to humans. Following ingestion, eggs develop into oncospheres which penetrate the intestinal mucosa and pass in the blood or lymphatics to host viscera including the liver (50–70%), lungs (20–30%), other organs, and peritoneal cavity. Oncospheres encyst in host viscera developing into mature larval cysts. These may be multiple and reach massive proportions (see Fig. 7.3).

Clinical features

Liver cysts grow ~1cm a year, presenting as masses, rather than abscesses. Patients may be asymptomatic or present with symptoms related to expansive growth of cysts, including abdominal pain, hepatomegaly, fever, and jaundice. Lung cysts may present when the cyst contents rupture into an airway and are coughed up.

Complications

Cyst rupture may be accompanied by life-threatening anaphylactic shock; conversely, other cysts collapse or disappear spontaneously. Cholangitis may occur due to rupture into the biliary tree. Pyogenic abscesses may form due to bacterial superinfection of cysts.

Diagnosis

The characteristic appearance of cysts on imaging (USS, CT, or MRI) is usually sufficient. Serology may aid diagnosis.

Management

- Most cysts are amenable to percutaneous aspiration-injection-reaspiration (PAIR) treatment (see Box 7.7). PAIR cure rates are >95%.
- In addition to PAIR, some authorities recommend albendazole 400mg bd oral for 1–6mths, starting before and continuing after drainage.
- Albendazole treatment alone not sufficiently reliable, although some individuals with multiple cysts are treated with prolonged courses.
- Surgical removal may be necessary for cysts not amenable to PAIR, especially if at risk of rupture or exerting pressure effects.

Alveolar hydatid disease

Occurs mainly in the northern hemisphere (hosts = foxes). *E. multilocularis* causes aggressive local tissue invasion by lateral budding of cysts and metastasis to other parts of the body (10% patients to CNS, lungs, bone, and eyes). Liver complications include cholangitis, Budd–Chiari syndrome, and portal hypertension. Due to the aggressive nature of the lesions, many are misdiagnosed clinically/radiologically as malignancy. Mortality untreated is high (>60% at 10yrs). Operable cases require wide surgical resection. Adjuvant albendazole is of benefit, and in inoperable cases, albendazole may provide arrest or cure in some patients.

Public health note: prevention of hydatid disease

- Education and hygiene to avoid exposure to/ingestion of dog faeces.
- In hyperendemic populations, periodic treatment of dogs (including wild and stray dogs) with praziquantel helps to prevent/control human disease.
- Strict control of livestock slaughtering and disposal of organs helps restrict the access of dogs to potentially contaminated viscera.

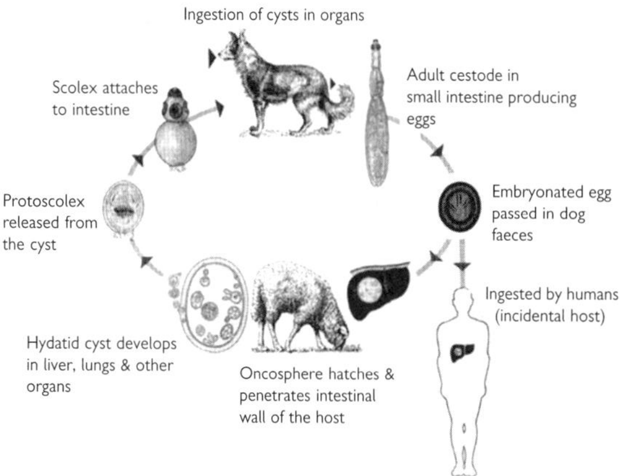

Fig. 7.3 Life cycle of *E. granulosus*.

Adapted from Piekarski, G, *Medical Parasitology in Plates*, 1962, with kind permission of Bayer Pharmaceuticals.

Liver disease

Jaundice

Jaundice (icterus) is visible if plasma bilirubin >35mmol/L. Causes may be pre-hepatic, hepatocellular, or post-hepatic/obstructive (see Box 7.9; for neonatal causes of jaundice, see 📖 Management of the sick child, Neonatal jaundice, p. 26). Sclerae and skin appear yellow. Do not confuse normal pale brown sclerae in dark-skinned people with jaundice. Carotinaemia (due to eating excess mangoes, tomatoes, or carrots) also → yellow skin, especially palms and soles, but the sclerae are white.

- *Pre-hepatic jaundice:* excess bilirubin production due to haemolysis, ↑ liver uptake, or ↓ conjugation leads to ↑ serum *unconjugated* bilirubin.
- *Hepatocellular jaundice:* hepatocyte damage +/– cholestasis.
- *Obstructive (cholestatic) jaundice:* bile excretion ↓ by intra- or extra-hepatic biliary obstruction ↑ *conjugated* bilirubin; pruritus common (look for excoriations, shiny fingernails). ↑ Urinary excretion of water-soluble conjugated bilirubin makes urine dark; stools pale as less bilirubin excreted in faeces. Steatorrhoea (fatty, pale, offensive stools that often float) may occur, and malabsorption of fat-soluble vitamins (A, D, E, K) may → osteomalacia and coagulopathy.

Assessment

Alcohol use, blood transfusions, sexual activity, tattoos, body piercing, jaundiced contacts, family history, and drugs, including herbal medicines. Examine for hepatomegaly and signs of chronic liver disease (CLD). Further investigations depend on clinical features, but include dipstick of urine for bilirubin; FBC, clotting, blood film, Coomb's test, U&Es, LFTs, hepatitis viral serology. Liver USS may show dilatated bile ducts (obstructive jaundice), gallstones, hepatic metastases, or pancreatic mass.

Hepatomegaly

Hepatomegaly is common in the tropics. Look for jaundice and signs of CLD. Palpate liver, noting texture, and percuss to define size (normal liver is <12cm in mid-clavicular line). Auscultate for hepatic bruit (typically in hepatocellular carcinoma, alcoholic hepatitis) or peritoneal rub over liver (may be present in metastases, liver abscesses).

Causes

Viral (e.g. Hep A-E, EBV, CMV, HIV), bacterial (e.g. leptospirosis, syphilis, severe typhoid, pyogenic liver abscess), protozoal (amoebic liver abscess), and parasitic (hydatid); CLD/cirrhosis (see Box 7.10); malignancy (metastases, hepatoma); infiltrative conditions (amyloid, sarcoid); Budd–Chiari syndrome; congestive cardiac failure; congenital Riedel's lobe; and polycystic liver.

Box 7.9 Common causes of jaundice (📖 Management of the sick child, Neonatal jaundice, p. 26)

Pre-hepatic jaundice

- Malaria.
- G6PD deficiency.
- Sickle cell disease.
- Gilbert's syndrome.
- Drugs (📖 Drug-induced hepatitis, p. 328).

Hepatocellular jaundice

- Viruses e.g. Hep A-E, EBV, CMV, yellow fever, Lassa fever).
- Other infections e.g. typhoid, leptospira, bartonella, syphilis.
- Alcoholic hepatitis.
- Chronic liver disease/cirrhosis.
- Drugs.
- Hepatic metastases.
- Hepatocellular carcinoma.
- Liver abscess.

Post-hepatic (cholestatic) jaundice

- Gallstones.
- Pancreatic CA.
- Porta hepatis lymph nodes.
- Cholangiocarcinoma.
- 1° biliary cirrhosis.
- Sclerosing cholangitis.
- Viral hepatitis (cholestatic phase).
- AIDS cholangiopathy.
- Ascariasis.
- Liver flukes.
- Choledochal cyst.
- Biliary atresia.
- Hydatid disease (rare).
- Drugs.

Box 7.10 Treatable causes of hepatomegaly without jaundice

Infections (= splenomegaly characteristically present)*

- Amoebic liver abscess.
- Schistosomiasis.*
- Miliary TB.*
- Malaria.*
- Visceral leishmaniasis.*
- Plague (*Yersinia pestis*).
- Trypanosomiasis.*
- Liver flukes.
- Toxocariasis.
- Hydatid disease.
- Bartonellosis.

Cardiac and nutritional

- Beriberi.
- Chagas disease.
- Kwashiorkor.

Viral hepatitis

Hepatitis A virus

Non-enveloped RNA picornavirus. Transmission is faeco-oral, e.g. ingestion of contaminated food or water. It is the commonest viral hepatitis worldwide and childhood infection is very common in areas of poor sanitation. In hyperendemic areas most adults have immunity (e.g. India 99%), thus HAV is an uncommon cause of acute hepatitis in adults in these settings. HAV frequently affects non-immunized travelers; 2° cases or outbreaks in resource-rich countries may follow importation of HAV.

Clinical features

- HAV severity is proportional to age.
- Asymptomatic infection is common in children, whereas fulminant hepatitis can occur in adults (<0.5%).
- A 1–6-wk incubation period → viraemic symptoms: malaise, anorexia, myalgia, headache, arthralgia, nausea, and fever.
- Symptoms improve as jaundice appears: this is often cholestatic and may last several weeks in adults.
- Hepatosplenomegaly, lymphadenopathy, or a rash may occur.
- Virus is excreted in the faeces 1–2wks before onset of jaundice and for 1–2wks after; some children may excrete virus for 1–2mths.
- Chronic carriage, relapses, and CLD do not occur.

Diagnosis

HAV IgM is detectable at symptom onset; HAV IgG rises 1–2wks later and remains detectable for life (= lifelong immunity). ALT/AST rise at the onset and typically settle in 2–6wks. ALP may take longer to settle, along with the cholestatic jaundice.

Treatment

Supportive Most infections are self-limiting. Avoid alcohol until LFTs return to normal.

Prevention

Improved sanitation ↓ transmission. Non-immune travellers to endemic areas should be vaccinated, as should household contacts in non-hyperendemic areas (see 📖 p. 910).

Hepatitis E virus

Hepatitis E virus (HEV) is a non-enveloped, RNA Herpes virus, which is endemic at a low level in many parts the world. Transmission and clinical features are similar to HAV. Pigs are infected with a similar virus, but human HEV is transmitted man-to-man. Unlike HAV, most adults are non-immune: thus outbreaks affecting adults have been described. In India, HEV accounts for >50% sporadic hepatitis in adults. Like HAV, most infections are self-limiting. Women in the 3rd trimester of pregnancy may have fulminant liver failure and death (>20%) for reasons that are poorly understood.

Diagnosis HEV-specific IgM is detectable at presentation in >90% cases; HEV-IgG rises thereafter. PCR may detect HEV RNA in blood or stool.

Treatment Supportive. No vaccine available. Pooled human immune globulin is not protective.

Hepatitis C

An enveloped, single-stranded RNA flavivirus, with six major genotypes and >50 subtypes. Transmission is predominantly blood-borne, and 2–5 million iatrogenic HCV infections occur annually. HCV prevalence among Egyptians >15%, mainly due to past mass parenteral anti-schistosomal treatment programmes. Less commonly, sexual and vertical transmission may occur. The risk of infection following needlestick injury from an HCV+ donor is 1–3%.

Natural history

1° infection usually gives no or mild, flu-like symptoms; however, 50–85% develop chronic HCV infection, with non-specific symptoms, e.g. malaise, nausea, and abdominal pain. Ongoing cycles of inflammation, necrosis, and apoptosis gradually → cirrhosis, which occurs in 2–20% over 20–30yrs. Progression is faster in males, those infected at an older age, HIV co-infection (especially if CD4 <200cells/mL) and/or HBV co-infection, and those with HCV genotype 1. Once cirrhosis present, the risk of hepatocellular carcinoma (HCC) is 1–4% per year. Extra-hepatic manifestations, which are uncommon, include glomerulonephritis, cryoglobulinaemic vasculitis, and lichen planus (see Fig. 7.4).

Diagnosis HCV IgG becomes detectable 6–8wks after infection. HCV RNA PCR is expensive and should only be done if treatment is available, at which point genotyping is also done.

Management

Avoid alcohol as this ↑ progression of cirrhosis. Specific therapy is costly and better (oral) agents are in development. Where available, use pegylated interferon and ribavirin combination therapy for 24wks. Genotypes 2 and 3 have been shown to have a better chance of treatment success (75–85%).

Contraindications to therapy

- Liver failure.
- Ongoing alcohol or substance abuse.
- Pregnancy.
- Co-existing conditions, e.g. uncontrolled seizures or autoimmune diseases.

HIV/HCV co-infected patients respond less well to HCV therapy. HAART improves the course of HCV and is the mainstay of therapy for co-infected individuals in resource-poor settings.

Hepatitis B virus

HBV is a double-stranded DNA hepadnavirus. It is an important cause of acute and chronic hepatitis and hepatocellular carcinoma. Worldwide 2 billion people show serological evidence of exposure and 400 million have active infection. Highest prevalence areas: sub-Saharan Africa, China, and Southeast Asia.

Transmission

HBV is in blood and (to a lesser extent) in semen, vaginal secretions, and saliva of actively infected individuals. Transmission occurs via infected blood products, unsterilized needles, sexually, and among children by close contact through mucosae or minor breaks in the skin. Vertical transmission from mother to child occurs perinatally. High-risk groups include health workers, haemophiliacs, IV drug users, haemodialysis patients, those in institutions, and homosexual men.

Natural history of acute HBV infection

Most HBV infections are asymptomatic, especially in young children. Symptoms occur after an incubation period of 1–4mths. Clinical features of HBV are indistinguishable from other acute viral hepatitides. Death from fulminant hepatitis occurs in ~1%; glomerulonephritis is a rare complication. Following acute HBV infection, there is either complete recovery (with long-term immunity) or persistent infection. The latter occurs in <5% infected as adults, 30% infected as children, and 90% infants infected at birth; it is more common in the immunocompromised. (See Fig. 7.5)

Serological markers of infection

Shown in Fig. 7.4. Following infection, there is marked viraemia. HBsAg becomes detectable after 4–10wks, followed by IgM anti-HBc. As the host immune response targets infected hepatocytes, ALT rises, and HBeAg (which is a marker of active viral replication) becomes detectable. Recovery with viral clearance is accompanied by disappearance of HBsAg and appearance of anti-HBs and anti-HBe antibodies. During the 'window' period between disappearance of HBsAg and appearance of anti-HBs, acute infection can be confirmed by the presence of anti-HBc.

Persistent infection Defined as presence of circulating HBsAg >6mths post-infection. There may be:

- Asymptomatic chronic HBV carriage (sub-clinical persistent viraemia, with normal ALT and normal/near normal liver histology); *or*
- Chronic hepatitis B (liver function and histology abnormal). Symptoms are usually non-specific and do not correlate with disease severity. 20% patients eventually develop cirrhosis, and there is a 100-fold increase in the risk of hepatocellular carcinoma (HCC).

Levels of HBV viraemia are usually lower in persistent infection and ↓ over time. Persistent HBeAg indicates higher levels of viral replication. Clearance of HBeAg may occur with development of anti-HBe, may be accompanied by a transient rise in ALT and clinical hepatitis (due to immune-mediated destruction of infected hepatocytes) and usually → ↓ viraemia. 1% of patients per year will clear the virus permanently and remain immune thereafter.

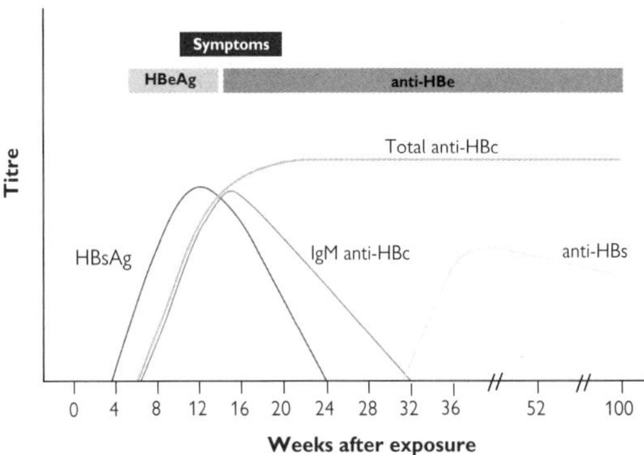

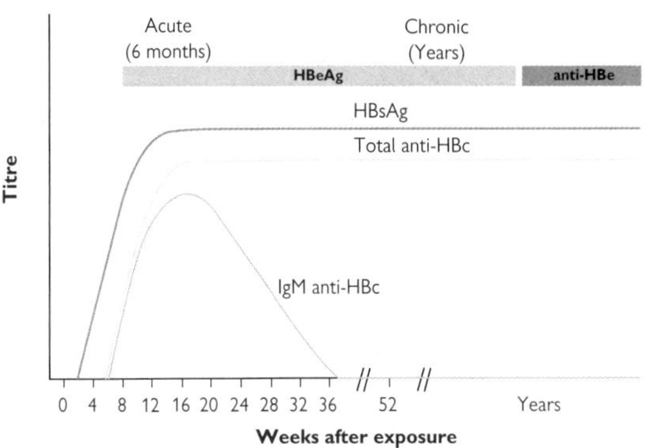

Fig. 7.4 Serological changes in hepatitis B infections. (HBsAg = HBV surface antigen; HBcAg = HBV core antigen; HBeAg = HBV e antigen; anti-HBsAg = antibody to HBsAg; anti-HBcAg = antibody to HBcAg; anti-HBeAg = antibody to HBeAg).

HBe –ve mutants

Most HBeAg –ve patients have low levels of viraemia. However, some have high viraemia despite being HBeAg –ve, due to a viral mutation which prevents HBeAg expression. Prevalence of these 'pre-core mutants' is higher in certain geographical areas (e.g. Asia 15–20%) and increases with infection chronicity. They appear to be associated with ↑ disease severity and ↑ risk of cirrhosis.

Management of acute HBV infection Supportive; avoid alcohol.

Management of chronic HBV

↓ Transmission risk and limit/prevent progression to cirrhosis and/or HCC. Measures include adequate nutrition, avoidance of alcohol (exacerbates liver damage) and drugs that ↑ viral replication (e.g. steroids, NSAIDs).

Where available, the goal of medical therapy for chronic HBV is to ↓ viraemia and liver damage; complete viral clearance occurs in <5% cases with current regimens.

Treatment options currently available

- Nucleoside analogues (e.g. lamivudine) interfere with HBV reverse transcriptase and inhibit viral replication. Lamivudine ↓ clinical progression in patients with chronic HBV and cirrhosis, ↓ risk of HCC. However, resistance is seen in >50% patients after 3yrs therapy. The future of HBV treatment is likely to be combination therapy (e.g. tenofovir, adefovir, entecavir, emtricitabine, famciclovir).
- Interferon-alpha showed modest benefit in clinical trials but is limited by side-effects.

Public health note: prevention of hepatitis B infection

- Immunization with hepatitis B vaccine recommended by WHO as part of expanded programme on immunization (EPI) schedule (see 📖 Immunization, p. 904). Studies in Taiwan showed that universal vaccination of children <5yrs ↓ incidence of hepatocellular CA.
- Post-exposure immunization should be given to babies born to mothers who are HBV carriers/had HBV during pregnancy; and to non-immune individuals exposed to HBV (e.g. needlestick injury).
- Passive immunization with hyperimmune hepatitis B immunoglobulin (HBIG)* within 12h of birth ↓ risk of developing the carrier state by ~ 70%; protective efficacy of 90% if combining HBIG with HBV vaccine.
- Give HBIG* plus HBV vaccine at day 0 and after 1 and 2mths, and a booster at 12mths (accelerated schedule). It is unclear whether the combination of HBIG and HBV vaccination provides significantly better protection than early (<24h) HBV vaccination alone, and practice varies between countries.

* HBIG doses: adults 500IU, children 5–9yrs 300IU, children <5yrs and infants 200IU.

Hepatitis D ('delta agent')

Hepatitis D (HDV) is a single-stranded RNA virus that can only replicate in the presence of HBV, and is transmitted by similar routes. 5% chronic HBV carriers are HDV co-infected, especially in the Mediterranean region, parts of eastern Europe, Africa, the Middle East, and South America. Co-infection leads to more severe acute HBV hepatitis or, in chronic HBV infection, accelerated hepatic failure and cirrhosis. Treatment and prevention is as for HBV (HBV vaccination prevents HDV co-infection).

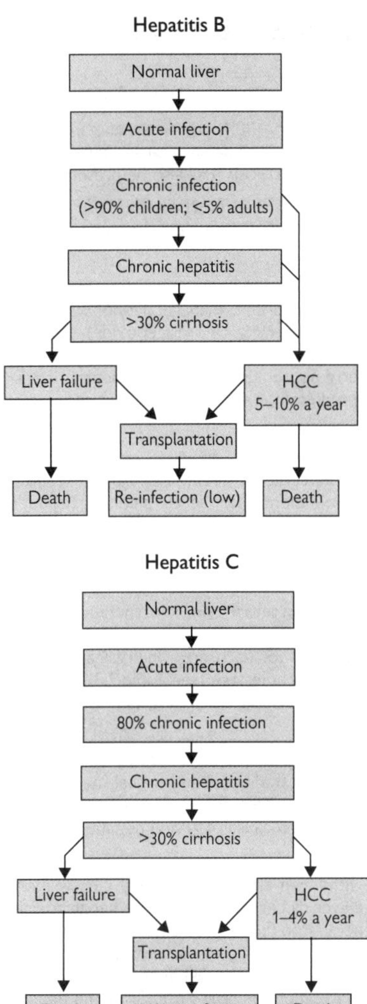

Fig. 7.5 Schematic comparing the natural history of hepatitis B and C infection.
Reprinted from *The Lancet*, 2006, 368: 896–7, with permission of Elsevier.

Alcohol and drug-induced hepatitis

Alcoholic hepatitis

Clinical features

Tender hepatomegaly, audible bruit in ~30%, jaundice, nausea/vomiting. The systemic inflammatory response to liver damage causes fever, malaise, anorexia, and ↑ WBC. Signs of CLD/cirrhosis may also be present.

Investigations ↑Liver transaminases (AST>ALT), ↑bilirubin, ↑ALP, ↑WBC. Alcohol excess *per se* may→ ↑γGT, ↑MCV, ↓platelets. ↓Hepatic synthetic function in cirrhosis → ↓albumin, ↑PT.

Management

Abstinence from alcohol is most important; manage alcohol withdrawal with reducing course of benzodiazepine (e.g. chlordiazepoxide). Optimize nutrition and give high-dose B vitamins (Pabrinex®) IV. Consider ascitic tap to rule out spontaneous bacterial peritonitis (SBP). If no evidence of sepsis and severe disease, consider prednisolone 40mg od for 5 days, tapered off during 2–4wks.

Prognosis

Scoring systems help to predict outcome (see Table 7.2). Abstinence from alcohol, good nutrition, and steroid therapy (for severe alcoholic hepatitis) have survival benefit: 7-yr survival was <50% in those who continued to drink, compared with >80% in those who abstain.

Drug-induced hepatitis

Drug-associated liver damage is commonly an idiosyncratic reaction = infrequent, occurs at therapeutic doses with variable latency period, and with a pattern that is consistent for each drug. Injury may result in hepatitis, cholangiohepatitis, or pure cholestasis (see Table 7.3). Steatosis, granuloma formation, and fibrosis may also occur. Women are at ↑ risk of drug-induced hepatitis.

Clinical assessment

Careful drug history including use of traditional and herbal medicines or over-the-counter drugs; timing of symptoms in relation to start of drug; alcohol abuse. Rule out other common causes e.g. viral hepatitis.

Management

The drug should either be withdrawn altogether, or very closely monitored for signs of progressive liver damage (e.g. nevirapine hepatotoxicity on instigating HAART). In general, stop the drug if ALT > 5× upper limit of normal OR ALT >3× upper limit of normal plus nausea, anorexia, vomiting, abdominal pain. A decision to re-challenge will depend on severity of the liver reaction and on the indication for drug's use. Risks and benefits of reintroducing a drug should be weighed up. For example, when deciding whether to re-challenge with antituberculous drugs, one should take into account strength of initial TB diagnosis and duration of TB therapy already received.

Table 7.2 Glasgow alcoholic hepatitis score (GAHS)

	Score		
Variable	**1**	**2**	**3**
Age (years)	<50	≥50	–
WCC ($\times 10^9$/L)	<15	≥50	–
Urea (mmol/L)	<5	≥5	–
PT ratio/INR	<1.5	1.5–2.0	>2.0
Total bilirubin	<125	125–250	>250

Table 7.3 Drugs causing hepatitis

Type of injury	Important drugs
Hepatocellular	Isoniazid, nevirapine, pyrazinamide, paracetamol
Cholestatic	Erythromycin, rifampicin, chlorpromazine
Allergic	Sulphonamides, sulphones, phenytoin, halothane
Granulomatous	Diltiazem, quinidine
Steatohepatitis	Stavudine, didanosine, tetracycline
Fibrosis	Methotrexate

Chronic liver disease and cirrhosis

CLD common in tropics due to alcohol consumption and frequent exposure to hepatitis viruses, parasites, bacteria, and toxins. Persistent liver injury causes cirrhosis: irreversible destruction of liver cellular architecture by fibrosis, with nodular regeneration of hepatocytes. Causes are shown in Box 7.11.

Clinical features Variable, according to degree of liver damage and compensation. Symptoms include malaise, pruritus, bleeding, abdominal swelling, and drowsiness (if encephalopathic). Ask about alcohol, blood transfusions, sexual activity, tattoos, body piercing, jaundiced contacts, family history, and drugs, including herbal medicines. May be hepatomegaly in early cirrhosis, although liver typically shrinks as fibrosis progresses. Examine for Dupuytren's contracture (associated with alcohol excess), jaundice, and extra-hepatic signs of CLD including portal hypertension (PHT) and hepatic encephalopathy:
- *CNS:* encephalopathy (drowsiness, flapping tremor, constructional apraxia = cannot copy a 5-pointed star).
- *Face and skin:* jaundice, hepatic fetor, excoriations.
- *Hands:* leuconychia, clubbing, palmar erythema, bruising.
- *Chest:* gynaecomastia, loss of body hair, spider naevi, bruising.
- *Abdomen:* splenomegaly, ascites, testicular atrophy.
- *Legs:* oedema (due to hypoalbuminaemia), muscle wasting.

Hyponatraemia occurs due to 2° hyperaldosteronism, and osteomalacia may occur due to ↓ 25(OH) vitamin D .

Diagnosis ↑ ALT/AST/ALP = hepatocellular damage (pattern often dependent on aetiology); ↓ albumin and ↑ PT = ↓ liver synthetic function. USS often shows characteristic cirrhotic liver architecture. Liver biopsy (check PT, platelet count, and Hb before biopsy) is mainstay of diagnosis.

Management and prognosis Depends on severity and underlying cause. Cirrhosis is irreversible; aim is to limit further damage, treat complications, and support patient.
- Avoid alcohol and hepatotoxic drugs (e.g. paracetamol).
- Treat dehydration and intercurrent infections.
- Ensure adequate nutrition.
- Treat ascites.
- Management and prevention of PHT (📖 p. 334) and variceal bleeds (📖 p. 304).
- Colestyramine 4–8g od oral if severe pruritus.
- If possible, treat underlying cause, e.g. peri-portal fibrosis in hepatic schistosomiasis is partially reversible with praziquantel treatment.

Box 7.11 Causes of chronic liver disease/cirrhosis
- Alcoholic liver disease.
- Viral hepatitis (HBV, HCV).
- Haemochromatosis.
- Autoimmune hepatitis.
- Cryptogenic.
- 1° biliary cirrhosis.
- Wilson's disease.
- Alpha-1-antitrypsin deficiency.
- Drugs.

Hereditary haemochromatosis

Inherited disorder of iron metabolism → ↑ intestinal iron absorption → iron deposition in multiple organs including liver, heart, pancreas, pituitary, adrenals, skin, and joints. Inheritance is usually autosomal recessive.

Clinical features

Classic triad of hyperpigmentation, hepatomegaly, and diabetes (30–50%). Fatigue and arthralgia are early symptoms. Cardiac involvement with heart failure and dysrhythmias is common, as is arthropathy; hypogonadism may occur 2° to pituitary involvement and/or cirrhosis. Presentation is usually in the 4th–6th decade, due to slow accumulation of body iron. Men are more frequently and severely affected, probably due to female menstrual iron loss. Complications include cirrhosis (9 × more likely in patients drinking >60g (= 6U) of alcohol/day) and hepatocellular carcinoma, which occurs in 30% of cirrhotic patients with haemochromatosis. Infections, e.g. bacteraemias are more likely because ↑ serum iron encourages bacterial growth.

Diagnosis

↑ Ferritin, ↑ transferrin ↑ saturation >80%, ↑ serum iron, ↓ TIBC. Check LFTs, blood glucose, ECG +/– echo. Joint X-rays may show chondrocalcinosis. Liver biopsy can assess severity of liver disease. Where available, genotype for mutations. Differential diagnosis includes haemosiderosis (see 📖 Haemosiderosis ('Bantu siderosis'), p. 332) and other causes of 2° iron overload (e.g. thalassaemia and sideroblastic anaemia); other causes of CLD (📖 Chronic liver disease and cirrhosis, p. 330); and porphyria cutanea tarda.

Management

Venesection ↓ morbidity/mortality of haemochromatosis

Remove 1U blood (500mL, 250g iron) weekly initially, until mildly iron deficient; then maintenance venesection of 1U every 2–3mths. Maintain serum ferritin <50ng/mL and transferrin saturation <50%. Treat cardiomyopathy and diabetes. Avoid vitamin C supplements, which ↑ iron mobilization and may worsen cardiomyopathy—ordinary intake of fruit and vegetables is not harmful. Screen 1st-degree relatives (check serum ferritin) and send for genotyping where available.

Haemosiderosis ('Bantu siderosis')

Haemosiderosis (a focal or general increase in tissue iron stores) occurs in southern Africa (and to a lesser extent in other areas) and is caused by chronic ingestion of traditional beer brewed in iron containers. Formerly called 'Bantu siderosis', condition is becoming less common as commercial products replace traditionally-brewed beer. Co-factors for CLD are commonly present, e.g. as high alcohol intake and HBV infection.

Clinical features Hyperpigmentation, hepatomegaly (portal fibrosis/cirrhosis), and cardiac failure occur. Ascorbic acid deficiency is often present. Associated osteoporosis may → vertebral collapse.

Management As for hereditary haemochromatosis, with regular venesection. Plastic containers for brewing and storage of beer → ↓ ↓ disease progression/occurrence.

Primary biliary cirrhosis

Chronic granulomatous cholangiohepatitis → destruction of interlobular bile ducts. Aetiology is autoimmune. 90% of primary biliary cirrhosis (PBC) patients are female. Associated with thyroid and pancreatic disease, Sjogren's syndrome, and scleroderma.

Clinical features Fatigue, hepatosplenomegaly, clubbing, xanthomata, xanthelasma, arthralgia, and features of cholestasis, cirrhosis (📖 Chronic liver disease and cirrhosis, p. 330), and portal hypertension (📖 Portal hypertension, p. 334).

Diagnosis Often diagnosed incidentally following discovery of abnormal LFTs. ↑ ALP, ↑ GGT, slightly ↑ AST/ALT; ↑ bilirubin in late disease. Perform liver USS to exclude extra-hepatic biliary obstruction. Antimitochondrial antibodies are highly specific. Liver biopsy and/or ERCP confirm diagnosis.

Management Symptomatic—colestyramine for pruritus, low-fat diet, and vitamin supplementation. Monitor for signs of portal hypertension. Death commonly occurs <5yrs in severe disease.

Wilson's disease

Rare, autosomal recessive disorder of copper excretion → toxic accumulation of Cu in liver and brain.

Clinical features Tremor, dysarthria, dyskinesias, parkinsonism, and eventually dementia; Kayser–Fleischer rings (greenish-brown pigment at corneoscleral junction) are pathognomonic, but may only be seen with slit lamp and often absent in young children.

Diagnosis ↓ Serum caeruloplasmin levels, ↑ 24h urinary Cu excretion. Liver biopsy shows ↑Cu (but also ↑ in chronic cholestasis). MRI may show typical changes in basal ganglia.

Management Lifelong chelation therapy with penicillamine. Screen 1st degree relatives.

Indian childhood cirrhosis

Affects children aged 1–3yrs in Indian subcontinent. It may follow a subacute, acute, or fulminant course, ranging from a viral type acute hepatitis to cirrhosis. Mortality is high, though progression to hepatocellular carcinoma is rare. Cause is unknown, although a high Cu intake (e.g. from milk stored in copper vessels), +/– an inherited defect of Cu absorption/metabolism has been implicated. No specific treatment.

Portal hypertension

PHT may be a sequel to any chronic liver disease, although cirrhosis and schistosomiasis are common causes in the tropics. Split causes according to the level of obstruction (see Box 7.12).

Clinical features

Signs of CLD should be present. ↑ portal pressure → splenomegaly and ascites; development of porto-systemic venous collaterals → oesophageal/gastric varices (most serious complication), caput medusae (distended collateral abdominal veins radiating from the umbilicus), and haemorrhoids.

Management

- Treat underlying cause where possible.
- Manage and prevent oesophageal variceal bleeds (see 📖 p. 304).
- Prompt treatment of SBP (see 📖 Spontaneous bacterial peritonitis, p. 334) and hepatorenal syndrome (see 📖 p. 336).
- Transjugular intrahepatic portosystemic shunting (TIPS) is an option where available, but expensive and shunt stenosis is common.

Ascites

Ascites occur in PHT due to a combination of Na^+ and water retention (splanchnic arterial vasodilation and ↓ splanchnic arterial pressure ↑ release of vasoconstrictors and antinatriuretic factors), ↑ portal hydrostatic pressure, and ↓ plasma oncotic pressure (↓ albumin) (see Box 7.13).

Management

Improve cirrhosis and PHT, give specific treatment to ↓ ascites:

- *Moderate ascites:* give low-dose diuretics (spironolactone 50–200mg od or amiloride 5–10mg od); if response poor or peripheral oedema present, add furosemide 20–40mg od for the 1st few days. Aim for 300–500g weight loss/day (800–1000g if peripheral oedema).
- *Massive ascites (rapid accumulation with abdominal discomfort):* drain ascites with plasma expander cover (e.g. 20% albumin 100mL IV per L drained); remove drain within 24h to minimize infection risk. High-dose diuretics are a less effective alternative (spironolactone 400mg od plus furosemide 160mg od oral). Irrespective of which method used, diuretics should be used to prevent re-accumulation.
- *Refractory ascites:* repeated ascitic drainage 2–4-weekly; consider TIPS.

Spontaneous bacterial peritonitis

Spontaneous infection of ascitic fluid, usually with intestinal pathogens (e.g. *E. coli*) occurs in 10–30% of patients with ascites. There may be abdominal tenderness or signs of sepsis, but often asymptomatic/non-specific presentation, ∴ consider in any patient with ascites who deteriorates. Hepatorenal syndrome complicates in up to 30% episodes.

Diagnosis Microscopy and culture of ascitic fluid: SBP defined as ≥250 polymorphonuclear cells/mm^3.

Treatment Broad-spectrum antibiotics, e.g. ceftriaxone, pending culture results. Consider 2° prophylaxis (e.g. ciprofloxacin 500mg od oral) as recurrent episodes common (70% at 1yr). Albumin (1.5g/kg initially and 1g/kg at 48h) ↓ the incidence of hepatorenal syndrome.

Veno-occlusive disease

Thrombosis of smaller hepatic veins due to toxins in certain herbal teas (e.g. *Heliotropium*, *Crotalaria*, and *Senecio*). It is an important cause of PHT in Jamaica, South Africa, Central Asia, and Southwest USA.

Box 7.12 Causes of portal hypertension

Pre-hepatic

- Hyper-reactive malarial splenomegaly (↑ portal blood flow).
- Portal vein occlusion (e.g. lymphoma, pancreatic cancer (CA)).
- Portal vein thrombosis (e.g. severe dehydration).
- Splenic vein occlusion (following neonatal umbilical sepsis).

Hepatic (sinusoidal)

- Cirrhosis.
- Schistosomiasis (*S. mansoni* or *S. japonicum*).
- HCC.
- Veno-occlusive disease.
- Congenital hepatic fibrosis.
- Drugs (e.g. dapsone).

Post-hepatic

- Congestive cardiac failure (e.g. rheumatic fever, TB pericarditis).
- Endomyocardial fibrosis.
- Inferior vena cava obstruction.
- Hepatic vein thrombosis (Budd–Chiari syndrome).

Box 7.13 Common causes of ascites

- Portal hypertension (see Box 7.12 for causes).
- Abdomino-peritoneal TB.
- Hypoproteinaemia (e.g. nephrotic syndrome).
- Right heart failure.
- Constrictive pericarditis.
- Chylous ascites.
- Malignancy (e.g. ovarian cancer).

Liver failure

In tropics, liver failure usually results from viral hepatitis or alcohol. Less common, but significant causes include drug-induced hepatitis (TB treatment or paracetamol overdose), other infections (e.g. leptospirosis), and acute fatty liver of pregnancy. Onset may be acute with no preceding illness or jaundice (fulminant hepatic necrosis). However, liver failure occurs more commonly in patients with pre-existing cirrhosis. Patients undergo chronic deterioration with infection, lethargy, GI bleeds, ↑ diuretic usage, and/or electrolyte disturbances.

Clinical features Include jaundice, fetor hepaticus (breath smells musty), hypoglycaemia, sepsis (which may be overwhelming), ascites +/– SBP, coagulopathy, hepatic encephalopathy, and hepatorenal syndrome.

Hepatic encephalopathy

Liver failure →↑ ammonia, which enters the brain where astrocytes clear it, producing glutamine in the process. ↑ Osmotic pressure due to excess glutamine causes fluid to enter cells → cerebral oedema and hepatic encephalopathy. Early signs include lethargy, asterixis (liver flap), constructional apraxia (e.g. inability to copy a 5-pointed star), and reversed sleep pattern with diurnal somnolence, which may → confusion, drowsiness, incontinence, ataxia, +/– ophthalmoplegia, extra-pyramidal signs, and eventually → coma.

Hepatorenal syndrome (HRS) Occurs in >10% patients with advanced cirrhosis and ascites, and is thought to be due to severe intravascular hypovolaemia causing renal vasoconstriction. Two types are recognized:

- *Type 1:* characterized by progressive oliguria and rapidly ↑ creatinine, often precipitated by SBP.
- *Type 2*: common in patients with refractory ascites, with gradually ↑ creatinine.
- *Prognosis poor:* median survival without treatment <1mth for type 1.
- Where available, vasopressin analogues (e.g. terlipressin 0.5–2mg bd IV) plus albumin may be effective in patients with type 1 HRS.

Management

- Monitor vital signs, neurological obs, blood glucose, urine output.
- Treat hypothermia and hypoglycaemia.
- Monitor FBC, U&Es, LFTs, and clotting.
- Control active bleeding with FFP/platelets; give Vitamin K 10mg od IV for 3d to correct PT (less effective in established cirrhosis).
- Insert NGT (unless oesophageal varices).
- Consider NG feeding.
- Avoid sedatives, hepatotoxic drugs, drugs metabolized by the liver, and NSAIDs (risk of GI bleed).
- Give lactulose (and/or neomycin) to ↓ammonia absorption from GIT.
- Manage coma in hepatic encephalopathy (Chapter 10) and monitor for signs of ↑ ICP (consider mannitol).
- Ensure careful control of fluid balance.
- Investigate and treat suspected infection promptly (e.g. SBP).
- Liver transplant, where available.

Hepatocellular carcinoma

Common, particularly in men aged 20–40yrs, causing ~1 million deaths/yr worldwide. Commonest cancer of men in sub-Saharan Africa, affecting up to 1/1000 men annually in Mozambique. Also common in parts of Asia and the western Pacific.

Aetiology and risk factors

- Chronic HBV and, to a lesser extent, HCV cause ~80% of HCC cases.
- *Aflatoxin B ingestion:* toxin produced by the plant mould *Aspergillus flavus*, which grows on groundnuts (peanuts), but also on maize, millet, peas, and sorghum. Levels of food contamination in Mozambique are the highest in world.
- Cigarette smoking.
- *Alcohol:* HCC is 5× more common in males who drink >80g alcohol (>8U)/d than in non-drinkers.

Clinical features

RUQ pain, weakness, and ↓ weight. Hepatomegaly in 90%, cachexia and ascites in 50%, abdominal venous collaterals in 30%, jaundice in 25%. Hepatic bruit is audible in half of cases. Bone metastases may cause pathological fractures. There may be evidence of CLD and PHT (e.g. bleeding from oesophageal varices).

Diagnosis Clinical. CXR may show a raised R hemidiaphragm. ALP and α-fetoprotein usually ↑ Other Ix: USS, CT scan, biopsy.

Management

HCC is a rapidly growing tumour, Treatment usually palliative. In tropics, presentation may be fulminant, with death occurring within weeks. Relieve pain and ↓ symptoms (e.g. anti-pruritic agents, drain ascites, transfusions for anaemia). Chemotherapy, radiotherapy, and transplantation are disappointing. Surgical resection is the only prospect for cure, although this is only possible in 2% of cases at presentation.

Prevention HBV vaccination and avoidance of risk factors (see 📖 Aetiology and risk factors, p. 337).

Secondary tumours of liver

Liver metastases are less common in the tropics than in the resource-rich regions. Clinical features may relate to the underlying 1° cancer or may be non-specific (e.g. malaise, lethargy, ↓ weight) (Box 7.14). The liver may have a characteristic knobbly feel on palpation or a rub on auscultation. Jaundice is relatively uncommon as a presenting feature.

Investigations

USS and biopsy are the best means of determining the cause of focal liver lesions, and whole-body CT scan may show the 1° tumour, although this is not likely to provide life-extending information except in diagnosing lymphomas.

Differential diagnosis of the irregular liver

- *Cystic lesions:* amoebic (or pyogenic) abscess. Both usually very tender in a febrile, toxic patient; congenital liver cysts, polycystic liver, or hydatid cyst. All non-tender, no fever unless 2° infection.
- *Solid lesions* are likely to be malignant. Surgical resection of small, solitary lesions may be attempted. If the patient is terminally ill, omit all investigations and concentrate on palliation.

Box 7.14 Primary cancers that cause liver metastases

		Rarer malignancies
• Stomach.	• Breast.	• Pancreas.
• Lung.	• Uterus.	• Leukaemia.
• Colon.	• Carcinoid.	• Lymphoma.

Liver flukes

Liver flukes (trematodes) are an important cause of human disease and prevalence is >50% in some endemic areas. All are transmitted by food contaminated with infective metacercariae.

Opisthorchiasis and clonorchiasis

~17 million people are infected by the closely-related human liver flukes *Clonorchis sinensis* (eastern Asia), *Opisthorchis felineus* (eastern Europe, northern Asia), *O. viverrini* (Thailand, Laos), and *O. guayaquilensis* (Ecuador). In Northeast Thailand, where the prevalence of *O. viverrini* infection reaches up to 25%, it contributes to the high incidence of cholangiocarcinoma (see Fig. 7.6).

Life cycle and transmission

Infection follows ingestion of raw or undercooked fish containing metacercariae (see Fig. 7.7). Adult flukes can live in the biliary tree for years. Pathology results from bile duct inflammation caused by large numbers of adult flukes.

Clinical features

RUQ pain, anorexia, dyspepsia, diarrhoea, and fullness common symptoms; fever, eosinophilia, obstructive jaundice, weight loss, ascites, and oedema occur in more severe cases. Some patients have a sensation of something moving within the liver. Asymptomatic hepatomegaly is common. USS may reveal gallbladder enlargement, sludge, gallstones, and poor function.

Complications

Gallstones and intrahepatic stones are common complications. Risk of cholangiocarcinoma due to *O. viverrini* infection is related to worm burden (5-fold increased risk for mild infection, 15-fold for heavy infection). Acute opisthorchiasis (*O. felineus*) causes fever, tender hepatomegaly, splenomegaly, and eosinophilia (up to 40% of WBC) soon after exposure to a large dose of metacercariae.

Diagnosis

Usually by detection of eggs in stool (may not be present if complete biliary obstruction or low worm burden). Adult worms may be identified by ERCP or during surgery. Percutaneous bile aspiration is not recommended: high risk of biliary peritonitis and haemorrhage. Serology (+/– stool antigen detection assays) available in some endemic areas.

Management Praziquantel 25mg/kg tid x 2d.

Public health note: Prevention of clonorchiasis/opisthorchiasis

- Improved sanitation and prohibition of the use of sewage ('night soil') in fishponds.
- Cook freshwater fish thoroughly; discourage consumption of raw fish.
- Saturated salt solution recommended for fish storage (but unproven).
- In non-endemic areas, suspect import of dried or pickled fish.
- Molluscicidal control of snail vectors is not feasible.

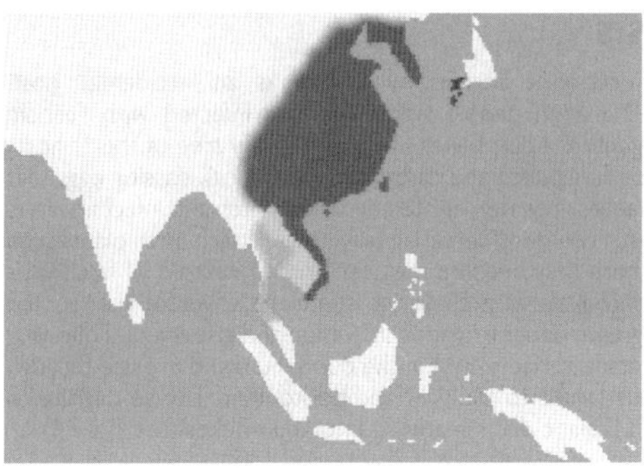

Fig. 7.6 Geographic distribution of *Clonorchis* and *Opisthorchis* (*C. sinensis*, black; *O. viverrini*, dark grey; *C. sinensis* and *O. viverrini*, light grey).

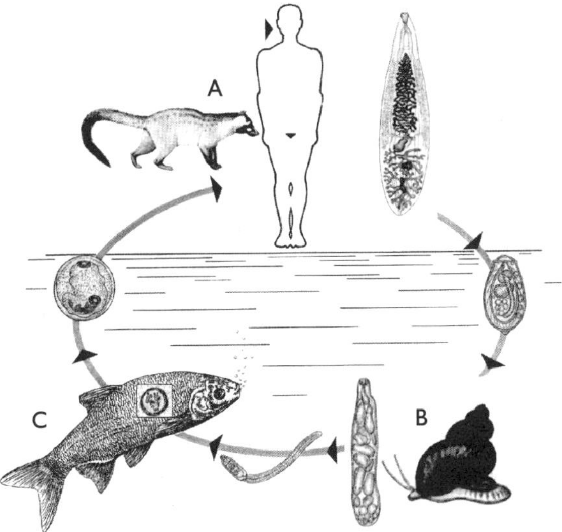

Fig. 7.7 Life cycle of *Opisthorchis* or *Clonorchis*: (A) adult flukes living in biliary tree of carnivorous host (e.g. man or palm civet) shed ova into bowel. Sewage contaminates fish ponds where freshwater snails (B) live. In snails, the parasites develop into miracidia, redia, then cercariae, infecting freshwater fish (C). Carnivore completes cycle, ingesting metacercariae in the flesh of uncooked fish.

Adapted from Piekarski, G, *Medical Parasitology in Plates*, 1962, with kind permission of Bayer Pharmaceuticals.

Fascioliasis

Primarily an infection of animals, with man as an 'accidental' host. Nevertheless, ~2 million people worldwide are infected with *Fasciola hepatica* or *F. gigantica*. Adult flukes live in the biliary tree of the 1° hosts (usually sheep for *F. hepatica* and cattle for *F. gigantica*), passing eggs that are excreted in faeces. In water, ciliated miracidia hatch and infect an intermediate snail host. Free-living cercariae leave snail, attaching to plants such as watercress where they become metacercaria. Outbreaks of fascioliasis have involved individuals who chew the stimulant leaves of khat (*Catha edulis*), which is grown under irrigation in Yemen and elsewhere. Following ingestion, the metacercariae excyst in the duodenum and migrate through the small intestinal wall into the liver and peritoneum. Larvae migrate to the common and hepatic ducts maturing into adult flukes (see Fig. 7.8).

Clinical features

Although many infections are asymptomatic, the pre-patent larval stage lasting 3–4mths may be accompanied by abdominal pain, weight loss, fever, and eosinophilia. During chronic or biliary stage fascioliasis, a small number of the adult flukes live in the bile ducts and shed eggs into the faeces. Patients are frequently asymptomatic, but may have symptoms and signs of biliary pain or obstruction.

Diagnosis

Eggs can usually be seen in the faeces < 2–4mths of infection (see Fig. 7.9). Serology is useful for diagnosis. There may be an eosinophilia, and USS +/– CT may be suggestive. As juvenile flukes migrate across liver to bile ducts, heterogenous hypodensities are seen on USS, which migrate with time. Similar anomalies are seen on CT. USS may show fluke within bile ducts. Dietary history is important, particularly in outbreaks and in returning travellers.

Management

Single-dose triclabendazole 10–20mg/kg oral is the treatment of choice, with ↓ incidence of side-effects. Give hyoscine to reduce GI spasm. The 2nd line drug is bithionol, which requires 10–15d treatment and causes side-effects in up to 50%. Praziquantel is *not* active against *F. hepatica*.

Public health note: prevention of fascioliasis

- Avoid eating raw watercress, khat, and other aquatic plants, especially from grazing areas.
- Exclude animals from commercial watercress and khat plantations.
- Avoid the use of livestock faeces to fertilize water plants.
- If practicable, treat livestock.
- Consider molluscicides to eliminate mollusks (not considered feasible in most settings).

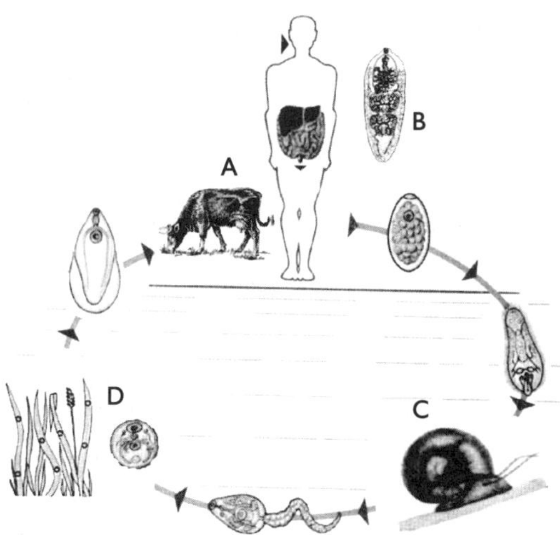

Fig. 7.8 Life cycle of *Fasciola hepatica*. Mammalian hosts (A), usually cattle, sheep, or man, become infected when ingesting aquatic plants (e.g. watercress) or grasses at edges of freshwater. The ingested metacercariae excyst to form young flukes, which migrate through the wall of the intestine and through capsule of liver and liver parenchyma until they reach a large bile duct. There adult fluke (B), 2–4cm long, lives for many years, passing its large (140µm) operculated eggs via the bile duct into the faeces. The eggs hatch in freshwater and undergo development in pond snails (C) into cercariae. These attach themselves to aquatic plants (D), which are ingested to complete the life cycle.

Adapted from Piekarski, G, *Medical Parasitology in Plates*, 1962, with kind permission of Bayer Pharmaceuticals.

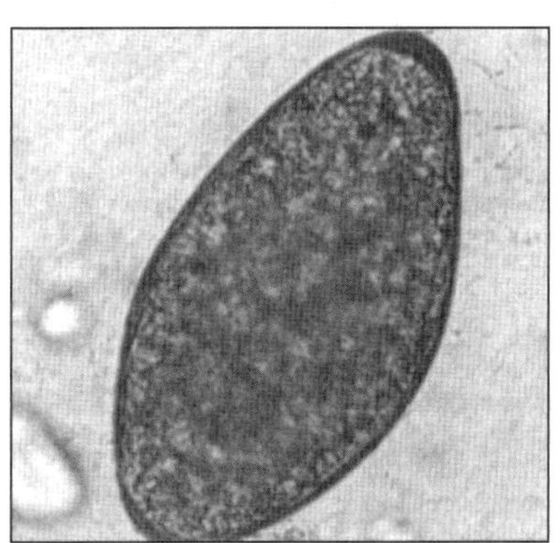

Fig. 7.9 *F. hepatica* egg in a faecal smear (7140 × 50µm).

Schistosomiasis (bilharzia)

Common, chronically debilitating, and potentially lethal disease affecting 200 million people worldwide (with 600 million people at risk), second only to malaria in socio-economic importance (see Fig. 7.10). Caused by infection with blood flukes (trematodes) *Schistosoma mansoni*, *S. japonicum*, *S. haematobium*, and, occasionally, *S. mekongi* or *S. intercalatum*. Most infections light or moderate. Usually a slow, insidious disease, but may → renal failure, colitis, periportal fibrosis, and bladder carcinoma.

Life cycle and disease burden

Transmission occurs when humans are exposed to water infested with the intermediate snail host while swimming, washing, or collecting water (Fig. 7.11). Schistosome cercariae released from the snails penetrate human skin losing their forked-tail to become schistosomules and enter blood vessels, passing via the lungs to the portal tract, where they mature into adults, pair and migrate to the vesical plexus (*S. haematobium*) or mesenteric veins (other species). Some schistosomulae continue to circulate in the systemic circulation and are the cause of acute schistosomiasis. The adults mate and may produce eggs for several years. Some of the eggs pass into the urinary tract (*S. haematobium*) or into the bowel (other species) before being excreted in urine or faeces. Other eggs lodge in bladder or bowel mucosa, or are carried in blood to ectopic sites (e.g. lungs, liver, CNS). Disease is caused by the granulomas around the eggs.

Adult worms do not multiply, so level of infection and disease is proportional to the exposure. Usually, there is a slow accumulation of egg granulomas; clinical illness occurs after several years. Infection peaks in early adult life with males/females equally affected. Infections may be very severe in those with regular exposure, e.g. fishermen on African rivers/lakes, rice farmers in Philippines. Prevalence and intensity of infection ↓ in older age groups due to ↓ water contact and ↑ acquired immunity.

Acute schistosomiasis

- Early reaction (swimmers' itch, cercarial dermatitis) occurs hours after infection. Pruritic papular rash with oedema, erythema, and eosinophilia caused by reaction to cercariae upon skin penetration. Resolves spontaneously within 10d and is rare in people living in endemic areas.
- Acute schistosomiasis is rare in endemic population, and occurs more commonly in travellers in the weeks following exposure. An immunopathological reaction due to hypersensitivity to circulating juvenile schistosomules, immune complex deposition, pro-inflammatory cytokine production and the toxic effects of eosinophilic proteins. Previously called Katayama fever, originally described as a result of infection with *S. japonicum*, now recognized to occur with *S. mansoni* and *S. haematobium* as well. Moreover, as fever is not a universal feature, the term Katayama fever is no longer used.
- *Clinical signs and symptoms:* fever, chills, sweating, fatigue, anorexia, headache, diarrhoea, dry cough, wheeze, hepatosplenomegaly, lymphadenopathy, and urticaria. Usually marked eosinophilia and ↑ immunoglobulins. Serial serology shows ↑ titres of anti-schistosomal antibodies, but may be −ve during early acute schistosomiasis. Ova are absent from urine or stool early in the course. Symptoms may persist for weeks, particularly fatigue.

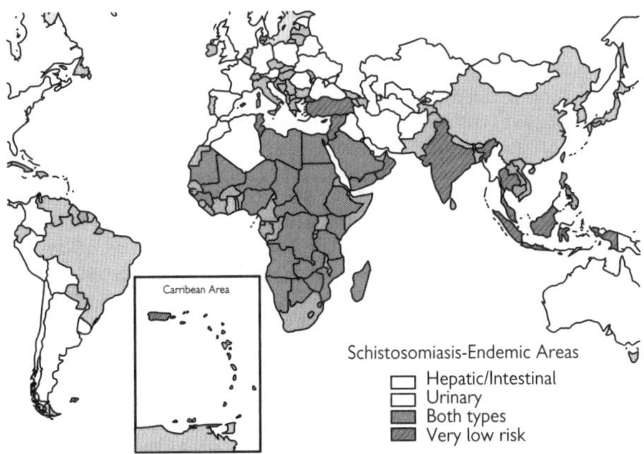

Fig. 7.10 Global distribution of schistosomiasis (2009). *Note:* schistosomiasis transmission is focal in many countries.

Reproduced from WHO – Global Health Observatory Map Gallery.

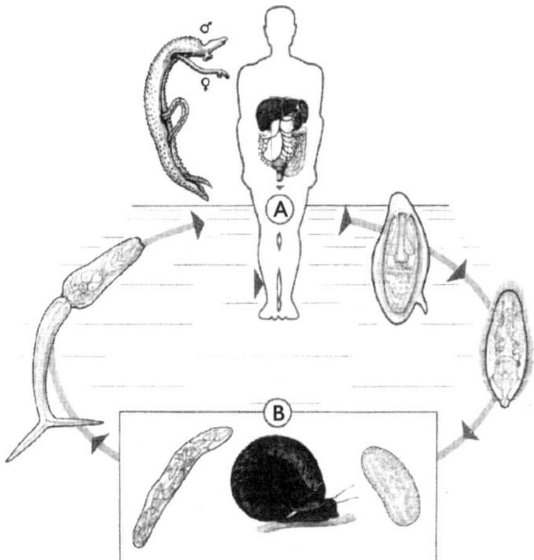

Fig. 7.11 Life cycle of schistosomiasis. Adult worms live in venous plexuses in pelvis; male wraps around female and encloses it in its gynaecophoral canal. Human host (A) sheds ova in stool or urine; these hatch, releasing miracidia, which infect freshwater snail host (B). After further development, cercariae are released into the water, which penetrate skin of humans during water contact.

Adapted from Piekarski, G, *Medical Parasitology in Plates*, 1962, with kind permission of Bayer Pharmaceuticals.

Chronic schistosomiasis

In chronic schistosomiasis, eggs induce granulomatous inflammation and fibrosis which may affect many organs:

- *Hepato-splenic disease (hepatic periportal fibrosis):* hepatosplenomegaly (often massive) and portal hypertension with porto-systemic collateral circulation, ascites, and oesophageal/gastric varices. Liver enzymes and albumin are usually normal, without liver failure until very late stages. Hypersplenism → pancytopenia. Characteristic USS appearance (pipe-stem fibrosis around portal veins, scarring of liver surface). Other causes of liver cirrhosis may co-exist, but in a mixed picture, always treat for schistosomiasis because established periportal fibrosis may improve substantially with treatment.
- *Intestinal disease:* eggs may reach both superior and inferior mesenteric venous plexuses (and superior haemorrhoidal veins in *S. japonicum* disease) and pass through to the intestinal mucosa to involve both small and large bowel. Chronic inflammation of large bowel may cause intermittent, bloody diarrhoea with tenesmus, pseudopolyp formation, hypoalbuminaemia, and anaemia, giving a clinical picture similar to that of ulcerative colitis or proctitis. A 'bilharzioma' is a mass of schistosomal eggs, which may be found in the omentum and/or mesenteric lymph nodes. Other features include protein-losing enteropathy, intussusception, and rectal prolapse.
- *Genitourinary disease:* chronic sequelae of *S. haematobium* infection include bladder fibrosis and calcification with ↓ capacity, and blockage of vesicoureteric orifice → ureteric obstruction, hydroureter, hydronephrosis, reflux, and 2° infection. Patients may have terminal haematuria (visible blood in last few drops of urine) or haemospermia. ↑ Risk of squamous cell carcinoma of the bladder at a relatively young age. Other pelvic structures, including fallopian tubes, may be affected. Granulomas on the cervix may mimic cervical cancer macroscopically.
- *CNS disease:* rare, but serious complication of ectopic egg deposition. Eggs of *S. japonicum* may embolize to brain causing meningoencephalitis or focal epilepsy. *S. mansoni* or *S. haematobium* eggs occasionally embolize to spinal cord, causing cauda equina syndrome, transverse myelitis, paraplegia, or bladder dysfunction.
- *Pulmonary disease:* embolizing eggs (especially *S haematobium*) occasionally occlude the pulmonary capillary bed, → pulmonary hypertension with breathlessness, fatigue, syncope, chest pain, and signs of RV failure (↑ JVP, tricuspid incompetence, peripheral oedema).
- *Other sites:* very rarely, there may be placental, genital, arthropathic, or cutaneous schistosomiasis.
- *Bacterial superinfection:* bacteria (e.g. *Salmonella* spp.) may colonize adult worms, providing a source for bacteraemic episodes.

Diagnosis

Always a history of exposure, but may be few clinical signs. Diagnosis usually by finding eggs (~150μ in length) in urine (*S. haematobium*) or faeces/rectal biopsy specimen (other species). Serology is accurate, but cannot distinguish current from past schistosomiasis. Urine dipstick for blood is a sensitive screening method for urinary schistosomiasis. Filtration or sedimentation of urine prior to microscopy ↑ yield. Thick faecal smears (Kato–Katz preparation) are examined under low (100×) magnification. Live ova have a flickering organelle ('flame cell') seen under high power. Collected eggs may be hatched in freshwater to demonstrate miracidia. Depending on the presentation and site of infection, other methods include liver biopsy and further radiological imaging. In biopsies, distinguish dead ova (calcified, partially collapsed, etc.), which persist for years, from viable ova which need treatment.

Management

Permanent cure is feasible in non-endemic areas, but not usually in endemic areas due to ↑ rate of re-infection. In cases where treatment does not achieve a full cure, egg production is ↓ by > 90%.

Acute schistosomiasis

Drugs are poorly active schistosomules. Give oral prednisolone to suppress the acute reaction, then praziquantel 40mg/kg oral (*S. haematobium* or *S. mansoni*) or 60mg/kg oral (*S. japonicum*) in divided doses over 1 day. Repeat 3mths after the last risk exposure so as to ensure maturation has occurred into the adult fluke against which praziquantel is active. Viable ova should no longer be excreted 6mths after effective treatment. Antibodies persist lifelong, ↓ antibody titres are not useful in indicating cure.

Chronic disease

- Praziquantel is effective against all schistosome species. For most species, give 2 doses of 20mg/kg oral during 1 day (3 doses of 20mg/kg for *S. japonicum*). If possible, take after food. *S. mekongi* may require repeated doses. For CNS disease, give 35mg/kg × 3 doses during 1d. Paediatric dosage is the same.
- Oxamniquine is an alternative for *S. mansoni* only. Contraindicated in pregnancy. Drug resistance is reported and availability limited.
- Metrifonate is an alternative for *S. haematobium* only. 3 doses are required, 2wks apart. Drug availability limited.

Surgical treatment is not recommended. Even chronic/fibrotic lesions will improve, especially in the young, and CNS disease may show resolution even after treatment.

Public health note: control of schistosomiasis

- Education and improved sanitation.
- Mass treatment of high-risk groups in high endemic areas (school-aged children, women of child bearing age, certain occupational groups).
- Personal protection, e.g. rubber boots for rice farmers.
- Avoid recreational swimming in at-risk areas.
- Rapid, vigorous drying following contact may kill cercariae that have not fully penetrated skin.
- Molluscicides (costly and have environmental consequences).

Ascariasis

Ascaris lumbricoides is a soil-transmitted roundworm infecting 25% of the world's population, with prevalence approaching 95% in parts of the tropics.

Life cycle

Eggs containing larvae are ingested and hatch in small intestine. Larvae penetrate intestinal wall and migrate via bloodstream through liver and heart to lungs, where they penetrate alveoli and ascend tracheobronchial tree to be swallowed. Returning to intestine they develop into mature worms, beginning egg production ~2mths after ingestion (see Fig. 7.12). Adult worms live 10–24mths and female worms lay ~200 000 eggs/d. Eggs passed in faeces persist in warm humid soil for up to 6yrs and are resistant to cold and detergents. Children in rural areas have highest burden of infection, as do communities using human faeces as fertilizer.

Clinical features

Most infections are asymptomatic. Heavy infection produces symptoms proportional to worm burden, especially in children:

- *Larval migration:* 1–7d after infection, larvae may → hypersensitivity response with cough, wheeze, eosinophilia, and patchy infiltrates on CXR (Löeffler's syndrome). Ectopic migration to the CNS occasionally → irritability, convulsions, meningism. Ocular granulomas, similar to those of *Toxocara canis*, may occur.
- *Adult worms:* mild infections usually asymptomatic, but may → ↓ appetite, abdominal discomfort, and dyspepsia. Heavier infections (particularly in children) may → anaemia and malabsorption of vitamins A and C, proteins, fats, lactose, and iodine. Growth retardation and cognitive impairment are frequently seen.
- A bolus of adult worms may cause bowel obstruction (usually near the ileocaecal valve), intussusception, volvulus, or perforation, which may occasionally be fatal. One study in Nigeria reported intestinal obstruction in 1:1000 infected children.
- Individual worms may enter common bile duct, pancreatic duct, or appendix, leading to colic and obstructive symptoms and 2° bacterial infections.
- If intestine is perforated, eggs released into peritoneum may cause granulomas and chronic peritonitis resembling TB peritonitis.
- High fever or exposure to anaesthetics can cause adult worms to migrate (e.g. to stomach). Worms are often vomited up by febrile patients; rarely they migrate to ectopic sites (e.g. Eustachian tubes).

Diagnosis

Marked eosinophilia occurs during larval migration; differential diagnosis of this stage includes toxocariasis, hookworm, strongyloidiasis, schistosomiasis, and TPE (see 📖 Tropical pulmonary eosinophilia, p. 212). Intestinal infection is diagnosed by identifying worms or eggs in faeces (colour plate 5). Worms may be seen on AXR or barium (Ba) studies as string-like or tramline shadows.

Management of ascariasis

- Albendazole 400mg oral stat (½ dose if <3yrs) kills adult worms. Alternatives in adults/children >1yr: mebendazole 500mg oral stat or 100mg bd for 3d; or pyrantel pamoate 11mg/kg oral stat (max 1g).
- Treat Löeffler's syndrome with prednisolone, followed by albendazole 2–3wks later to kill adult worms.
- Intestinal or biliary obstruction is best managed conservatively (analgesia, NGT, antispasmodics, IV fluids, liquid paraffin) followed by antihelminthic treatment once the acute phase is over.
- Laparotomy may be necessary for worsening/persistent obstruction, appendicitis, or intestinal perforation. Sometimes the bolus of worms can be 'milked' into the colon by the surgeon.

Public health note: prevention of ascariasis

- *Education:* improve hygiene and protect food from dirt.
- *Sanitation:* prevent soil contamination by faeces (e.g. latrines).
- *Mass treatment:* indicated when prevalence of infection >50% or frequency of heavy infection (>50 000 eggs/g faeces) ≥10% in pre-school children. Give single-dose albendazole or mebendazole to women (annually) and pre-school children (2–3 × per year).

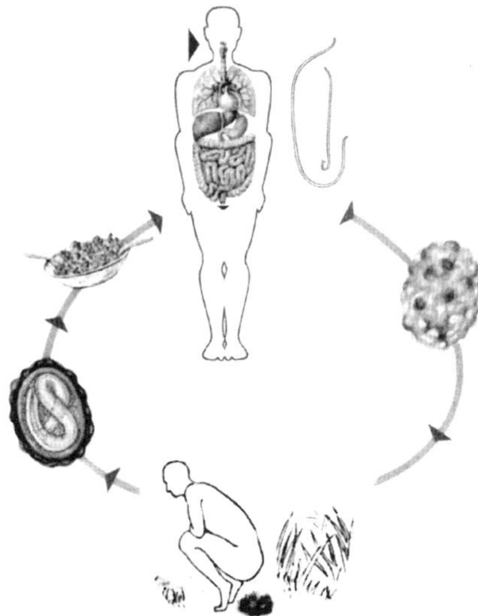

Fig. 7.12 Life cycle of *A. lumbricoides*. Vegetable gardens are faecally contaminated by eggs, which become embryonated (infectious) after 1–7wks in the soil. Ingested eggs hatch in the intestine, larvae migrate through lungs (see text), are then swallowed to become adult worms (females up to 40cm, males smaller).

Adapted from Piekarski, G, *Medical Parasitology in Plates*, 1962, with kind permission of Bayer Pharmaceuticals.

Hookworm

Infection caused by soil-transmitted helminths *Necator americanus* and *Ancylostoma duodenale*. As with ascariasis, hookworm infections often occur where human faeces are used as fertilizer or where open-field defecation occurs. High-intensity hookworm infections occur among both children and adults (see Fig. 7.13 for lifecycle). Most serious effects are anaemia and protein deficiency caused by blood loss at site of intestinal attachment of adult worms. When children are continuously infected by many worms, loss of iron and protein can ↓ growth and mental development.

Diagnosis Suspect in individuals with microcytic anaemia (see 🕮 Haematology, p. 493). Hookworm ova are often abundant in stool.

Treatment Albendazole 400mg od oral × 3d or mebendazole 100mg bd oral × 3d are both effective, as is mebendazole 500mg oral × 1 dose. Iron supplements can also be given for anaemia.

Prevention Provide latrines to ↓ people defecating outdoors.

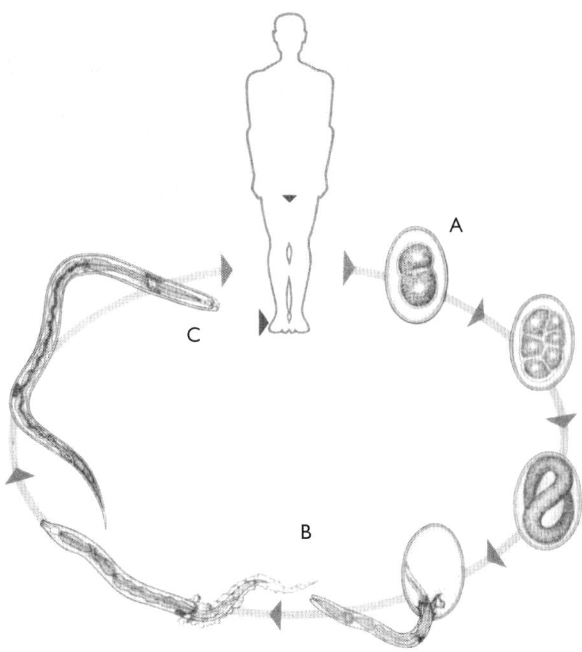

Fig 7.13 Life cycle of hookworm – best under moist, warm, shady conditions. Eggs are passed in stool (A) and larvae hatch in 1–2d, releasing rhabditiform larvae (B), which, after 5–10d, become infective filariform larvae (C), which can survive 3–4wks in favourable environmental conditions. On contact with human host, infective larvae penetrate skin and are carried through blood vessels to heart and then lungs. They penetrate into pulmonary alveoli, ascend bronchial tree to pharynx, and are swallowed. Larvae reach small intestine, where they mature into adults. Adult worms can survive several years attached to the intestinal wall with resultant blood loss by the host.

Toxocariasis

The canine and feline roundworms *Toxocara canis* and *T. cati* have a worldwide distribution. Humans are an accidental host: adult worms do not develop in humans, yet larvae migrate around the body and may persist for >10yrs, causing visceral larva migrans and ocular disease.

Life cycle Eggs excreted in dog or cat faeces (particularly from puppies) become embryonated in soil and are later ingested by humans (see Fig. 7.14). Larvae hatch in stomach, penetrate intestinal mucosa and enter circulation via mesenteric blood vessels, from where they may migrate to brain, eye, and other organs.

Clinical features

Depend upon density of infection:

- Visceral larva migrans, occurs predominantly in children <5yrs, and is characterized by heavy infection. Asymptomatic infection may occur. Typical features are: fever, hepatomegaly and splenomegaly, bronchospasm, and eosinophilia. CNS involvement (seizures, encephalopathy, and/or neuropsychiatric symptoms), myocarditis, and nephritis are described. In most cases, the disease resolves spontaneously <2yrs, although it can be fatal, particularly if there is CNS involvement.
- Ocular toxocariasis usually manifests in slightly older children (5–10yrs) and is an important cause of ↓ visual acuity in the tropics. Usually presents with unilateral visual impairment. Peripheral involvement of the retina by subretinal granulomata and choroiditis resembles retinoblastoma in the early stages. Diffuse endophthalmitis or papillitis and 2° glaucoma can occur.
- Co-infection with *Ascaris* and *Trichuris* may also occur. 2° infection with gut bacteria carried by the larvae is common.

Diagnosis Clinical suspicion; history of exposure, particularly to puppies; fever and organ involvement, eosinophilia, ↑ gamma globulins.

ELISA using recombinant antigens to 2nd stage larvae has >92% specificity and reasonable sensitivity (>78% for titre 1:32). CXR may show mottling in lung disease. Demonstration of larvae is very difficult, though they are sometimes present at the centre of granulomatous lesions at biopsy or post mortem.

Management Albendazole 400mg oral bd for 5d; alternatively, thiabendazole 50mg/kg oral daily in 3 divided doses for 7–28d; or diethylcarbamazine 3mg/kg oral bd for 21d. Steroids may be required for ocular disease.

Public health note: prevention of toxocariasis

- Educate pet owners; avoid contamination of soil by dog and cat faeces near houses and child play areas.
- Control stray dogs and cats.
- Regular de-worming of cats and dogs beginning at 3wks of age.

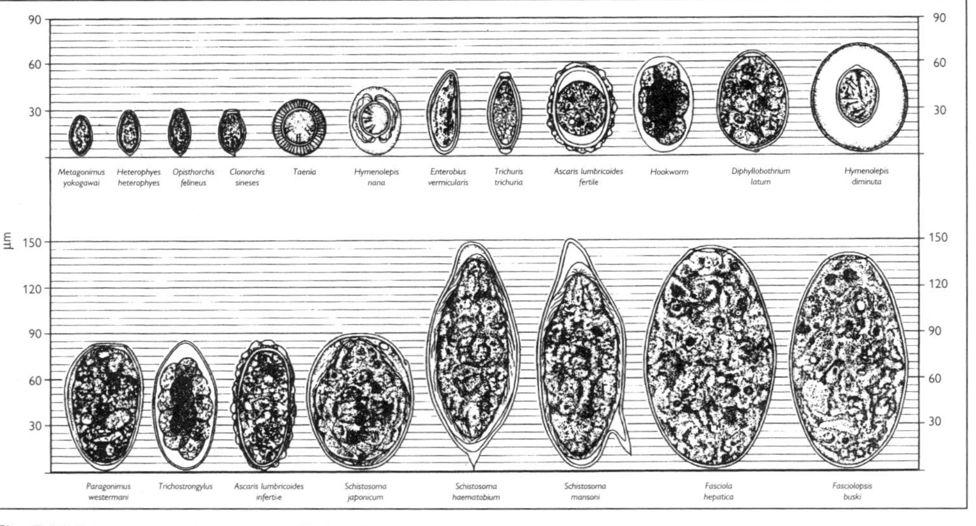

Fig. 7.14 Relative size and appearance of helminth eggs.

Reproduced with permission by the WHO from WHO Bench Aids for the Diagnosis of Faecal Parasites.

**Schistosoma mekongi* and *Schistosoma intercalatum* have been omitted. Eggs of *S.mekongi* measure 51–78µm; eggs of *S.intercalatum* measure 120–240µm long.

Lower GI bleeding

Less frequent than upper GI bleeding and presents with passage of red blood per rectum. (Rarely, very brisk upper GI bleeds may result in passage of red blood pr, rather than malaena.)

Causes

In absence of diarrhoea, most frequent cause is haemorrhoids. Other causes include colonic malignancy, diverticular disease, angiodysplasia, IBD, typhoid fever, schistosomiasis, and amoebic or bacterial dysentery (📖 Acute diarrhoea with blood, p. 238). Other causes in HIV+ individuals include TB, disseminated fungal infection (e.g. histoplasmosis), and intestinal KS.

Diagnosis and immediate management

- Resuscitate as for upper GI haemorrhage (📖 Upper gastrointestinal bleeding p. 304).
- Detailed history and examination, including rectal examination. Stool colour gives an indication of the level of pathology in the GI tract (in general, the darker the stool, the higher the cause). Be alert for symptoms and signs of typhoid fever and constitutional symptoms of TB.
- Proctoscopy and rigid sigmoidoscopy +/– biopsy where appropriate.

Further management

Depends on cause. In many cases, bleeding will cease spontaneously with bed rest. Prolonged bleeding will necessitate further investigation (e.g. colonoscopy). Consider keeping patient nil by mouth (give IV fluids) if urgent surgery may be required. For large bleeds, involve a surgical team at an early stage.

Diverticular disease

A diverticulum is an out-pouching of the gut wall, which may be congenital, but is more commonly acquired due to ↑ intra-luminal pressure (e.g. 2° to straining at stool due to constipation), which forces the mucosa to herniate through the muscular layers of the gut wall. Condition less common in many parts of tropics, probably due to a diet high in fibre. Patients typically report altered bowel habit, LIF colic (relieved by defecation), and painless rectal bleeding. Diverticula may become infected (diverticulitis), → fever, ↑ white blood cell count (WBC), ↑ ESR. Treat with bed rest, high-fibre diet, and (if infected) antibiotics. Monitor for signs of perforation (>40% mortality).

Colorectal carcinoma

Relatively uncommon in the tropics.

- *Risk factors*: high-fat, low-fibre diet; prolonged colonic transit time; polyposis coli; and ulcerative colitis. Tumours may be annular, polypoid, or ulcerous.
- *Clinical features*: altered bowel habit, blood/mucus pr, tenesmus, and non-specific features of malignancy (↓ weight, ↓ appetite, ↑ lethargy,

etc.). Anaemia and/or faecal occult blood may suggest lower GI bleeding. Abdominal or rectal examination may reveal a palpable mass.
- *Late presentation*: may be with bowel obstruction or perforation. Perform lower GI endoscopy + biopsy where available (proctoscopy/sigmoidoscopy/colonoscopy, as available). With complete surgical resection, the prognosis of carcinoma confined to the bowel wall is good.

Inflammatory bowel disease

Rare in tropics outside of resource-rich areas. Present with ↓ weight and diarrhoea with blood and mucus. Severe disease may present with intestinal obstruction or toxic dilatation of the colon. Anorectal fissures/fistulae and oral or perineal ulceration may complicate Crohn's disease. Associated extra-intestinal manifestations include erythema nodosum, pyoderma gangrenosum, anterior uveitis, arthritis, sacroiliitis, 1° sclerosing cholangitis, renal stones, malnutrition, and amyloidosis.

Diagnosis Sigmoidoscopy/colonoscopy and biopsy.

Management Acute cases with systemic steroids (or topical prednisolone enemas if disease is localized to the rectum). Exclude infective aetiology (e.g. amoebic dysentery) as best as possible first. 5-ASA drugs, e.g. sulfasalazine and mesalazine form the backbone of maintenance therapy. Severe cases may require surgery.

Haemorrhoids (piles)

Prolapsing anal cushions, normally associated with constipation and/or childbirth; varicosities of the anal canal may also occur in severe portal hypertension. Presentation with bright red pr bleeding, prolapse, and/or discomfort (pain may be severe if thrombosis).

Prevention High-fibre diet; avoid straining during defecation. Classified and treated as follows:
- *First degree:*
  - prolapse down anal canal, but not out, recognized at proctoscopy
  - *treatment*—sclerotherapy, inject 2mL of 5% phenol in oil.
- *Second degree:* prolapse through the anus, but reduce spontaneously. Treatment is sclerotherapy or rubber band ligation.
- *Third degree:* as above, but requires digital reduction.
- *Fourth degree:*
  - remain permanently prolapsed
  - *treatment*—rubber band ligation or haemorrhoidectomy.
- *Thrombosed piles:* treat with analgesia and bed rest. The clot may be expressed under local anaesthetic, usually relieving the pain.

Paediatric note: childhood causes of rectal bleeding

Age (most common)	Characteristics
Neonate	
Swallowed maternal blood	Tarry red blood; check maternal nipples
Haemorrhagic disease of the newborn	Coagulopathy, haemorrhage elsewhere
Ano-rectal fissures	Painful defecation, withholding stool, see fissure on examination
Necrotizing enterocolitis (NEC)	Usually preterm, likely very unwell, with systemic signs and abdominal distension
Malrotation with mid-gut volvulus	Bile-stained vomitus, pain, obstruction Life-threatening emergency
Hirschsprung's disease	Delayed passage of stool after birth (>48h) and abdominal distension
1mth–2yrs	
Milk or soy protein intolerance	Occult bleeds due to sensitivity to protein in cow's milk or soy; may be with formula feeds, but can also occur with breastfeeding if mother ingests allergens
Intussusception	Usually 6–36mths
Anorectal fissures	History of painful defecation, see fissure on examination
Bleeding Meckel's diverticulum	Congenital; painless; anaemia. Common at 2yrs; boys:girls 2:1
Henoch–Schönlein purpura (HSP)	Pain, arthralgia, haemolytic anaemia
HUS	Diarrhoea usually a prominent feature
Haemangioma/telangiectasia	Congenital; may be cutaneous lesions
Children	
Infective diarrhoea	
Juvenile polyps	Painless bleeding, benign hamartomas occur between 2 and 8yrs
HUS and HSP	As above
Other (IBD, peptic ulcer, varices, etc.)	As for adults

Around the anus

Pruritus ani

Peri-anal itching/discomfort may be caused by:

- *Skin infection or damage:* e.g. due to enterobiasis, tinea cruris, psoriasis, contact dermatitis, lichen planus, lichen sclerosis, leukoplakia, *Corynebacterium minutissimum* (the causative agent of erythrasma).
- *Surgical conditions:* e.g. haemorrhoids, fissure-in-ano, fistulae, skin-tags, polyps, malignancy.

Enterobiasis (threadworm, pinworm)

The soil-transmitted helminth *Enterobius vermicularis* is a common infection of young children worldwide.

Life cycle

Transmission is usually faeco-oral (pruritus ani → scratching → eggs transferred on fingers or under fingernails from anus to mouth; eggs may also be carried on contaminated bed linen or fomites) or by retro-infection in which larvae hatching at the anus migrate back upwards into the bowel. Ingested ova hatch in the stomach and larvae migrate to the appendix and caecum where they invade the crypts and mature into adult worms (9–12mm long by 2–4mm wide). Female migrates through anus (usually at night) and bursts, depositing eggs on perianal skin and perineum, which are then carried on faeces or picked up under fingernails during scratching. No multiplication inside body. Cycle takes ~ 2–4wks (see Fig. 7.15).

Clinical features

In the majority of cases, infected individuals are asymptomatic until female deposits her eggs perianally. Induces intense pruritus. General symptoms include insomnia, restlessness, loss of appetite, and weight; children are often irritable and frequently have enuresis. Worms can enter the vulva, and cause a mucoid discharge and pruritus. Worms may also occasionally be found in ears and nose. Very rarely, worms gain access to abdominal cavity and cause chronic peritonitis and granulomata. 2° bacterial infection of skin damaged by scratching may occur.

Diagnosis Requires detection of eggs on swabs from either perianal region (use Sellotape), under fingernails, or (less commonly) in faeces. Occasionally, adult worms may be seen around anus at night.

Management Really only beneficial in symptomatic individuals, since reinfection is virtually inevitable in most cases, unless there is change in behaviour. Where possible, treat whole family and school members. A single dose of albendazole 400mg oral (children 12–24mths 200mg) or mebendazole 100mg repeated after 2–3wks.

Public health note: prevention of recurrent infection

- Education to improve personal hygiene.
- Scrub children's hands before meals and after defecation.
- Keep fingernails short.
- Wash bedclothes, underwear, and nightclothes regularly at ≥55°C for several days after treatment.

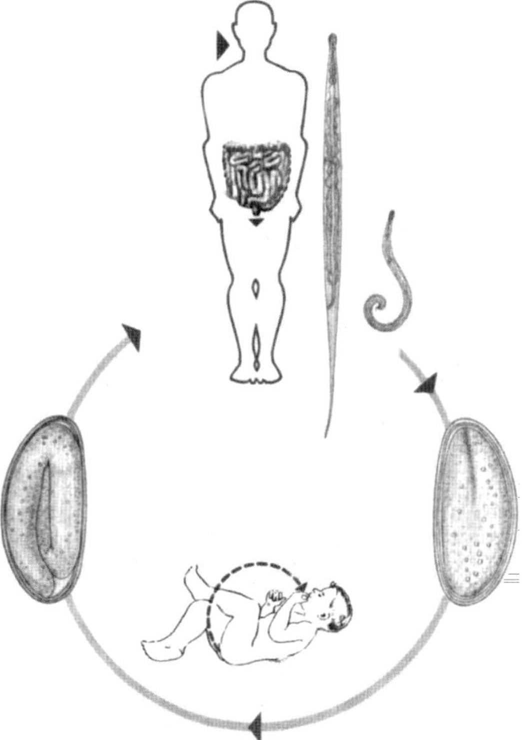

Fig. 7.15 Life cycle of threadworm *(Enterobius vermicularis)*. Eggs are ingested (e.g. from fingers which have scratched itchy perianal skin). Larvae hatch in intestine, develop, and penetrate mucosa. Male and female worms mate in intestine and smaller males die; gravid females (about 12mm long) migrate through anus and deposit up to 10 000 eggs on perianal skin.

Adapted from Piekarski, G, *Medical Parasitology in Plates*, 1962, with kind permission of Bayer Pharmaceuticals.

Visible 'worms' in stool

Some helminth infections may present following direct observation of worms in the stool. These include *Ascaris lumbricoides* (📖 p. 348), *Taenia saginata* and *Taenia solium* (the beef and pork tapeworms), and *Hymenolepsis nana* (the dwarf tapeworm) (see Fig. 7.18 for sizes of worms).

Taenia saginata (the beef tapeworm)

Despite being called 'beef' tapeworm, humans are only definitive hosts of the tapeworm—larval (cyst) form affects bovines. *Taenia saginata* is common wherever raw beef is eaten, e.g. Ethiopia. Adult worm typically 3–5m long (although some reach 10m) and attaches, via suckers, to upper small intestine wall. Adult worms may shed up to 50 000 eggs/d (contained in proglottids, or sometimes in stool) for >10yrs; see Fig. 7.16) Mature proglottids are highly motile and conspicuous in the faeces of infected individuals. Occasionally, proglottids (white, 16 × 8mm, flat, motile) may be felt emerging independently from the anus, causing embarassment. Patients may have vague abdominal pain, distension, anorexia, and nausea, although infection is often asymptomatic.

Diagnosis

Eggs may be seen on faecal microscopy, but are often absent because they are contained within proglottids—if stool is –ve, ask patient to collect proglottids to show you. Intact proglottids can be speciated according to number of uterine branches. Eosinophilia is not usually a feature.

Management Praziquantel 10mg/kg oral as a single dose.

Prevention Avoid eating undercooked beef (cysts destroyed >48°C). Improve sanitation. Avoid cattle grazing in areas of open-field defecation.

Taenia solium (the pork tapeworm)

Cysts are eaten in poorly cooked pork (the intermediate host) and mature in the small intestine. The adult tapeworm attaches to the mucosal surface by two encircling rows of hooklets, measuring 2–3m (up to 8m). Unlike *T. saginata*, humans are also readily infected by larval form of tapeworm after ingesting eggs excreted by a human carrier (often auto-infection from faecal-oral contamination), causing human cysticercosis. Symptoms of adult worm infection are as for *T. saginata*. Proglottids are smaller (712 × 6mm) and less motile.

Management Praziquantel 10mg/kg oral as a single dose.

Hymenolepsis nana (the dwarf tapeworm)

H. nana is slender, 3–4cm (Fig. 7.18), and worm seldom seen in the stool, but may give rise to abdominal symptoms like other tapeworms. However, unlike other tapeworms, *H. nana* has both larval and adult stages in humans and does not require intermediate hosts. Infection with several hundred worms is common. Since encystation occurs within small intestinal villi, there is immune stimulation, resulting in eosinophilia. Characteristic eggs are seen on faecal microscopy (see Fig. 7.17).

Management: Praziquantel 20mg/kg oral as a single dose.

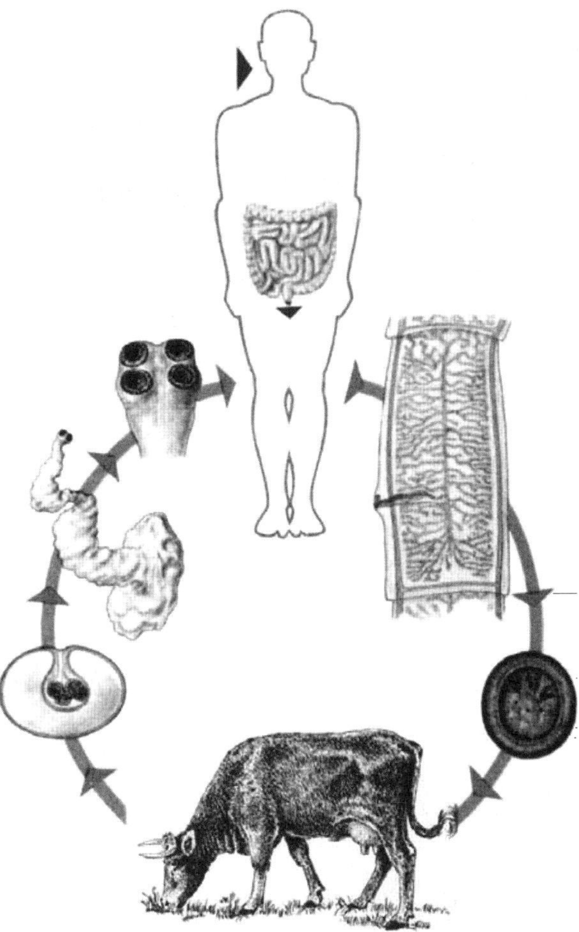

Fig. 7.16 Life cycle of *T. saginata*. Man ingests cysticercus in beef, which evaginates, and scolex attaches to wall of intestine. Adult worm grows to several metres length in intestine, releasing gravid segments (proglottids) and some free eggs. Cattle become infected when grazing on grass contaminated with faeces.

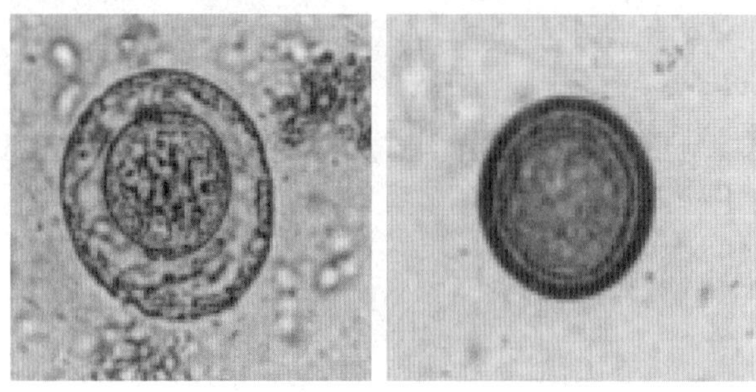

Fig. 7.17 Egg of *H. nana* (30 × 45μm) and of *T. solium* (30 × 45μm diameter).

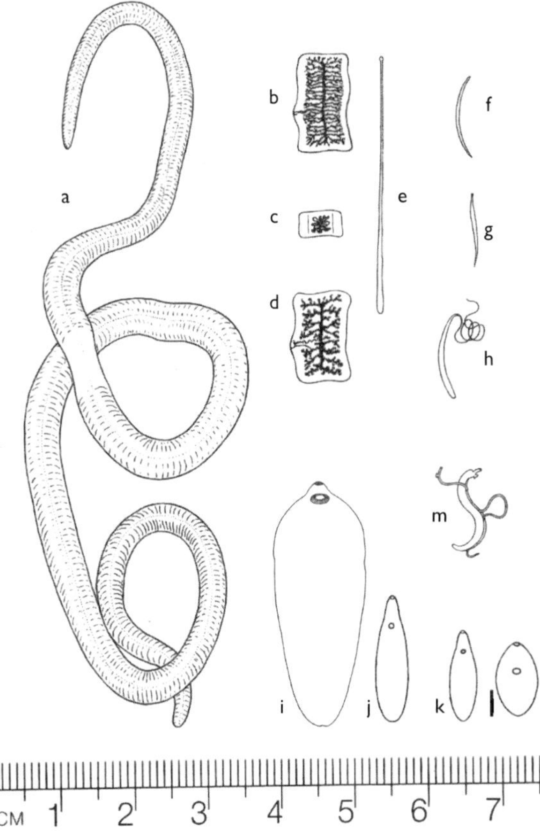

Fig. 7.18 Sizes of mature worms. a = *Ascaris lumbricoides*; b = proglottid of *Taenia saginata*; c = proglottid of *Diphyllobothrium latum*; d = proglottid of *Taenia solium*; e = *Hymenolepis nana*; f = *Ancylostoma duodenale*, *Necator americanus*; g = *Enterobius vermicularis*; h = *Trichuris trichiura*; i = *Fasciola hepatica*; j = *Clonorchis sinensis*; k = *Opisthorchis felineus*, *O. viverrini*; l = *Paragonimus westermani*; m = Male and female *Schistosoma*.

Chapter 8
Cardiovascular medicine

Invited author **Bongani Mayosi**

Cardiology in resource-poor countries

The pattern of cardiovascular disease is changing in resource-poor countries. Although infectious diseases still dominate clinical medicine in many countries (especially in sub-Saharan Africa), increasing urbanization, with its attendant risk factors of smoking, hypertension, and obesity lead to a pattern of disease that includes stroke, diabetes mellitus, and ischaemic heart disease (IHD).

'Metabolic syndrome' is term given to a cluster of some of the most important risk factors: diabetes and ↑ fasting plasma glucose, abdominal obesity, ↑ triglycerides, and ↑ BP. The cause of metabolic syndrome is unclear, with insulin resistance, central obesity, genetics, physical inactivity, ageing, a pro-inflammatory state and hormonal changes all being implicated. While IHD is increasing in Latin America, India, and China, it is still rare in rural parts of Africa, India, and South America. Rheumatic heart disease, TB pericarditis, and infectious (e.g., Chagas' disease and HIV) and other cardiomyopathies remain major contributors to cardiovascular disease in many resource-poor countries.

Acute rheumatic fever and rheumatic heart disease still disable young patients and are the most common causes of heart failure in children and young adults. HIV co-infection has led to many more cases of TB pericarditis, carrying a mortality of 40% in HIV+ individuals. The cardiomyopathies are endemic in many resource-poor countries. Peripartum cardiomyopathy is highly prevalent in parts of Africa; endomyocardial fibrosis occurs in the peri-equatorial tropical regions of Africa, America, and India.

Chagas' disease is a major cause of 2° disability in young adults in Latin American countries. Congestive heart failure caused by Chagas' cardiomyopathy is the most frequent and severe clinical manifestation of *Trypanosoma cruzi* infection, and associated with poor prognosis and ↑ mortality compared with heart failure due to other causes.

Advanced life support protocols

Most sudden deaths result from arrhythmias associated with acute MI or chronic IHD. Successful resuscitation following a cardiopulmonary arrest is most likely if:

- The arrest is witnessed.
- Basic life support (BLS) is started promptly.
- Defibrillation (if appropriate) is carried out as early as possible.

Basic life support

The purpose of BLS is to maintain adequate ventilation and circulation until a means can be obtained to reverse the underlying cause of the cardiac arrest.

- Remember A, B, and C—Airway, Breathing, and Circulation.
- Ensure that it is safe to approach the patient.

Airway Remove foreign bodies from the airway (including false teeth); use suction if necessary. Tilt the head back (unless a neck injury is suspected) or do jaw thrust.

Breathing Is the patient breathing? If not, assist via a mask (with 100% O_2) and bag ventilation if available, or mouth-to-mouth resuscitation until intubation is possible. If there is upper airway obstruction, a cricothyrotomy may be needed. If there is a tension pneumothorax, relieve it before proceeding further.

Circulation

Is there a pulse in the carotid arteries? If not, begin external cardiac massage until defibrillation (under the guidelines in Fig. 8.1) is possible.

If you are alone and the patient is unconscious, assess whether going/calling for help would be of more benefit than attempting resuscitation alone. It is hard to leave an injured/unconscious person, but their only realistic hope of survival may be if you go straight for help.

Advanced life support treatment algorithms for cardiopulmonary arrest

The algorithm shown in Fig. 8.1 is a summary of methods used in the advanced life support (ALS) training scheme. Methods involve skilled procedures, which should only be attempted by qualified staff, since improper use of defibrillators could result in more harm being done to patient, as well as harm to those carrying out resuscitation. It is strongly recommended that all medical staff read the ALS (or equivalent) course book and practise arrest protocols in 'mock' arrest scenarios.

Note Intubation and IV access should take <30s. If difficult, they should be delayed until next loop of cycle. If defibrillation remains unsuccessful, consider changing the paddle positions or the defibrillator. If, at any stage, a spontaneous pulse is felt, defibrillation should stop, BP checked and 12-lead ECG performed, and ventilation continued as appropriate.

ALS protocols are presented with kind permission of the Resuscitation Council (UK) Ltd., and are also given on the inside back cover of the book for easy reference in emergency.

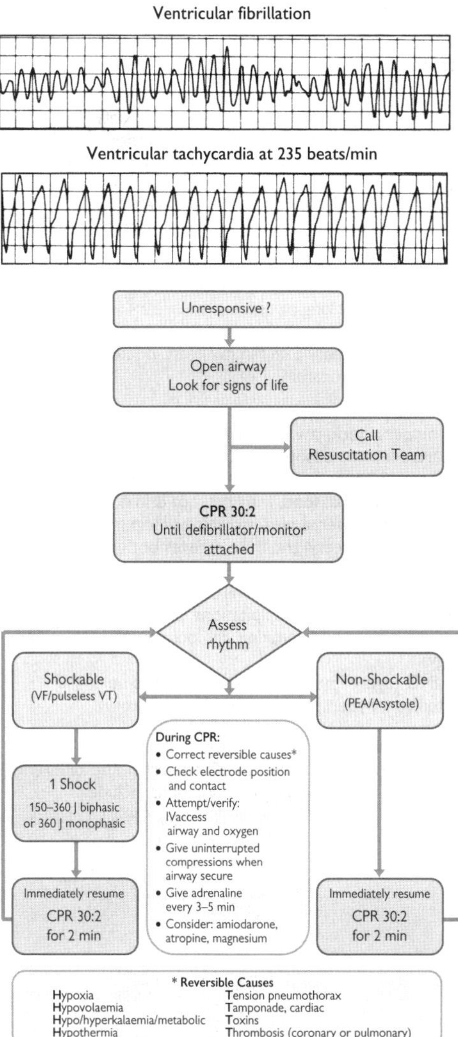

Fig. 8.1 Adult cardiac arrest algorithm.

Reproduced with kind permission of Resuscitation Council (UK) Ltd.

Chest pain

Central chest pain

Nature

- A constricting pain suggests angina, oesophagitis, or anxiety.
- A sharp pain may be from the pleura or pericardium (both may be exacerbated by deep inspiration, chest movement, or change in positions or posture).
- Prolonged, crushing, tight ('like an elephant on my chest'), intense pain unrelated to position or breathing suggests myocardial infarction (MI).
- The pain of aortic dissection is often felt in the back.

Pains that are unlikely to be cardiac in origin include:

- Short, sharp, stabbing or pricking pains.
- Pains lasting <30s, however intense.
- Well-localized left submammary pain ('in my heart, doctor').
- Pains of continually varying location.

Ask about

- Radiation (to shoulders, neck, jaw, or arms, especially left; suggests lesion of the heart, aorta, or oesophagus).
- Precipitating and exacerbating factors (exercise, emotion, or palpitations suggest ischaemia; food, lying flat, hot drinks, or alcohol suggest oesophagitis. However, a meal may also precipitate angina).
- Alleviating factors (*Note:* glyceryl trinitrate relieves both cardiac pain and oesophageal pain, but acts much more rapidly in the former). Pericardial pain improves on leaning forward.
- Associations (e.g. dyspnoea and/or palpitations, pallor, sweating, feeling of impending doom, nausea and vomiting; can occur with both an MI and GI pathology).
- Risk factors for IHD (age >55yrs, previous angina/MI, smoking, diabetes, hypertension, hyperlipidaemia, and family history).

Non-central chest pain

May still be cardiac in origin, but other conditions enter the differential diagnosis (see Box 8.1). The more common conditions include:

- Pleuritic pain.
- Musculoskeletal pain.
- Gallbladder disease.
- *Varicella zoster* (shingles).
- Pancreatitic disease.

Box 8.1 Causes of chest pain

Cardiovascular

- Angina
- Myocardial infarction
- Aortic dissection
- Aortic aneurysm
- Large pulmonary embolus
- Tumours (primary)

Pleuro-pericardial

- Pericarditis
- Pleurisy
- Pneumothorax
- Pneumonia

Airway

- Intubation
- Central bronchial carcinoma
- Inhaled foreign body
- Tracheitis

Chest wall

- Rib fracture
- Rib tumour
- Muscular strain
- Thoracic nerve compression
- Costochondritis
- Thoracic varicella zoster
- Coxsackie B infection

Mediastinal

- Oesophageal spasm
- Oesophagitis
- Mediastinitis
- Sarcoid or TB lymphadenopathy
- Lymphoma

Other

- Anxiety, hyperventilation
- Panic attacks
- Tabes dorsalis
- Gallbladder disease
- Pancreatic disease

Shock

Shock is inadequate perfusion of vital organs due to hypotension.

Clinical features

Tachycardia (unless on β blockers) with thready pulse, hypotension, especially postural in early stages, although in fit adults there may be >10% blood loss before ↓ BP; pallor, faintness, sweating, and cold peripheries with slow capillary refill.

Causes of shock

Cardiogenic shock

Failure of heart to pump sufficient blood around circulation. May occur rapidly or after progressive heart failure. Carries a high mortality and may be due to arrhythmias, pericardial tamponade, pneumothorax, MI, myocarditis, endocarditis, PE, aortic dissection, drugs, hypoxia, sepsis, and acidosis.

Management Treat cause, if known. Give O_2 by mask if hypoxic. Monitor ECG, urine output, ABGs, U&Es, central venous presure (CVP). Consider inotropes to keep the systolic BP >80mmHg. Refer to specialist if possible.

Anaphylactic shock See Box 8.2.

Endocrine failure See 📖 Addison's disease, p. 555, and hypothyroidism (📖 Thyroid disease, p. 550).

Septic shock See 📖 Shock, p. 734.

Hypovolaemic shock

Due to sudden loss of blood (e.g. trauma, ruptured aneurysm, or ectopic pregnancy) or body fluid (e.g. cholera).

Management

Prevent further blood loss and aim to restore circulatory volume as quickly as possible until PR ↓ and BP starts to ↑. Give whole blood where possible (cross-matched if there is time, otherwise use Rh –ve blood). Whilst waiting for blood to arrive, give warmed crystalloids, such as Hartmann's solution or a synthetic colloid.

For the last two causes of shock, the immediate need is rapid IV fluid replacement.

For guidance on treatment of shock in children see 📖 Circulation and shock, p. 10 and 📖 Management of shock in children with severe malnutrition, p. 12.

Points on fluid resuscitation

- Use the largest vein and cannula possible.
- Add pressure to the fluid bag to speed the infusion.
- If access is difficult, it may be necessary to cut down to a vein (e.g. 2cm above and anterior to the medial malleolus).
- If this fails, intraosseous infusion is possible using specific cannulae below and medial to the tibial tuberosity; useful in children (📖 Intraosseous needle insertion, p. 13).

- Give extra fluid if there are fractures: ribs 150mL, tibia 650mL, femur 1500mL, pelvis 2000mL.
- Double these estimates if there are open fractures.
- Remember to splint fractures and apply traction to ↓ blood loss.

Box 8.2 Anaphylaxis

Anaphylactic shock requires prompt energetic treatment of laryngeal oedema, bronchospasm, and hypotension. May be caused by exposure to insect venom (bee stings), food (eggs, peanuts), drugs (antibiotics, aspirin; especially if given IV), and other medicinal products (e.g. vaccines, antivenom, incompatible blood transfusion.

Management

- Stop infusion if this has caused the anaphylaxis.
- Secure the airway, give O_2.
- Give adrenaline 0.5mg (0.5mL of a 1:1000 solution) IM.
- Repeat every 5min until BP and pulse both ↑. (Patients on non-cardioselective β-blockers may not respond to adrenaline in usual doses; they may need salbutamol IV for 48h.)
- Give an antihistamine (e.g. chlorphenamine 10–20mg by slow IV injection). Continue this orally for 48h.
- Continuing deterioration requires additional treatment with IV fluids and IV aminophylline or nebulized salbutamol. Assisted ventilation and emergency tracheostomy (for laryngeal oedema) may be required.
- Give hydrocortisone 100–300mg IV slowly; may need oral steroids tapered for a few days depending on the antigen.

If there is doubt about the adequacy of the patient's circulation, it may be necessary to give the adrenalin IV as a dilute solution. This should be done by staff experienced in the use of IV adrenaline infusions, ideally in a high dependency or intensive care setting; refer to specialist protocols.

Anaphylactic reactions require prior exposure to antigen. Anaphylactoid reactions appear clinically similar, but occur when large quantities of allergen are infused IV (e.g. horse serum antivenoms). Prior skin testing does not exclude possibility of a subsequent anaphylactoid reaction since reaction is dependent on quantity of antigen injected. Always have adrenaline already drawn up when injecting antivenoms.

Hypertension

Hypertension (HT) is an ↑ problem in tropics. A major risk factor for MI, stroke, renal and heart failure, and peripheral vascular disease (PVD). Treatment of HT aims to ↓ incidence and complications.

Clinical features Usually asymptomatic until irreversible damage has occurred.

Symptoms Dizziness, fatigue, headache, palpitations.

Signs ↑ BP (although BP may be normal if heart failure); if 2° HT, there may be signs of the 1° disease; end-organ damage (e.g. LV hypertrophy, heart failure, retinopathy, proteinuria, uraemia). *BP should be checked* with correct sized cuff, sitting (supine and erect in elderly/suspected postural drop) after at least 5 and preferably 15min relaxing, and checked twice.

Who to treat?

- Where BP is >180mmHg systolic or >95mmHg diastolic, confirmed on three separate occasions over 1–2d, treatment should be started. If severe or in presence of associated conditions (e.g. heart failure), treat immediately (see Box 8.3).
- Where the initial BP is >140/90 over several weeks:
  - if no vascular or end organ complications and no diabetes, advise non-drug treatment and reassess in 3mths
  - if BP still high, start drug therapy
  - if vascular or end organ complications, or diabetes are present, start drug therapy.
- Isolated systolic hypertension (systolic BP >160mmHg, diastolic BP <90mmHg) in persons >60yrs should be monitored over 3mths and treated if it persists, preferably with low-dose thiazide diuretic +/– low-dose β-blocker.
- HT during pregnancy can be treated with methyldopa; β-blockers and Ca^{2+} channel blockers can be used during the 3rd trimester.
- In diabetics and patients with vascular risk factors or chronic kidney disease, aim for BP <130/80.

Investigations
Recheck the BP on at least three separate occasions. Search for cause (particularly in the young). Depending on resources, do U&E, Cr, glucose, plasma lipids, mid-stream urine, urinalysis, renal USS, 24h urinary catecholamines/urinary vanillylmandelic acid (VMA), ECG, CXR, fundoscopy.

Specific indications/agents and contraindications

- *Carotid atherosclerosis:* Ca^{2+} channel blockers.
- *CHF:* ACE inhibitor, β-blocker, ± spironolactone (depending on severity).
- *Chronic kidney disease:* ACE inhibitor or angiotensin receptor blocker (ARB).
- *Diabetes:* ACE inhibitor or ARB.
- *ECG left ventricular hypertrophy:* ARB or ACE inhibitor.
- *IHD:* β-blockers, long-acting Ca^{2+} channel blockers.
- *Resistant HT:* spironolactone.

- *2° Prevention of stroke:* ACE inhibitor plus diuretic or ARB.
- *Reserpine:* still used; cheap, effective, keep dose <0.5mg/day.
- *PVD:* avoid β-blockers as these exacerbate PVD.
- *Gout:* diuretics may exacerbate/trigger gout.

Accelerated HT

Rapidly ↑ BP with end-organ damage. Heralded by sudden onset heart failure, renal failure, encephalopathy (convulsions/coma), or a diastolic BP >140mmHg. Untreated, mortality is 90%; treated, it carries a 5yr survival of only 60%. See Box 8.3 for management.

Box 8.3 Management of HT

Aim to ↓ incidence of stroke, heart and renal failure, and MI.

- *Non-drug therapy:*
  - stop smoking (not itself a risk factor for HT; only for MI/stroke)
  - ↓ Na^+, alcohol intake, weight if obese
  - ↑ intake of K^+, fresh vegetables, and fruit
  - ↑ exercise.
- *Drug therapy:* explain that the patient may need to be on tablets for life, even though they have no symptoms, and may even feel worse. Encourage patient to return to a doctor if there are unacceptable side-effects and not simply to stop taking the medication.

Suggested approach

- Start with a thiazide diuretic (e.g. bendroflumethiazide 2.5mg od oral) as 1st-line therapy. Use low dose; check plasma K^+ 4wks after starting therapy).
- If not controlled, start either an ACE inhibitor (e.g. captopril 6.25mg tds), or ARB if ACE inhibitor intolerant, use a long-acting Ca^{2+} channel blocker (e.g. modified-release nifedipine 10–40mg oral bd) as 2nd- or 3rd-line therapy.
- If still uncontrolled, add a β-blocker (e.g. atenolol 25–50mg oral od) as 4th-line treatment.
- If the HT is still not resolved (<10% will not respond to one or a combination of these drugs), seek expert help before starting centrally acting antihypertensives (e.g. moxonidine, clonidine) or vasodilator agents (e.g. hydralazine).
- Always try to stop ineffective drugs.

Management of accelerated HT

- Bed rest, use of IV furosemide 40–80mg, IV glyceryl trinitrate infusion 5–10 micrograms/min, nifedipine 5mg.
- Maintenance therapy is with same drugs listed above for HT.
- Patients need close monitoring; may need specialist evaluation or opinion. Dihydralazine should be used with caution.
- Aim to reduce BP over days/hours, not minutes (increased risk of stroke).
- Do not lower BP in acute stroke unless >220/120. If so, lower slowly by 15–20% every 24 h.

Angina

Classically, this is central, crushing chest pain that may radiate to jaw, neck, or one or both arms. May be felt only in jaw or arm, or be felt as tightness across the chest. Represents myocardial ischaemia and may be precipitated by exertion, anxiety, cold, or a heavy meal, and be associated with dyspnoea, pallor, and faintness. Relieved by rest and nitrates. In most cases, caused by coronary artery disease, but may be due to valvular heart disease (aortic stenosis, aortic regurgitation, mitral stenosis), hypertrophic cardiomyopathy, hypoperfusion from tachyarrhythmias, arteritis, or anaemia. Indigestion is the most common differential diagnosis. IHD is particularly common in people of Asian, Melanesian, Polynesian origin (who also have high incidence of type 2 diabetes). The incidence is also higher in black than in white Americans. Angina is graded clinically using the Canadian Cardiovascular Society (CCS) grading system (see Box 8.4).

Diagnosis

On the ECG look for ST depression, flattened (or inverted) T waves, and evidence of old infarcts (Q waves). If available, do an exercise ECG 48h after the angina settles. Take blood for FBC and ESR to exclude non-atheromatous causes (see above), and cardiac enzymes, as available, to exclude myocardial infarction.

Management

Risk factor modification Stop smoking, prudent diet (↓ lipids and ↑ fruit and vegetable intake), ↓ weight, ↑ exercise. Look for hypertension, diabetes, and hyperlipidaemia and treat as appropriate. Start aspirin 75–150mg od.

Anti-anginal therapy Start with glyceryl trinitrate (GTN) 300–600micrograms either sublingually or as a spray at 0.4mg per dose prn up to every hour. If inadequate, switch to triple therapy:

- *β-blockers:* e.g. atenolol 50–100mg oral od (contra-indicated in asthma).
- *Slow-release calcium antagonists:* e.g. nifedipine MR 30–90mg oral od; felodipine 5–10mg/day, diltiazem 60mg oral 2–3 × daily, increasing to max 360mg daily (contra-indicated in fertile women). Short-acting Ca^{2+} blockers ↑ cardiac events.
- *Isosorbide mononitrate or dinitrate (as available):* mononitrate 10–60mg/d (od or bd); dinitrate 10–60mg tds. *Note:* need nitrate-free interval of 7h in every 24h. When drugs fail to control angina (CCS Class II–IV, see Box 8.4), coronary angiography is indicated to consider revascularization either by percutaneous coronary intervention (PCI) or by coronary artery bypass grafting (CABG) for relief of symptoms.

Unstable angina

New onset angina of at least CCS III severity (see Box 8.4), or angina that is rapidly worsening and present on minimal exertion or at rest or within 30 days of MI.

Management

Aspirin, clopidogrel, β-blocker, and bed rest. Give unfractionated heparin 7500–10,000 IU IV q4h to keep APTT twice control, if monitoring is available. (If available, low molecular weight heparin does not require monitoring.) If pain persists or recurs or TIMI risk score ≥5 (see Box 8.4) refer for specialist assessment/angiography/revascularization.

Box 8.4 Grading of angina pectoris by the CCS

- *Class I:* angina occurs only with strenuous, rapid, or prolonged exertion.
- *Class II:* slight limitation of ordinary activity: angina occurs on walking or climbing stairs rapidly, walking uphill, walking or stair climbing after meals, or in cold, or in wind, or under emotional stress, or only during the few hours after awakening.
- *Class III:* marked limitation of ordinary physical activity: angina occurs on walking 1 or 2 blocks on the level and climbing one flight of stairs in normal conditions and at a normal pace.
- *Class IV:* inability to carry on any physical activity without discomfort—anginal symptoms may be present at rest.

Risk of myocardial infarction or death

(Thrombolysis in myocardial infarction (TIMI) IIB trial risk score*)

Prognostic variable	Point
>2 angina events within 24h	1
Use of aspirin within 7d	1
Age ≥65yrs	1
>3 coronary risk factors	1
Known coronary obstruction	1
ECG: ST-segment deviation	1
Elevated cardiac enzymes	1
Total	7

*Risk of adverse outcome (death, repeat MI) ranges from 5 (score 0 or 1) to 41% (score 6 or 7)

Myocardial infarction

This is the irreversible necrosis of part of the heart muscle, almost always due to coronary artery atherosclerosis.

Clinical features

The pain is usually of greater severity and duration (>30min) than angina, though similar in nature and usually associated with nausea and vomiting, sweating, pallor, and distress. In the elderly and diabetics, small MIs may be painless. There may be tachycardia, tachypnoea, cyanosis, mild pyrexia (<38.5°C). The BP may be ↑, normal, or ↓. There may also be features of complications (e.g. dyspnoea, basal lung crepitations, pericardial rub, or pan-systolic murmur of mitral incompetence or ventriculoseptal defect (VSD)).

Diagnosis

ECG and cardiac enzymes. Diagnosis is based on (i) history (ii) ECG changes, and (iii) cardiac enzymes in order to allow the classification into ST-elevation myocardial infaction (STEMI) or non-ST-elevation MI (NSTEMI). Troponins, where available, are the investigations of choice.

Other tests

- CXR—look for features of heart failure, change in cardiac size (ventricular aneurysm), or aortic dissection.
- Measure Hb, WBC, and platelet count; urea, creatinine, Na^+, K^+, and glucose.

ECG changes in MI

An initially normal ECG → tall T waves and ST elevation (>2mm in two chest or >1mm in two adjacent limb leads for a diagnosis of STEMI). Alternatively, patient may develop new onset LBBB. Within 24h, the T wave inverts as ST elevation begins to resolve. Pathological Q waves (>1 small square in width and >2mm in length) form within a few days. These may persist or completely resolve in 10%. T-wave inversion may or may not persist. If ST elevation persists, suspect ventricular aneurysm (see Figs 8.2 and 8.3).

Site of infarct

- *Anterior:* changes occur in V2–5.
- *Septal:* changes in V1–3.
- *Inferior:* changes in II, III, and aVF.
- *Lateral:* changes in I, aVL, and V6.
- *Posterior:* look for the reciprocal (i.e. inverted) changes in the anterior leads V1–3: dominant R wave (= inverted Q wave) and ST depression (= inverted ST elevation) with the clinical features of an infarct. May be associated RV infarct — ask for V4R ECG lead (lead V4 placed in mirror image position over right chest) which will show ST elevation.

Non-Q-wave infarcts: (formerly called 'subendocardial infarcts') do not involve the whole thickness of the myocardium and, thus, have the ST changes but not the Q waves.

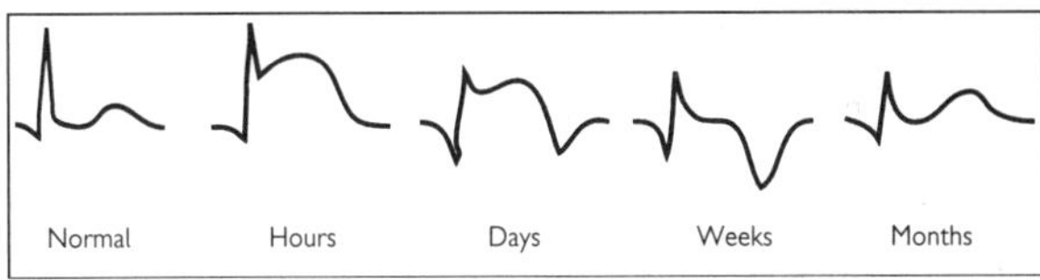

Fig. 8.2 ECG changes following MI.

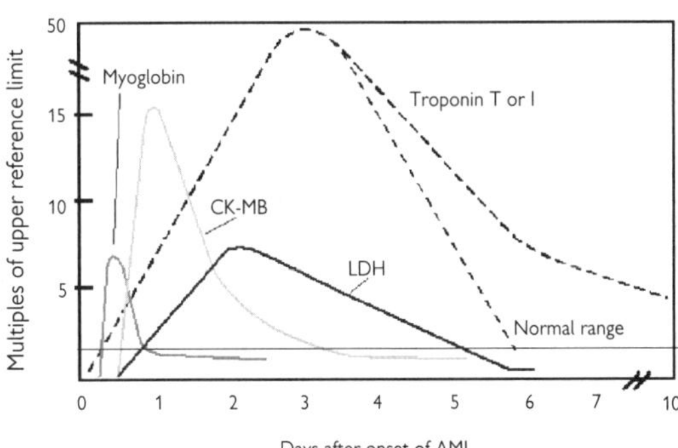

Fig. 8.3 Release patterns of cardiac markers.
Wu, A.H., *Journal of Clinical Immunoassay* 1994; 17: 45–8.

Immediate management of MI

The greatest risk of death is in the 1st hour. *Prompt action saves lives.*

- Relax and reassure the patient.
- Give O_2 by face mask if hypoxic or left ventricular failure (LVF)/ pulmonary oedema suspected. Finger pulse oximetry to monitor arterial O_2 saturation.
- Insert an IV line and give pain relief (morphine 10mg by slow IV injection, followed by further 5–10mg doses as necessary; half the dose in elderly or frail patients).
- Give GTN 0.3–0.6mg sublingual tablet or spray.
- Give aspirin 300mg po stat, then 75mg od, thereafter. Confers a 24% risk reduction even if given alone in situations where thrombolysis and PCI are not available.
- Give clopidogrel, initially 300mg, then 75mg oral daily on admission, in conjunction with aspirin.
- If STEMI, refer to a centre for primary PCI if this can be achieved within 3 hours of onset of pain, otherwise give streptokinase if within 6–12 hours of onset of pain (see Box 8.5, 📖 p. 382).
- Give a β-blocker (e.g. atenolol 5mg IV over 5min, 50mg oral 15min later, then 50mg bd) unless the patient has heart failure or asthma. It will ↓ cardiac O_2 demand, infarct size, and ↓ risk of arrhythmias and septal rupture.

- Start the patient on an oral ACE inhibitor 24h after the infarction. Titrate dose against BP.
- Start statin in hospital in all patients regardless of initial cholesterol level.
- Tightly control blood sugar with insulin in patients with both type 1 and type 2 diabetes in the peri-infarction period.
- Prohibit smoking.
- At least 24h bed rest with continuous ECG monitoring and qds temp, pulse, RR, BP. Perform frequent clinical examination for complications (see 📖 Complications of MI, p. 381).
- Daily ECG, cardiac enzymes, U&Es (and CXR if there is breathlessness) for the subsequent 2–3d.

Post-infarct management

If the post-MI period is uncomplicated, the patient may be mobilized by day 2 or 3. If there are no complications, the patient can usually be discharged by day 3 and gradually ↑ the amount of exercise done over 1mth. The patient should not drive during this period. Strongly discourage smoking and give dietary advice.

Prognosis

Depends upon the degree of LV dysfunction, presence of significant arrhythmias, heart size on CXR, presence of post-MI angina, and the presence of pulmonary oedema. In the UK, mortality rates for the 1st year after discharge are 6–8% with over half these deaths occurring in the first 3mths.

Box 8.5 Thrombolysis

Streptokinase is the most widely available thrombolytic agent. Give 1.5 million units streptokinase in 100mL 0.9% saline IV over 1h. Carries ~1% risk of stroke. Other side effects include hypotension (usually responds to slowing or stopping infusion), nausea, vomiting, haemorrhage, anaphylaxis (rare). tPA, rPA, and tNK are more expensive thrombolytics than streptokinase, but slightly more effective and cause less hypotension.

Contraindications to thrombolytic therapy

A thrombolytic agent should *not* be given if the patient:

- Has had a stroke or active bleeding (e.g. peptic ulcer) < 2mths.
- Has systolic BP >200mmHg.
- Has had surgery or trauma in the past 10d.
- Has a bleeding disorder or uses anticoagulants.
- Is pregnant.
- Is menstruating.
- Has had previous streptokinase treatment between 4d and 1yr previously (in the case of streptokinase).

Long-term treatment

Patients with no complications and good prognostic indices should be discharged and followed by the general practitioner. All patients should modify their risk factors. All patients should ideally take aspirin (indefinitely), clopidogrel (for at least 9–12mths), β blocker (for >18mths), an ACE inhibitor (indefinitely), and a statin (indefinitely).

Complications of MI

Post-infarct angina: (within 30 days of MI)

Is associated with ↑ mortality and occurs in up to 30%. Treat vigorously with nitrates, β-blockers, Ca^{2+} channel blockers, heparin, and aspirin. Angiography is indicated.

Arrhythmias

See 📖 Cardiac arrhythmias, p. 384.

- *Sinus bradycardia:* may be due to infarct or medication (β-blocker). Usually no action is required if the patient is haemodynamically stable.
- *Supraventricular tachycardia:* a sinus tachycardia is common post-MI. Atrial fibrillation (AF) occurs in 10% and should be rapidly controlled to avoid the onset of ventricular tachycardia (VT) and infarct spread. Use β blockade. AF is usually transient, but, if necessary (in presence of heart failure or hypotension, or refractory to other treatments), conversion back to sinus rhythm can be achieved by DC cardioversion or IV amiodarone (see 📖 Atrial fibrillation, p. 385).
- *Ventricular arrhythmias:* most common in the first few hours post-MI and may be heralded by ventricular premature beats. VT >120bpm may → ventricular fibrillation (VF). Treat with an IV β-blocker. Correct low serum K^+. Amiodarone (300mg IV over 20–60min; then 900mg over 24h) may be added if VT recurs. VF may occur in the 1st few hours to days, and needs emergency treatment. It carries a poor prognosis in the presence of cardiogenic shock or failure. Accelerated idioventricular rhythm can occur after any MI with reperfusion (following thrombolysis)—it is usually benign, not affecting cardiac output, and needs no treatment.
- *Nodal rhythms:* have a narrow QRS complex, normal axis usually, but have no associated P wave (or it may come after the QRS). They are usually intermittent and self-limiting, but in a large MI may ↓ both cardiac output and BP. Treat with atropine or a temporary pacemaker.
- *Conduction disturbances:* all degrees of AV block may occur, most commonly in inferior MIs (20%). 1st-degree block needs no treatment. 2nd-degree block is usually Wenckebach and only requires treatment if there is symptomatic bradycardia. 3rd-degree block often follows 2nd-degree block and is usually temporary. Again, treat with atropine or isoprenaline if symptomatic. In extensive anterior MIs, damage to the conducting system will cause complete and progressive AV block that will require pacing, possibly permanently. Heart block in inferior MIs is usually temporary, lasting <5d.

Myocardial dysfunction

- *Left ventricular failure:* see 📖 Left ventricular failure, p. 388).
- *Cardiogenic shock:* severe LV failure causing hypotension, tachycardia, oliguria, distress, and peripheral shutdown. It may be due to: acute mitral regurgitation (MR), severe LV dysfunction, cardiac rupture, VSD, arrhythmias, RV infarct. Treatment is with face mask O_2, IV diuretics (if LVF), fluids (if RV infarct), inotropes. Evidence from clinical trials supports invasive intervention in cardiogenic shock post-MI.

Right ventricular infarct

Occurs in 1/3 of inferior infarcts, but is clinically significant in less. There is ↓ BP and ↑ JVP with clear lung fields on auscultation. Lead V4R (see 📖 Site of infarct, p. 378) on the ECG may show ST elevation. Treatment is with IV fluids to ↑ LV filling. Inotropes may be useful.

Mechanical defects

- *Papillary or septal rupture:* occurs in <1% of all MIs and may occur 1–7d after anterior or inferior MI (MR most commonly after infero-lateral MIs, VSD after septal MIs). Listen for new murmurs and basal crackles; watch for clinical deterioration. Urgent surgery indicated for papillary muscle rupture with acute MR; early closure of VSD advised.
- *Left ventricular aneurysm:* occurs in 10–20% of anterior MIs. Apex beat diffuse; there may be atypical/stabbing chest pain, accompanied by ST elevation lasting 4–8wks. Rarely rupture, but associated with emboli, arrhythmias, and CCF. Patients may require lifelong anticoagulation. Surgical removal of aneurysm is indicated in intractable heart failure, recurrent VT, and frequent embolism in spite of anticoagulation.
- *Cardiac rupture:* usually → rapid death 2–7d post-MI. Occurs in <1% of MIs. A small or incomplete rupture may be sealed by the pericardium, forming a pseudoaneurysm that needs prompt surgical repair.

Pericarditis

20% of patients have a pericardial rub after 24h. Chest pain, relieved by sitting up and varying with respiration. Usually self-limiting, but a single-dose NSAID (e.g. indomethacin 100mg per rectum) may be very effective, avoiding the need for long-term therapy.

Dressler's syndrome An autoimmune pericarditis occurring 1–10wks post-MI in 5% of patients. There is fever, leukocytosis, and, occasionally, pericardial or pleural effusion. Treatment is with NSAIDs +/– corticosteroids.

Mural thrombus Is common in large MIs and may cause arterial emboli, leading to strokes, gut/limb/renal infarcts. Usually diagnosed by echocardiography; needs warfarin for ≥3mths.

Public health note: preventing IHD

The prevention of IHD applies to three groups:

- Cardiovascular health promotion in children and adolescents: promote healthy diet, no smoking, and ↑ physical activity.
- 1° prevention in adults without overt features of cardiovascular disease.
- 2° prevention in adults with established cardiovascular disease (i.e. IHD, peripheral vascular disease, or stroke).

Interventions

- *Diet:* ↑ consumption of a variety of fruits, vegetables, whole grains, dairy products, fish, legumes, poultry, and lean meat. Fat intake is unrestricted <2yrs. After age 2, limit foods high in saturated fats (<10% of calories/d), cholesterol (<300mg/d), and *trans*-fatty acids. Limit salt intake to <6g/d.
- *Smoking:* avoid beginning cigarette smoking and exposure to environmental tobacco smoke, and complete cessation for those who smoke.
- *Physical activity:* >60min/d of moderate to vigorous physical activity, and sedentary time must be limited (e.g. limit TV time to <2h/d).
- *Weight management:* aim for a body mass index of 18.5–24.9kg/m^2, and waist circumference of <101.6cm in men and <88.9cm in women.

The following 1° prevention interventions are of proven cost effectiveness in adults who do not have overt cardiovascular disease:

- Prudent diet, smoking cessation, and physical activity.
- Identification and treatment of hypertension, diabetes, and familial hyperlipidaemia.
- Statins in patients with diabetes and hypertension with multiple risk factors.

The following 2° prevention interventions are of proven value and cost effectiveness in adults with overt cardiovascular disease:

- Prudent diet, smoking cessation, and physical activity.
- Statins in patients with IHD, stroke, PVD, and diabetes.
- ACE inhibitors for all patients with MI, PVD, stroke.
- Cardiac rehabilitation following MI.
- Influenza vaccination.

Cardiac arrhythmias

Most commonly occur in an acute MI (📖 Complications of MI, p. 383), but may also occur in chronic ischaemia.

Clinical features Usually 'funny turns', collapse, and palpitations. Distinguish from epilepsy — a witness may help in this.

Investigations FBC, U&E, Ca^{2+}, glucose, TFTs, CXR (see Fig. 8.4), ECG. Echocardiography if cardiomyopathy or valvular disease suspected.

Tachyarrhythmias

Tachyarrhythmias may be divided into wide-complex tachycardia (QRS≥0.12s) or narrow-complex tachycardia.

- Wide-complex regular tachycardias are commonly due to VT.
- Narrow complex tachycardias are commonly due to atrial fibrillation (AF; irregular, no P waves), atrial flutter (regular P waves visible before each QRS), or AV junctional re-entry tachycardia due to AV nodal re-entry or accessory pathway (regular tachycardia with no P waves seen or P waves just after QRS).

Management of tachyarrhythmias

Acute symptomatic tachyarrhythmias are a common medical condition in the emergency unit. Direct current (DC) cardioversion is the 1st-line therapy in wide-complex tachycardia, atrial flutter, and in patients with haemodynamically unstable tachyarrhythmias. Patients with haemodynamically unstable tachyarrhythmia, any wide-complex tachycardia or atrial flutter are managed with DC cardioversion (see Box 8.6).

Patients with haemodynamically stable tachycardia thought to be due to paroxysmal re-entry are managed initially with vagal manoeuvres (i.e., carotid sinus massage and/or Valsalva manoeuvre). If this is unsuccessful, give verapamil 5–10mg IV; or adenosine 6mg IV followed by 12mg ±, a further 12mg if tachycardia persists. If the tachycardia persists, the patient is electrically cardioverted (see Box 8.6).

Patients with AF are managed according to the underlying condition. Only patients with acute (<24h) haemodynamically unstable atrial fibrillation are electrically cardioverted. (see 📖 p. 387).

Common causes of arrhythmias and conduction disturbances

- IHD, especially post-MI.
- Drugs (mostly those used to treat arrhythmias).
- Cardiomyopathy.
- Myocarditis.
- Thyroid disease.
- Electrolyte disturbances.

Atrial fibrillation

AF is an irregular atrial arrhythmia, resulting in irregular ventricular contraction. Common causes are MI, ischaemia, mitral valve (MV) disease, hyperthyroidism, hypertension, and excess alcohol. Also cardiomyopathy (especially alcoholic), pericarditis, sick sinus syndrome, CA bronchus, endocarditis, atrial myxoma, and haemochromatosis. It is a significant risk factor for stroke.

Clinical features

An irregularly irregular pulse with a 1st heart sound of varying intensity and apex rate > radial rate. The patient may be breathless and complain of palpitations. ECG shows a chaotic baseline with no P waves and irregularly irregular QRS complexes.

Therapeutic strategy

The therapeutic goals in patients with AF are:

- Identify and treat the underlying cause or risk factor for AF.
- Restore and maintain sinus rhythm (rhythm control) or accept arrhythmia and control ventricular rate (rate control).
- Assess thrombo-embolic risk and give antithrombotic treatment for patients at risk. Anticoagulation with warfarin is superior to antiplatelet therapy but requires monitoring and carries a higher risk of bleeding.

Identification of the underlying cause

1st step in management of all patients with AF. Address any underlying cause prior to or at same time as initiating specific treatment for AF.

Rhythm control

Using DC cardioversion, drugs, ablation, or surgery may be particularly useful in younger patients with structurally normal hearts and paroxysmal AF, or persistent AF of recent onset. Both electrical and chemical cardioversion carry risk of embolization of atrial thrombus, so should only be attempted <48h of new AF onset, or in patient adequately anticoagulated for >6wks, or if pre-cardioversion transoesophageal echo shows no thrombus.

Rate control

- Appropriate in elderly patients with hypertension or structural heart disease and persistent or permanent arrhythmia, especially if this can be tolerated symptomatically.
- Use drugs (usually β or Ca^{2+} channel blockers with or without digoxin) or, occasionally, AV node ablation and implantation of a permanent pacemaker.

Antithrombotic treatment

Anticoagulation with warfarin is indicated in patients with AF (paroxysmal or persistent) listed below. Warfarin carries a risk of bleeding which should be balanced against its likely benefits and discussed with the patient in each case.

- Previous stroke or transient ischaemic attack.
- Valvular or other structural heart disease.
- Hypertension.

- Diabetes.
- Age >65yrs.
- Left ventricular dysfunction and/or left atrial enlargement on echo.

Bradycardia

If bradycardia is acute and symptomatic (usually post-MI):

- Treat/remove underlying cause (e.g. β-blockers, including eye drops).
- Give atropine 0.3–0.6mg slowly IV, repeating to a max. of 3mg in 24h.
- Alternatively, try isoprenaline 1–4micrograms/min IV (↑ to 8micrograms/min if necessary for Stokes–Adams attacks).
- Temporary pacing may be needed for unresponsive bradycardia.
- Chronic bradycardia due to complete heart block is an absolute indication for permanent pacing.

Box 8.6 DC cardioversion

A safe DC cardioversion protocol is as follows:

- All cardioversions should be performed in a cubicle with full resuscitation equipment on hand.
- Patient sedated with aliquots of IV midazolam, via a drip in situ, until he/she is asleep and does not respond to his/her name.
- Flumazenil readily available to reverse sedation.
- O_2 given by face mask.
- Defibrillator placed into synchronized mode (this is important as unsynchronized shocks may precipitate VF in this scenario). After application of electrode jelly, right paddle is placed under right clavicle, adjacent to the sternum, and left paddle against left lateral chest. Firm pressure is applied.
- Initial energy setting is 50J. Energy is doubled after each unsuccessful shock to a maximum of 360J. Note that some defibrillators require the syncronized mode to be reselected after each shock.
- Patient observed in high-care area post-cardioversion.
- 12-lead ECG performed pre- and post-cardioversion.

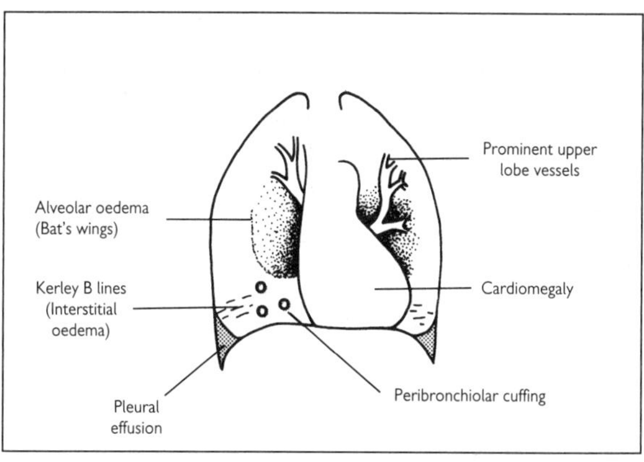

Fig. 8.4 CXR changes in heart failure.

Heart failure

Heart failure is a clinical syndrome of effort intolerance which is due to a cardiac abnormality and is usually associated with neurohumoral adaptations → salt and water retention. Thus, heart failure is a syndrome and not a diagnosis, i.e. the patient may have features consistent with heart failure, but always ask what is the cause?

Causes of heart failure

- Hypertension – systemic or pulmonary.
- IHD.
- *Heart muscle disease:* cardiomyopathy, myocarditis, infiltrative diseases (haemochromatosis, sarcoid, amyloid), Chagas' disease, beriberi.
- *Valvular heart disease:* aortic stenosis/regurgitation, mitral stenosis/regurgitation.
- Pericardial disease: effusive/effusive-constrictive/constrictive pericarditis.
- Congenital heart disease.
- *Other causes:* prolonged tachycardia, thyrotoxicosis, alcohol and other toxins (e.g. chemotherapy, cocaine), pregnancy, severe anaemia, Paget's disease, arteriovenous fistula, phaeochromocytoma.

Fluid overload involves pushing the myocardium too far over the Starling length–tension relationship (initially, stretching results in ↑ contractile force, but beyond the apex of the curve, further stretch results in ↓ force), resulting in ↓ cardiac output. The neurohumoral activation of the renin-angiotensin-aldosterone system → salt and water retention.

Based on clinical manifestations, heart failure may be classified as left, right, or biventricular failure.

Left ventricular failure

Dominated by pulmonary oedema, resulting in exertional dyspnoea, orthopnoea, paradoxical nocturnal dyspnoea, wheeze, cough, and fatigue. May also be accompanied by cardiogenic shock.

- *Signs:* tachypnoea, tachycardia, basal lung crackles, third heart sound, pulsus alternans, cardiomegaly, peripheral cyanosis, pleural effusion, ↓ peak expiratory flow.
- *CXR signs:* see Fig. 8.4.
- *ECG:* changes will depend on the specific cause.
- *Echocardiography:* may differentiate valvular and pericardial lesions.

Right ventricular failure

RVF causes dependent oedema (i.e. in the legs if standing, in the sacrum if supine), abdominal discomfort, nausea, fatigue, and wasting. Usually 2° to chronic lung disease ('cor pulmonale') or LVF.

Signs ↑ JVP, hepatomegaly (may be pulsatile if tricuspid regurgitation is present), and pitting oedema.

Management

Identify and treat cause if possible:

- Treat reversible exacerbating factors (e.g. anaemia, arrhythmia, electrolyte disturbance, infection, non-adherence to treatment).
- Restrict salt and alcohol intake.
- Avoid NSAIDs as they cause fluid retention. They may also interact with diuretics and ACE inhibitors → renal failure.
- *Drug treatment:*
  - *start with a diuretic (ceiling, e.g. furosemide)*—monitor weight daily; adjust dose to achieve 'dry weight' with optimal symptoms
  - once stabilized, begin an ACE inhibitor (see Box 8.7)
  - Consider low-dose spironolactone (25–50mg od) if available and patient not hyperkalaemic, and/or adding inotrope e.g. digoxin
  - *β blockers*—introduce cautiously once patient is clinically stable (not in acute severe heart failure), starting at low dose and titrating up dose slowly ('start low, and go slow')
  - *ARBs*—indicated in patients who do not tolerate ACE inhibitors (e.g. cough, angioedema)
  - combination of isosorbide dinitrate and hydralazine has been shown to be effective add-on treatment in African-American patients.

Resistant heart failure

Search for other causes and check patient compliance with drug regimes and daily weighing:

- Admit to hospital for bed rest, anti-DVT stockings, heparin 5000U sc tds, IV furosemide, and training in the use of the weight scale in fluid and symptom management.
- Increase the ACE inhibitor or venodilator dose to the maximum tolerated; consider metolazone where available. Often adding a thiazide to a loop diuretic will cause synergistic diuresis.
- In extreme circumstances, consider using IV inotropes for a short time only (e.g. dobutamine, starting at 2.5–10micrograms/kg/min, or dopamine starting at 2–5micrograms/kg/min; increasing both according to response up to a maximum of 40micrograms/kg/min (dobutamine) or 20–50micrograms/kg/min (dopamine)).
- Sometimes, a degree of peripheral oedema and exercise limitation must be accepted in order to avoid unacceptable symptoms of low output.

Box 8.7 Starting an ACE inhibitor

- Watch for hypotension after the 1st and 2nd doses.
- *Check BP:* if <100mmHg systolic, give the 1st doses in hospital if possible.
- Ensure the patient is not salt or volume depleted (e.g. due to D&V).
- Check for aortic stenosis or mitral stenosis (relative contraindication), and renal artery stenosis.
- If there is symptomatic hypotension, give 0.9% sodium chloride infusion (plus atropine if the patient is bradycardic).
- *Contraindications:* significant hypotension, angioedema, renal artery stenosis, pregnancy, porphyria.

Other precautions

- Check U&Es and creatinine routinely and stop ACE inhibitor if there is significantly ↓ renal function. However, urea and Cr will often ↑ when ACE inhibitors or diuretics are 1st used. This is not necessarily a reason to stop—levels will usually plateau and drop later. Monitor closely; stop if Cr/urea increase >20% or continue to ↑.
- Weigh patient regularly to monitor response and train patient to maintain ideal 'dry weight' by adjusting the diuretic dose as needed.
- Monitor WBC and urine protein if there is co-existent connective tissue disease.
- Beware of other interactions: Li^+ (levels ↑), digoxin (levels may ↑), NSAIDs (urea and K^+ ↑), anaesthetics (BP ↓).
- Watch for K^+ derangement (usually ↓) through diuretic action. Mild hypokalaemia is well tolerated without the need for K^+-sparing diuretics as long as: (i) the K^+ is >3.5mmol/L, (ii) there is no predisposition to arrhythmias, and (iii) there are no other K^+-losing conditions (e.g. cirrhosis, chronic diarrhoea).

However, do not be put off trying a patient on an ACE inhibitor by these cautions. Most patients tolerate them very well and gain a significant benefit from them.

Rheumatic fever

Rheumatic fever (RF) is an important cause of cardiovascular morbidity and mortality in resource-poor regions. Group A β-haemolytic streptococcal (*Streptococcus pyogenes*) pharyngitis leads, in 3–6% of cases, to rheumatic fever, due to an immune cross-reactivity between the bacteria and connective tissue.

A disease of the poor, overcrowded, and poorly housed, with children being chiefly affected. Disease is often more severe in resource-poor countries. Severity reflects failure of health services to prevent recurrences of acute RF. If these recurrences can be prevented, many patients who have carditis in their 1st attack will eventually lose their murmurs and have normal or near normal hearts.

Clinical features

- *Arthritis:* occurs in 80% of RF cases. Typically an asymmetrical and migratory 'flitting polyarthritis' affecting large joints; the pain is severe while swelling is often modest. Onset is acute and subsides over a week; as one joint improves, a second gets worse. This process may continue for 3–6wks. There is a dramatic response to aspirin.
- *Carditis:* occurs in 40–80%. It is the most serious manifestation of acute RF, causing death acutely in <1% of cases. It may affect only the endocardium (valvulitis, often MR +/– AR, 'mild carditis'), or the myocardium and pericardium may also be involved ('severe carditis').
- *Chorea:* occurs in 10% after a longer incubation period. Sydenham's chorea is emotional lability and involuntary movements (face, limbs, especially hands). More common in girls; one-third have no cardiac involvement. Seldom affects those with arthritis.
- *Erythema marginatum:* <5% cases.
- *Subcutaneous nodules:* now rare.

Diagnosis Based upon the revised Jones criteria (see Box 8.8) and requires (i) evidence of recent streptococcal infection plus (ii) either two major criteria, or one major and two minor criteria.

Management

- Bed rest until child feels better.
- Anti-inflammatory drugs to suppress the inflammatory process:
  - aspirin 20–25mg/kg oral qds. Continue for 3–6wks if heart is not involved; 3mths in mild carditis; 4–6mths in severe carditis
  - prednisolone 0.5mg/kg qds may be given for 2wks in severe carditis.
- Treat heart failure.
- Treat chorea with sodium valproate 7.5–10mg/kg oral bd for 3mths for chorea (alternative haloperidol 0.05mg/kg od).

Primary prevention of rheumatic fever

There is good trial evidence to show that the treatment of suspected streptococcal pharyngitis in children with one dose of IM benzathine benzylpenicillin ↓ the risk of developing RF by 80%. Sixty children need to be treated to prevent 1 episode of RF.

Secondary prophylaxis is essential for all patients

Give benzathine benzylpenicillin 1.2 million units (children <30kg, 600 000U) IM every 2–4wks, duration as follows:

- For 5yrs after the last attack of rheumatic fever or until age 18yrs, whichever is the longer, for patients without proven carditis.
- For 10yrs after the last attack of rheumatic fever or until age 25yrs, whichever is the longer, for patients with mild mitral regurgitation or healed carditis.
- Lifelong prophylaxis is recommended for patients with severe valvular heart disease and after valve surgery (WHO, 2004).

(Alternative for penicillin-allergic patients is erythromycin 250mg bd oral.) Any effort that will make the IM injection less painful (such as use of lidocaine as diluent for penicillin injection), and therefore less frightening for the child, will make 2° prophylaxis more successful.

Box 8.8 Revised Jones criteria

Diagnosis of RF requires

- Evidence of recent streptococcal infection *plus*
- Either two major criteria, or one major and two minor criteria.

Evidence of recent group A β-haemolytic streptococcal infection

- Positive throat culture or streptococcal antigen test.
- Elevated or ↑ streptococcal antibody titre.

Major manifestations

- Carditis.
- Polyarthritis.
- Chorea.
- Erythema marginatum.
- Subcutaneous nodules.

Minor manifestations

Clinical findings

- Arthralgia.
- Fever.

Laboratory findings

- Elevated acute-phase reactants (ESR or CRP).
- Prolonged PR interval.

Infective endocarditis

Fever + regurgitant murmur = infective endocarditis until proven otherwise.

50% of infective endocarditis (IE) is on normal valves. When it is caused by highly pathogenic bacteria like staphylococci, pneumococci, and β-haemolytic streptococci, endocarditis follows an acute course, often with serious emboli, heart failure, and death. The course is subacute if *Streptococcus viridans* affects valves previously damaged by RF or other causes. Endocarditis often occurs on prosthetic valves (2%), in which case the involved valves often need replacing.

Pathogenesis

Any bacteraemia may expose the valves to colonization. This usually occurs spontaneously, or less often following dental procedures, GU manipulation, or surgery. Gum or tooth infections do not generally lead to endocarditis, whereas intestinal lesions occasionally do - especially colon cancer in the case of *Strep. bovis*. Viridans streptococci, *Enterococcus faecalis*, and *Staphylococcus aureus* are common. Rarely fungi, *Coxiella*, or *Chlamydia* sp. infect valves. Gram –ve bacteria (e.g. *E. coli*) almost never cause infective endocarditis. Rare non-infective causes include SLE and malignancy. Right-sided disease (especially with *Staph. aureus*) is more common in IV drug users → pulmonary abscesses.

Clinical features

Include evidence of:

- *Infection:* fever, rigors, malaise, night sweats, finger clubbing, splenomegaly, anaemia.
- *Heart murmurs:* especially regurgitation of aortic or mitral valves; sometimes murmurs change from day to day — not because the vegetation is changing rapidly, but because fever accentuates the murmur and because valve function may suddenly deteriorate. Usually, the murmurs deteriorate until treatment is effective.
- *Embolic events*: vegetations on valves may cause embolic events (e.g. strokes or acute limb ischaemia). Occasionally, embolic abscesses or mycotic aneurysms form.
- *Vasculitis*: microscopic haematuria, splinter haemorrhages, Osler nodes (painful lesions on finger pulps), Janeway lesions (painful red patches on the palms), Roth spots (on fundoscopy), and renal failure.

Diagnosis

Take three blood cultures from different sites at different times. It is not necessary to time cultures with fever spikes, as bacteraemia is relatively constant. Always take blood cultures before starting antibiotics, delaying antibiotics for a few hours is seldom critical, and culture result will guide therapy. At least one culture will be +ve in 99% of cases. The commonest cause of culture –ve endocarditis is that the patient has received even a single dose of antibiotic prior to taking cultures. Check ESR, FBC, U&E, Cr; echocardiography may show the vegetations on valves. Perform urinalysis for haematuria.

Management

For highly susceptible streptococcal infection (mean inhibitory concentration (MIC) to penicillin ≤ 0.1microgram/mL), give benzylpenicillin 1.2g IV every 4h plus synergistic doses of gentamicin 60–80mg IV bd for 2wks. Less sensitive streptococcal isolates require 4–6wks of penicillin plus gentamicin for 2–6wks. For *S. aureus* infections, give flucloxacillin 2g IV every 4–6h and gentamicin as above for 2wks, then IV flucloxacillin for a further 2–4wks. Use vancomycin or teicoplanin if meticillin-resistant *Staphylococcus aureus* (MRSA) suspected. For *S. epidermidis* infections, e.g. on prosthetic valve, use vancomycin, gentamicin and rifampicin for ≥4wks.

If 'blind' empirical therapy is required, give benzylpenicillin and gentamicin, and add flucloxacillin if the endocarditis is acute in onset. Change treatment according to blood culture results. This recommendation is based on streptococcal infections being the most common cause of endocarditis. Alter these recommendations according to the local circumstances.

Prognosis

30% mortality in the UK from staphylococcal endocarditis, and 6% with sensitive streptococci.

Prevention

The value of antibiotic prophylaxis is being questioned. The American Heart Association has revised its guidelines for patients with underlying heart conditions at risk of IE. Changes include: prophylaxis for dental procedures only indicated in patients with underlying cardiac conditions associated with the highest risk, for procedures involving manipulation of gingival tissue or the periapical region of teeth, or perforation of the oral mucosa. Prophylaxis not required for patients with underlying cardiac conditions undergoing genitourinary of gastrointestinal procedures if antibiotics solely for prevention of infective endocarditis (*http://www.ncbi.nlm.nih.gov/pubmed/17446442/*). Traditional guidelines are given in Box 8.9.

Antibiotics

- Amoxicillin 3g oral 1h before procedure under local anaesthetic.
- If allergic to penicillin or >1 course of penicillin in last month, give clindamycin 600mg oral 1h before procedure.
- For procedures under general anaesthetic, give amoxicillin 3g oral 4h before procedure and again as soon as possible after procedure.
- For procedures under general anaesthetic in patients at high risk (antibiotics in the previous month, prosthetic valve, or allergic to penicillin), refer all procedures to hospital. Amoxicillin plus gentamicin (or vancomycin in penicillin-allergic patients) can be used for such patients.

Box 8.9 Traditional guidelines for IE prophylaxis

Traditional guidelines indicated that:

Prophylaxis required for:

- Previous history of endocarditis.
- Prosthetic valves.
- Congenital heart disease (except secundum atrial septal defect (ASD)).
- All acquired valvular heart disease.
- Hypertrophic cardiomyopathy with mitral regurgitation.
- Mitral valve prolapse with regurgitation.
- Surgically corrected shunts/conduits.

Prophylaxis not required for:

- Previous CABG.
- Pacemakers/implanted cardio-defibrillators.
- Mitral valve disease without regurgitation.
- Previous rheumatic fever without valve defects.
- 'Innocent' murmurs.

Procedures requiring prophylaxis:

- Any dental procedure that causes bleeding from gingiva, mucosa, or bone.
- Tonsillectomy.
- Rigid bronchoscopy.
- Incision of abscess.
- Vaginal delivery with chorioamnionitis.
- 'Dirty' surgery/procedure.

Procedures not requiring prophylaxis:

- Natural shedding of teeth.
- Caesarian section.
- Vaginal delivery without infection.
- 'Clean' procedures.

Pericardial disease

Pericarditis

In the tropics, this is commonly due to TB or pyogenic infection.

- *Tuberculous pericarditis:* is especially important in HIV+ individuals. Spread is probably from the adjacent lymph nodes and pleura. The effusion may be massive in HIV; echocardiogram may show strands of fibrin floating in the effusion.
- *Acute pyogenic pericarditis:* results from generalized bacteraemia from a 1° focus elsewhere.
- *Other causes:* any infection (especially coxsackie virus), malignancy (such as KS in AIDS patients), uraemia, MI, Dressler syndrome, trauma, radiotherapy, connective tissue diseases, and hypothyroidism.

Clinical features

Pericarditis

A sharp constant sternal pain, which may radiate to the left shoulder, down the left arm, or to the abdomen. It is relieved by sitting forward, and made worse by lying on the left, coughing, inspiring, or swallowing. Auscultation may reveal a scratchy superficial pericardial rub, loudest at the left sternal edge. In a large effusion, the rub is generally lost, and heart sounds are heard faintly.

Pericardial effusion

Depends on the speed at which it is formed. If formed quickly, the pericardium cannot stretch → pressure rises and compression of the heart producing cardiac tamponade. There is ↓ cardiac output (↓ BP), ↑ JVP, Kussmaul sign (JVP rises with inspiration), tachycardia, impalpable apex, pulsus paradoxus, peripheral shut down, and quiet heart sounds. In more chronic effusions, signs of heart failure predominate with severe ascites and hepatomegaly. Percussion reveals ↑ cardiac dullness in the retrosternal and right parasternal areas, and the apex beat is impalpable or felt within the area of dullness. Impending tamponade or restriction is first indicated by ↑ JVP; however, JVP may be so high that patient must be examined sitting or standing upright. Patients with pyogenic pericarditis are extremely unwell with signs of severe sepsis.

Diagnosis

ECG classically shows upwardly concave (saddle-shaped) ST segments in all leads except lead AVR, with no reciprocal changes. In pericardial effusions, CXR shows a large globular heart (and may show pleural effusions). ECG has low voltages and changing QRS complexes (electrical alternans = a changing axis beat-to-beat). See Fig. 8.5. Echocardiography is diagnostic with an echo-free zone showing the heart surrounded by effusion. In exudative effusions, fibrinous strands are clearly seen within the fluid. Differentiate from an MI and PE.

Constrictive pericarditis

Encasement of the heart in a non-expansive pericardium, usually following TB. Features are as for chronic effusion; however, the heart is small on CXR and may show calcification, especially on lateral CXR. Onset is usually insidious, with ascites, oedema, hepatomegaly, proteinuria being found. The patient may or may not be breathless. Often JVP is so far elevated that it is missed on routine inspection of the neck.

Management

Pericarditis:

- Find and treat cause.
- Give analgesia with NSAIDs if pericardial pain is present.
- For TB pericarditis, commence anti-TB treatment for 6mths and perform HIV test. Whilst effectiveness of adjunctive steroids is uncertain, some use them in an attempt to reduce risk of death or constriction: prednisolone 2mg/kg/day, tapering over over 6–8 wks.
- *Pericardial effusion:* find and treat cause (e.g. antibiotics for bacterial infections; anti-TB drugs for TB).
- *Tamponade:* requires urgent drainage. Aspirate with a 50mL syringe, fitted with a long needle and two-way tap, inserting upwards and to the left of the xiphisternum. Patient should be propped up 45°. Watch the ECG monitor to know if the myocardium is touched. Steroids are often effective in reducing the re-accumulation of pericardial fluid.
- *Recurrent pericardial effusion:* especially of pyogenic origin, requires surgery draining through a pericardial window or pericardiotomy.
- *Constrictive pericarditis:* requires surgical excision of the pericardium.

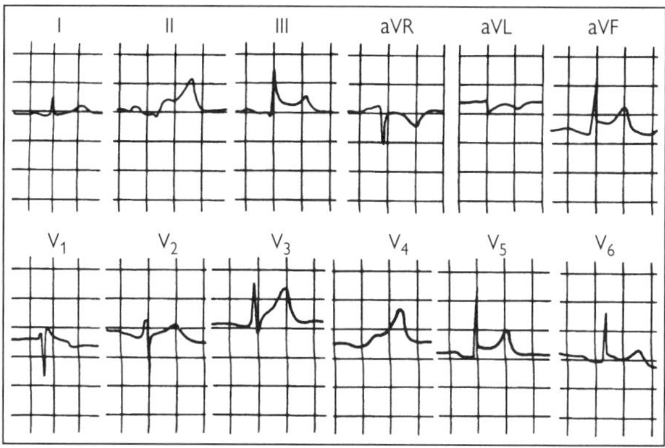

Fig. 8.5 ECG changes in pericarditis.

Cardiomyopathies

Disease of the myocardium → cardiac dysfunction → heart failure, arrhythmia, and sudden death.

Dilated (congestive) cardiomyopathy

Cause may not be identifiable, but recognized causes include alcohol, unrecognized HT, pregnancy, HIV, previous myocarditis, or familial/genetic cause.

Clinical features

- Are of heart failure.
- Apex diffuse and displaced, often functional valvular incompetence and murmurs.
- May be AF (especially in alcoholics) and associated emboli.
- Typically, patient is male 40–50yrs.
- HIV cardiomyopathy occurs in younger patients.

Diagnosis and management

Echocardiography shows a dilated hypokinetic heart with involvement of all cardiac chambers. However, in HIV-associated cardiomyopathy the left ventricle may be of normal size, but severely hypokinetic. Evaluation is in three stages:

- *Non-invasive clinical evaluation:* reversible causes including HT, alcohol, thyrotoxicosis, infiltration (iron, amyloid, sarcoid), tachycardia-induced cardiomyopathy, DM, myocarditis, and phaeochromocytoma must be excluded.
- *Invasive evaluation:* coronary angiography and endomyocardial biopsy in patients with risk factors for IHD or ECG suggestive of MI or when infiltrative disorders or myocarditis are suspected.
- *Family evaluation:* if no cause found, screen 1st degree relatives by ECG and echo to exclude familial dilated cardiomyopathy.

Full evaluation yields a cause in 50–75% cases. Cause linked to prognosis; investigation important when possible. Mortality of idiopathic dilated cardiomyopathy high — 40% by 5yrs.

Peripartum cardiomyopathy

Dilated cardiomyopathy beginning in last month of pregnancy or <5mths postpartum, with no other history of heart failure and with no discernible cause for heart failure.

Risk factors

High parity, age, low socio-economic status. Myocarditis found in ~50%, but mechanism unclear. Cultural practices, such as eating Na^+-rich foods in hot climates in the puerperium may have a role. The combination of increased circulatory demand (+/– anaemia), heat (→ peripheral vasodilatation), and high salt load might lead to a high output cardiac failure.

Investigation and management

As for heart failure. In ~50% cases there is irreversible cardiac dysfunction. Arrhythmias, persistently dilated heart, and systemic or pulmonary emboli mark poor prognosis. Consider *sterilization* in patients with irreversible cardiac dysfunction beyond 6mths follow-up.

Restrictive cardiomyopathy/endomyocardial fibrosis

Due to endomyocardial stiffening, resembling constrictive pericarditis. Often due to endomyocardial fibrosis in which hypereosinophilia (possibly triggered by helminthic infection, especially filariasis) damages the myocardium. Mural thrombus formation produces a fibrotic mass. Rare causes are amyloid or carcinoid.

Clinical features

May begin with a febrile illness, facial oedema, and dyspnoea that may → death within months. Most patients are seen in chronic stage with heart failure. There may be features of LV and/or RV failure. LV disease consists of mitral regurgitation (MR; never mitral stenosis or atrial regurgitation cf. RF) with an S_3, and progressive pulmonary hypertension. RV disease (usually tricuspid regurgitation) → gross ascites and markedly ↑ JVP, but often minimal peripheral oedema. May be exophthalmos, central cyanosis, delayed puberty, ↓ pulse pressure, and AF. Murmurs may be heard (cf. pericardial disease). Pericardial effusion common in endomyocardial fibrosis.

Diagnosis

CXR varies from massive cardiac shadow (aneurysm of R atrium, or pericardial effusion) to almost normal. Echo and Doppler studies show fibrosis of inflow tracts with involvement of ventricles and regurgitation of mitral and tricuspid valves. Pericardial effusion and thrombi in the atria or ventricles also seen.

Management

Acute treatment is supportive. If there is hypereosinophilia, look for and treat cause. In established disease, resist the temptation to drain the ascites, since it may cause the patient to lose protein. Digoxin may control ventricular rate if there is AF.

Hypertrophic cardiomyopathy

Hypertrophic cardiomyopathy is unexplained ventricular hypertrophy (i.e. hypertrophy in absence of HT, aortic stenosis, DM, obesity, or other cause) → obstruction of the LV outflow tract in 20% cases (i.e. hypertrophic obstructive cardiomyopathy, HOCM). Over 90% of cases show autosomal dominant inheritance. Genetic counselling and screening of 1st degree relatives essential.

Clinical features

Dyspnoea, angina, syncope, palpitations. May be a double impulse at apex, jerky pulse, S_4, late systolic murmur. ECG almost always abnormal, showing left ventricular hypertrophy (LVH), Q waves, and deep T-wave inversion. ECG abnormalities precede the echocardiographic onset of cardiac hypertrophy, which manifests from adolescence onwards.

Management

β-blockers for angina and treat arrhythmias. Uncontrolled AF needs anticoagulation. Consider high-risk patients (i.e. family history of sudden death, syncope, abnormal BP response to exercise) for implantable cardioverter defibrillator.

Acute myocarditis

Inflammation of myocardium, may present like an MI.

Causes

Viral (*Coxsackie* virus), diphtheria, RF, drugs, other infections; angina, dyspnoea, arrhythmia, tachycardia, and heart failure. Exclude MI, pericardial effusion. Management is supportive.

Left atrial myxoma

Rare benign tumour, developing from atrial septum → left atrial obstruction (as in MS), emboli, AF, fever, ↓ weight, and ↑ ESR. May be a family history. Rarely, a tumour 'plop' on auscultation. 2:1 female excess. Differentiate from MS by occurrence of emboli without AF or on echo.

Treatment Excision—the lesion may recur.

Chapter 9
Renal medicine

Invited authors **Sally Hamour**
Dwomoa Adu

Assessing renal function

The kidneys:

- Regulate fluid, electrolyte, and acid base balance
- Eliminate potentially toxic substances
- Produce renin and erythropoietin.

The renal tubules synthesize 1,25-dihydroxycholecalciferol (vitamin D3).

Serum creatinine

Simple to measure and widely available. However, serum creatinine concentration remains in the normal range until glomerular filtration rate (GFR) has ↓ by ~40 %→ not a useful measure of *early* renal impairment.

Glomerular filtration rate

Normal range for GFR is 88–174mL/min in men and 87–147mL/min in women. A complex formula can be used to calculate GFR. See http://www.renal.org/eGFRcalc/GFR.pl for a useful online GFR calculator. To avoid a 24-h urine collection, the Cockroft Gault equation can be used to estimate creatinine clearance.

Calculated creatinine clearance

Calculated creatinine clearance (ml/min) =

1.2 × [140 – age (yrs) × weight (kg)]/ plasma creatinine (μmol/L)

In females, the result is × 0.85 to account for ↓ creatinine production.

Urine analysis

- *Colour:* if pale, consider over hydration, diabetes insipidus or post-obstructive diuresis. If dark consider bilirubin, blood, haemoglobin, myoglobin, beetroot or drugs. Rarely melanoma, ochronosis, porphyrins.
- *Transparency:* cloudiness may be due to blood, pus, chyle, or crystals.
- *Smell:* commonly due to a UTI (bacteria split urea → ammonia). Also antibiotics or vitamins.

Chemical analysis

- *pH:* urine is normally acidic (range 4.5–8.0).
- *Protein:* see 📖 Proteinuria, p. 406).
- *Glucose:* usually = DM, but may also be normal variant or part of renal tubular disease.
- *Ketones:* diabetic ketoacidosis, starvation.
- *Nitrites:* suggests a UTI .
- *Blood:* intact RBCs → punctate staining, while free Hb or myoglobin → homogeneous colour. Confirm by urine microscopy—intact RBC will be seen in haematuria, but not haemoglobinuria or myoglobinuria.
- *Leukocyte esterase:* +ve in UTIs, but not specific as may be present in systemic inflammation.

See Box 9.1 regarding abnormal urinary sediment.

Box 9.1 Abnormal urinary sediment

Urine is centrifuged, supernatant poured off, and sediment examined microscopically.

Cells

- *Red cells:* see 📖 Haematuria, p. 407).
- *Leukocytes:* usually indicates a UTI. May also occur in glomerulonephritis and interstitial nephritis. If a sterile pyuria persists, consider TB of the urinary tract.

Casts

- *Hyaline casts or fine granular casts:* non-specific mucoprotein—in normal urine, febrile illnesses, after exercise, in concentrated urine, and in renal disease.
- *Coarse granular casts:* usually pathological = glomerulonephritis.
- *Red cell casts:* glomerular bleeding = glomerulonephritis.
- *White cell casts:* pyelonephritis.

Proteinuria

Normal protein excretion is <150mg/d. Dipsticks are very sensitive to albumin, but insensitive to Bence–Jones protein and light chains in urine in myeloma.

- *Micro-albuminuria:* daily excretion of 30–300mg albumin/24h. Not detected by dipsticks. Abnormal and early feature of diabetic nephropathy.
- Dipsticks become +ve for protein when albuminuria is >300mg/24h (macro-albuminuria).

If persistent proteinuria is present, quantify this by urine albumin/creatinine ratio, urine protein/creatinine ratio, or 24-h urine protein excretion.

Causes of persistent proteinuria

- Renal disease.
- *Postural (orthostatic) proteinuria:* absent proteinuria after overnight rest, → mild proteinuria after 2h of standing/walking. Patients are asymptomatic and have no haematuria; other investigations are normal. Renal Bx is not indicated and long-term prognosis excellent.
- *Other causes:* exercise induced, CCF.

Chyluria

Chyle in the urine resembles milk; must be differentiated from pyuria, phosphaturia, and lipuria. Results from rupture of lymphatic varices → fistula between lymphatic system and urinary tract. Rose/pink colour of urine means there is also haematuria. Chyluria in tropics, often 2° to lymphatic filariasis. Other causes rare; usually involves stenosis or obstruction of the thoracic duct (e.g. neoplastic infiltration, trauma, TB).

Clinical features

Usually relapsing and remitting. Main symptom is passage of milky white urine; also loin pain, ureteric colic, passage of clots (may cause retention), and fever.

Diagnosis

Urine microscopy → chylomicrons and fat globules. IVU, cystoscopy (2h after a fatty meal) to detect site of lesion; lymphography may be useful. Measure 24h urine, protein excretion, and serum proteins (may be useful to assess albumin loss).

Management

>50% resolve spontaneously; treat filariasis, although some lesions may be irreversible. A low-fat diet and high fluid intake ↓ risk of urinary stasis and clot formation. If chyluria is severe or accompanied by episodes of dysuria, colic, retention, or weight loss, consider surgical repair.

Haematuria

Blood in the urine always requires investigation. It may be:

- *Microscopic:* with ≥5 RBC/high-power field, *or*
- *Macroscopic:* i.e. can be seen with the naked eye.

While ~50% patients presenting with haematuria in the West have neoplastic lesions, in resource-poor regions, a large number of other diseases → bleeding from the urinary tract.

Causes

- *Surgical:* renal stone disease; transitional cell or squamous carcinoma (CA) of the bladder, ureter, or pelvis; renal cell CA; trauma; benign prostatic hyperplasia; AV malformations.
- *Medical:* UTI, schistosomiasis, TB, glomerular disease (IgA nephropathy, glomerulonephritis, SLE), polycystic kidneys (PCK), infarction, bleeding diatheses.

Investigating haematuria

Look for stones, malignancy, UTIs, and schistosomiasis (in endemic areas) before considering rarer medical causes. Ask the following questions:

- *Is it true haematuria?* Check other causes of red urine (haemoglobinuria, myoglobin, porphyrins, beetroot; Box 9.2).
- *What is its timing in relation to micturition?* Early haematuria → low (urethral/genital) bleeding site, late haematuria (i.e. at the end of voiding) → bladder site; red colouration throughout micturition → ureteric or renal lesion.
- *Is the haematuria painful?* CA and schistosomiasis tend to be painless, Cystitis, obstruction (e.g. stones), and infection are commonly painful.
- *Is there dysuria and fever (UTI), poor stream (urethral/bladder neck lesion), loin pain (ureteric obstruction due to tumour, stone, or clot), family history (PCK), or a history of trauma?*

Diagnosis Urine microscopy (RBC casts and dysmorphic RBCs suggests glomerular bleeding), culture, cytology; USS; IVU; cystoscopy, FBC.

Box 9.2 Is it true haematuria?

Haemoglobinuria

Is caused by intravascular haemolysis due to toxins/venoms, falciparum malaria, incompatible blood transfusions, glucose 6-phosphate dehydrogenase (G6PD) deficiency, paroxysmal nocturnal haemoglobinuria, chronic cold agglutinin disease, microangiopathic haemolytic anaemia, march haemoglobinuria.

Myoglobinuria

Is caused by rhabdomyolysis (muscle destruction) after muscle injury, excessive contraction (convulsions, tetanus, hyperthermia, very heavy exercise), viral myositis (influenza, Legionnaires' disease), and drugs/toxins (alcohol, snake venoms). Myoglobinuria may be idiopathic.

Urinary schistosomiasis (bilharzia)

Caused by *Schistosoma haematobium* in Africa and parts of the Middle East. *S. intercalatum* and hybrid species can produce atypical clinical pictures, with ectopic localization of worms. For distribution and life cycle, see 📖 Schistosomiasis (bilharzia), p. 344. Worm eggs → a T-cell-mediated immune response → eosinophilic granulomata in the bladder, uterus, and genitals. Eggs may also affect the GI tract, lungs, liver, skin, and CNS.

Transmission

Requires:

- Human (definitive host) availability and freshwater contact.
- *Bulinus* snails (intermediate host).
- *S. haematobium.*

Peak prevalence 15–30yrs, then ↓ due to age-related changes in water-contact, ↑ immunity, and death of adult worms.

Clinical features

- *Egg deposition:* begins 3mths after infection → painless haematuria, which may persist for months or years, +/– dysuria, pain, malaise, and mild fever.
- *Established infection:* haematuria often ↓ in chronic stage, unless there is infection, ulceration, or malignancy. Fibrosis and calcification of bladder → ↓ volume → frequency and dribbling (see Fig. 9.1). Other complications include perineal fistulae and bacterial infection. In severe cases → urinary retention, stasis, stone formation, and renal failure. In men, involvement of seminal vesicles → eggs shed in semen ('lumpy' semen); prostate, epididymis, and penis uncommonly affected. In women, ulcerating, polypoid, or nodular lesions may be seen in the vulva, vagina, and cervix. The ovaries, fallopian tubes, and uterus rarely affected. *S. haematobium* infection may → ectopic pregnancies and infertility. Heavy/lifelong infection predisposes to squamous bladder CA.

Diagnosis

- *Microscopy:* parasite eggs in urinary sediment, bladder biopsies, or rectal mucosal snips. Schistosome ova large (150 × 50 um); require low-power only (see Colour plate 7). Distinguish viable ova by flickering 'flame cell' visible in wet preparation, by observing eggs hatching in water, or by being uncalcified with intact organelles in biopsies.
- *Serology:* antibodies to *Schistosoma* develop 6–12wks post-exposure.
- *Imaging:* USS → bladder wall thickening or hydronephrosis. Heavy infections may → bladder calcification on AXR ('foetal head' sign); IVU may show hydronephrosis, hydroureter.

Treatment

See 📖 Schistosomiasis (bilharzia), p. 344. Praziquantel is effective against all species of schistosomes; dose of 40–60mg/kg oral given in divided doses over 1d usually curative. Follow-up at 2 and 6mths for urinalysis and clinical assessment. If in doubt, do cystoscopy to exclude bladder CA.

S. haematobium and bladder cancer

Association between bladder CA and chronic heavy *S. haematobium* infection well-recognized. Lag period of >20yrs between infection and development of CA. 75% of patients (with squamous bladder CA) in Egypt are <50yrs; by contrast, in non-schistosome areas, most patients (with adenoCA) are >65yrs. ↑ Common in males, smokers, and those working with aromatic amines (e.g. in the rubber industry).

Clinical features

Haematuria, cystitis, and obstruction. Spread is local → pelvic structures, via the lymphatics → iliac and para-aortic nodes, and via the blood → liver and lungs.

Investigation

Urinalysis, FBC. AXR may show a calcified bladder wall. Perform IVU, cystoscopy, and biopsy.

Management

Cystoscopic diathermy for superficial tumours. Intra-vesicular chemotherapy or BCG administration, radical surgery and radiotherapy or palliation (long-term catheterization) depending on stage.

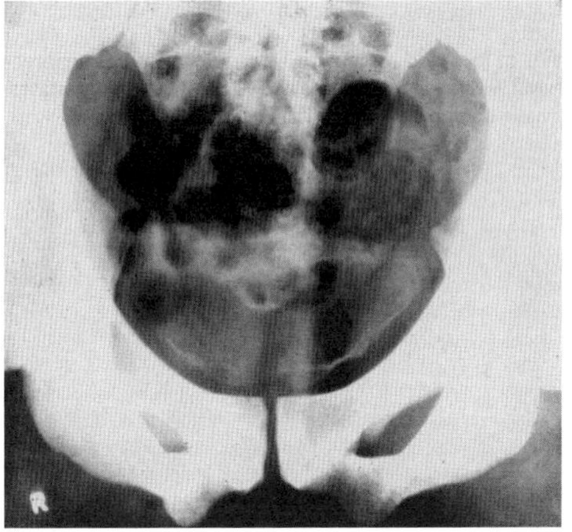

Fig. 9.1 Bladder calcification in urinary schistosomiasis — the 'foetal head' sign. Such patients commonly have well-preserved bladder function.

Renal masses

Enlarged kidneys tend to bulge forwards, whilst perinephric abscesses or collections tend to bulge backwards. With chronic obstructed states and tumours, mass is usually better defined and less tender. Bilateral, irregular kidneys suggest polycystic renal disease (Box 9.3).

Kidney tumours

Three main types of renal tumours:

- *Nephroblastoma (Wilms' tumour):* undifferentiated mesodermal tumour of children; may be sporadic or familial; 95% are unilateral.
- *Urothelial tumours:* arise in renal pelvis, ureters, urethra, or bladder. In Europe and America, transitional cell CA accounts for 90% of urothelial malignancies, in Africa squamous CA predominates due to urinary schistosomiasis. Tumours may → chronic urethral strictures, obstruction, and recurrent infection.
- *Renal CA (hypernephroma):* majority of renal cell CAs are clear cell CAs. Classic symptoms are loin pain, a mass, and frank haematuria. Anaemia and hepatic dysfunction are common, sometimes with polycythaemia due to ↑ erythropoietin secretion. Tumours are often discovered incidentally on USS.

Diagnosis USS or CT scan; CXR (for metastases); urine cytology; histology.

Management

Standard treatment of localized tumours is by radical unilateral nephrectomy. Five-yr survival with localized disease is 90%, but <10% if metastases. Drug treatments have been disappointing so far.

Box 9.3 Polycystic kidney disease

Autosomal dominant polycystic kidney disease occurs in ~1 in 1000 individuals and is a major cause of chronic kidney disease.

Clinical features

Renal pain, gross haematuria, and urinary infections, but sometimes incidental finding of abdominal mass. HT common; treatment ↓ progression of renal failure. Cysts are common in liver and pancreas. Some families have intracerebral aneurysms that may → intracerebral or subarachnoid haemorrhage. >50% of patients develop chronic renal failure (CRF) in later life.

Diagnosis USS shows enlarged kidneys with characteristic multiple cysts. Look for a family history.

Management

Supportive. Treat hypertension and UTIs. For infected cysts, co-trimoxazole and ciprofloxacin have good penetration. Manage bleeding conservatively. CRF usually causes death unless there is access to dialysis or transplantation. Consider screening family members for asymptomatic disease. Most affected individuals have cysts by 20y.

Autosomal recessive polycystic disease

Occurs in ~1 in 20 000 children; can cause death *in utero* or in the neonatal period from pulmonary atresia. CRF and fibrosis develop in those children who survive.

Renal calculi and renal colic

Renal and ureteric calculi are less common in resource-poor countries, and are seen less frequently in Africa than Asia and the Middle-East. M:F ratio is 2.5:1. Factors such as diet, affluence, climate, and metabolic factors are significant. Congenital renal abnormalities (e.g. polycystic disease, horseshoe kidney), schistosomiasis, and TB predispose to stones. 80% of stones are calcium oxalate; triple phosphate stones (staghorn calculi) are associated with UTI, usually *Proteus* spp.; uric acid and cysteine stones are uncommon.

Clinical features

Stones in the ureter → renal colic with sudden onset of agonizing paroxysms of pain. Pain radiates from loin → groin and patient often cannot lie still. Kidney stones may cause loin pain with abdominal/loin tenderness and haematuria. Bladder stones cause strangury—urgent desire to pass something that will not pass. Common sites of obstruction are vesico-ureteric and pelvi-ureteric junctions.

Diagnosis

- Kidney-ureters-bladder (KUB) X-ray for calculi (90% of urinary stones are radio-opaque).
- Dipstick for blood.
- Screen for UTI.
- USS or IVU to look for stone and obstruction.
- *Blood tests:* U&E, uric acid, Ca^{2+}, bicarbonate.

Management

- ↑ Fluid intake. Treat infection.
- *Give pain relief:* NSAIDs (beware renal impairment) or opiates for severe colic (beware opiate addicts fabricating symptoms).
- Most stones will pass spontaneously. >70% of ureteric stones <4mm wide will pass spontaneously in 1yr; <10% of stones >8mm wide will pass. Stones likely to pass without complications can be managed conservatively.
- If there is obstruction, infection, or bilateral involvement, seek urgent urological advice. Decompress renal tract before renal failure occurs. Stones can sometimes pass once broken up by extracorporeal shock wave lithotripsy or surgery.

Prevention

Avoid oxalate-rich foods (spinach, beetroot, green peppers, almonds, cashew nuts, cocoa, grapefruit juice, orange juice, black tea, cola drinks) and excessive dietary protein. High risk of recurrence.

Urinary tract infection

UTIs may progress rapidly in the tropics and complications are common, especially in malnourished individuals. Infection commonly due to Gram –ve organisms, most often *E. coli* (70%). More common in women.

Clinical features

- *Cystitis:* abrupt onset of frequency, dysuria, urgency, suprapubic pain, and tenderness; occasionally haematuria, incontinence, retention. Consider whether dysuria represents a UTI or urethritis from an STI. Absence of urethral discharge important in UTIs. Terminal haematuria in schistosomiasis is not usually painful.
- *Acute pyelonephritis:* features of cystitis, plus high fever +/– rigors, loin pain, nausea, and vomiting.

Ask about Previous infections including STD, recent urinary instrumentation, diabetes, childhood UTI, known urinary tract abnormalities, renal colic, renal stones, obstructive uropathy.

Examine for Loin tenderness, renal mass, large prostate, meatal ulcers, urethral or vaginal discharge, pelvic mass on vaginal examination.

Is it a complicated UTI?

UTI in a male is usually 2° to prostatic hypertrophy, sometimes with prostatitis. UTIs in pregnant women may → pyelonephritis and may → premature labour. Complicated UTIs are often associated with:

- Urinary tract abnormality (congenital, obstruction, calculi).
- Reflux.
- Neurogenic bladder.
- Recent urinary instrumentation.
- Female genital mutilation.
- Diabetes predisposes to UTIs.

Diagnosis

Clean-catch MSU specimen. Visually inspect urine for turbidity and haematuria. Test urine for leukocytes and nitrites (blood and protein alone have low specificity/sensitivity). Send specimens for microscopy (pyuria, bacteria, epithelial cells) and culture. Pyuria with a growth $>10^5$ cfu/mL urine, of a single recognized urinary pathogen, confirms UTI. However, genuine mixed growth may occur in complicated UTI and lower counts may be significant, particularly in men and with slow-growing organisms.

Perform further investigations:

If recurrent UTI in women, first UTI in men, UTI in children (see 🕮 Paediatric note, p. 416), overt or persistent haematuria, sterile pyuria.

Further investigations

Include USS, IVU, micturating cystourethrogram and DMSA scan for scars in children (Paediatric note, 🕮 p. 416).

Sterile pyuria

Consider partially-treated UTI, TB chlamydia, candida, calculi, bladder tumour, prostatitis, papillary necrosis (the elderly, over-use of NSAIDs), polycystic kidneys, appendicitis.

Management of UTI

- ↑ Fluid intake, frequent voiding, double micturition, and post-coital voiding.
- Start antibiotic treatment empirically, guided by local sensitivities.
- Except for pregnant women, asymptomatic bacteriuria does not usually require antibiotics.

Lower tract infection (cystitis) 3–5d of any of trimethoprim 200mg bd oral; ciprofloxacin 500mg bd oral; cefalexin 500mg bd oral.

Upper tract infection (pyelonephritis) or complicated UTI 2wks of antibiotics. Start with IV 3rd generation cephalosporin (e.g. ceftriaxone 2g od) or IV ampicillin 1g qid plus oral ciprofloxacin 500mg bd; with clinical improvement, change to an oral agent for lower tract UTI (ideally guided by microbiology), but continue for 2wks total.

If urinary tract is obstructed (urethral valves/stricture, prostate, stones), urgent decompression is required (urinary catheter; suprapubic catheter; nephrostomy, guided by USS).

Recurrent UTIs Emphasize frequent voiding and double micturition. 3–6mths of prophylactic antibiotics (e.g. trimethoprim 100mg nocte) may break cycle of infection. In young women, cefalexin 500mg after sexual intercourse helps ↓ UTIs.

Paediatric note: UTI in children

- UTIs are common in children, but in a minority they may be a sign of underlying renal tract abnormalities including vesico-ureteric reflux (VUR). Recurrent UTI in infants, particularly with VUR, may → progressive renal failure.
- UTIs in children can present with varied symptoms; have a low index of suspicion in a child with fever. Symptoms in young children incl. vomiting, being off feeds, lethargy and irritability. In children <3mths UTIs are often associated with sepsis. Older children may have dysuria and frequency. Assess for risk factors for abnormalities (including family history, previous UTIs, ↓ urine flow, recurrent fevers, spinal lesions, poor growth, ↑ BP, constipation, enlarged bladder, difficulty voiding, abdominal mass, known renal abnormality).
- Obtain a urine specimen before treatment. Dipstick +ve for both nitrites and leukocyte esterase indicates UTI. However, in children <3yrs dipstick tests are unreliable; if possible, sample should be sent for microscopy and culture.
- Treatment with IV broad spectrum antibiotics for all children <3mths (e.g. ampicillin 50mg/kg IV qds plus gentamicin 7mg/kg od (4mg/kg od for neonates)). Children who are unwell and/or have signs of upper tract infection may need IV treatment before switching to oral therapy to complete 10-d course. Lower tract infections, e.g. cystitis may be treated with 3-d course of oral antibiotics, e.g. trimethoprim 4mg/kg oral bd.
- Investigations are the subject of debate and also limited by resources in tropical settings. Investigation should be according to risk. USS is non-invasive, and more readily available and should be undertaken on all children <6mths, or children with recurrent or atypical UTI (e.g. non-*E. coli* infection, seriously ill, failure to respond to treatment, sepsis, ↑ creatinine, ↓ urine flow, abdominal mass). MCUG and DMSA may be indicated based on risk (recurrent UTI, age, atypical illness, abnormal USS). NICE (UK) guidelines available at: http://www.nice.org.uk/nicemedia/live/11819/36030/36030.pdf

Glomerular disease

Glomerulonephritis (GN) more common in tropics than temperate regions, especially infection-associated GN is higher.

Clinical features

GN may present with:

- Asymptomatic microscopic haematuria or frank haematuria.
- Proteinuria.
- Nephrotic syndrome.
- Acute nephritis (haematuria, proteinuria, oliguria).
- Acute kidney injury (rapidly progressive glomerulonephritis).
- CRF.
- Hypertension.

GN may be idiopathic or 2° to infection or autoimmune disease (see Table 9.1). >70% of all GN is idiopathic. A careful search for infections is important.

Diagnosis

- *Urine:* proteinuria; dysmorphic RBCs (and RBC casts in proliferative GN) on microscopy; albumin/creatinine or protein/creatinine ratios.
- *Blood:* serum creatinine, albumin, lipid profile, U&E, FBC, ESR.
- *Serology:* (to help determine the cause) anti-nuclear antibodies (ANA), dsDNA, complement C3 & C4 (immune disease); HBsAg, anti-DNAase B, ASOT, Hep C and HIV antibody (infections); ANCA (vasculitis); anti-GBM Ab (Goodpasture's disease).
- *Radiology:* renal USS.
- *Renal biopsy:* where available.

Management of GN

Depending on aetiology, histology, and chronicity, GN may be amenable to treatment. Ina resource-poor setting, where histological classification is unavailable, management usually based on clinical syndrome (Box 9.4).

General principles

- Salt restriction.
- ACE inhibitors or ARBs (check creatinine and potassium 2wks after starting and after each dose increase).
- Careful use of diuretics.
- Aim for a BP of <130/80mmHg.
- Avoid further renal insults, e.g. nephrotoxins, NSAIDS.

Specific treatment

Idiopathic GN is usually treated with steroids and immunosuppression. However, these carry significant risks, and require experienced supervision. In addition, ensure that the patient does not have chronic infection (e.g. strongyloides, amoebiasis, viral hepatitis, or HIV) that might be exacerbated by such treatment.

Table 9.1 Glomerular histology and associated aetiology

Glomerular histology	Aetiology
Minimal change nephropathy	Usually idiopathic; lymphoma (rare), NSAIDS
Focal segmental glomerulosclerosis	Can be idiopathic; ↓ renal mass, *S. mansoni*, HIV-associated nephropathy, sickle cell anaemia
Membranous nephropathy	Majority idiopathic; hepatitis B infection, lupus, CA, *S. mansoni*, syphilis, leprosy, filariasis
Proliferative glomerulonephritis	Streptococci, *S. mansoni*, leprosy, lupus, *Wuchereria bancrofti*, onchocerciasis; can be idiopathic
Mesangiocapillary glomerulonephritis (membranoproliferative glomerulonephritis)	Lupus, sickle cell anaemia, *S. mansoni*, onchocerciasis, hepatitis C; can be idiopathic

Box 9.4 GN summary

Minimal change GN

- Presents with nephrotic syndrome and is less common in children in tropical areas.
- Treatment is with steroids and long-term prognosis is excellent. In adults, time to remission is slower and rate of remission is lower.

Focal segmental glomerulosclerosis

Common in children and adults in tropical areas. 40–60% of patients respond to 6mths treatment with steroids.

HIV-related nephropathy

Ranges from HIV-associated nephropathy with proteinuria to the nephrotic syndrome. The typical histological lesion is a collapsing focal segmental glomerulosclerosis. Other lesions include HIV immune complex disease, membranous nephropathy, mesangial hypercellularity, post-infectious glomerulonephritis and IgA nephropathy. Treatment as for other causes of GN, in particular ACE inhibitors; commence ART.

Hepatitis B-associated glomerulonephritis

Occurs mainly in children who are carriers for hepatitis B. Most patients are male; age of onset is 2–12yrs. Histological lesion is of membranous nephropathy. Most children → spontaneous remission but adults often → renal failure. Manage conservatively in children, but anti-viral treatment in adults.

'Quartan malarial nephropathy'

The previously suggested association between chronic *P. malariae* infection and nephrotic syndrome is no longer seen.

Acute glomerulonephritis

Acute GN most often post-streptococcal in the tropics; occurs 2–3wks after a β-haemolytic streptococcal throat, ear, or skin infection (impetigo, infected scabies, or infected eczema).

Clinical features

Haematuria, oliguria, fluid retention (with mild oedema, ↑ JVP), hypertension, and (sometimes) uraemia.

Complications Include hypertensive encephalopathy, pulmonary oedema, ↓ renal function; rarely, rapidly progressive GN.

Diagnosis

Haematuria, +/– RBC casts, proteinuria, ↑ blood urea and ↑ creatinine, ↓ creatinine clearance, and ↑ anti-DNAase B, ASOT. Culture throat and skin lesions for streptococcus. CXR may show pulmonary oedema.

Management of acute nephritis

- If oliguric (urine output < 0.5mL/kg/h) restrict fluid intake to urine output over past 24h plus 500mL.
- Restrict salt and K^+ in diet.
- Give diuretics (e.g. furosemide) IV or oral and antihypertensive treatment (not β-blockers which may → pulmonary oedema).
- To eradicate residual streptococcal infection, give oral penicillin 500mg qds for 10d; or single dose of benzathine benzylpenicillin 900mg IM; or if allergic to penicillin, erythromycin 250–500mg qds.

Nephrotic syndrome

The nephrotic syndrome is characterized by ↑ proteinuria (>3g/24h or albumin/creatinine ratio >300), ↓ serum albumin, oedema, and ↑ serum cholesterol. Most cases in the tropics are idiopathic; some are 2° to:

- Infections, including HIV, hepatitis B, hepatitis C.
- Diabetic nephropathy.
- Autoimmune diseases, e.g. SLE, HSP.
- Neoplasia (especially CA).
- Amyloid (leprosy, tuberculosis), sickle cell disease.

Clinical features

Facial and peripheral oedema; with ascites and pleural effusions if severe. Urine is frothy. Complications include:

- *Venous thromboembolism:* suspect renal vein thrombosis if sudden ↓ renal function with haematuria, especially with back pain. Treat with anticoagulants.
- *Infection:* especially 1° peritonitis (e.g. pneumococcal). Consider prophylaxis with penicillin V 500mg bd while oedematous; treat infections.
- *Hypercholesterolaemia:* treat in chronic cases.
- *Hypovolaemia:* check postural BP, monitor urine output.

Management

- ↓ Salt intake.
- Give diuretics to relieve oedema. Use cautiously since volume depletion may be present (postural drop in BP, low urine output).
- Monitor U&E and creatinine, and weigh daily.
- Use ACE inhibitors to ↓ proteinuria.
- Treat hypercholesterolaemia with statins if chronic.
- Consider prophylaxis with penicillin V during oedematous state
- Treat the cause in 2° GN. Use steroids +/– 2nd-line immunosuppression in idiopathic GN depending on histology, with caution.

Renal oedema

Oedema often presenting feature in both nephrotic syndrome and acute nephritis (see 📖 Acute glomerulonephritis, p. 420; and 📖 Nephrotic syndrome, p. 421). Can occur in acute kidney injury (AKI) and CRF.

- *Nephrotic syndrome:* mechanism of oedema in nephrotic syndrome is unclear. Glomerular damage → large protein loss in urine → hypoalbuminaemia → transudation of fluid from capillaries to the extracellular fluid compartment → oedema; ↓ intravascular volume → activation of the renin-angiotensin-aldosterone system → hyperaldosteronism with retention of salt and water → ↑ oedema. However, only one-third of patients are hypovolaemic and the others are normovolaemic or hypervolaemic.
- *Acute nephritis:* glomerular inflammation → ↓ glomerular filtration → retention of Na^+ and water → ↑ intravascular volume → ↑ hydrostatic pressure within capillaries → oedema due to transudation of fluid into extracellular fluid compartment.
- *Renal failure:* in AKI or CRF volume overload → oedema because Na^+ and water intake exceeds the kidney's capacity to excrete.
- *Other causes of generalized oedema:* CCF, pericardial disease, cirrhosis, malnutrition, hypothyroidism, drugs (NSAIDs, Ca^{2+} channel blockers, oestrogens, and steroids), pregnancy, and idiopathic oedema.

Acute kidney injury

The term 'acute kidney injury' has replaced 'acute renal failure'. Causes of AKI are ~60% medical, ~25% surgical, and ~15% obstetric. If AKI is part of multiple-organ dysfunction, it has a poor prognosis. The prognosis is better when the AKI is isolated, e.g. following haemolysis or malaria.

- *Pre-renal AKI:* ↓ volume or hypoperfusion (dehydration, shock, blood loss, hypotension, or septicaemia) → AKI, oliguria, concentrated urine. Requires careful fluid resuscitation, watching the JVP, to restore normal BP. Hypovolaemia best shown by postural hypotension: the ↓ in BP on standing is proportional to the severity of hypovolaemia.
- *Intrinsic renal disease:* e.g. leptospirosis, falciparum malaria, massive intravascular haemolysis from G6PD deficiency, snake bite, post-streptococcal GN, rhabdomyolysis, history of drugs, toxins, IV contrast.
- *Post-renal AKI (obstruction):* distended bladder, palpable kidneys (hydronephrosis), pelvic mass, large prostate. USS is diagnostic. A urinary catheter will relieve lower tract obstruction.

Clinical features

- ↑ Blood urea, creatinine, and K^+.
- Oliguria (<500mL/day or <0.5mL/kg/h) or anuria.
- Patient may be dehydrated *or* fluid overloaded.
- Anorexia, nausea and vomiting, confusion, pericardial rub.
- *Acidosis:* Kussmaul breathing (deep, sighing breathing).
- Bruising, GI bleeding due to uraemic platelet dysfunction.

Diagnosis

- *Examine urine:* absence of urinary sediment suggests a pre-renal cause; proteinuria, RBCs and RBC casts suggest GN.
- *Blood:* urea, creatinine, electrolytes, ABG (acidosis), FBC.
- *Radiology:* USS kidneys to exclude obstruction; CXR for pulmonary oedema.
- *Renal biopsy:* if expertise available and cause unclear.

Course and progress

Oliguria lasts up to 6wks with ↑ urea and creatinine, often → polyuric recovery phase which requires careful balance of fluid and electrolytes.

Management

- *Examine patient:* assess volume status (JVP, skin turgor, peripheral perfusion, mucous membranes, pulmonary crepitations, peripheral oedema, heart rate, postural BP).
- *Optimize fluid balance:* give fluids if dehydrated; no proven benefit from furosemide, but may be worth trying if fluid overloaded and there are no dialysis facilities.
- *Catheterize to exclude lower tract obstruction:* monitor urine output. Remove after 24h if anuric. Arrange renal tract USS.
- *Consider urgent dialysis:* e.g. peritoneal dialysis, if pulmonary oedema, K^+ >6.5mmol/L, severe uraemia, or acidosis. see Box 9.5.

- Prevent GI bleeding, e.g. with ranitidine 150mg bd.
- Record fluid input and output, daily weight, daily U&E.
- Once fluid replete, limit fluids to 500mL + previous days' losses.
- Treat sepsis.
- Avoid nephrotoxic or K^+ sparing drugs; adjust doses of other drugs.
- Start a low K^+ diet.
- During polyuric recovery phase, avoid dehydration and hypokalaemia.

Complications

See Boxes 9.5 and 9.6 for pulmonary oedema and hyperkalaemia.

Metabolic acidosis If pH <7.1, cautiously give slow IV bicarbonate. Optimize hydration and attempt to establish a urine output.

Box 9.5 Pulmonary oedema

Requires specialist treatment and/or dialysis. Sit upright, lower legs, give O_2. Offload with IV nitrate and furosemide. If no response, urgent dialysis needed for removal of fluid. Consider emergency venesection before dialysis, if very severe.

Prognosis is usually good. Proteinuria and abnormal urinary sediment may persist for up to 2yrs. If it persists for longer, consider biopsy.

Box 9.6 Hyperkalaemia

- If ECG changes are present or potassium >6.5, protect heart with 10–20mL of 10% calcium gluconate by slow IV injection with ECG monitoring (this will not alter serum potassium). Repeat if ECG changes persist.
- Give soluble insulin 5–10U with 50mL of 50% glucose by IV infusion over 15min.
- Give nebulized salbutamol 5mg (salbutamol shifts K^+ intracellularly). Side effects are tremor, tachycardia, and anxiety.
- In refractory hyperkalaemia, particularly if anuric, dialysis is required.
- Cation exchange resins (Calcium Resonium®, polystyrene sulphate) 15g qds oral or as enema ↑ faecal K^+ excretion. Give with lactulose to ↓ constipation. Furosemide will ↑ K^+ loss if the patient is well-filled and passing urine.
- Remember to stop medications that ↑ K^+ and ↓ dietary K^+ intake.

AKI in pregnancy

Common causes are post-abortion septicaemia, pre-eclampsia and eclampsia, HELLP syndrome (Haemolysis, Elevated Liver enzymes, Low Platelet count), antepartum and postpartum haemorrhage, *abruptio placentae*, and puerperal sepsis.

Chronic kidney disease

Chronic kidney disease (CKD) results from progressive and irreversible loss of renal function. Kidneys can support life with as little as 8% of their original nephrons functioning. Below this level, patients develop uraemic symptoms and need dialysis (see Box 9.7) and/or transplantation is required for survival. The prevalence of CKD in tropical countries is unknown, but likely to be >10%. In tropical countries, GN, hypertension, and diabetic nephropathy are major causes of CKD, as is obstructive uropathy (e.g. chronic urinary schistosomiasis affecting ureters).

Clinical features

Few symptoms of CKD until GFR is ↓ to <20%, when tiredness due to anaemia develops → fluid overload and hypertension. Uraemia may → anorexia, vomiting, hiccups, peripheral neuropathy, confusion, and drowsiness.

- *Hyperkalaemia and acidosis:* onset with GFR <20mL/min. In most patients, salt and water balance is maintained until GFR <15% of normal; this may occur earlier in diabetes.
- *Bone disease:* ↓ vitamin D → ↑ parathyroid hormone (PTH) → renal osteodystrophy (osteomalacia, bone erosions, osteitis fibrosa.
- *Anaemia:* ↓ erythropoietin → ↓ Hb when GFR <30mL/min.

Diagnosis

- *Blood:* measure urea, creatinine, electrolytes, Hb, FBC, Ca^{2+}, PO_4, urate, glucose, ESR, serum proteins (do electrophoresis if myeloma suspected).
- *Urine:* analysis, microscopy, culture, urine albumin/creatinine ratio.
- *Imaging:* USS (for renal size, obstruction).
- *Renal biopsy:* especially in patients with normal-sized kidneys and mild to moderate CRF, when the cause of CRF is unknown.

Pathophysiology of CKD

- Nephron loss → glomerular hypertrophy → glomerular hypertension, hyperperfusion and hyperfiltration → progressive glomerular sclerosis, tubulointerstitial atrophy, scarring.
- ↓ Intraglomerular pressures by good BP control with angiotensin blockade, ↓ progression of renal failure in CKD.

Management

See Box 9.7.

Treat cause and reversible contributing factors

- Relieve obstruction.
- Avoid nephrotoxic drugs, e.g. NSAIDs.
- Treat urinary infections.

Prevent progression

- Maintain good glucose control in DM.
- *Control BP:* aim for 125/75mmHg in patients with a urine albumin/creatinine ratio >100 or proteinuria >1g/24h.
- Use ACE inhibitors or ARBs to ↓ progression of renal failure, especially when there is proteinuria.
- Low-salt diet if oedematous/hypertensive; low-K^+ diet if hyperkalaemia.

Manage anaemia

- Consider erythropoietin when Hb falls to <9.0g/dL. However, first, exclude other causes of anaemia (e.g. deficiency of Fe, folate, B12); investigate as appropriate. Fe supplements are frequently required.
- A major side-effect of erythropoietin is hypertension; monitoring BP is essential.

Manage bone disease

- Start a calcium-containing phosphate binder when serum phosphate is >1.6mmol/L. To be taken with meals 2–3×/d.
- If serum parathyroid hormone (PTH) is >2x the upper limit of normal, start alfacalcidol 0.25mcg per day and increase.
- Once patient established on calcium supplements or alfacalcidol, monitor calcium and phosphate 3-monthly and PTH 6-monthly.

Manage cardiovascular risk

- CKD ↑ risk of cardiovascular disease so ↓ risk factors, e.g. smoking, exercise, BP, and lipids.
- To ↓ cholesterol, statins are generally safe, but fibrates contraindicated.

Starting angiotensin inhibitors or ARBs

- Check creatinine and K^+ 2wks after starting drug and after any ↑ in dose. There is usually slight ↓ in GFR. Discontinue only if GFR ↓ by >20% and consider referral to exclude renal artery stenosis.
- In patients with ↓ renal function on these drugs, do not use K^+ sparing diuretics (spironolactone/amiloride) or NSAIDS because of risk of hyperkalaemia.

Treat hyperkalaemia (K^+ 5.5–6.0) with furosemide and recheck in 2wks. Discontinue angiotensin inhibitors if K^+ ≥6.0mmol/L.

Box 9.7 Dialysis

Many countries cannot offer chronic dialysis programmes. However, short-term peritoneal dialysis (PtD) or haemodialysis (HD) can be life-saving in AKI. HD requires specialist equipment and expertise; PtD is more affordable and requires less training.

Intermittent peritoneal dialysis

Instill 1–2L of dialysate over 10min into the peritoneal cavity via a PtD catheter. Keep the dialysate within the peritoneal cavity for 30min before allowing it to drain out by gravity over 30min. Dialysate may be pre-prepared or formulated locally.

Complications of dialysis

Infection, including line sepsis, PtD peritonitis, exit site infection, remains the most significant complication. Additional complications include bleeding, thrombosis, or air embolism in HD and catheter blockage and fluid leaks in PtD.

Chapter 10
Neurology

Invited authors

Nguyen Thi Hoang Mai
Jeremy Farrar
David Warrell (Rabies)
Charles Newton (Epilepsy)
Diana Lockwood (Leprosy)

Impaired consciousness

Patterns of arousal and awareness are complex and variable, and range from full consciousness to coma. Although various terms have been applied to these intermediate states, overlap inevitably occurs.

Acute confusional state and delirium

Clinical features

May fluctuate and include:
- Globally impaired cognition and clouding of consciousness.
- Short attention span.
- Easy distractability.
- Disorientation in time and place.
- Bewilderment.
- Impaired recall and memory.

Delirium More florid and may be accompanied by frightening hallucinations and/or delusions, irritability and/or aggressive behaviour.

Check carefully

For signs of ↓ consciousness, particularly drowsiness. This may be a warning of impending coma. Psychiatric causes of confusion (e.g. schizophrenia, paranoid state) and early dementia do not cause drowsiness.

Management

- If possible identify and treat cause (see Box 10.1). Common causes vary with age and geography. Look carefully for focal signs of infection (including chest, urinary tract, surgical wounds, IV cannula sites, CSF).
- Give 50mL of 20% glucose IV if hypoglycaemia suspected.
- At night, turn the lights on to improve the patient's orientation.
- Treat disturbed behaviour with chlorpromazine (25–50mg IM/po tds) or haloperidol (0.5–3mg po tds; or 2–10mg IM, repeated as necessary every 4–8h to a maximum daily dose of 18mg).
- Avoid benzodiazepines as they may worsen confusion.

Nursing is very important If possible use a well-lit room with familiar staff. Attempt to reassure the patient.

Coma

Coma is a state of unresponsiveness in which the patient lies with eyes closed and cannot be aroused to respond appropriately to stimuli. Coma is usually defined as a GCS ≤8 (see Box 10.2). The three broad categories of coma and common associated signs are:
- *Metabolic:* normal pupil responses; normal or absent eye movements (depending on the depth of coma); suppressed, Cheyne–Stokes, or ketotic respiration—drug overdoses often → suppressed respiration; symmetrical limb signs, usually hypotonic.
- *Intrinsic brainstem disease:* from the outset there may be abnormal pupil responses and eye movements; abnormal respiratory pattern; bilateral long tract and cranial nerve signs.
- *Extrinsic brainstem disease: due to compression:* papilloedema and hemiparesis *with progressive* loss of pupillary responses, loss of eye movements, abnormal respiratory pattern, long tract signs.

Box 10.1 Common causes of acute confusion/delirium at presentation (they may all progress to coma)

- *CNS infection:* malaria, meningitis including TBM, encephalitis; HIV-related.
- *Systemic infections:* with or without focal signs of infection.
- *Electrolyte disturbances:* ↑Na^+, ↓Na^+.
- *Respiratory failure:* ↓PaO_2, ↑$PaCO_2$.
- *Other metabolic causes:* e.g. ↓ or ↑ glucose, uraemia, hepatic encephalopathy.
- *Nutritional:* Wernicke's encephalopathy.
- *Toxins:* carbon monoxide, methanol, poisons, lead, cyanide, thallium.
- *Alcohol:* excess or withdrawal.
- *Drugs:*, e.g. steroids, efavirenz.
- Head injury/concussion.
- Stroke (📖 Stroke, p. 460).
- ↑ Intracranial pressure (📖 Raised intracranial pressure p. 438).
- Epilepsy (post-ictal) (📖 Epilepsy, p. 472).
- Chronic subdural haematoma (📖 Subdural haemorrhage, p. 466).
- Urinary retention (especially in elderly).

Management of the unconscious patient

Initial assessment

- ABC: ensure adequate airway, oxygenation, breathing, and circulation. Check for life-threatening injuries.
- Obtain a reliable history from witnesses: how rapidly did the patient become unconscious? Sudden onset suggests vascular aetiology, hypoglycaemia, etc. Progression to coma over days suggests e.g. CNS infection; progression over weeks suggests e.g. space occupying lesion (SOL). Any relevant past medical history, e.g. diabetes, alcohol abuse, or drug overdose?
- *General exam including:*
  - temp (?fever/hypothermia)
  - BP (hypertension may be due to stroke)
  - O_2 saturation and respiration
  - neck stiffness (meningitis or subarachnoid haemorrhage (SAH), 📖 Subarachnoid haemorrhage, p. 465)
  - signs of head injury (if suspicious, immobilize cervical spine; blood in external auditory meatus, from nose or over mastoid area is sign of base of skull fracture)
  - signs of liver or renal disease including venepuncture marks (IV drug addict might have septicaemia, brain abscess)
  - hemodialysis shunt.
- Check blood glucose.
- Assess level of coma: use GCS or BCS (see Boxes 10.2 and 10.3). Check corneal and brainstem reflexes, Doll's eye movements. Do caloric tests if brain death is suspected.

- *Check pupillary light reflex:*
  - unilateral, fixed, dilated pupil suggests 3rd nerve compression due to uncus herniation or posterior communicating aneurysm
  - bilateral, fixed, dilated pupils suggest brainstem pathology (herniation, massive overdoses of atropine)
  - bilateral small pupils suggest opioid overdose, pontine haemorrhage or organophosphate poisoning.
- *Fundoscopy:* for retinopathy (hypertensive, diabetic) and papilloedema.
- *Look for focal neurological signs:* search for asymmetry, e.g. in response to pain or in the face during expiration. If response to pain is asymmetrical, the side with ↓ response is the abnormal side (e.g. hemiparesis).
- *Identify coma due to brainstem compression:* since urgent surgery might be required. Progressive deterioration +/– focal neurology suggests possible brainstem compression.

Investigations

Depend on clinical picture and include Hb, WBC, U&E, glucose, Ca^{2+}, Mg^{2+}, LFT, thyroid function tests, PT, ABG; blood cultures if febrile; LP if intracranial infection suspected. (Beware ↑ ICP); malaria test if potential malaria exposure; toxicology screen if overdose/poisoning suspected; skull X-ray if trauma; ECG; CXR; CT/MRI head if indicated and available.

Determine the cause and treat

- *Urgent neurosurgery and/or management of ↑ICP* (📖 Raised intracranial pressure, p. 438): may be required for coma with focal signs, e.g. due to subdural or extradural haematoma or SOL.
- *Treat hypoglycaemia:* 50mL of 20% glucose IV; give thiamine 100mg IV before glucose if history of alcohol abuse or severely malnourished.
- *Manage suspected serious infection:* e.g. cerebral malaria (📖 Severe malaria, p. 42), meningitis (📖 p. 440).
- *Treat suspected poisoning:* see 📖 Poisoning and envenoming, p. 871.

Ongoing care

Nurse comatose patients in the intensive care unit or high dependency unit. Monitor every 15min to 4h depending on clinical state, including vital signs; level of consciousness (GCS or BCS); pupil size, equality, and response to light. Pay special attention to respiration, circulation, skin, bladder, and bowels.

Prognosis

Depends mainly on cause, depth, and duration of coma. The combination of absent pupillary light reflex and corneal and brainstem reflexes at 24h, or the persistence of deep coma for greater than 72h, indicate a grave prognosis.

Box 10.2 Glasgow coma scale

Use GCS for adults and children who are able to talk (usually >5yrs). Assess on admission and then at regular intervals to follow progress and predict prognosis.

Best motor response

6 Carries out request (obeys a command)
5 Localizes pain
4 Withdraws limb in response to pain
3 Flexes limb in response to pain
2 Extends limb in response to pain
1 Does not respond to pain

Best verbal response

5 Orientated in time and place
4 Responds with confused but understandable speech
3 Spontaneous speech but inappropriate and not responsive
2 Speech but incomprehensible
1 No speech

Eye opening

4 Opens eyes spontaneously
3 Opens eyes in response to speech
2 Opens eyes in response to pain
1 Does not open eyes

Box 10.3 Blantyre coma scale

A modification of the GCS for use with children too young to talk. A score of ≤2 indicates 'unrousable coma'. The maximum score is 5.

Best motor response

- 2 localizes pain
- 1 withdraws limb from pain
- 0 no response or inappropriate response

Best verbal response

- 2 cries appropriately to pain
- 1 moans or abnormal cry to pain
- 0 no vocal response to pain

Best eye movement

- 1 watches or follows
- 0 fails to watch or follow

Dementia

Unlike confusional states and delirium, there is no disturbance of consciousness in dementia. It is a chronic or progressive condition characterized by ↓ higher mental function (e.g. memory, reasoning, comprehension), and emotional and behavioural changes. Common causes are Alzheimer's disease and multiple strokes (vascular dementia). Uncommon, but treatable causes include communicating hydrocephalus; vitamin B12 or B1 deficiency; hypothyroidism; syphilis; neurocysticercosis; brain tumour; chronic subdural haematoma. HIV can cause a dementia that is variably responsive to antiretroviral therapy (📖 Antiretroviral therapy, p. 112).

Management

Identify the few patients with treatable causes. Aim to supply others with general support to give highest quality of life possible.[1]

Remember that the family will also need support. Information useful to Alzheimer's disease patients and their carers is available at www.alz.org.

[1] Guidance on dementia assessment and management is given in: WHO, mhGAP intervention guide for mental, neurological and substance use disorders in non-specialized health settings: mental health Gap Action Programme (mhGAP). WHO: Geneva 2010. Available free from: http://www.who.int/mental_health/evidence/mhGAP_intervention_guide/en/index.html

Headache

Brain parenchyma is insensitive to pain. Headaches result from distension, traction, or inflammation of the cerebral blood vessels and dura mater. Pain is referred from the anterior and middle cranial fossae to the forehead and eye via the Vth nerve, and from the posterior fossa and upper cervical spine to the occiput and neck via C2–3 nerve roots. Both infratentorial and supratentorial masses can → frontal headaches by causing hydrocephalus.

Causes of a headache

Primary headache

1° headache is likely in patients with a long history of similar attacks, free of symptoms between attacks, otherwise well and no sinister symptoms or clinical signs. Three most common causes of 1° headache are:

- *Migraine:* headaches that occur at intervals (not daily) associated with nausea and vomiting, anorexia, photophobia, phonophobia, and in 20% of cases, visual, mood, sensory, or motor disturbances. Most 1st attacks occur while young; often a family history. Identify and avoid precipitating factors; give analgesia (paracetamol, NSAIDs, or codeine) plus metoclopramide 10mg (avoid in children; dose 5mg in adolescents aged 15–19). If simple analgesia inadequate, use a $5HT_1$-receptor antagonist ('triptan'). Ergotamine seldom used, because of side effects. Chemoprophylaxis (propranolol, etc.) may work for regular migraines.
- *Tension headache:* most common cause of headache. Normally a benign symptom due to an identifiable cause (e.g. overwork, family stress, lack of sleep, emotional crisis). Often a daily occurrence unlike migraine headache, getting worse as the day goes on. Visual disturbances, vomiting, and photophobia do not occur. Management involves thorough examination and reassurance of its benign course, analgesia (usually paracetamol 1g qds), and rest. Ask about drugs, caffeine, and alcohol. Amitriptyline starting at 10mg at night, increasing by 10mg each week up to 75mg, is often of benefit. Tension headaches may be part of depression—check for other signs or symptoms such as mood change, ↓ appetite, ↓ weight, ↓ libido, or disturbed sleep pattern.
- *Cluster headaches:* very severe orbital/supra-orbital/temporal headaches that are strictly unilateral, usually last ~1h associated with ipsilateral eye or nasal symptoms, and may recur every other day up to many times a day. Nocturnal attacks are common. Diagnostic criteria have been proposed (see International Headache Classification, http://ihs-classification.org/en). Oxygen, triptans and verapamil are the treatments of choice.

Secondary headache

In 2° headache, headache is the sign of a disease. Need to identify any warning features in the history.

- *SAH* (Subarachnoid haemorrhage, p. 465): acute thunderclap headache (intense headache with abrupt onset). CT scan without constrast can detect recent bleeds. LP should be performed to look for xanthochromia if SAH is suspected and if the results of CT are inconclusive.

- *Giant-cell arteritis (temporal arteritis):* more common in women, mean age of onset ~70yrs. Presents with fever, tender engorged occipital or temporal artery, +/– bruits. Blindness may occur rapidly due to ischaemic optic neuropathy so diagnosis is a medical emergency. ESR markedly ↑. Temporal artery biopsy may confirm diagnosis, but do not delay treatment while awaiting biopsy. Start prednisolone 40–60mg od oral as soon as diagnosis suspected; consider higher dose, e.g. 80mg/kg or 1mg/kg in complicated cases with visual symptoms.
- *Intracranial neoplasm:* headache with symptoms of ↑ ICP (📖 Raised intracranial pressure, p. 438). Progressive neurological deficit (progessive weakness, sensory loss, ataxia) correlated with the location of the tumour. CT scan can detect most tumours, but MRI is even more sensitive as it can detect both infiltrating and very small tumours.
- *Intracranial infection (meningitis or encephalitis):* caused by bacteria, viruses, fungi: headache with fever, +/– signs of meningism, vomiting, ↓ consciousness. LP aids diagnosis, including aetiology of the infection.
- *Analgesic-overuse headache:* also called analgesia rebound headache and chronic daily headache; follows long-term inappropriate use of analgesia. History reveals increasing and frequent use of multiple analgesics, especially codeine. *Management*—reassurance followed by stopping all forms of analgesia; may benefit from amitriptyline as above. The headache initially worsens before improving.
- *Acute glaucoma* (📖 Acute glaucoma, p. 581): ocular emergency. Symptoms include sudden eye pain, seeing halos around lights, red eye, nausea, vomiting, sudden decreased vision. Very high intraocular pressure (>30mmHg).
- *Sinusitis:* causes pressure-like pain +/– tenderness in a specific area of face or head, worse in the morning and exacerbated by sudden head movements, bending forwards, and sudden temperature change. *Causes*—viral and/or bacterial upper respiratory tract infection; allergy.

Neuralgias

- *Trigeminal neuralgia:* characterized by paroxysmal attack of (usually unilateral) facial pain—intense, sharp, stabbing, or like an electric-shock, and lasting from a few seconds to several minutes/hours. May be spontaneous or triggered, e.g. by eating, talking, shaving or touch (trigger zones). Most cases believed to be caused by compression of the Vth nerve root by blood vessels; CT/MRI imaging may demonstrate cause. Carbamazepine and gabapentin are 1st line for relieving pain. Carbamazepine should be tried initially and dose increased gradually to achieve pain control. Other treatments include antidepressants, muscle relaxants, and pharmacological nerve blockade. Surgery may be indicated in patients who have failed medical therapy.
- *Post-herpetic neuralgia:* may occur as a complication of herpes zoster (see 📖 Varicella Zoster virus, p. 616). Uncommon in young patients, but common in older age (up to 50% patients >50yrs). Similar shooting pain to trigeminal neuralgia. Treatment includes amitriptyline, gabapentin and topical capsaicin. Prompt treatment of herpes zoster with antivirals (and possibly amitriptyline) ↓ risk of post-herpetic neuralgia.

Raised intracranial pressure

Clinical features

- *Headache:* often worse in the morning due to CO_2 retention during sleep → cerebrovascular dilatation, possibly waking the patient from sleep; made worse by coughing, straining, standing up; relieved by paracetamol in the early stages.
- *Vomiting:* may relieve headache; sometimes 1st sign of ↑ ICP.
- *Altered level of consciousness:* drowsiness → coma.
- *Hypertension, bradycardia, irregular respiration:* Cushing's reflex.
- *Papilloedema:* classical sign, but frequently not present; see Fig. 10.1.

Failing vision and decreasing consciousness are ominous signs.

Causes and pathophysiology

SOL; cerebral oedema; hydrocephalus (📖 Hydrocephalus, p. 470). Cerebral oedema may complicate tumours, infection (cerebral malaria, encephalitis), trauma, or hypoxic cell death. Mechanisms such as ↓ CSF volume initially compensate for slow ↑ in ICP (e.g. slow-growing tumour). However, if ICP continues to ↑ or increase is acute and compensatory mechanisms overwhelmed, brain often becomes laterally displaced and pushed towards foramen magnum at skull base. Medial temporal lobe (uncus) may be forced down through the tentorial hiatus, or a cerebellar tonsil forced through the foramen magnum, causing the brainstem to become compressed (coning). See Fig. 10.2 for anatomy. This → the following progressive changes:

- Level of consciousness decreases, drowsiness → coma.
- Pupils dilate and become unresponsive, 1st ipsilaterally then bilaterally.
- Posture becomes decorticate, then decerebrate.
- Slow deep breaths → Cheyne–Stokes breathing → apnoea.

Beware of false localizing signs due to ↑ ICP in the absence of focal intracranial pathology: unilateral or bilateral VIth cranial nerve palsy most common; also IIIrd and IVth cranial nerve palsies; uncal herniation may rarely cause an ipsilateral hemiparesis and/or contralateral homonymous hemianopia).

Management

- Sit patient up at 30° to ↑ venous drainage from the brain.
- Ensure adequate oxygenation and optimal ventilation. Aim to keep $paCO_2$ 4–4.5kPa. Ventilate if necessary.
- Give 20% mannitol 5mL/kg IV over 30–60min to ↓ cerebral oedema.
- Steroids may → rapid improvement within 24h in patients deteriorating with a brain tumour or abscess: give dexamethasone 8–16mg by slow IV injection if severe oedema, or 4mg IM qds for less severe oedema. Steroids are not recommended for ↑ ICP due to head injury.
- Control seizures if present.
- Image brain (CT/MRI) to establish cause of ↑ ICP (if GCS ≤ 8 intubate to protect airway before scanning).

- Institute specific treatment for proven/suspected aetiology:
  - manage for cerebral malaria if malaria blood film positive (📖 Severe malaria, p. 42)
  - If SOL suspected, refer to a neurosurgeon. If ↑ ICP progresses rapidly, urgent decompression with burr holes may be life-saving - see 📖 Space-occupying lesions, p. 469.

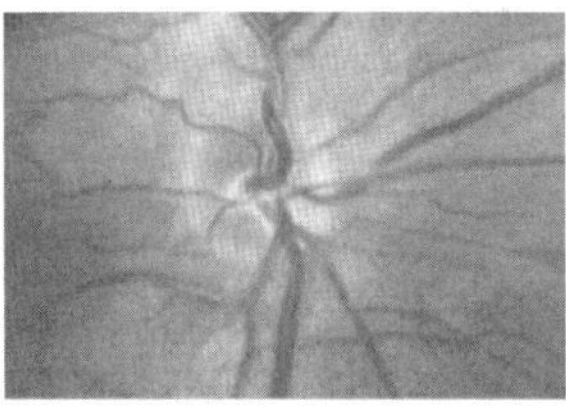

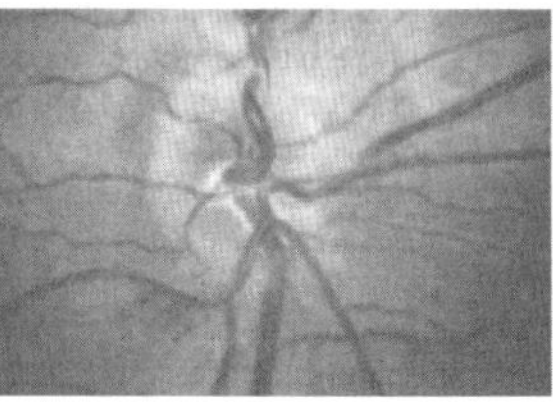

Fig. 10.1 Early stages of papilloedema (Left eye). Early nerve fibre layer oedema is first seen superiorly and temporally (left), then inferiorly and nasally (right).

Reproduced with permission from Spalton DJ, Hitchings, RA, Hunter PA, *et al. Atlas of Clinical Ophthalmology*. Philadelphia: Elsevier Mosby 2005.

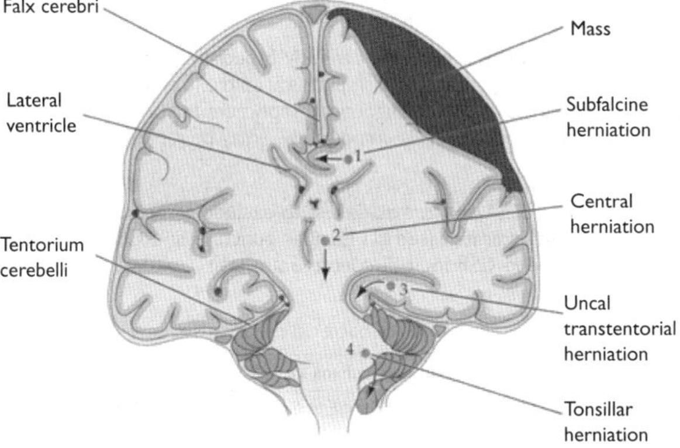

Fig. 10.2 Anatomy of brain herniation syndromes.

Reproduced from Blumenfeld, H, *Neuroanatomy through Clinical Cases*, 2002, with permission from Sinauer Assoc. Inc.

Acute bacterial meningitis

Pyogenic (bacterial) meningitis is the most important since it has a high fatality rate and is readily treatable. All febrile patients with a history of headache should be examined for meningism (see Box 10.4).

Aetiology

Aetiology varies according to age (Table 10.1) and geographically. *Streptococcus pneumoniae* (Gram +ve diplococci) most common cause overall, although pneumococcal conjugate vaccine should ↓ incidence; risk factors include previous head injury, sinusitis, otitis media and pneumonia. Hib (Gram −ve coccobacilli) meningitis remains common in regions without Hib immunization. *Neisseria meningitidis* (Gram −ve intracellular diplococci) causes most disease in patients aged 2–18yrs in many regions, as well as epidemics (📖 Epidemic meningococcal disease, p. 444). *Streptococcus suis* is an important cause in Southeast Asia; *Listeria* in pregnant women and the immunosuppressed; *E. coli* and *Klebsiella* spp. in elderly patients and diabetics; *S. aureus* following head trauma.

Clinical features

Headache, fever, N&V, lethargy, impaired consciousness, delirium, meningism (stiff neck, photophobia, Kernig's sign; see Box 10.4). Acute complications include ↑ ICP, seizures, sepsis, syndrome of inappropriate antidiuretic hormone secretion (SIADH), subdural empyema and cerebral abscess (may cause focal neurological signs; lower cranial nerve palsies and urinary retention more common in TBM).

Check the conjunctivae and skin carefully Especially back, buttocks, and soles of feet) for any petechiae/rash/purpura; cold extremities and leg pain may also be early signs of meningococcal septicaemia. If present or unsure treat for meningococcal sepsis immediately—may be rapidly fatal.

Diagnosis

Blood culture, FBC, U&E, (± malaria test to exclude cerebral malaria). Do LP unless contraindicated (see 📖 Lumbar puncture and CSF interpretation, p. 442). Send CSF for cell count, Gram stain, culture, protein and

Table 10.1 Common causes of bacterial meningitis

Age	Most common organisms
<1mth	Group B streptococcus, *E. coli*, *Salmonella* spp., *Klebsiella* spp., *L. monocytogenes*
1–3mths	*E. coli*, Group B streptococcus, *S. pneumoniae*, *H. influenzae*, *N. meningitides*, *L. monocytogenes*
3mths–18yrs	*N. meningitides*, *S. pneumoniae*, *H. influenzae*
18–50yrs	*S. pneumoniae*, *N. meningitidis*, (*S. suis* – especially Southeast Asia)
>50yrs	*S. pneumoniae*, *N. meningitidis*, *L. monocytogenes*, Gram negative bacilli, (*S. suis* – especially Southeast Asia)

glucose estimation, if available; plus AFB microscopy, TB culture, and India ink stain or CRAG (+/– serum CRAG) if differential diagnosis includes TBM or cryptococcal meningitis (e.g. immunocompromised, subacute/chronic history). Guidance for interpretation of CSF indices is shown in Table 10.2.

Box 10.4 Neck stiffness

Involuntary neck stiffness ('nuchal rigidity') is a sign of meningeal irritation/inflammation ('meningism'). In severe cases there may be arching backward of the spine ('opisthotonus'). Patients with meningitis or SAH characteristically lie still not willingly moving their heads, and often complain of a sore head, rather than a sore neck. Clinical signs of meningism may be absent in infants. Other causes of meningism include streptococcal sore throats, pneumonia, and pyelonephritis.

To test for neck stiffness

- Lie patient flat in bed (remove the pillows) and inform them of what you are doing and reassure them.
- Ask the patient to nod their head so their chin is on their sternum. If a child, you can also ask them to 'kiss their knees'. If the patient can do this, it is unlikely you will find a stiff neck in the next step.
- Facing patient, hold the head securely by putting your hands over the mastoids (behind the ears). Slowly rotate the neck all the way from side to side—this will relax the patient, and enable you to compare rotation (which is not stiff in meningitis) to flexion (which is). Slowly rock head forward to assess for stiffness; repeat this a few times until you are sure. In mild meningitis, it is only the final part of flexion which is stiff – 'terminal rigidity'. If neck does not flex fully (chin does not touch sternum), flex head still further forwards and watch whether you can lift patient's shoulders away from bed.

Kernig's sign

Detects painful/inflamed nerve roots ('spinal meningitis') and is similar to straight leg raising. It is sensitive in meningitis, but not very specific. Lie the patient supine and passively flex the knee and hip on one side to 90°. Try passively to straighten knee, until patient winces and knee cannot be straightened further. Pain felt in in low back is suggestive of meningitis; pain felt in hamstrings is less specific. Repeat on other side—result should be the same.

Brudzinski's sign

Little used. In presence of meningeal irritation, neck flexion in an infant sometimes causes involuntary flexion of hips and knees.

Lumbar puncture & CSF interpretation

Indications to LP include suspected meningitis, suspected SAH (📖 p. 465) and symptomatic relief in cryptococcal meningitis (📖 p. 100).

Contraindications: Avoid LP if prolonged fits, focal CNS signs (e.g. due to SOL), pupillary dilatation, signs of skin or soft tissue infection at LP site, known or suspected bleeding disorder, or signs of focal neurology or ↑ ICP (📖 p. 438). Focal signs or ↑ ICP ≥ risk of brain herniation (see Fig. 10.1). If possible perform CT prior to LP to look for evidence of brain shift if any of these signs is present. If CT not available consider mannitol and review clinical signs. Do not delay antibiotics while awaiting CT if meningitis suspected.

Interpretation If possible measure opening pressure. If no manometer available, attach an IV giving set, hold the tube vertically allowing it to fill and measure height of CSF column using a ruler or tape measure. Normal range ~10–20 cm CSF; raised in many conditions; may be very high in cryptococcal meningitis). A guide to CSF analysis is given in Table 10.2. Other useful CSF tests include CRAG (cryptococcal meningitis), VDRL/RPR (syphilitic meningitis), cytology (malignancy).

Table 10.2 Typical CSF indices in cerebral infections of different aetiology

Cause	Normal CSF	Pyogenic bacteria	TB	PAM	Virus	Cryptococcus
Appearance	Clear and colourless	Cloudy or purulent	Clear, yellowish, slightly cloudy	Clear or slightly cloudy	Clear	Clear or slightly cloudy
White cells (majority)	<5/mm^3	>200/mm^3 (neutrophils)	>10/mm^3 (mononuclear)	>200/mm^3 (neutrophils)	>10/mm^3 (mononuclear)	>10/mm^3 (mononuclear)
Glucose	2.5–4mmol/L (45–72mg%)	Markedly ↓ or absent	Low	Normal or slightly ↓	Normal	Low
Total protein	0.15–0.4g/L	Raised	Raised	Normal or slightly ↓	Raised	Raised
Microscopy	None	Gram: pus	ZN: AFB present	Wet: motile amoebae	None	India ink +ve

Prognosis

Mortality 10–80%; varies with age and organism—highest in the very young and elderly and in patients with co-existent septicaemia. Long-term complications include deafness, paralysis, visual loss, epilepsy, cognitive impairment.

Management

Antibiotics

- Give immediately if diagnosis suspected. See Box 10.5 for doses.
- Ceftriaxone is the preferred 1st line empiric Rx in children and adults.
- *Alternatives in adults:* if ceftriaxone not available ampicillin plus co-trimoxazole; or chloramphenicol (see Box 10.6) plus co-trimoxazole.
- *Alternatives in children:* if ceftriaxone not available ampicillin (or penicillin) plus gentamicin; or chloramphenicol (see Box 10.6).
- Add ampicillin for *Listeria* if <3mths, >50yrs old or immunosuppressed.
- Add vancomycin if available and high prevalence of penicillin-resistant pneumococci.
- Benzylpenicillin is 1st line drug for meningococcal meningitis.
- For meningitis following neurosurgery use vancomycin plus ceftazidime.

Supportive care

Give fluids, O_2. Maintain normal electrolytes, pain relief, and tepid sponging to ↓ temperature.

Dexamethasone

0.15mg/kg IV qds for 2–4d is beneficial in developed countries in children with Hib meningitis and adults with pneumococcal meningitis. Evidence in developing countries is conflicting.

Box 10.5 Antibiotic doses for meningitis

- *Ceftriaxone:* 2g IV bd; children <50kg, 50mg/kg (avoid in neonatal jaundice); IM alternative if no IV access.
- *Benzylpenicillin:* 2.4g IV every 4h for 7d; neonates 75mg/kg tds; children >1mth old 50mg/kg 4–6-hourly (max 2.4g every 4h).
- *Ampicillin:* 2g IV every 4h for 10d; neonates 50mg/kg bd (<7d old) or tds (7–21d old), or qds (21–28d old); children >1mth old 50mg/kg 4–6-hourly (max 2g every 4h).
- *Co-trimoxazole:* only in combination therapy as above. 10–20mg/kg (based on trimethoprim component) IV daily in 2–4 divided doses.
- *Chloramphenicol:* 12.5–25mg/kg qds; child >1mth old 12.5mg/kg tds; neonate 14–28d old 12.5mg/kg 2–4 daily; neonate <14d old 12.5mg/kg bd; avoid in prematurity/LBW (see Box 10.6).
- *Gentamicin:* in combination with ampicillin or penicillin for childhood meningitis. 7.5mg/kg IV od (where resources allow dose may be adjusted according to serum levels).
- *Vancomycin:* 1g IV bd; neonates and children 15mg/kg tds (max. 2g daily). If possible monitor plasma levels; adjust dose accordingly.
- *Ceftazidime:* 2g IV tds; neonates 50mg/kg od (<7d old), bd (7–21d old), tds (>21d old); children 50mg/kg tds (max. 6g daily).

Epidemic meningococcal disease

There are at least nine serogroups of *Neisseria meningitidis* (meningococci), of which 3 (groups A, B, and C) cause meningitis outbreaks. Serogroup A causes large epidemics every 2–10yrs across the 'meningitis belt' of Africa and hyperendemic meningococcal disease between epidemics in the same region (Fig. 10.3). Types A and C have both been responsible for large outbreaks in the rest of the world. Some strains appear to be more virulent than others. Large epidemics occur when such strains encounter populations of non-immune individuals in areas of poverty during particular climatic conditions (e.g. dry season, dust storm). In between epidemics, the bacteria survive in the community in the nasopharynx of carriers.

WHO advice on surveillance and epidemic control is available at: www.who.int/csr/resources/publications/meningitis/WHO_EMC_BAC_98_3_EN/en.

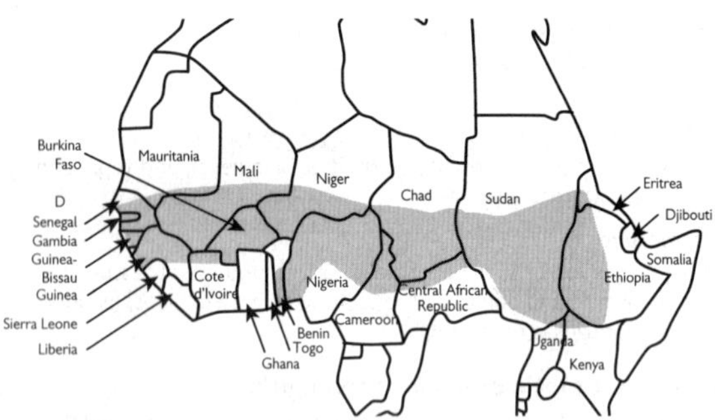

Fig. 10.3 African meningitis belt.

Reproduced with permission from Control of Epidemic Meningococcal disease: WHO practical guidelines, 2nd edn.

Treatment

Benzylpenicillin is treatment of choice (see Box 10.5). Oily chloramphenicol (3g IM stat; children 100mg/kg (max. 3g) stat; repeated after 24–48h if required) is a logistically simple alternative if health resources are stretched in an epidemic (Box 10.6).

Vaccination

Is essential to halt an epidemic once it has begun; kits for vaccination campaigns available from WHO.

Chemoprophylaxis

Is indicated for household contacts: ciprofloxacin 500mg oral stat; child 2–5yrs 125mg, 5–12yrs 250mg.

Alternative Rifampicin 600mg (children 10mg/kg, infants <1yr 5mg/kg) oral bd for 2d.

Box 10.6 Chloramphenicol

Chloramphenicol has one serious toxicity—aplastic anaemia—with a frequency of ~1 in 10 000 to ~1 in 70 000 courses of therapy (similar to risk of death due to penicillin anaphylaxis: ~1 in 40 000 courses). After due consideration of the risks and benefits, the WHO Expert Committee on Use of Essential Drugs concluded chloramphenicol is essential for modern medical practice in all countries, reaffirming its value in severe bacterial infections such as meningitis.

Viral meningitis

Enteroviruses (e.g. ECHO and coxsackie viruses) are important causes of epidemic viral meningitis worldwide, while arboviruses (📖 Arboviruses and viral hemorrhagic fever, p. 804) cause sporadic disease in endemic regions. Other causes of sporadic viral meningitis include polio, mumps virus, EBV, HIV, VZV, CMV, and HSV, especially HSV-2. Clinical features are usually less severe than bacterial meningitis. Diagnosis is by CSF examination (📖 Lumbar puncture and CSF interpretation, p. 442), but interpretation may be difficult, particularly if the patient has already received antibiotic treatment. If in doubt, treat with antibiotics to cover bacterial meningitis (📖 Acute bacterial meningitis, p. 440). The causative virus may be apparent during epidemics. In sporadic cases, peripheral signs may suggest the aetiology such as genital or rectal lesions (HSV), skin blisters (VZV), orchitis (mumps, lymphocytic choriomeningitis virus), rashes (enterovirus), parotid swelling (mumps). Treatment is symptomatic. The prognosis is usually good, with complete recovery. HSV may cause recurrent viral meningitis ('Mollaret's meningitis').

Chronic meningitis

TBM or *Cryptococcus neoformans*, other disseminated fungal infections, and cysticercosis in children typically present with a longer history (>7d), headache, and low-grade fever. Confusion and drowsiness are common and may be due to hydrocephalus. Papilloedema, visual symptoms, and nerve lesions (particularly VI, VII, and urinary retention) may occur.

Tuberculous and cryptococcal meningitis

Cryptococcal (📖 Cryptococcal meningitis, p. 100) and TB meningitis 📖 pp. 133, 158) occur commonly in immunosuppressed patients, particularly AIDS, but they also occur in previously healthy individuals. Although 'chronic' meningitis, these are still medical emergencies, as delayed therapy → significantly worse prognosis.

Diagnosis

By clinical presentation and CSF examination, including AFB microscopy +/– TB culture; India ink stain; and cryptococcal antigen test (CRAG) on CSF and/or serum (📖 Cryptococcal meningitis, p. 100). Look for signs of infection in other sites (e.g. CXR). In HIV+ patients the CSF cellular response to TBM may be neutrophilic causing confusion with pyogenic meningitis.

Management

Tailor to likely aetiology. If clinical and CSF picture fits TBM, and best available test for *Cryptococcus* is –ve, start TB treatment. Adjunctive steroids reduce mortality in TBM, e.g. dexamethasone IV 0.4mg/kg/day in divided doses reduced over 4wks to 0.1mg/kg/day and then stopped.[1]

Eosinophilic meningoencephalitis

Follows CNS infection with the nematodes *Angiostrongylus cantonensis*, *Gnathostoma spinigerum*, or *T, solium* (📖 Cysticercosis, p. 476). CSF examination shows eosinophilic pleocytosis.

Angiostrongyliasis

Results from the ingestion of *Angiostrongylus cantonensis* larvae in infected snails or contaminated shrimps, fish, and vegetables that are eaten raw or inadequately cooked. The larvae migrate to the brain, where they induce an immune response to dead parasites, and then to the eyes and lungs. Initial presentation is of acute, intermittent intense headache without fever; malaise; N&V; cranial nerve palsies; +/– meningism. If severe, there may be fever, ↓ GCS, and spinal cord involvement. The eyes are sometimes involved (papilloedema, retinal damage, occasionally larva seen in vitreous). Give sedatives and analgesia. The headache responds well to LP every 3–7d. Consider albendazole and steroids—role of antihelminthics and steroids remains controversial as dying parasites can elicit a strong immune reaction that can be fatal and the disease is normally self-resolving.

[1] Thwaites GE, Nguyen DB, Nguyen HD, *et al.* Dexamethasone for the treatment of tuberculous meningitis in adolescents and adults. *N Engl J Med* 2004; 351:1741–51.

Spinocerebral gnathostomiasis

Is usually acquired by eating inadequately cooked, infected fish, or shrimps, following which *Gnathostoma spinigerum* larvae migrate to the CNS. It frequently presents with intensely painful radiculitis followed by rapidly advancing myelitis → paraplegia with urinary retention or quadriplegia, or as a cerebral haemorrhage in a previously healthy person. Treatment is as for angiostrongyliasis with albendazole and steroids.

Primary amoebic meningoencephalitis

1° amoebic meningoencephalitis (PAM) is a rare, but potentially fatal infection that follows intranasal infection with *Naegleria fowleri* while swimming in warm fresh water. The amoebae invade the CNS through the cribiform plate → extensive tissue necrosis. Headache occurs first, then fever, meningism, coma, convulsions. The CSF shows neutrophils, red cells, and amoebae on wet microscopy. The prognosis is poor. *Acanthamoeba* cause a similar syndrome, granulomatous amoebic encephalitis, in immunosuppressed individuals.

Management

Amphotericin 1mg/kg IV; also give amphotericin intrathecally (via a reservoir). Start with 0.025mg, then increase to 0.25–1mg (*total* intrathecal dose, *not* per kg) on alternate days.

Other causes of chronic meningitis

The following illustrates wide range of possible causes; important to make a definitive microbiological diagnosis whenever possible.

- Fungi (e.g. histoplasmosis, coccidiomycosis, candidiasis).
- Cysticercosis.
- Borreliosis (Lyme disease).
- Brucellosis.
- Syphilis.
- Malignancy.
- Sarcoidosis.
- Autoimmune diseases (e.g. Behçet's disease).

Meningitis may also occur 2° to, or along with, other focal CNS infections or encephalitides.

Encephalitis

Encephalitis is inflammation of brain parenchyma. Aetiology is most commonly viral (Table 10.3). Seasonal epidemics occur in many parts of the world causing death and disability in the young and elderly. HSV encephalitis is the most important cause of sporadic viral encephalitis worldwide since it is treatable and ∴ should be considered in all cases. However, Japanese encephalitis far outstrips HSV in actual numbers. This and other arboviruses are discussed elsewhere (📖 Arboviruses and viral haemorrhagic fever, p. 804). African trypanosomiasis is an important non-viral cause of encephalomyelitis in endemic areas (📖 African trypanosomiasis, p. 782).

Clinical features

High fever, headache, N&V, followed by convulsions, confusion, and altered conscious level. Meningism (meningoencephalitis), focal neurological signs, abnormal behaviour, and/or ↑ ICP may be present. Severe cases may cause prolonged coma, hemiparesis, dystonia, decorticate/decerebrate posturing, and respiratory failure. Neurological sequelae include mental retardation, hemiparesis, and behavioural problems, and are particularly common after Japanese encephalitis, untreated HSV encephalitis, and post-infectious/vaccination encephalomyelitis.

Diagnosis LP (see 📖 Lumbar puncture and CSF interpretation, p. 442, for contraindications). CSF usu. shows lymphocyte predominant pleocytosis, ↑ protein, normal/slightly ↓ glucose. Where available PCR of CSF may confirm specific viral aetiology.

Management Supportive, except for HSV encephalitis (aciclovir (see next paragraph)), CMV encephalitis (ganciclovir or foscarnet) and HIV encephalitis (ART). Control seizures and pyrexia. Beware respiratory failure and ↑ ICP (📖 Raised intracranial pressure, p. 438). The role of steroids to prevent cerebral oedema is unclear.

Herpes simplex virus encephalitis

Always consider HSV in a patient with encephalitis—it is the only encephalitis for which there is effective treatment. Neurological signs relate to frontal and temporal cortex, and limbic system; they include changes in behaviour, seizures, and focal CNS signs. Where available, MRI shows temporal lobe enhancement. Diagnosis is confirmed by detection of HSV in CSF by PCR. If PCR not available and there is clinical suspicion of HSV infection then treatment should be started immediately. Untreated HSV encephalitis has a mortality of 40–70% and many survivors have neurological sequelae. Aciclovir decreases mortality and the incidence of sequelae. Delayed treatment greatly increases the risk of a poor neurologic outcome.

Equine encephalitis

Three alphaviruses—western, eastern, and Venezuelan equine encephalitis viruses (EEVs)—cause widespread epizootics of encephalitis in horses in the USA, Central America, and northern South America. The EEVs are not common causes of human encephalitis, but Venezuelan EEV has caused

Table 10.3 Important viral causes of encephalitis

Virus family	Examples of viruses causing encephalitis
Adenoviruses	Adenovirus
Alphaviruses	Western, eastern and Venezuelan encephalitis viruses
Arenaviruses	Lymphocytic choriomeningitis, Lassa, Machupo viruses
Bunyaviruses	Rift Valley fever virus
Enteroviruses	Polio, coxsackie and ECHO viruses
Filiviruses	Marburg, Ebola viruses
Flaviviruses	Japanese encephalitis, West Nile, dengue
Herpes viruses	HSV, VZV, EBV, CMV, HHV-6, HHV-7
Orthomyxoviruses	Influenza
Paramyxoviruses	Measles, mumps, Nipah virus, Hendra virus
Retroviruses	HIV
Rhabdoviruses	Rabies, Lyssavirus
Togaviruses	Rubella

large epidemics in both horses and humans in Colombia and Venezuela. Rodents and birds are the 1° hosts; the virus is amplified during horse infections and may subsequently → human encephalitis. Transmission to humans is via *Culex*, *Culiseta*, and *Aedes* mosquitoes. Most infections are subclinical.

There may be a short febrile illness with rigors (in Venezuelan EEV also sore throat, features of URTI, and diarrhoea). Occasionally, illness is biphasic with encephalitis following recovery from febrile phase. Neurological sequelae are unusual in adults, but common in infants and young children with encephalitis, among whom mortality is >10%.

Nipah virus encephalitis

Nipah virus caused an outbreak of encephalitis in Malaysia and Singapore, and appears to now be endemic in South Asia (Bangladesh). Causative agent was a new paramyxovirus named Nipah, closely related to Hendra virus described in Australia, and potentially a new genus. Nipah virus is a zoonosis infecting pigs and fruit bats. No specific treatment.

Post-infectious post-vaccination encephalomyelitis

On rare occasions, infection or vaccination may elicit an antiviral immune response → CNS immunopathology and an encephalitic picture. When this occurs it usually follows infection with measles, rubella, herpes zoster, mumps, or influenza and after vaccination with the Semple form of the rabies vaccine (prior to availability of newer tissue/cell culture rabies vaccines this small risk was usually outweighed by the benefits of vaccination).

Rabies

Human rabies encephalomyelitis is a fatal zoonosis caused by rabies virus genotype 1 (classical dog rabies and all bat rabies in the Americas) and four genotypes of rabies-related bat lyssaviruses. Most of the world is enzootic for rabies (Fig. 10.4) and continuing recognition of bat lyssaviruses in new areas makes the concept of 'rabies-free' countries misleading. Rabies causes ~60 000 human deaths each year (15 000–20 000 in India alone). Prolonged anxiety in those exposed to rabies → considerable morbidity.

Transmission

To humans is by mammal bites and saliva-contaminated scratches with viral entry though mucosae and broken skin. Domestic dogs are the major reservoir and vector of human rabies throughout most of Africa, Asia and Latin America. Wildlife vectors and/or reservoirs include cats, wolves, foxes, jackals, skunks, mongooses, raccoons, vampire bats (Caribbean and Latin America only), and fruit- and insect-eating bats. Rodents pose negligible, if any, risk. Human-to-human transmission has been documented only through infected corneal and solid organ grafts from unsuspected rabies-infected donors. Vertical transmission is vanishingly rare; inhalation was documented in a single laboratory accident.

Clinical features

The virus spreads from the wound along nerve axons to reach the CNS causing fatal encephalomyelitis. The incubation period is usually a few months, but varies from 4d to many years. The first symptom is often itching at the site of the healed bite. Within a few days, symptoms of either furious or paralytic rabies develop.

Furious rabies

This is the more common presentation. Symptoms include headaches, fever, confusion, and fluctuating periods of excitation with hallucinations together with hydrophobia. This fear of water is pathognomonic of the condition: attempts to drink water induce jerky spasms of the inspiratory muscles +/– painful laryngopharyngeal spasms associated with indescribable terror. Spasms may precipitate convulsions leading to cardiorespiratory arrest. Other features include cranial nerve defects and signs of autonomic/hypothalamic hyperactivity, such as hypersalivation, lacrimation, and fluctuating BP and temperature. Complications during intensive care include pneumonitis, myocarditis, cardiac arrhythmias, pneumothorax, haematemesis, ↑ ICP, diabetes insipidus, and rarely SIADH.

Paralytic or dumb rabies

Presents as ascending flaccid paralysis, accompanied by pain, fasciculations and mild sensory disturbances progressing to paraplegia, sphincter involvement, and fatal paralysis of bulbar and respiratory muscles.

Diagnosis

Suggested by neurological symptoms following a mammal bite in an endemic area. Laboratory confirmation in a patient during life is by PCR

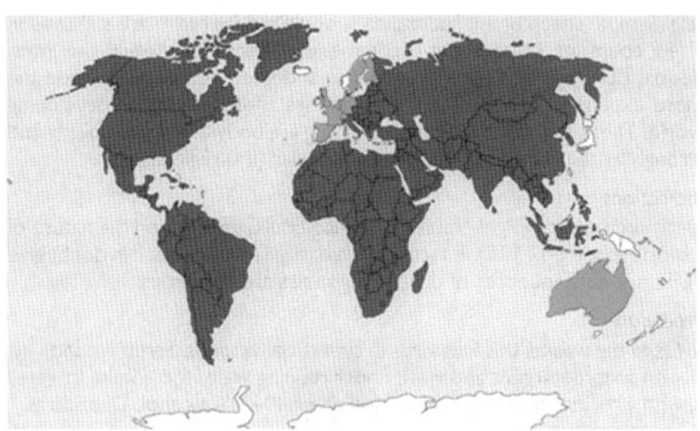

Fig. 10.4 Global distribution of rabies viruses. Black areas: rabies in terrestrial mammals and bats; Grey areas: no rabies in terrestrial mammals but rabies-related viruses in bats; White areas: no rabies reported.

(saliva, skin biopsy), virus isolation (saliva, brain, CSF), and immunofluorescence of viral antigen (skin punch biopsies). Neutralizing antibody response is absent or delayed.

Prognosis and treatment

Rabies encephalomyelitis is almost invariably fatal within a few days in the furious form and within 30d in the paralytic form. There are <10 documented survivors from rabies encephalomyelitis, most with devastating sequelae. Recent successes have been attributed to a combination of intensive care, sedation and a cocktail of antiviral drugs and vitamins ('Milwaukee protocol'), which remains unproven. Experience suggests that intubation and intensive care is appropriate only for patients with early symptoms of encephalomyelitis after infection with American bat rabies virus, especially if rabies neutralizing antibody is detectable. In most places, the best that can be offered is palliative treatment with sufficient analgesia and sedation to relieve pain and terror.

Prevention

Vaccination of domestic dogs, and, in some countries, wild foxes, jackals, raccoons, skunks, etc., is key to control. In humans, pre- and post-exposure prophylaxis has proved highly effective (see the next paragraph and 📖 Expanded programme on immunization recommended vaccines, p. 904).

Rabies post-exposure prophylaxis (PEP)

PEP, consisting of immediate wound cleaning, and modern tissue/cell culture vaccine and rabies immune globulin initiated within a few days of exposure, is extremely effective in preventing rabies encephalomyelitis. The old, less effective and highly reactogenic nervous tissue vaccines (e.g. Semple sheep brain, Fuenzalida suckling mouse brain) are still used in a few countries, but are not recommended. Economical multi-site intradermal (ID) regimens have proved safe and effective and have made the more expensive tissue/cell culture vaccines affordable in the developing world. These regimens induce neutralizing antibody at least as quickly and strongly as the standard 5-dose intramuscular (IM) regimen.

Indications

Decision to start PEP +/– rabies immunoglobulin depends on the nature of exposure (see Box 10.7). Intact skin is a barrier to infection. If in doubt give PEP since consequences of developing rabies are disastrous.

Procedure

- *Clean the wound:* this kills virus in superficial wounds. Scrub wound with soap/detergent and wash under running water for >5min. Irrigate with virucidal agent—povidone iodine or 40–70% alcohol. Debride as necessary, but delay suturing if possible.
- Give anti-tetanus toxoid.
- Consider prophylactic antibiotics.
- *Give vaccine:* various regimens given in Boxes 10.8, 10.9, and 10.10.
- *Give rabies immunoglobulin:* human rabies immunoglobulin 20IU/kg or equine rabies immunoglobulin 40IU/kg. If possible infiltrate whole dose into all bite wounds, diluting if necessary; inject residual RIG IM—distant from vaccination sites.

Box 10.7 Indications for post-exposure vaccine and rabies immunoglobulin (RIG)

Minor exposure

Nibbling (tooth contact) with uncovered skin, or minor scratches or abrasions without bleeding:

- Start vaccine immediately.
- Stop treatment if the animal can be observed and remains healthy for 10d.
- Stop treatment if animal's brain proves –ve for rabies by appropriate investigation.

Major exposure

Single or multiple bites or scratches that break the skin, or licks on broken skin, or licks/saliva on mucosae, or physical contact with bats:

- Immediate rabies immunoglobulin and vaccine.
- Stop treatment if animal remains healthy for 10d.
- Stop treatment if animal's brain proves –ve for rabies by appropriate investigation.

Box 10.8 Vaccines and intramuscular/intradermal regimens for rabies PEP

Tissue culture vaccines

Note: vaccine dose (mL) per injection depends on the vaccine:

- *Verorab® (Sanofi-Pasteur):* reconstitute to 0.5mL (ID dose 0.1mL/site).
- *Rabipur®/Rabavert® (Novartis):* reconstitute to 1mL (ID dose 0.2mL/site).

Regimens

- *Standard 5-dose IM method (1–1–1–1–1): whole ampoule into single IM site (deltoid) on days 0, 3, 7, 14, 28; or*
- *4-site ID method (4–0–2–0–1):*
    - *day 0*—divide whole ampoule (0.5 or 1.0mL*) between 4 sites (2 × deltoids and suprascapular or thighs)
    - *day 7*—give ID dose (0.1 or 0.2mL*) in two sites (2 × deltoids)
    - *day 28*—give ID dose (0.1 or 0.2mL*) in 1 site (deltoid); *or*
- *2-site ID method (2–2–2–0–2):* give ID dose (0.1 or 0.2mL*) at each of 2 sites (deltoids) on days 0, 3, 7, and 28. This regimen should be given only by experienced staff together with RIG.

Intradermal regimens

Require use of 1mL syringes and must raise a bleb (*peau d'orange*) immediately, exactly as with administration of BCG vaccination or Mantoux test. If given too deep, withdraw needle and repeat at adjacent site.

Box 10.9 Pre-exposure rabies vaccination

Rabies vaccination is strongly recommended for inhabitants and travellers in rabies enzootic countries. It confers long lasting recall of antibody levels in response to boosting after subsequent exposure (see Box 10.10). Using any of the available vaccines give 0.1mL ID or the whole ampoule IM on days 0, 7, 28. The 3rd dose can be given any time from day 21 if there is insufficient time before travel. There have been no reported failures of the following protocol when combined with boosting on exposure.

Box 10.10 Rabies post-exposure vaccine regimens in those who have had rabies vaccine pre-exposure

- Give whole ampoule IM at single site on days 0 and 3; OR
- Give 0.1 or 0.2mL* ID at single site on days 0 and 3; OR
- Using any of the available vaccines give 0.1mL ID at 4 sites on day 0 (deltoids/subscapular/thighs).

* See note in Box 10.8 regarding ID doses (mL) for each vaccine.

Tetanus

Contamination of a wound with the bacterium *Clostridium tetani* can → severe neurological sequelae due to endotoxin production. The toxin tracks up nerves innervating local muscles, entering the CNS; it also enters the blood and passes to other muscles where it is again transported via peripheral nerves to the CNS. There it blocks release of inhibitory neurotransmitters → widespread activation of both motor and autonomic nervous systems. Muscles of the jaw, face, and head are involved first because of the shorter axonal paths, but all muscle groups become involved in most cases. Activation of opposing groups → rigidity. Protracted uncontrolled muscular spasms of the chest → ineffective breathing and hypoxia. Death is due to respiratory complications, circulatory failure, or cardiac arrest. In patients with access to ITU support, autonomic instability and arrhythmias become the most common causes of death.

Tetanus is easily prevented by vaccination

Its incidence worldwide is directly related to immunization coverage. Where immunization coverage is high it is rare, but in regions where coverage is low it is a common condition, particularly of neonates who become infected at birth. Currently, >800 000 people die each year. Immunization of pregnant women prevents neonatal tetanus.

Transmission

C. tetani spores are ubiquitous in the environment and can infect even the most trivial cuts, typically on feet, legs, and hands. Neonatal infection occurs via the cut umbilicus from the use of a dirty knife or the practice of applying dung to the stump.

Incubation period

Is usually 7–10d, but varies; many patients cannot recall the injury. *Period of onset* (between 1st symptom and onset of spasms) varies between 1 and 7d and is a good prognostic indicator—the shorter the interval the more severe the disease.

Clinical features

The first symptom is often trismus (masseter rigidity → difficulty opening mouth). As disease progresses, other muscle groups become rigid, including muscles of face (→ characteristic look: *risus sardonicus*), skeleton (→ difficulty in breathing; opisthotonos; rigid limbs), and swallowing (→ aspiration). Spasms are an exaggeration of underlying rigidity and occur in more severe disease, either as reflex response to stimuli (touch, sounds, sights, emotions) or spontaneously. May be brief and mild, or prolonged and very painful. Prolonged thoracic spasms may → respiratory failure; laryngeal spasms → death from anoxia. In severe disease fever, tachycardia, and cardiovascular instability are common, mainly due to involvement of the autonomic nervous system—see Box 10.11.

Neonatal cases

Present with inability to suckle → characteristic opisthotonos (see 📖 Neonatal tetanus, p. 31).

Diagnosis is made on clinical features alone.

Box 10.11 Grading of tetanus severity*

- *Grade I (mild):* mild to moderate trismus; general spasticity; no respiratory problems; no spasms; little or no dysphagia.
- *Grade II (moderate):* moderate trismus; well-marked rigidity; mild to moderate, but short-lasting spasms; moderate respiratory failure with tachypnoea >30–35/min; mild dysphagia.
- *Grade III (severe):* severe trismus; generalized spasticity; reflex and often spontaneous prolonged spasms; respiratory failure with tachypnoea >40/min; apnoeic spells; severe dysphagia; tachycardia >120/min.
- *Grade IV (very severe):* features of grade III plus violent autonomic disturbances involving the cardiovascular system. These include: episodes of severe ↑ BP and tachycardia alternating with relative ↓ BP and bradycardia; severe persistent ↑ BP (diastolic >110 mmHg); severe persistent ↓ BP (systolic <90).

* Thwaites CL, Yen LM, Glover C, *et al.* Predicting the clinical outcome of tetanus: the tetanus severity score. *Trop Med Int Hlth* 2006; 11(3): 279–87.

Complications of tetanus

- *Respiratory:* collapse; aspiration, lobar or bronchopneumonia (often due to Gram –ve organisms); anoxia due to prolonged laryngeal spasm; severe hypoxia and respiratory failure in severe tetanus if patient is not paralysed and ventilated; unexplained tachypnoea and respiratory distress; ARDS. Complications also include those of tracheostomy and prolonged ventilation.
- *Cardiovascular mostly mediated by autonomic nervous system:* persistent tachycardia, ↓ BP or ↑ BP; labile BP; severe peripheral vasoconstriction → shock-like state.
- Autonomic storms characterized by sudden sinus tachycardia + severe ↑ BP → sudden bradycardia and ↓ BP. They may precede cardiac arrest. ↑ vagal tone is shown by sudden bradycardia—sucking out of the trachea may lead to an arrest. Dysrhythmias include supraventricular tachycardia (SVT), junctional rhythms, atrial and ventricular ectopics, short bursts of self-resolving VT. Hyperthermia may occur (hypothermia is rare).
- *Sudden death:* caused by many of the above complications, massive PE, or unidentified event.
- *Sepsis:* most commonly nosocomial.
- *Renal insufficiency.*
- *Mid-thoracic vertebral fracture:* occurs during severe spasms; there are usually few sequelae (the muscle stiffness prevents painful movements) and healing occurs without incident.

Prevention

By active vaccination of children and pregnant women (📖 Tetanus immunization, p. 909); good wound toilet and passive vaccination following injuries; provision of clean facilities for childbirth.

Management of tetanus

Management of severe tetanus can be extremely difficult, particularly in the open ward where conservative management has an appalling mortality rate. Ideally, ALL patients should be treated in an ITU setting. However, careful management of the patient with particular attention to critical care and ventilatory support can markedly improve the prognosis where an ITU is not available.

The overall aims of care are:

- To maintain adequate arterial PaO_2 and O_2 saturation.
- To maintain fluid, electrolyte, and acid-base balance.
- To maintain circulatory support in grade IV hypotensive patients.

A central venous line is very useful if available. If ventilators are limited, they should be kept for patients with:

- Grade IV disease.
- Grade III disease uncontrolled by sedatives.
- Serious respiratory complications.

On admission all patients should receive:

- *Antiserum (antitoxin):* preferably human tetanus immunoglobulin 150U/kg IM in multiple sites; otherwise equine antiserum 10 000U by slow IV injection, but *be prepared for an anaphylactic reaction* in all patients receiving equine antiserum and have treatment ready.
- *Antibiotics:* metronidazole 500mg oral or IV tds for 7–10d (poorer alternative: benzylpenicillin 1.2g IM or IV tds for 8d).
- *Local infiltration of antiserum:* of uncertain efficacy, but recommended in some parts of the world.
- *Magnesium:* can help reduce need for muscle relaxants and sedatives and may be helpful in reducing autonomic dysfunction. Give loading dose of $MgSO_4$ 40mg/kg IV over 30min; followed by IV infusion of 2–3 g/h for patients >45kg and 1.5g/h for patients ≤45kg until control of spasms achieved.
- *Wound debridement:* performed after other steps, to remove necrotic tissue. Delay suturing.
- *Tetanus vaccination:* before discharge, as an attack of tetanus does not immunize the patient.
- Prevent, detect, and promptly treat any infection.

Critical care and nursing is essential

- *Detect early hyperpyrexia:* treat with paracetamol and wet cloths.
- ↓ *External stimuli:* physical examination must be gentle.
- *Keep airway patent:* use *gentle* suction to remove saliva and secretions at the back of the throat.

- *Take exquisite care of the tracheostomy:* gently and frequently change patient's posture.
  - *use physiotherapy to keep lungs patent* – give small IV bolus of diazepam before physiotherapy
  - in paralysed patient perform physiotherapy when the action of pancuronium (or gallamine) is at its maximum.
- Keep up patient's nutrition: give 3500–4000cal/d (including >100g protein) by NGT.

Subsequent management

Depends on the severity of the condition.

Grade I

- Beware complications of septic wound.
- Observe carefully - grade I can → more severe disease.
- For sedation/muscle relaxation give diazepam, e.g. 5mg oral/IV tds (children 0.1–0.3mg/kg every 1–4h). Alternative: chlorpromazine 50–150mg (adult), 25mg (child), or 12.5mg (neonate) IM qds (phenobarbital can be added if essential).

Grade II

Treat as for grade I, but ↑ sedation/muscle relaxation:

- ↑ Diazepam dose up to 4-fold in adults (do not exceed 80–100mg/d because of respiratory depression). Give by slow IV infusion over 24h. The ideal sedative/muscle-relaxant schedule ensures continuous sedation such that patient can sleep, but can be woken up to obey commands. Objective guide is relaxation of abdominal muscles.
- Perform a tracheostomy (may prevent death due to prolonged laryngeal spasm and anoxia).
- If laryngeal spasm occurs, promptly give chlorpromazine 50mg IV (alternative: diazepam 10–20mg IV).

Grade III

Treat as for grade II, but also paralyse and ventilate:

- ↓ Diazepam dose (e.g. to 30–40mg over 24h for adults). Give pancuronium 2–4mg (poorer alternative: gallamine 20–40mg) IV, titrated for each patient to give sufficient neuromuscular blockade for efficient ventilation. Initially, give every 1–1.5h (1st 1–2wks), then extend interval as the patient improves. Check with periodic arterial blood analysis, if available.
- Spasms still occur under paralysis, but they need not affect ventilation; pancuronium can be stopped when spasms cease.
- Continue ventilation until patient can be weaned off.

Grade IV

Treat as for grade III, with addition of drugs that act on the cardiovascular system (CVS) if deemed ***essential*** for grossly deranged haemodynamics:

- If ↓ BP – give IV fluids; if ineffective or contraindicated, use dopamine to keep systolic BP >100mmHg.
- If ↑ BP (systolic >200, diastolic >100mmHg) give propranolol 5–10mg po or nifedipine 5mg sublingual.
- Treat bradyarrhythmia or persistent tachyarrhythmias.

Stroke

A rapidly developing focal loss of cerebral function that lasts >24h, with no history of recent head injury. In industrialized world usually caused by thrombosis/embolism leading to cerebral infarction (>80%). The situation differs in the developing world (see Box 10.12). ~20% of stroke patients die within the 1st month; mortality is higher after haemorrhagic stroke than following thrombosis.

Transient ischaemic attack (TIA) Acute loss of focal cerebral or monocular function lasting < 24h. TIAs are associated with ↑ risk of stroke (>5%/yr) and death 2° thromboembolic events (stroke or MI, >10%/yr).

Risk factors for stroke Include hypertension, IHD, atrial fibrillation, TIAs, peripheral vascular disease, DM, smoking.

Clinical features

History of sudden event is crucial in establishing diagnosis. Neurological deficits vary according to the anatomy of stroke (see Table 10.4; Fig. 10.5). Possible to relate clinical features to known anatomy of particular cerebral blood vessels, but collateral blood supply may make this difficult. Infarcts affecting cerebral hemisphere may cause contralateral hemiparesis (→ upper motor neurone paralysis after initial spinal shock), sensory loss, homonymous hemianopia, and/or dysphasia. Infarcts affecting subcortical structures, e.g. thalamus and basal ganglia, can cause mixed or isolated motor and/or sensory defects or ataxia. Brainstem infarcts can have profound effects: quadriplegia, visual and/or respiratory problems, locked-in syndrome. There is often a transient hypertension that settles.

Management

- Ensure adequate airway, oxygenation and circulation.
- If ↓ BP, consider bolus normal saline 250–500mL.
- Determine exact time of onset—critical to establish eligibility for acute thrombolysis if available (see Box 10.13).

Box 10.12 Main causes of stroke in sub-Saharan Africa

- Hypertension (haemorrhagic stroke).
- Atherosclerosis (thrombotic stroke).
- Rheumatic heart disease (embolic from left atrium),
- *Others:*
  - haemoglobinopathies (including sickle cell disease)
  - HIV
  - subarachnoid haemorrhage
  - unexplained (mainly young persons).

Table 10.4 Overview of stroke anatomy

Vascular territory affected by stroke	**Clinical manifestations**
Middle cerebral artery (MCA)	Contralateral hemiplegia, hemianaesthesia, homonymous hemianopia, gaze preference to ipsilateral side. Global aphasia (when dominant hemisphere involved). Constructural apraxia, general or unilateral neglect, dysarthria.
Anterior cerebral artery (ACA)	Paralysis of opposite foot and leg, paresis of opposite arm, cortical sensory loss over toes, foot and leg, urinary incontinence, contralateral grasp reflex, hypertonia.
Anterior choriodal artery (AChA)	Contralateral hemiplegia, hemianaesthesia, homonymous hemianopia.
Proximal posterior cerebral artery (PCA)	3rd nerve palsy with contralateral ataxia or contralateral hemiplegia.
Distal PCA	Contralateral homonymous hemianopia with macular sparing, disturbance in memory.
Vertebral-basilar artery	Unilateral or bilateral motor/sensory deficits, accompanied by cranial nerve and brainstem signs.

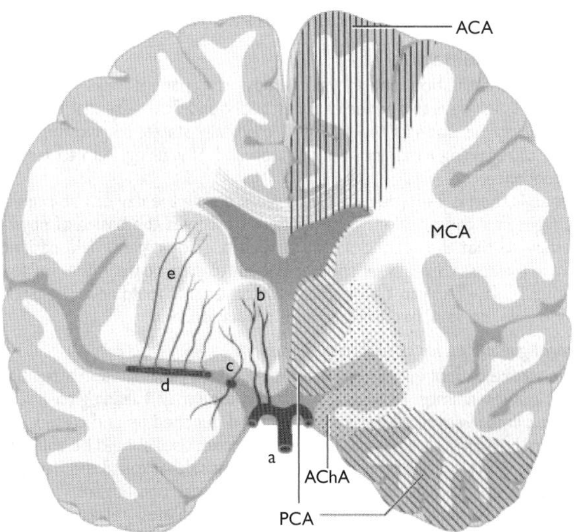

Fig. 10.5 Coronal view of the cerebral hemispheres: ACA: anterior cerebral artery, MCA: middle cerebral artery, PCA: posterior cerebral artery, AChA: anterior choroidal artery, a: basilar artery, b: thalamoperforator, which originate in the PCA, c: AChA, d: MCA, e: lenticulostriate arteries.

Do a non-contrast head CT scan to rule out haemorrhage. *If CT shows no blood* consider thrombolysis (see Box 10.13). If thrombolysis not indicated or available give aspirin 150mg daily.

- Slowly and carefully lower BP by no more than 10–20% if very high (>120 diastolic; >220 systolic).
- Take great care of the airway in the unconscious patient.
- Turn the patient every 4h to avoid bedsores.
- Ensure adequate nutrition and hydration.
- Look for and treat any treatable cause (e.g. cardiac source of emboli, giant-cell arteritis).
- Watch out for causes of neurological deterioration — see Box 10.14.
- If evidence of cerebral oedema, consider mannitol.
- ***Think about rehabilitation*** early in the patient's illness (see 📖 Stroke rehabilitation, p. 460). Do not ignore this issue until the patient has developed joint contractures that will prevent physical recovery.

Stroke prevention

Recovery for most patients is rarely complete and 1° prevention is important. ↓ Risk of strokes by controlling risk factors, particularly hypertension and smoking. In patients who have had TIAs or previous strokes, it is particularly important to control BP and ↓ risk of further thrombotic events by giving aspirin 75mg oral od. Assuming no contraindications, and the availability of safe, reliable monitoring of INR (often not available in low resource settings), anticoagulation is recommended for patients with AF, pro-coagulant clotting disorders, or recurrent DVT.

Stroke rehabilitation

Without rehabilitation and physiotherapy, the patient risks spending the rest of her days in a wheelchair or bedbound. It is essential to start physiotherapy as soon as the patient is medically stable, to give the best chance of regaining hand and arm function and of walking. Aim to regain independence.

Rehabilitation is 24-h process. Good work during the day can be ruined by a night in a bad position. Teach patient's relatives the basics of physiotherapy so that they can look out for bad positioning and help patient perform exercises. Initially, encourage patient to participate in therapy for ~20min, 3x/day. This can ↑ with time. Physiotherapy should never be painful. 'No pain, no gain' has no place in rehabilitation.

General guidelines for stroke rehabilitation

- The stroke patient initially has ↓ tone. At onset, rehabilitation attempts to ↑ power in limbs. However, over time, tone may ↑ leading to spastic limbs with fixed deformities. A hand bunched up and curled under the arm is useless. Gentle repetitive exercises should be able to ↓ tone. Work on opposite movements to those that cause the hand to bunch up—extension at shoulder, elbow, wrist, and fingers.
- Normal movement is easier if the person is completely relaxed. This is accomplished by supporting the whole body (see Fig. 10.6).

Box 10.13 Thrombolysis for acute non-haemorrhagic stroke

Thrombolysis with recombinant tissue plasminogen activator (tPA) is licensed for treatment of acute ischaemic stroke within the first 3h after stroke onset. It has been shown to ↓ mortality and ↓ morbidity despite a small ↑ risk of intracranial haemorrhage. It should only be considered in centres with appropriate clinical and neuro-imaging expertise, ∴ not appropriate in most low resource settings. Contraindications include delayed presentation, recent surgery, head trauma, GI or urinary haemorrhage, seizure at stroke onset, bleeding disorder, severe uncontrolled hypertension.

Box 10.14 Causes of neurological deterioration after stroke

- *Local:* extension of thrombus; recurrent embolism or haemorrhage; haemorrhagic transformation of the infarct; post-haemorrhage vasoconstriction; further ischaemia; cerebral oedema; brain shift and herniation; hydrocephalus; epileptic seizures.
- *General:* hypoxia (pneumonia, PE, cardiac failure); hypotension; infection; dehydration; hyponatraemia; hypoglycaemia or hyperglycaemia; drugs; depression.

- Aim of stroke rehabilitation is normal movement. Some patients will neglect one side—ensure that patient is able to see both arms and hands at all times. Reinforce message that they are symmetrical. The patient can practise actions with weak limbs (e.g. picking up a cup, stepping from one foot to the other while sitting) by carefully noting action with normal limb, and then copying this with weak limb.
- Repetition of a movement over a period reinforces plastic adaptation. After a stroke, the brain has to relearn how to do things. It needs to practise. However, repetition can strengthen both bad and good habits, so it is essential to get the practised movements right.

Early stage

- Support and position the patient carefully, paying particular attention to the hemiplegic shoulder to ↓ risk of injury. Fig. 10.6, nos. 1–3, show how to cushion the patient.
- Relatives or nurses should roll patient carefully (no. 4). As patient becomes stronger, teach rolling from side to side, and then to get up from lying (nos. 5 and 6). Patient will often need help.
- Frequent changes in position are good.
- Aim to maintain muscle length (prevent contractures) with *gentle* passive/active movements into extension, taking particular care over Achilles tendon, and flexors of elbow, wrist, and fingers.
- Encourage selective and controlled movements. It is better to work slowly to get good control of arm and hand movements than to be able rapidly to regain function with gross abnormal limb movements.

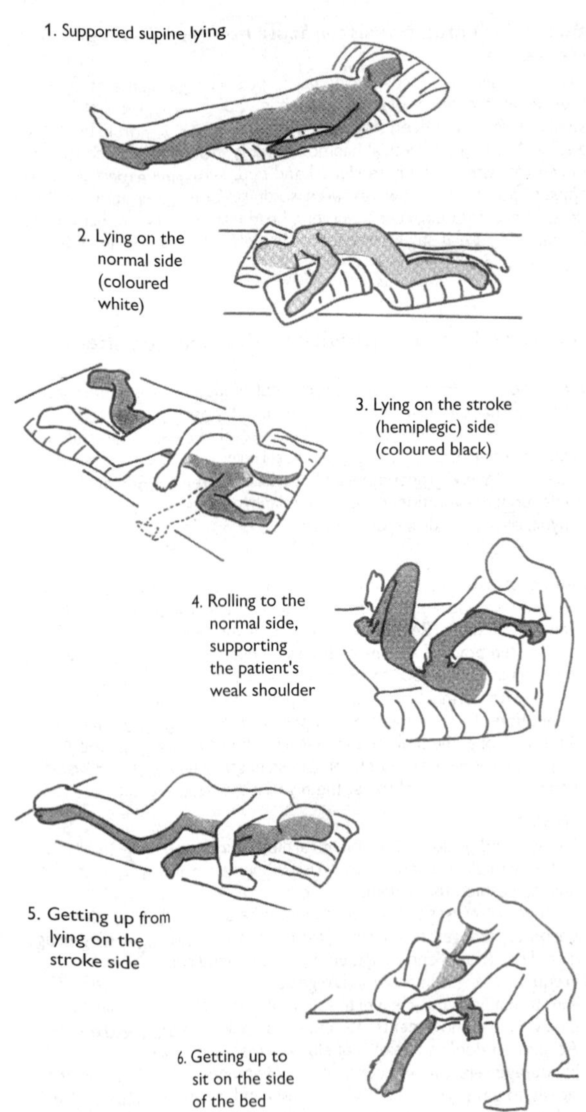
1. Supported supine lying
2. Lying on the normal side (coloured white)
3. Lying on the stroke (hemiplegic) side (coloured black)
4. Rolling to the normal side, supporting the patient's weak shoulder
5. Getting up from lying on the stroke side
6. Getting up to sit on the side of the bed

Fig. 10.6 Patient support and positioning in stroke rehabilitation.

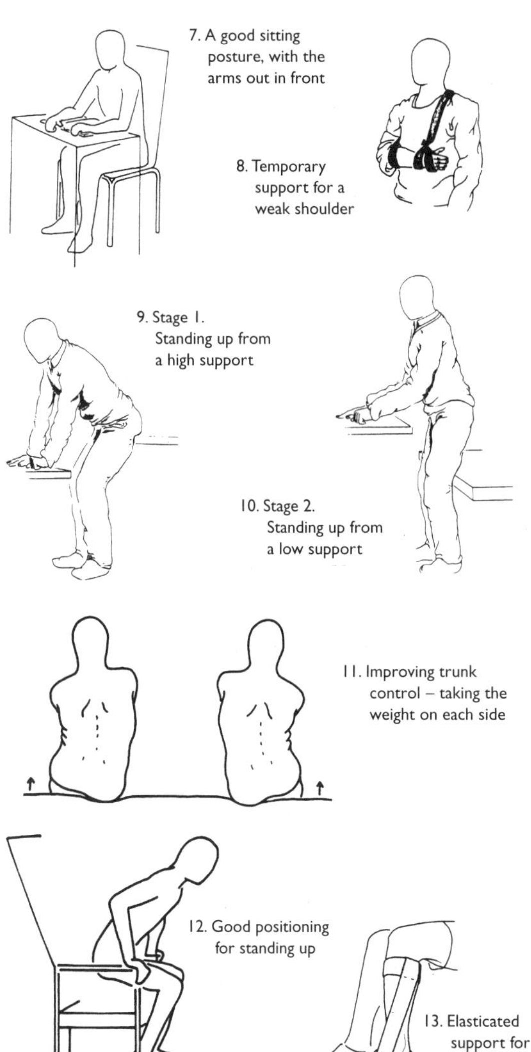

7. A good sitting posture, with the arms out in front
8. Temporary support for a weak shoulder
9. Stage 1. Standing up from a high support
10. Stage 2. Standing up from a low support
11. Improving trunk control – taking the weight on each side
12. Good positioning for standing up
13. Elasticated support for foot drop

Fig. 10.6 *(continued)*

Basic principles for this early stage

- Aim for symmetry: sit patient in a good position with adequate support. Set arms forward. Sit patient out for short periods if trunk control is poor. Practice transferring weight from side to side → easier for her to shift weight from one leg to the other while learning to walk again.
- *Aim for good control of movement:* patient needs to be able to control transfer of body weight in sitting/standing. Patient needs to lean forward to get up, using a high seat initially. With progress, seat can be lowered, before trying a chair.
- *Aim for trunk control:* in sitting, before trying to stand and especially during sitting → standing.
- *Aim for balance:* in standing and stepping before walking.

Walking stage

- *Aim for normal gait:* equal stride length and equal time on both sides.
- The patient may require support on one or both sides.
- Start walking with the *unaffected* leg. This means that patient must have already learned to shift weight from leg to leg.
- *Walking aids:* use a wheeled frame/rollator or a normal walking stick (a quadruped stick should be a last resort).
- Patient may require help with a 'drop foot'.
- Use mime, gestures, repeating and rephrasing movements, and physical prompts to help the patient. Allow time for slow synapsing.
- Little and often is a better way to build stamina and sustain carry-over from one session to another.

Some 'don'ts' for stroke rehabilitation

- *Do not ask the patient to try harder:* **avoid** effort as it ↑ tone and gross patterns of movement.
- *Do not ask the patient to squeeze a ball:* this encourages arm flexors that are already too strong.
- *Avoid a painful shoulder:* do not make any arm movements unless whole shoulder, including the scapula, is relaxed and supple. *Support for a weak arm* may be useful temporarily (e.g. while concentrating on walking).
- *Never lift under stroke arm or pull it:* muscles that hold the shoulder are weak and joint easily dislocated.
- *Prevent dislocation:* support forearm and hand forwards with natural weight through the elbow.

Subarachnoid haemorrhage

An acute bleed into the subarachnoid space → a sudden intense headache ('like being hit on the back of the head'), sometimes accompanied by nausea and vomiting. Most cases of SAH are caused by ruptured aneurysms. Other causes are mycotic aneurysms (due to endocarditis) and arteriovenous malformations; 15% have no identified cause. Some SAH are preceded by minor herald bleeds that also elicit an intense headache +/– meningism or back pain. If suspected, refer for evaluation since surgical treatment at this time may prevent a later severe bleed. Re-bleeding occurs in >30% of cases; it is a common cause of death.

Clinical features

The conscious level may be ↓. The more severe the bleed, the lower the conscious level, and the worse the prognosis. Other features include: headache with meningism; vomiting; seizure. Focal signs are rare. The patient is often irritable and drowsy; the headache may last for weeks. Complications include vascular spasm → cerebral ischaemia.

Beware

↓ Conscious level, the appearance or worsening of a neurological deficit (e.g. development of hemiparesis, dilatation of a pupil), or systemic changes such as ↑ BP that may indicate ↑ ICP.

Diagnosis

Is by clinical findings with LP (and early CT scan if available). The CSF is uniformly blood stained in the first few days. Xanthochromia (straw-coloured supernatant) may be present from 6h after bleed onset up to 14d. Do not delay LP if differential diagnosis includes meningitis.

Management

Often involves neurosurgery to evacuate an intracerebral haematoma or clip the aneurysm. Medical treatment involves extended bed rest, analgesia, sedation (beware masking of ↓ conscious level), and cautious control of hypertension. Give IV hydration (3L/day). Nimodipine (60mg po every 4h for 2–3wks, starting within 4d of haemorrhage) ↓ the incidence of vascular spasm.

Subdural haemorrhage

A slow venous bleed that follows damage to veins crossing from the cortex to venous sinuses. May even occur after minor trauma in those predisposed: elderly, alcoholics, people with clotting disorders, epileptics. Presentation can occur months after the forgotten accident as chronic bleeding slowly ↑ size of the haematoma (see Fig. 10.7).

Clinical features

Common acute symptoms include headache, vomiting, fluctuating levels of consciousness; less commonly, mood changes, irritability, incontinence, drowsiness. Signs may include changes in pupil size, distal limb weakness, and increased reflexes; less commonly, seizures and dysphasia.

Management

Requires a neurosurgical opinion and, if possible, a CT scan → evacuation through burr holes in most cases (Box 10.15). Minor haematomas may resolve spontaneously. With appropriate management outcome is good in all ages: >90% return to normal, so it is important to consider the diagnosis in a confused elderly person.

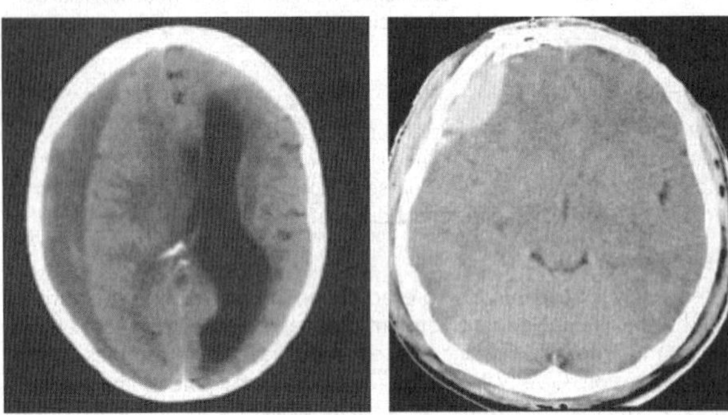

Fig. 10.7 Typical crescent-shaped hypodense chronic subdural haematoma (left); typical lens-shaped acute extradural haematoma (right).

Box 10.15 How to do a burr hole

Incision (see Fig. 10.8)

- Shave scalp if there is time.
- Local anaesthetic not usually necessary.
- Make a 4-cm incision over the site of fracture or injury: this is usually in the temporal region (just above the zygomatic arch), where a curved incision is made so that it can be enlarged.
- Incise right down to the bone. Do not stop to control bleeding.

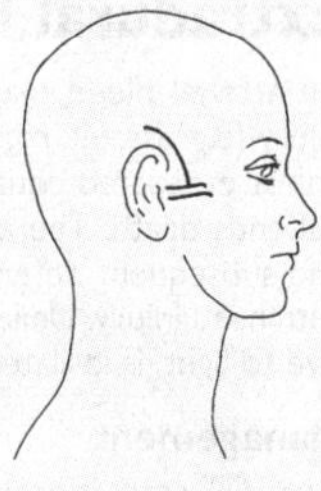

Fig. 10.8 Incision.

Scrape back the pericranium (periosteum) using a periosteal elevator (or similar instrument) to expose skull. Insert a mastoid retractor—this will stop all bleeding (see Fig. 10.9). Leave retractor in.

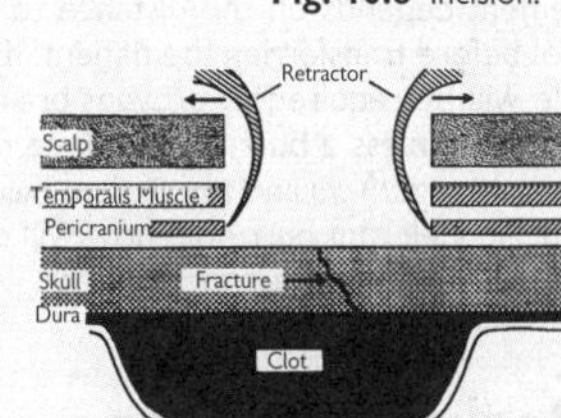

Fig. 10.9 Scrape pericranium.

Perforate the bone using a perforator

- Dark blood will ooze out.
- The dura will not be seen as it is stripped away by the blood clot.
- Do no more than *just* perforate the skull (see Fig. 10.10).
- This will create a conical hole.

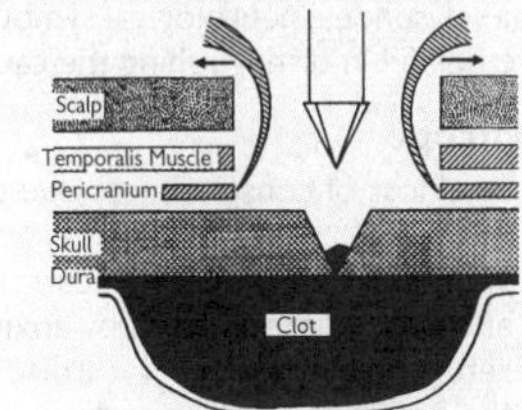

Fig 10.10 Perforate bone.

Enlarge the perforation using a burr

- The burr will enlarge the hole so that it is nearly cylindrical.
- ***The blood clot will immediately ooze out.***
- Suck blood away by applying a sucker to the burr hole but do not insert sucker into cavity. This will cause more bleeding and might damage brain. (See Fig. 10.11)

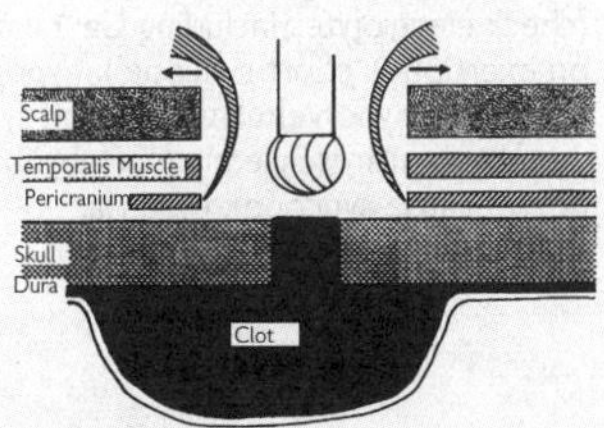

Fig 10.11 Enlarge perforation.

Aftercare

- It is now safe to transfer the patient to a neurosurgical unit.
- Leave the scalp retractor in; organize for its return.
- Leave in the endotracheal tube and leave a drip up.

Extradural haematoma

An arterial bleed that normally results from a skull fracture after head injury (e.g. assault, road traffic accident). Haematoma enlarges rapidly and, unless evacuated equally rapidly, there is high risk of brain herniation and patient's death. There is often a lucid interval between initial head injury and subsequent deterioration. Suspect when conscious level ↓ in patient with head injury. Unilateral dilation of pupil, which is sluggish or unresponsive to light, is ipsilateral to side of haemorrhage.

Management

Do a CT scan, if possible, to localize the expanding lesion. Further management depends on the distance to a neurosurgeon. If close, give mannitol before transferring the patient. If the neurosurgeon is remote, a burr hole will be required to prevent brain herniation (see Box 10.15). In this situation, unless a burr hole is done rapidly, the patient will die or suffer brain damage. You and the patient have nothing to lose, and everything to gain. An inelegant burr hole now will do much more good than an elegant operation one hour or more later.

Blackouts/syncope

The most common causes of blackouts are epilepsy and syncope. A detailed history including any prodromal symptoms (e.g. palpitations, chest pain, dyspnoea, neurological symptoms), and a reliable eyewitness account are helpful in distinguishing the cause.

Syncope

- Brief loss of consciousness due to an acute reduction in cerebral blood flow.
- Most common cause of recurrent episodes of disturbed consciousness and may be precipitated by anxiety or pain. It is due to ↓ venous return to the heart → ↓ cardiac output, or an inadequate response of the heart when ↑ demand requires ↑ cardiac output.
- Causes include ↓ BP (including postural hypotension), vagal slowing of the heart (vasovagal syncope), autonomic neuropathy, dysrhythmias (check electrolytes including Ca^{2+} and Mg^{2+}), aortic stenosis (may occur on exertion – 'effort syncope'), hypoglycaemia, hypoxia, carotid-sinus syndrome, hyperventilation, cough syncope, micturition syncope, vertebrobasilar ischaemia (vertebrobasilar TIAs, although most TIAs do not cause syncope), hysteria.

Space-occupying lesions

Classically present with focal neurological signs, ↑ ICP, or seizures. Focal neurological signs may help localize the mass but beware false localizing signs due to ↑ ICP (see 📖 Raised intracranial pressure, p. 438).

Causes

- *Infection:* tuberculoma, toxoplasmosis, cysticercosis, echinococcosis, bacterial or amoebic brain abscess, paragonimiasis, schistosomiasis, fungal granulomata.
- *Tumour:* glioma, meningioma, metastases, lymphoma, pituitary adenoma, cysts.
- *Others:* aneurysm, haematoma.

Brain abscess

Brain abscesses may occur due to spread from a contiguous focus (e.g. meningitis, subdural empyema) or septic emboli. Infection is often mixed with streptococci, *S. aureus*, and anaerobes. Diagnosis is confirmed by CT brain with contrast which shows ring-enhancing lesion(s).

Empiric antimicrobial therapy should be chosen to cover the most likely pathogens based on the 1° infection site. When no preceding infection can be found, ceftriaxone plus metronidazole ± vancomycin is a reasonable regimen. Surgical drainage is indicated when the size of the abscess is >3 × 3cm.

Hydrocephalus

In older children and adults, the skull will not expand if ↑ ICP. Blockage of CSF flow through the ventricles or failure to reabsorb CSF → build-up of pressure or hydrocephalus. While producing ↑ head circumference in young children, it → ↑ ICP with dilatation of the ventricular system in older persons that will need urgent management. It exists in two forms:

- *Non-communicating hydrocephalus:* due to blockage of CSF flow through the ventricles, normally at foramina or aqueduct between ventricles and/or basal cistern. Caused by any SOL, such as tumour or cyst, or stenosis of the aqueduct. Location of blockage must be identified and blockage removed surgically, or a ventriculo-peritoneal shunt placed to relieve pressure.
- *Communicating hydrocephalus:* due to CSF obstruction in basal cisterns or subarachnoid space (CSF still flows out of ventricular system, but it cannot be reabsorbed in arachnoid villi). It may result from intracranial haemorrhage or meningitis (acute pyogenic or chronic meningitis, especially TB or cryptococcal meningitis); cause is often unknown. It may present with a triad of dementia, incontinence, and gait disturbance. (This condition is also called normal pressure hydrocephalus.) Treatment of any underlying cause with repeated LPs may be sufficient. Medical therapy with a combination of furosemide (adults 40mg, children 1mg/kg daily) and acetazolamide (adults 10–20mg/kg, children 30–50mg/kg daily) has also been recommended as an option for initial treatment in communicating hydrocephalus complicating TBM. Shunting may be required.

Epilepsy

Epilepsy is the continuing tendency to have seizures—spontaneous paroxysmal discharges of neurons that result in clinical symptoms. It is common, affecting ~70 million people worldwide. Its incidence is higher in the developing world than the industrialized world: 1–2% of the population has epilepsy due to higher incidence of brain injury and CNS infections. It is associated with considerable stigma, ↓ education and employment opportunities, and ↑ mortality. Unfortunately, at present only 15% of cases are treated adequately and many people suffer unnecessarily. There is a need to ↓ its incidence in the developing world (by ↓ the number of head injuries and infections and improving obstetric services) and find ways of providing adequate supplies of affordable effective anti-epileptic drugs to poorer countries.

Epilepsy

Usually defined as at least two unprovoked seizures, needs to be distinguished from acute symptomatic seizures, which do not need long-term anti-epileptic drugs.

Acute symptomatic seizures

Are events, occurring in close temporal relationship with an acute CNS insult, which may be metabolic, toxic, structural, infectious, or due to inflammation. Unlike epilepsy, the cause of these seizures is identifiable, e.g. CNS infections, head trauma, eclampsia (urgent delivery is required), and alcohol (particularly withdrawal).

Febrile convulsions

Seizures that occur in children aged 6mths to 6yrs in response to an extracranial infection. They have a better prognosis than seizures described above (see 📖 Febrile convulsions, p. 16).

Causes of epilepsy

No cause is identified in ~70% cases (some may be due to hamartomas—very small areas of focal dysgenesis). Among the remaining ~30% cases causes include:

- *Infection:* cysticercosis, tuberculoma, schistosomiasis, paragonimiasis, sparganosis, hydatid disease, toxoplasmosis, toxocariasis, cerebral malaria, cerebral amoebiasis, syphilitic gumma, HIV. Epilepsy can also be a late consequence of almost any meningeal or brain parenchyma infection.
- *Brain injury:* including antenatal or perinatal brain injury and head injury (e.g. assault or road traffic accident).
- *Other:* including brain tumour or metastases, cerebrovascular disease, metabolic causes (especially ↓Na^+), degenerative disorders, inherited diseases, and drugs.

Clinical features and classification of seizures

Pragmatic definition is based on origin and spread of seizure. This is important for deciding on further investigations and choice of drug therapy (see 📖 Management, p. 473; Box 10.16). Classification usually based upon description of seizure (usually only a history is available), although electroencephalography (EEG) can help detect focal seizures and epileptic syndromes.

- *Focal (partial) seizures:* remain localized to their area of origin, and have signs and symptoms referable to a part of one hemisphere. Distinguishing between simple and complex partial seizures is not thought to be useful but it is important to document ↓ consciousness (see 📖 Secondarily generalized seizures, below).
- *Secondarily generalized seizures:* are focal seizures that subsequently spread from their region of origin to involve whole brain leading to ↓ consciousness.
- *Generalized seizures:* originate in centrally positioned cells and activate all parts of brain simultaneously leading to ↓ consciousness. They do not have features that are referable to only one hemisphere. Types of generalized seizure include:
  - *Absence seizures*—typically these are brief (<10s) pauses, e.g. stops talking mid-sentence, carries on where left off. Classically, has pathognomic 3Hz activity on EEG (*petit mal*). Atypical absences may last for longer or may be associated with myoclonus.
  - *Tonic-clonic (grand mal) seizures*—sudden onset with loss of consciousness, body stiffens for up to 1min before jerking, with post-ictal drowsiness. Tonic or clonic seizures can occur in isolation.
  - *Myoclonic and akinetic* seizures.

Important points to elicit in the history are:

- *Events before the seizure:* an aura or warning, or abnormal behaviour before the attack suggests a focal origin.
- Movement of the head (localizing sign).
- ↓ Consciousness (indicates generalized seizure).
- Stiffening (tonic) or jerking (clonic/convulsive).
- Tongue biting and incontinence of urine (rarely faeces).
- Post-ictal confusion, drowsiness, or headache; and failure to remember the onset all suggest diagnosis of a seizure if there is uncertainty.

Management

If the seizure appears to have a focal onset, look for a treatable underlying cause (see 📖 Causes of epilepsy, p. 472). If available, do CT or, preferably, MRI).

The decision to start treatment should be made in consultation with the patient and their family. This will depend upon the frequency (usually >2 seizures in a year), cultural, educational, and social consequences of having seizures, and cost and availability of drugs. Patients should be warned not to drive and to avoid swimming; discuss occupational hazards, e.g. working at heights, using power tools, etc.

First-line drugs

- *Phenobarbital:* 1st choice for partial and generalized tonic-clonic seizures. Start at 1–1.5mg/kg po od (30–60mg in adults) building up as required to usual maintenance dose of 2.5–4mg/kg od or bd daily (max. 180mg daily). Side-effects in children appear at higher doses.

- *Carbamazepine:* 1st choice for tonic-clonic seizures in association with partial seizures; reserve drug for partial seizures alone. Start at 100mg po bd, building up to 600mg bd if tolerated (children 5mg/kg up to 20mg/kg/day).
- *Sodium valproate:* 1st choice for typical absences, myoclonic and akinetic seizures, and tonic-clonic seizures in association with typical absences. Start at 300mg po bd, building up to 750mg bd (max = 2.5g/day) as required (children 5mg/kg/day up to 40mg/kg/day).
- *Phenytoin:* reserve drug for tonic-clonic and partial seizures (not for absences). Start at 3–4mg/kg (adults) or 1.5–2.5mg/kg (children) oral od; adjust according to response and plasma levels; usual dose 200–500mg (adults); max dose in children 300mg daily. It is a toxic drug and plasma levels should ideally be monitored.
- *Other drugs:* include clonazepam, ethosuximide, lamotrigine, and newer drugs (vigabatrin, gabapentin, levetiracetam).

Changing drugs

Persist with one drug until it has been used at its maximum dose or causes intolerable side effects before considering a change. Introduce the new drug at its starting dose and slowly ↑ to its mid-range; then start to slowly ↓ the dose of the old drug.

Stopping drugs

It is unclear how long any person needs to stay on anti-epileptic drugs once the seizures have been controlled. In general if a patient has not had a seizure within the last 2yrs, discuss with them whether they would like to discontinue treatment, balancing the risk of recurrence vs. gravity of the side-effects.

Box 10.16 Principles of anti-epileptic drug therapy

- Establish a clear clinical diagnosis.
- EEG may help classify the seizures and/or syndrome if available.
- Choose a drug, considering the:
  - seizure type(s)
  - interaction with other drugs
  - patient's age
  - possibility of pregnancy
  - price.
- Start with one drug and aim to control seizures with monotherapy.
- Begin with low-modest dosage, ↑ slowly over 2–3mths.
- Give full information to the patient concerning:
  - names and alternative names of the drug supplied
  - the main side-effects of the drug
  - the need for adherence with instructions
  - possible interactions with other medications.
- Monitor progress, seizure frequency, and side-effects.
- Ensure adequate supplies of anti-epileptic drugs.

Status epilepticus

Status epilepticus is defined as at least 15min of continuous seizures or >2 discrete seizures without regaining consciousness. Status epilepticus can → death, permanent neurological damage, or the onset of chronic epilepsy—risk factors for such sequelae include aetiology, duration of seizure, and systemic complications.

Aetiology

The most common causes are acute CNS infection (particularly in children), head injury, and known epilepsy. Other causes include pesticide poisoning, stroke, and eclampsia.

Principles of management

- Remove patient from potential danger.
- Stop seizures quickly.
- Prevent complications.
- Find and control the underlying causes.

Management

- Secure the airway, preferably with oral airway, give O_2.

Note Do not attempt to intubate if the jaw is clenched. Wait for sedation to have its effect.

- Give glucose 20% as 50mL IV bolus unless hypoglycaemia excluded.
- Give thiamine 250mg by slow IV infusion over 20min if patient alcoholic or malnourished: note risk of anaphylaxis.
- Give diazepam 10mg in 2–4mL IV or PR at a rate of 5mg/min (children <12yrs old 0.3–0.4mg/kg, or 1mg per year of age; max 10mg). This should control >80% of patients. Repeat once after 10min if necessary. Beware respiratory depression following bolus diazepam. Lorazepam or midazolam may be used as alternatives if available.

If convulsions continue after giving diazepam:

- ***Manage the patient in ICU if possible.***
- ***Give phenytoin*** 10–15mg/kg as IV infusion at <50mg/min through a separate giving set. Once seizures are controlled, maintain with phenytoin 100mg po or IV q6–8h. Alternatively, give phenobarbital 10–20mg/kg as an IV infusion, at <100mg/min to a maximum of 1g. Phenobarbital is preferred for seizures associated with poisoning. Clomethiazole is another alternative. Do not give more diazepam.
- ***Beware respiratory depression and hypotension.***
- ***Check for and treat*** ↑ ICP.

If convulsions continue after phenytoin:

- Exclude pseudo-status (i.e. pseudo-seizures).
- Check drugs have been given correctly.
- Then give general anaesthetic and ventilate, whilst treating causative condition. Give thiopental 75–125mg (3–5mL of a 2.5% solution) IV over 10–15s. Give further doses according to response. Beware hypotension. If large amounts of thiopental are infused over a long period, it will accumulate and delay recovery.

Cysticercosis

This condition, caused by the pork tapeworm *Taenia solium*, is a common cause of epilepsy worldwide. Humans normally become infected with the tapeworm stage by eating cysts in undercooked pork meat - see life cycle in Fig. 10.12. Accidental human ingestion of eggs from human faeces → disease in which humans act as the alternative host with involvement of the CNS, muscles, skin, and eye. The symptoms are caused by the inflammatory reaction to the living and dying parasites (active disease), and long-term effects of the inflammatory reaction to the cysts—fibrosis, calcification, and granulation (inactive disease).

Clinical features

- CNS involvement (neurocysticercosis) normally manifests as epilepsy. However, since the number and localization of cysts vary greatly, neurocysticercosis can also → hydrocephalus, dementia (frontal lobe involvement; often in children).
- Infarcts (due to vasculitis).
- Basal meningitis; cranial nerve defects; spinal symptoms.
- Subcutaneous and muscular cysts (small, round, painless, firm nodules) occur in 25% of CNS cases, but may also occur in isolation.
- Calcified cysts resembling rice grains may be an incidental finding on X-ray. Rarely, cardiac involvement can → conduction defects. Ocular cysticercosis may → blurring of vision and the sensation of something in the eye. If untreated, it may → blindness and eye atrophy.

Diagnosis Active CNS lesions can be identified by CT or MRI (see Fig. 10.13); calcified inactive lesions can be seen on CT (and sometimes on X-ray). Serology.

Management

- Control of seizures with anticonvulsants is the priority.
- Cysts that appear to be living, particularly those that are large and demonstrate no inflammatory reaction, are most likely to benefit from anti-parasitic therapy. Options include:
  - *albendazole* 15mg/kg/day oral in 2 doses for 8–30d plus oral dexamethasone 0.4mg/kg/day for 10d *or*
  - *praziquantel*—either as 1-d regimen of 25mg/kg in 3 doses 2h apart, or 15-d regimen using 50mg/kg/day orally in 3 divided doses. (1-d regimen should only be used for a single or low cyst burden).
- Surgery is usually reserved for subarachnoid and intraventricular cysts causing hydrocephalus or cord compression.
- Ocular infection in isolation should not be treated with drugs. Ocular cysts may need to be treated surgically.

Prevention

Health education and public health measures to improve personal hygiene, meat inspection, adequate cooking of pork, sanitation on farms, and sewage disposal to prevent pigs consuming human faeces. Mass chemotherapy including praziquantel mass treatment for schistosomiaisis may also have a role in control at the population level.

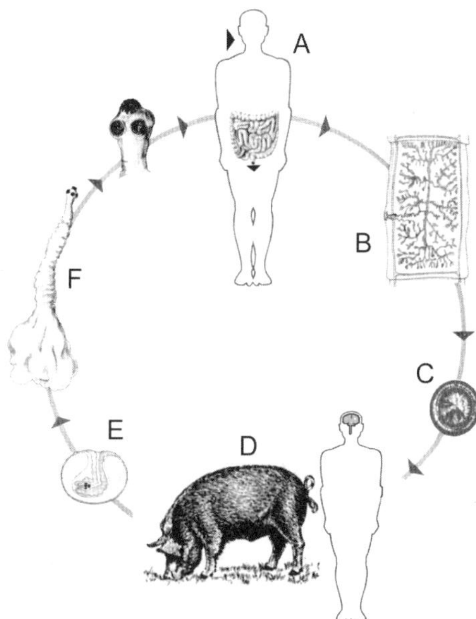

Fig. 10.12 Life cycle of *Taenia solium*. Man (A) is the definitive host, with a tapeworm 3–4m long in the small intestine. Proglottids (segments; B) of the tapeworm detach and are shed in the faeces, each containing a branching uterus and thousands of eggs (C). When human faeces are ingested by man or pig (D) these eggs, which contain an embryo, develop into a larval stage (the cysticercus, E) in muscles, brain or other tissues. When man ingests uncooked pork containing cysticerci, these evaginate (F) in the human small intestine to form the head of the tapeworm; this elongates and forms new segments, completing the life cycle.

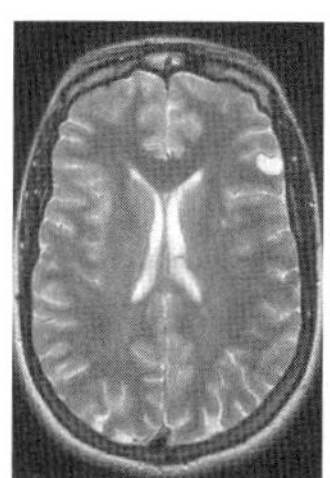

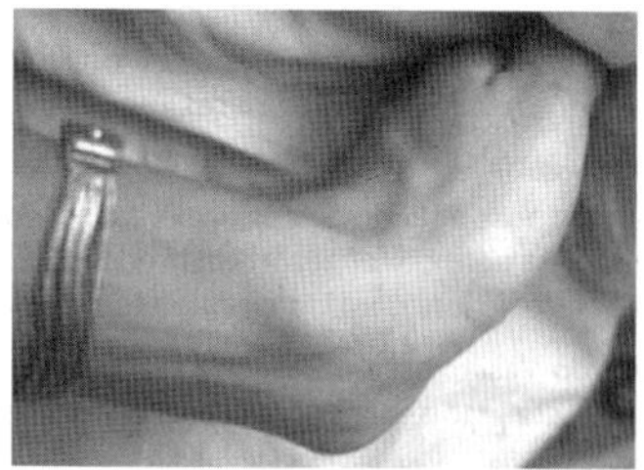

Fig. 10.13 MRI of cysticercus in left fronto-pariental cortex of a 35-yr-old woman who presented with focal seizures. A cystercus was also visible under the skin of her left wrist. Both lesions disappeared after 4wks of albendazole treatment.

Weak legs and spinal cord disease

Causes of weak legs include upper motor neurone (UMN) and lower motor neurone (LMN) pathology (see Box 10.17). There may be mixed UMN and LMN signs in some conditions (e.g. spinal cord compression accompanied by nerve root compression; conus medullaris lesions; motor neuron disease). A careful history and examination will suggest the most likely anatomical location and differential diagnosis in each case.

It is important to establish:

- Is the weakness bilateral (= paraparesis) or unilateral?
- Was the onset gradual or sudden?
- Is the tone spastic (suggesting UMN pathology) or flaccid (suggesting LMN pathology)?
- Is there sensory loss, in particular a sensory level? A sensory level is a strong clue to spinal cord disease.
- Is there any loss of sphincter control (bowels or bladder)?
- Is there normal sensation around the sacrum and good anal tone?

The differential diagnosis then depends on the presentation:

Sudden weak legs with spasticity

Cord compression—an emergency

- Consider especially when rapid progression of leg weakness and/or sphincter failure.
- Causes include:
  - spinal or paraspinal infection (e.g. TB, Brucella, pyogenic abscess)
  - tumours (metastases, Hodgkin's/Burkitt's lymphoma, myeloma)
  - disc prolapse
  - Paget's disease
  - vertebral collapse 2° avascular necrosis in sickle cell disease)
  - trauma.
- Image spine (X-ray and/or CT/MRI if available).
- Treat cause.
- If malignancy, give dexamethasone 4mg qds IV immediately and consider surgery, radiotherapy, chemotherapy).
- Drain epidural abscesses and treat with appropriate antibiotics according to suspected aetiology.
- Early intervention ↓ risk and severity of longer-term neurological sequelae due to spinal cord compression.

Transverse myelitis

- Infectious or post-infectious: back pain, fever, double incontinence, sensory loss at defined level surmounted by a zone of hyperaesthesia.
- Multiple sclerosis less common in the tropics.

Cord infarction Vasculitis, anterior spinal artery thrombosis, trauma, compression, dissecting aortic aneurysm, surgery; tumours.

Box 10.17 Causes of weak legs

Upper motor neuron causes
- Spinal cord pathology (extrinsic compression or intrinsic disease).
- Brainstem pathology.
- Cortical disease (*Note:* stroke usually causes unilateral weakness).
- Parasagittal meningioma (rare).

Lower motor neuron causes
- Radiculopathy (nerve root pathology due to extrinsic compression or intrinsic disease).
- Cauda equina syndrome.
- Peripheral neuropathy.

Acute flaccid paralysis

See Table 10.5 for comparison of conditions in the differential diagnosis of acute flaccid paralysis (AFP). Causes include:
- *Cauda equina compression*—a neurosurgical emergency: ask about back and radicular leg pain, bladder and bowel sphincter control. Check perineal area for loss of sensation (saddle anaesthesia). Do PR to assess anal sphincter tone. Causes include tumour; disc prolapse; canal stenosis; TB; cysticercosis; schistosomiasis. Management is similar to spinal cord compression (see 📖 p. 480)—focus on treating the cause.
- Poliomyelitis (📖 Poliomyelitis, p. 482).
- Guillain–Barré syndrome (📖 Guillain–Barré syndrome, p. 485).
- *Other:*
  - acute cord trauma/infarction
  - myelitis (in early stages)
  - rabies (📖 Rabies, p. 450)
  - lumbosacral nerve lesion; hypokalaemic periodic paralysis.

Chronic spastic paraparesis/weak legs

- *Cord compression:* spinal degenerative disease (e.g. cervical spondylosis); many of the causes listed for acute spastic paraparesis, p.481.
- *Human T lymphotrophic virus (HTLV-1):* associated myelopathy/tropical spastic paraparesis (HAM/TSP)—progressive spastic paraparesis, which usually presents in middle age. Described in several regions including Caribbean, Japan, equatorial Africa, South America.
- Subacute combined degeneration of the cord (📖 Vitamin B12 deficiency, p. 718).
- *Konzo:* myelopathy linked to chronic cyanide consumption in cassava.
- *Lathyrism:* linked to excessive chick pea consumption (e.g. in India).
- *Other causes:*
  - motor neuron disease (often mixed UMN and LMN signs, but no sensory loss)
  - syphilitic taboparesis (mixed UMN and LMN signs and sensory loss)
  - syringomyelia
  - intrinsic cord tumours.

Chronic flaccid paraparesis/weak legs

- *Peripheral neuropathies and myopathies:* check for arm involvement.
- *Tabes dorsalis:* see section on tertiary syphilis, 📖 Syphilis, p. 666).

Causes of absent knee jerks with extensor plantar responses

- Friedreich's ataxia.
- Motor neuron disease.
- Subacute combined degeneration of the cord.
- Diabetes mellitus.
- Syphilis.

Principles of management of paraplegia

- Emergency management of acute spinal cord or cauda equina compression (if applicable): imaging, consider surgical decompression, ± steroids.
- Prevention of pressure sores by turning every 2h.
- Attention to bladder and bowels (urinary catheter if incontinent).
- Ensure adequate hydration and nutrition.
- Prevent complications: aspiration and pneumonia (ensure adequate swallowing), DVT (support stockings/heparin), contractures (physiotherapy), malaria (mosquito net).
- Identify and treat the underlying cause.

Poliomyelitis (polio)

This disease, usually of young children, is caused by the poliovirus, an enterovirus. The virus selectively infects and destroys anterior horn cells in the spinal cord → acute flaccid paralysis (AFP), the cardinal sign of polio. The clinical disease is relatively uncommon, however: 99% of infected people show no paralytic manifestations.

Epidemiology

A worldwide effort is under way to eradicate polio by a combination of high immunization coverage, effective surveillance, and a rapid, vigorous response to the occurrence of new cases. Since 1988 the global annual incidence of polio has ↓ by 99% and the number of countries that remain polio endemic has ↓ from 125 to 4: Afghanistan, India, Nigeria, and Pakistan. In early 2012 India also announced interruption of wild poliovirus transmission, with no recorded new cases during the preceding year.

Transmission Via ingestion of faecally contaminated food or water, or via droplet spread from the respiratory tract.

Clinical features

Polio and other conditions in the WHO differential diagnosis of acute flaccid paralysis are summarized in Table 10.5. Prodromal symptoms of polio are common to many infections and practically indistinguishable: fever, malaise, headache, drowsiness, sore throat. In a minority, CNS disease (pre-paralytic disease) follows with abrupt onset of fever, headache, body pains, sensory disturbances, and neck stiffness, due to poliovirus meningitis. Flaccid paralysis then occurs in 65%, developing asymmetrically over a variable time, particularly affecting lower limbs with no sensory loss (although pain is characteristic). The paralysis rarely progresses for >3d or after the temperature falls. There is then some recovery of function over the following weeks or months, as some damaged anterior horn cells recover. Death is relatively uncommon, but results from aspiration or airway obstruction (bulbar paralysis) or respiratory failure (respiratory paralysis). A rare complication is slow deterioration of function after many years—the post-polio syndrome.

Diagnosis Is clinical, with retrospective serological analysis. Isolation of wild poliovirus from the stools confirms a case.

Management

Supportive. Paralytic polio is made worse by IM injections (e.g. of antibiotics) during pre-paralytic phase or by muscles becoming fatigued (e.g. after exercise), so a high index of suspicion in endemic regions is important to prevent polio being made worse. Avoid injections. Bed rest essential. Give analgesia, sedation. Patients must be carefully observed during onset of paralysis for signs of life-threatening bulbar and respiratory paralysis. Nurse patients with poor swallowing on their side. Good nursing care, including frequent suction and observations, may delay need for a tracheostomy. However, perform a tracheostomy early in serious cases.

Prevention Vaccination; improved sanitation, hygiene, and water supply.

Polio rehabilitation

Acute stage

- *Treatment:* based on rest and positioning.
- Support the wrist and hands (if affected) in a functional position with a splint or other support (e.g. pillow).
- Support the ankle (if affected) at 90° and avoid excessive inversion or eversion.

Subacute stage

- Progress from passive movements → active assisted movements→ active movements within the normal range.
- Progress → standing and walking with assistance—use walking aids if necessary (e.g. stick, crutches).
- Avoid:
  - muscle shortening
  - malformation due to muscle imbalance.

Table 10.5 WHO differential diagnosis of acute flaccid paralysis

	Polio	Guillain–Barré syndrome	Traumatic neuritis	Transverse myelitis
Onset of paralysis	24–48h, from onset to full paralysis	Hours to 10d	Hours to 4d	Hours to 4d
Flaccid paralysis	Usually acute, asymmetrical, principally proximal	Usually acute, symmetrical, and distal	Asymmetrical, acute, affecting one limb only	Acute, affecting lower limbs, symmetrical
Muscle tone	Reduced or absent in the affected limb	Global hypotonia	Reduced or absent in the affected limb	Hypotonia in lower limbs
Deep tendon reflexes	Decreased to absent	Globally absent	Decreased to absent	Absent in lower limbs early, increased late
Sensation	Severe myalgia, backache, no sensory changes	Cramps, tingling, hypoanaesthesia of palms/soles	Pain in gluteus muscles, hypothermia	Anaesthesia of lower limbs, sensory level
Cranial nerve	Only when bulbar involvement is present	Often present, affecting nerves VII, IX, X, XI, XII	Absent	Absent
Respiratory insufficiency	Only when bulbar involvement is present	In severe cases; worsened by bacterial pneumonia	Absent	Sometimes
CSF findings	Inflammatory	Albumin-cells dissociation	Normal	Normal or a few cells
Bladder dysfunction	Absent	Transient	Never	Present

Guillain–Barré syndrome

Guillain-Barré syndrome is an acute poly-radiculitis that symmetrically affects the spinal nerve roots and often the cranial nerve roots as well. GBS may be a consequence of preceding infection but in 60% cases no cause is identified. *Campylobacter jejuni* is the most commonly identified antecedent infection; other infectious causes include EBV, *Mycoplasma pneumonia*, *Herpes zoster*, Lyme disease, and diphtheria, usually preceding the onset of GBS by 1–2wks. GBS develops over a few hours (rarely), to several weeks, and is a medical emergency. Respiratory arrest may occur without notice in severe cases; sudden death may also be caused by the cardiovascular consequences of autonomic nervous system involvement. GBS patients need constant observation, in an ITU if possible.

Clinical features

Usually ascending weakness, which includes progressive symmetrical limb weakness of <4wks duration; distal paraesthesia (less often sensory loss) usually with total absence of deep tendon reflexes. Back and limb pain may be occasionally present. Also cranial nerve palsies (particularly VII); autonomic nervous system disturbances; ileus.

Management

Prognosis for spontaneous recovery is good. Treatment generally limited to supportive nursing care and prevention of complications. Monitor respiratory function and heart rhythm. Cases with rapid progression and respiratory insufficiency should be treated with plasma exchange or high-dose immunoglobulin 0.4g/kg on 5 successive days, if available; this ↓ hospital stay. Corticosteroids provide no benefit. Recovery occurs over several weeks or months with re-myelination of peripheral nerves.

Peripheral neuropathy

Peripheral neuropathy may affect individual peripheral or cranial nerves (mononeuropathies), or multiple nerves (polyneuropathies). Involvement of multiple individual nerves simultaneously is termed 'mononeuritis multiplex'.

Mononeuropathies

May arise from trauma (e.g. fractured fibula → common peroneal nerve palsy), compression (e.g. median nerve in carpal tunnel syndrome), diabetes or leprosy. Diabetes and leprosy may also → mononeuritis multiplex or widespread peripheral polyneuropathy.

Polyneuropathies

Usually affect the peripheries initially (the longest nerves are the most vulnerable to damage), producing a symmetrical glove and stocking distribution. In the tropics, environmental toxins and nutritional deficiencies are important causes (see Box 10.18). They may be seen in epidemic form after toxins are released into the environment by industry or in an endemic form in particular regions. Some toxins are used in traditional medicines or they may contaminate food, liquor, etc. They frequently produce a recognizable syndrome. As always, there is no replacement for local clinical experience. In these situations, treatment involves removal of the toxin and/or supplementation with the deficient nutrient. The effects of many neuropathies are permanent.

Causes of unilateral foot drop

Common peroneal nerve palsy (see causes of mononeuropathy); stroke; prolapsed vertebral disc; motor neuron disease; organophosphate poisoning; idiopathic.

Box 10.18 Causes of polyneuropathy

- *Vitamin and micronutrient deficiencies:* vitamin B1, B6, and B12; plus a variety of multiple nutrient deficiencies (see 📖 Chapter 17, Nutrition).
- *Toxins:*
  - *heavy metals*—including lead (motor involvement), thallium (found in rodenticides → alopecia), arsenic (Mee's nail lines, changes in skin pigmentation, skin cancers)
  - *drugs*—including isoniazid, ethambutol (affects optic nerve), sulfonamides, clioquinol, metronidazole, phenytoin, didanosine, stavudine
  - *industrial chemicals/solvents*—e.g. triorthocresyl phosphate
  - *pesticides*, particularly organophosphorous (OP) compounds
  - *excessive consumption of certain foods*—e.g. cassava containing a cyanogenic glycoside) can cause tropical ataxic neuropathy.
- *Metabolic diseases:* DM, renal/liver failure, alcohol, hypothyroidism.
- *Infections:* leprosy, HIV, syphilis.
- *Other:* genetic diseases, malignancy, connective tissue disease.

Leprosy

Leprosy (Hansen's disease) still elicits immense stigma in many communities. It is a chronic inflammatory disease affecting skin and peripheral nerves caused by *Mycobacterium leprae*. Presentation and progress are determined by the host cell-mediated immune response to the mycobacterium. Most people (>95%) develop an effective immune response and clear *M. leprae*. A minority are unable to do so and develop clinical leprosy. The clinical features then form a spectrum determined by the immune response, from tuberculoid (TBd) to lepromatous (LL) leprosy (see Table 10.6). At the TBd pole there is a strong immune response to the bacteria that limits bacillary growth (TBd is paucibacillary), but damages peripheral nerves and skin. At the LL pole, there is cellular anergy towards *M. leprae* with abundant bacillary multiplication (LL is multibacillary). Between these two poles are the borderline patients—borderline tuberculoid (BT), borderline (BB), and borderline lepromatous (BL)—reflecting the spectrum of immune response and bacterial load. The polar groups (TBd, LL) are stable, but the borderline groups are unstable and experience tissue-damaging reactions. The immune-mediated reactions that complicate leprosy are difficult to manage and require immune-suppresssion.

Transmission

Untreated lepromatous patients discharge bacilli from the nose. Infection occurs when *M. leprae* invades via the nasal mucosa with haematogenous spread → skin and nerve. Leprosy bacilli can survive for several days in the environment. People in close contact with infected people have a greater, but still small, chance of becoming infected. The incubation period is 2–5yrs for TBd cases and 8–12yrs for LL cases. HIV infection does not appear a risk factor for the development of leprosy.

Clinical features

- *Skin:* most common lesions are anaesthetic macules or plaques; more rarely, papules and nodules, or diffuse infiltration. Indeterminate leprosy is an early form of disease often found in screening programmes; lesions can last for months before resolving or progressing to established leprosy.
- *Nerve enlargement and damage:* occurs in peripheral nerve trunks (e.g. great auricular nerve (neck), ulnar nerve (elbow), radial-cutaneous nerve (wrist), median nerve (wrist), lateral popliteal nerve (neck of the fibula), and posterior tibial nerve (medial malleolus)), producing typical patterns of regional sensory and motor loss. Small dermal nerves also involved, producing patches of anaesthesia in TBd/BT lesions, and glove and stocking sensory loss in LL patients.
- *Other organ involvement:* eyes (may → blindness); bones (dactylitis, resorption); testes (orchitis, sterility); nasopharynx (nasal collapse).

Clinical presentations

Include skin lesions, weakness, and/or numbness due to peripheral neuropathy, or a burn/ulcer in an anaesthetic hand or foot. Borderline patients may present in reaction with nerve pain, sudden palsy, multiple new skin lesions, pain in the eye, or systemic febrile illness. The ulceration and digit loss seen in leprosy is due to 2° damage in neuropathic hands and feet and is not an intrinsic disease feature.

Diagnosis

Leprosy is present when one of three features is detected:

- A typical skin lesion (loss of sensation in TBd/BT patients).
- Thickened peripheral nerves.
- Skin smear from lesion edge/ear lobe positive for mycobacteria.

Test skin lesions for sensation. Palpate peripheral nerves to assess enlargement/tenderness. Assess nerve function by testing the small muscles' power and sensation in hands/feet. Many patients are unaware of their anaesthesia. Eye function should be checked (visual acuity, corneal sensation, and eyelid closure). Serology is not helpful.

Table 10.6 Clinical features of leprosy

Classification	Skin lesions	Nerve involvement
Indeterminate	Solitary hypopigmented 2–5cm lesion. Centre may show sensory loss although both doctor and patient are often uncertain about this loss. May become TBd-like.	None clinically detectable.
TBd	Lesions with well-defined borders and anaesthesia . The patch is dry (loss of sweating) and hairless.	May have one peripheral nerve affected. Occasionally presents as a mononeuropathy.
BT	Irregular plaques with raised edges and anaesthesia. Satellite lesions at the edges.	Asymmetrical peripheral nerve involvement
BB	Many lesions with punched out edges. Satellites are common.	Widespread nerve enlargement. Sensory and motor loss.
BL	Many lesions with diffuse borders and variable anesthesia.	As above.
LL	Numerous nodular skin lesions in a symmetrical distribution. Lesions are not dry or anaesthetic. There are often thickened shiny earlobes, loss of eyebrows, and skin thickening.	As above.

Management of leprosy

Chemotherapy to treat the infection

WHO regimens combine monthly supervised drug treatment with daily self-administration of a additional drug(s) (Table 10.7). More than 16 million people have been treated with these regimens. Relapse rates are 0.1%/yr. Clinical improvement is rapid and adverse reactions are rare. These drugs are considered safe during pregnancy and breastfeeding. Patients are classified for treatment by the number of skin lesions present: paucibacillary have 1–5; multibacillary >5.

Educate the patient about leprosy

Within 72h of starting chemotherapy, they are non-infectious and can lead a normal social life. No limitations on touching, sex, sharing utensils. Leprosy is not a curse from God or a punishment. Gross deformities are not inevitable endpoint of disease. Care and awareness of limbs are as important as chemotherapy.

Prevent disability

Monitor sensation and muscle power in patient's hands, feet, and eyes as part of routine follow-up, so that new nerve damage is detected early. Treat any new damage with prednisolone 40mg daily, reducing by 5mg/day each month. Patient self-awareness is crucial in minimizing damage. Patients with anaesthetic hands or feet need to inspect hands and feet (using a mirror) daily for injuries or infection and dress wounds immediately. Protect hands and feet from trauma ('trainers' are excellent shoes for anaesthetic feet). Identify the cause of any injury so that it can be avoided. Soak dry hands and feet in water and then rub with oil to keep skin moist.

Manage complications

Ulcers in anaesthetic feet are the most common cause of hospitalization. Ulceration is treated by rest and cleaning. Ulcers should be carefully probed to detect osteomyelitis and sinuses that require surgical debridement. Unlike ulcers in diabetic or ischaemic feet, ulcers in leprosy heal if they are protected from weight-bearing. No weight-bearing is permitted until ulcer heals. Ensure appropriate footwear to prevent recurrence.

Support the patient socially and psychologically.

Table 10.7 WHO recommended multi-drug therapy regimes

Leprosy type	Drug treatment		Duration
	Monthly plus supervised	Daily self-administered	
Paucibacillary (1–5 skin lesions)	Rifampicin 600mg	Dapsone 100mg	6mths
Multibacillary (>5 skin lesions)	Rifampicin 600mg + Clofazimine 300mg	Dapsone 100mg + Clofazimine 50mg	12mths

Reactions

Immune-medicated, tissue-damaging phenomena that may occur before, during, or after treatment. Reactions are important because they are common, recurrent and require prompt treatment to prevent serious nerve damage. Presentation and management of reactions are summarized in Box 10.19. Do not stop chemotherapy during a reaction. Patients with difficult reactions should be discussed with an expert in leprosy (e.g. regional government leprosy officers, international leprosy non-governmental organization (NGOs)).

Box 10.19 Reversal reaction (type 1 reaction)

Due to delayed type hypersensitivity and occurs in 30% patients with borderline leprosy. Skin lesions become erythematous; peripheral nerves become tender and painful. Loss of nerve function can be sudden, with foot-drop occurring overnight. Neuritis may occur without skin lesions or in a clinically silent form without nerve tenderness.

Management

For severe reactions, prednisolone 40–60mg po od reduced every 2–4wks over 20wks. A few patients may require 15–20mg prednisolone daily for many months. Response rates vary depending on the severity of initial damage but even promptly treated nerve damage will only improve in 60% cases.

Erythema nodosum leprosum (ENL) (type 2 reaction)

This is due to immune complex deposition and occurs in 20% LL and 5% BL patients. It manifests with malaise, fever, and crops of painful red nodules that become purple and then resolve. If severe, plaques may form with necrosis and ulceration. Iritis is common; other signs are bone pain and swollen joints, painful neuritis, lymphadenopathy, iridocyclitis, orchitis, nephritis (rarely).

Management

In moderate and severe cases (systemic features or painful nerves), treat in hospital with one of:

- Prednisolone 60–80mg po od, reduced after 2wks by 5–10mg every 2wks (best for short episodes).
- Thalidomide 400mg nightly for 4wks. Once a satisfactory response, ↓ by 50mg every 2–4wks (best drug, but contraindicated in women of childbearing age and often not available; causes drowsiness).
- Clofazimine 300mg daily, reduced after 3mths (preferred drug for premenopausal women; takes 3–4wks to have full effect so should be combined with prednisolone initially). Causes brown skin staining.
- Treat iridocyclitis with steroid and homatropine eye drops.

ENL is difficult to treat. Some patients develop a chronic relapsing form, which may last for up to 5yrs, but will then resolve.

Chapter 11
Haematology

Invited authors **Sara Ghorashian**
Subarna Chakravorty

Anaemia

Introduction

Anaemia (see Table 11.1) affects ~ 70% of children and pregnant women in resource-poor countries. A slight ↓ in Hb is a physiological response to pregnancy, due to an ↑ in the plasma:RBC ratio. Anaemia in pregnancy is associated with 25–40% of maternal deaths.

Causes of anaemia

Anaemia is due to ↓ red blood cell (RBC) production or ↑ RBC loss/haemolysis (see Tables 11.2 and 11.3); More than one cause may be present. Younger RBCs (reticulocytes) appear 'bluer' on a blood film → polychromasia. Reticulocytes ↑ if RBC loss and ↓ if RBC production is impaired. The blood film morphology, degree of reticulocytosis, and the size of RBCs (i.e. mean cell volume—MCV) are helpful in determining the cause (see Box 11.2).

Severe anaemia is usually multifactorial. Infections (HIV, bacteraemia, malaria, hookworm), nutritional deficiency (vitamins B12, A, Fe) and blood loss are most common associated causes of severe anaemia.

Table 11.1 WHO definitions of anaemia

Age	Hb (g/dL)
6–59mths	<11.0
5–11yrs	<11.5
12–14yrs	<12.0
Non-pregnant women	<12.0
Pregnant women	<11.0
Men	<13.0

Table 11.2 Causes of anaemia due to ↓ RBC production

Aetiology	Clinical findings	Laboratory tests
Iron, folate, and B12 deficiency		
Iron	Koilonychia, angular stomatitis, oesophageal webs	↓ MCV, MCH, MCHC, RBC count, ferritin, serum Fe, transferrin saturation; ↑ TIBC. Blood film: pencil cells.
Folate and vitamin B12	Glossitis, ↑ skin pigmentation, sub-acute combined degeneration of the cord (vitamin B12 only)	↓ Platelets ↓ WCC↑ MCV, MCH; normal MCHC. Blood film: oval macrocytes, hypersegmented neutrophils
↓ Erythropoietin		
Renal failure		Normocytic anaemia
		Blood film: 'burr cells'
Anaemia of chronic inflammation		
	Features specific to the underlying condition	Normocytic anaemia, ↓ serum Fe, TIBC; ↓/normal transferrin saturation/ normal ferritin
Bone marrow suppression or dysfunction		
Drugs (e.g. cytotoxics), aplastic anaemia, malignant infiltration, alcoholism, hypothyroidism, myelodysplasia	Features specific to underlying condition	↓ Platelets and WBC normal/↑ MCV

Table 11.3 Causes of anaemia due to ↑ RBC loss and haemolysis

Aetiology	Clinical findings	Laboratory tests
↑RBC loss		↑ Reticulocyte count, polychromasia (unless acute)
Haemorrhage		
Acute (e.g. post-partum, trauma)	Shock (tachycardia, hypotension, cold extremities)	MCV normal, Hb, and HCT initially normal
Chronic, (e.g. peptic ulcer, hookworm, schistosomiasis)	Black stools, haematuria	Fe deficiency, ↑ platelets, stool/ urine for parasites
Haemolytic anaemias	Jaundice, dark urine	↑ Bilirubin and LDH
Inherited		
Haemoglobinopathies, e.g. sickle cell disease, thalassaemia	FHx anaemia, ↓ growth, hepato-splenomegaly, gallstones, leg ulcers	Blood film, haemoglobin electrophoresis, high performance liquid chromatography (HPLC)
Enzymopathies, e.g. G6PD deficiency	FHx, gallstones, infection or recent drug ingestion	Intravascular haemolysis, e.g. ↓ haptoglobins, haemoglobinuria, haemosiderinuria
Membranopathy, e.g. hereditary spherocytosis	FHx, splenomegaly, gallstones	Extravascular haemolysis (↑conjugated bilirubin, urobilinogen); blood film (spherocytes)
Acquired: immune		
Allo-immune, e.g. post-transfusion, haemolytic disease of the newborn	Transfusion <10d	Blood film (spherocytes), +ve direct Coombs' test RBC antibodies
Auto-immune, e.g. antibody-mediated, drug-induced	Underlying infection, lymphoma, auto-immune disease, discoloured extremities (cold antibody)	Blood film (spherocytes), +ve direct Coombs' test RBC antibodies, RBC agglutination (cold antibodies)
Acquired: non-immune		
Infections, e.g. malaria, bartonellosis, parvovirus B19, clostridial sepsis	Underlying infection	Blood film (malaria, bartonella)
Others, e.g. micro-angiopathic haemolysis, burns, snake bite		Blood film (RBC fragmentation), thrombocytopenia, renal failure

Clinical features of anaemia

History

Symptoms of anaemia depend on the rapidity of onset and severity. Chronic anaemia may be asymptomatic because of a compensatory ↑ in cardiac output. Symptoms are usually non-specific: fatigue, headache, dizziness, syncope, dyspnoea, palpitations, ↓ work or intellectual capacity. Anaemia may also exacerbate pre-existing intermittent claudication or angina.

The history is important in determining the cause(s) of anaemia:

- Previous and family Hx of anaemia suggests an inherited disorder, e.g. haemoglobinopathy or G6PD deficiency.
- Haemolysis may be suggested by splenomegaly, jaundice, and dark urine, and may be precipitated by infections.
- Blood loss can be revealed from colour of stools, haematuria, and menstrual history. Ask about recent surgery, childbirth, or trauma.
- Occupation may be important, e.g. fishermen may be prone to schistosomiasis and rice farmers to hookworm infection.
- Poor diet may suggest a nutritional deficiency.
- Chronic infections, such as HIV and TB, renal failure, rheumatoid arthritis, or drugs used to treat these conditions may be associated with anaemia.

Examination

Clinical assessment has low sensitivity and specificity for mild–moderate anaemia. Signs include:

- Pallor of mucous membranes or nail beds (sensitivity 50–70% for moderate to severe anaemia).
- A compensatory hyperdynamic circulation (tachycardia, bounding pulse, cardiomegaly, systolic flow murmur).
- Severe, decompensated anaemia → shock (i.e. thirst, sweating, cold extremities, hypotension, and cardiac failure). These signs warrant fluid replacement or, where it can be performed safely, blood transfusion (see 📖 Blood transfusion, p. 518).

Laboratory diagnosis of anaemia

Measure the Hb or PCV (or haematocrit) of venous or capillary blood. For capillary samples from a finger or heel prick, the first few drops of blood should be wiped away to encourage free flow. Avoid squeezing—tissue fluid causes dilution (Box 11.1).

Box 11.1 Measuring Hb

- Hb can be measured photometrically, but this requires laboratory equipment and skill.
- The HemoCue Hb301 system is portable, battery-operated, and designed for accurate measurement of Hb in tropical conditions. It uses whole blood, and is simple and rapid.
- The WHO Hb colour scale can be used where no power or equipment is available and an approximate Hb estimation is adequate. The colour of a drop of blood on chromatography paper is matched against a colour scale representing blood of Hb in 2g/dL increments (range 4–14g/dL). It is simple and cheap, but the correct filter paper must be used and it must be read under good light.
- Measurement of PCV or haematocrit (HCT) requires a microhaematocrit centrifuge and electricity but can be carried out by non-technical staff. Blood is taken into capillary tubes from a finger prick and centrifuged for 5min. This separates cells and plasma and the ratio of the length of RBC column to the total length of the blood sample = HCT (%). Where only HCT available, Hb (g/dL) may be crudely estimated as ~1/3 of the HCT (%).The accuracy of this estimation varies with age and Hb level, and is least accurate in children < 5yrs.

Box 11.2 Classification of anaemia according to RBC size*

Microcytic (low MCV)

- Iron deficiency
- Thalassaemia
- Anaemia of inflammation
- Lead poisoning
- Sideroblastic anaemia

Normocytic (normal MCV)

- Acute blood loss
- Anaemia of inflammation
- Marrow hypoplasia or infiltration
- Chronic infection
- Renal failure

Macrocytic (high MCV)

- Folate deficiency
- B12 deficiency
- Drugs affecting DNA metabolism
- Rare enzyme defects
- No megaloblasts in bone marrow
- Myelodysplasia
- Alcohol
- Liver dysfunction
- Hypothyroidism
- Haemolytic anaemia
- Neonate (normal)
- Megaloblasts in bone marrow

* Normal MCV = 76–96fL

Iron-deficiency anaemia

This is one of the most common causes of anaemia worldwide.

Causes of iron (Fe) deficiency

- ↑ *Fe losses:* menstrual, gastrointestinal infections (e.g. hookworm, whipworm, amoebiasis), peptic ulceration, carcinoma, oesophageal varices, haemoptysis, haematuria.
- ↑ *Fe requirements:* lactation, puberty, infancy (Box 11.3).
- ↓ *Intake:* ingestion of only milk (human or cow's) beyond 6mths of age; lack of red meat and/or legumes.
- ↓*Fe absorption:* ingesting inhibitors of Fe absorption with meals (tea, milk, phytates present in grain); achlorhydria, malabsorption.

Clinical features

Brittle nails, koilonychia, angular stomatitis, glossitis, dysphagia (Plummer–Vinson syndrome = Fe def anaemia + oesophageal web).

Laboratory features

(See Box 11.1). Low serum ferritin (<20micrograms/L) is specific, but can be insensitive as it is an acute phase protein. Ferritin >100micrograms/L generally excludes Fe deficiency, even in the setting of infection.

Management

- Ferrous sulphate 200mg tds. Expect ↑ in Hb 1–3g/dL after 4wks of therapy if Fe deficiency is the cause of anaemia (this can be used as a diagnostic test). Continue Fe therapy for 3mths after normalization of Hb to replenish stores.
- Identify and treat the underlying cause and any other haematinic deficiencies (e.g. folate).
- Severe anaemia + signs of heart failure may require blood transfusion.

Notes

- Severely malnourished children should not receive Fe supplements until at least 15d into a feeding programme because ↑ risk of bacterial sepsis and toxicity related to free radicals.
- To improve absorption, oral Fe preparations should be taken between meals and with vitamin C (e.g. orange juice, ascorbic acid tablets).
- Oral Fe should not be taken with antibiotics or antacids.
- Side-effects include GI upset (try lower dose or take with meals), constipation, green/black stools.

Box 11.3 Maternal and infant anaemia

Fe deficiency particularly affects children, and pregnant or breastfeeding women. Mothers are at risk of anaemia during pregnancy, delivery, and lactation. Supplementary maternal iron or iron + folic acid can prevent anaemia and iron deficiency at term. If the mother has sufficient Fe stores, a neonate is born with enough stores to last 6mths. After 6mths, Fe requirements must be met from the diet; requirements ↑ with rate of growth. Useful guidance on reproductive health topics are at:
http://apps.who.int/rhl/pregnancy_childbirth/en/
http://apps.who.int/rhl/newborn/en/

Prevention of iron deficiency

- *Nutritional advice:* eat meat and legumes with vitamin C (e.g. orange juice) and avoid tea, dairy products, or cereals as these ↓ Fe absorption.
- *Prophylactic Fe supplements:* the WHO recommends these for women of child-bearing age and children >6mths where the prevalence of anaemia is >40%. However, these guidelines are controversial because of ↑ malaria and other infections when supplements given to children in malarial areas, and an absence of studies investigating improved clinical outcomes in pregnancy. Supervised weekly/twice weekly supplementation is effective for the prevention of Fe deficiency in school children.
- *Anti-helminthics:* empiric treatment may be helpful in those with anaemia where helminth infections are common.

Anaemia of inflammation

This anaemia is associated with chronic inflammatory or malignant disease. There is ↓ RBC production, abnormalities of Fe utilization, and ↓ erythropoietin levels and/or response. These abnormalities are mediated by inflammatory cytokines and production of hepcidin, which blocks the release of Fe from enterocytes and macrophages.

Causes of chronic inflammatory disease

- *Infectious:* e.g. TB, HIV, lung abscess, osteomyelitis, pneumonia, SBE.
- *Non-infectious:* e.g. RA, SLE, other connective tissue disorders, sarcoidosis, Crohn's disease.
- *Malignancy:* e.g. carcinoma, lymphoma, sarcoma.

Differential diagnosis: anaemia of chronic renal failure, hypothyroidism, hypopituitarism, other microcytic anaemias (see Box 11.2).

Clinical features Are of anaemia, as well as those relating to underlying diagnosis.

Diagnosis Laboratory features: mild normocytic (occasionally microcytic), normochromic anaemia. Low reticulocyte count for degree of anaemia. ↓ serum Fe and TIBC. Normal or ↑ serum ferritin and a low/normal transferrin saturation. ↑ ESR, CRP.

Management

- *Treat underlying cause:* blood transfusions are a last resort, but may be more practical in the field. Fe overload may complicate repeated transfusions (see 📖 Blood transfusion, p. 518).
- Anaemia of inflammation may be complicated by another form of anaemia (e.g. Fe, vitamin B12, or folate deficiency), renal failure, bone marrow failure, hypersplenism, or endocrine abnormality.
- Ferritin <100micrograms/L may suggest concomitant Fe deficiency, but there is little response to oral Fe because of the block of Fe uptake in the small bowel. IV Fe may be required (Box 11.4).

Box 11.4 Intravenous iron

Failure to respond to oral Fe may be due to malabsorption, poor compliance, ongoing Fe loss, concomitant anaemia of chronic disease, or an erroneous diagnosis. The first three may respond to IV iron thereby preventing the need for transfusion. The first dose should be given slowly because of the risk of adverse reactions (e.g. anaphylaxis, local irritation). IM iron injections are not recommended because they are painful, there is a risk of abscess formation, and absorption is unpredictable.

Macrocytic anaemias

Folate deficiency

Folic acid is present in green vegetables and fruits. It is absorbed in the duodenum and jejunum. The body's stores of folate are limited and clinical deficiency occurs <2mths. States of rapid cell division (e.g. pregnancy, haemolytic anaemia) ↑ folate utilization and require prophylaxis. ↓ dietary intake (e.g. in alcoholics, the malnourished) can also → deficiency. Combined B12 and folate deficiency is common (see Table 11.4).

Vitamin B12 deficiency

Vitamin B12 is present in meat or dairy products. The complex absorption of vitamin B12 requires proteases and binding factors released in the stomach and combination with intrinsic factor before uptake in the terminal ileum. Deficiency may result from a block at any stage. Stores of vitamin B12 take 2–3yrs to deplete. Vitamin B12 is essential for DNA production. Folate acts as a co-factor, hence, similarity of their deficiency states. There are unique neurological manifestations of B12 deficiency.

Clinical features

Mild jaundice, glossitis, angular stomatitis, purpura (↓ platelets), sterility, skin pigmentation, and ↑ susceptibility to infections. Neuropathy, subacute combined degeneration of the cord (↓ vibration sense, hypertonia, weakness, and sensory ataxia see 📖 Neurology, p. 429), psychosis, and dementia are specific to a lack of vitamin B12.

Laboratory findings

↑ MCV and MCH, normal MCHC, ↓ reticulocyte count, ↓ WCC and ↓ platelets in severe cases.

Blood film

Oval macrocytes, hypersegmented neutrophils. Mildly ↑ unconjugated bilirubin and ↑ LDH because of ineffective erythropoiesis. ↓ serum B12 and folate levels (though mildly low levels may be misleading). Measuring RBC folate, homocysteine and methylmalonic acid levels ↑ accuracy.

Management

Replacement therapy

- *Folic acid 5mg oral od for 4mths*; maintenance requirements depend on underlying disease. Consider co-existing B12 deficiency and replace empirically if necessary (replacing folate alone may → neurological complications in combined deficiency).
- *Hydroxocobalamin (vitamin B12):* 6 injections of 1mg IM over 1–2wks and maintenance with 1mg every 3mths. Oral vitamin B12 can be given if malabsorption is excluded. Anaemia should resolve over months.

Prophylaxis

Improve diet. Consider prophylactic treatment (e.g. folic acid 400micrograms/day) in pregnancy, severe haemolytic anaemia, after partial gastrectomy and ileal resection.

Table 11.4 Causes of folate and B12 deficiencies

	Folate	Vitamin B12
↓ Intake	Seasonal shortage Boiling bottle feeds Prolonged storage of food Anorexia Famine Inappropriate weaning foods Prolonged cooking/reheating Feeding infants with goat's milk Alcoholism	Breastfeeding by B12-deficient mothers Strict veganism Alcoholism
Malabsorption	Diarrhoea in infancy Acute enteric infections *Giardia lamblia* Systemic infections (TB, pneumococcus) Strongyloides Coeliac disease Crohn's disease	Pernicious anaemia Gastrectomy Chronic *G. Lamblia* HIV infection Ileocaecal TB Strongyloides Tropical sprue Crohn's disease Fish tapeworm
↑Physiological demands	Growth Pregnancy/lactation	
↑Pathological demands	Haemolysis Malignant disease	
Metabolic		Nitrous oxide Chronic cyanide Intoxication (Cassava)

Haemolytic anaemias

In haemolysis, RBCs are broken down and their components metabolized in the reticuloendothelial system (RES), in the hepatic and splenic sinusoids. Under certain circumstances (e.g. sickling crisis, severe oxidative damage), RBC lyse within the circulation. RBC normally remain in the circulation for ~120d, but their lifespan can be ↓ due to abnormalities inside the RBC (e.g. haemoglobinopathies, enzymopathies), in/on their membrane (e.g. structural defects, deposition of antibody or complement), or due to mechanisms arising outside the RBC. Normally, the bone marrow is able to compensate up to 5× faster RBC turnover (compensated haemolysis); if haemolysis exceeds this or there are haematinic deficiencies or associated disease, anaemia results.

Laboratory findings

- ↑*RBC destruction:* unconjugated hyperbilirubinaemia, ↑ LDH, ↑ urinary urobilinogen, ↑ faecal urobilinogen.
- ↑ *RBC production:* polychromasia, reticulocytosis causing ↑ MCV.
- *Intravascular haemolysis:* ↓/absent haptoglobins, ↓ haemopexin, ↑ ↑ haem/methaemoglobin, +ve Schumm's test (methaemalbumin), haemosiderinuria, haem/methaemoglobinuria.

Genetic abnormalities of RBCs are common in the tropics. Despite the disadvantage of haemolytic anaemia in homozygotes, they persist in populations because the heterozygous state provides some protection against severe malaria. This is by altering the environment within the RBC or by conferring resistance to various stages in the parasite's lifecycle.

Red cell membranopathies

Conditions may provide a degree of protection against malaria due to ↓ penetration of the RBC by merozoites.

Hereditary spherocytosis

Usually autosomal dominant. Mainly found in North Europeans.

- *Clinical features variable:* +ve family history, mild anaemia (8–12g/dL), intermittent jaundice, splenomegaly, cholelithiasis.
- *Diagnosis:* blood film shows spherocytes, ↑ MCH, ↑ reticulocytes, ↑ lysis in osmotic tests, membrane protein analysis by SDS-PAGE, ve direct antiglobulin test.
- *Management:* folic acid 5mg/d. Splenectomy for those most severely affected (see 📖 Splenomegaly, p. 528).

Hereditary elliptocytosis

Autosomal dominant. Usually asymptomatic; haemolysis may be severe in homozygotes. There may be episodes of jaundice and moderate splenomegaly following infections.

- *Diagnosis:* elliptical RBCs, parental studies, membrane protein analysis by SDS-PAGE.
- *Management:* is not usually required; folic acid supplements and splenectomy may help if haemolysis is significant.

Southeast Asian hereditary ovalocytosis Autosomal dominant. Common in Malaysia, Indonesia, Philippines, Papua New Guinea, and Solomon Islands. Not associated with haemolytic anaemia (Box 11.5).

Box 11.5 Acquired haemolytic anaemia

- *Drug-induced immune haemolytic anaemia:* occurs when drugs bind to RBCs (e.g. high-dose penicillin), form new RBC antigens (e.g. quinidine), or provoke auto-antibodies (methyldopa, mefenamic acid, levodopa). A careful drug history (incl. herbal preparations) is crucial.
- *Autoimmune haemolytic anaemia:* can be caused by cold (IgM) or warm (IgG) antibodies. They may be 1° (idiopathic) or 2° to lymphoproliferative disorders, malignancy, autoimmune diseases, or infections. The direct anti-globulin (Coombs' test) test is positive because the patient's RBCs are antibody-coated.
- *Warm AHA:* presents as chronic or acute haemolytic anaemia with splenomegaly. Treat any underlying causes. Specific therapy is with steroids (e.g. prednisolone 1mg/kg daily) until Hb>10 g/dL, then gradually reduce. Splenectomy is an option if steroids fail. Blood transfusion may be required in severe cases.
- *Cold AHA:* presents as chronic anaemia made worse by cold; associated with Raynaud's phenomenon and acrocyanosis. Management involves treating underlying cause; steroids are not helpful. Advise the patient to keep warm. Chlorambucil can be helpful if underlying lymphoma. Splenectomy does not usually help as IgM-coated cells are removed in the liver.
- *Paroxysmal cold haemoglobinuria:* may occur after mumps, measles, chickenpox, syphilis, especially in children.

Glucose-6-phosphate dehydrogenase deficiency

G6PD deficiency predisposes to oxidative damage of the RBC and haemolysis. Fig. 11.1 shows world distribution of G6PD deficiency, which affects 400 million people. Superimposed are three zones where different G6PD variants occur: zone I (GdMediterranean), zone II (GdMediterranean, GdCanton, GdUnion, GdMahidol), and zone III (GdA). These have different severities. GdA causes moderate, intermittent haemolysis, whereas GdMediterranean and GdCanton are more severe. G6PD deficiency is x-linked, so more common in males.

Clinical features Most affected people are asymptomatic, but episodic haemolysis may be severe and intravascular in nature, particularly in non-African mutations. Chronic haemolysis is unusual. In Africa, adults with G6PD deficiency usually only suffer mild haemolysis but neonates may develop severe hyperbilirubinaemia and kernicterus. Haemolytic episodes are precipitated by infection and, to a lesser extent, drugs.

Diagnosis

- *Between attacks:* tests of G6PD enzyme activity detect hemizygous males and heterozygous women.
- *During a crisis:* blood film may show 'bite' and 'blister' cells. Testing during a crisis often unhelpful because haemolysis eliminates older RBCs, which have lowest G6PD activity, so only youngest RBCs (which may have normal G6PD activity) remain. Following crisis, delay testing for 6wks. In more severe variants, a greater proportion of RBCs have low G6PD.

Management

- *Treat underlying infection:* avoid drugs that precipitate haemolysis (Box 11.6).
- Withdraw any drug that could have precipitated the crisis.
- Maintain a high urine output
- Give folic acid supplements if recurrent haemolysis
- *G6PD-deficient babies are prone to neonatal jaundice:* phototherapy and exchange transfusion may be necessary.

Box 11.6 Examples of drugs to be avoided in G6PD deficiency

- *Antimalarials:* primaquine, Fansidar®, Maloprim®.
- *Sulfonamides/sulphones:* co-trimoxazole, sulfanilamide, dapsone, sulfasalazine, sulfamethoxazole.
- *Antibiotics:* nitrofurans, nalidixic acid.
- *Analgesics:* phenacetin.
- *Antihelminths:* naphthol, stibophen, nitrodazole.
- *Miscellaneous:* naphthalene, fava beans, methylene blue, trinitrotoluene, amylnitrates, phenylhydrazine.

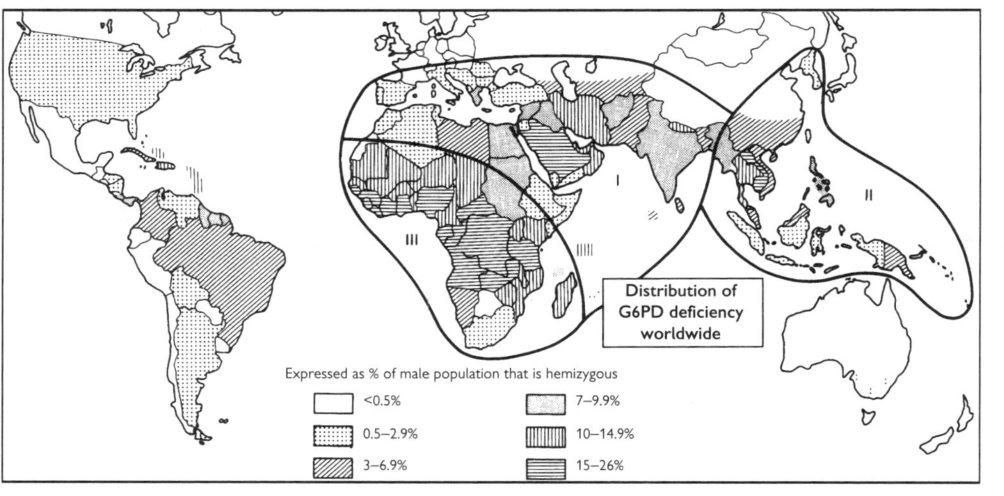

Fig. 11.1 Global distribution of G6PD deficiency.

Sickle cell anaemia

The sickle gene is common in equatorial Africa (frequency up to 25%), Saudi Arabia, and southern Asia, but less common in the Mediterranean and the mixed populations of the Americas (frequency 5%) (see Fig. 11.2). Due to single point mutation in Hb β-globin gene chain. When deoxygenated, HbS molecules polymerize into elongated structures causing RBCs to deform and haemolyse. Sickled RBCs are rigid and block the microcirculation in various organs → infarcts (see Fig. 11.3).

The heterozygous (sickle trait; HbAS) is generally asymptomatic; it provides protection against malaria. Sickle cell disease occurs with homozygous inheritance (HbSS) or co-inheritance of another β-globin chain disorder such as HbC (see 📖 Other sickling syndromes, p. 510). Sickle cell disease and G6PD deficiency may occur together because of the high prevalence of both conditions in some regions.

Other sickling syndromes

- *HbSC disease* occurs in west Africa. There is less haemolysis than with HbSS. May present only in adulthood. Splenomegaly is common. Anaemia is less severe than in HbSS but vaso-occlusive complications (e.g. avascular necrosis, proliferative retinopathy) are prominent and may → significant disability in adulthood. Electrophoresis shows two haemoglobin bands, HbS and HbC. The blood film has many target cells and irregularly contracted cells.
- *HbSB^0 thalassaemia:* occurs mostly in North Africa, Sicily, and mixed populations of the Americas. Clinically similar to HbSS, there is a lower incidence of stroke. The blood film shows hypochromic microcytic RBCs and target cells. Hb electrophoresis shows HbS, absence of HbA, and elevated HbA2 and HbF. Definitive diagnosis can be made by parental studies or DNA analysis.
- *HbSB$^+$ thalassaemia:* most commonly seen in West Africa. The clinical course and degree of anaemia is milder than HbSS. Proliferative retinopathy occurs. Definitive diagnosis with Hb electrophoresis shows HbA 5–30%, HbS 70–95%.
- *HbSD^{Punjab} and HbSO^{Arab}:* as severe as HbSS. HbD occurs in Sikh and mixed populations.
- *HbSE, HbS^{Lepore}, and HbSHPFH:* (hereditary persistence of foetal haemoglobin). All these conditions have a mild clinical course compared to HbSS.

Clinical features of sickle cell anaemia

Severe haemolytic anaemia punctuated by severe pain crises. Young patients alternate periods of good health with acute crises. Later, chronic ill health supervenes due to organ damage. Symptoms begin after 6mths of age as the HbF level ↓. The first signs are often of acute dactylitis due to occlusive necrosis of the small bones of the hands and feet, → digits of varying length. The long bones are affected in older children and adults. Anaemia (Hb 6–8g/dL; reticulocytes 10–20%) is well–tolerated because of cardiac compensation and a lower affinity of HbS for O_2.

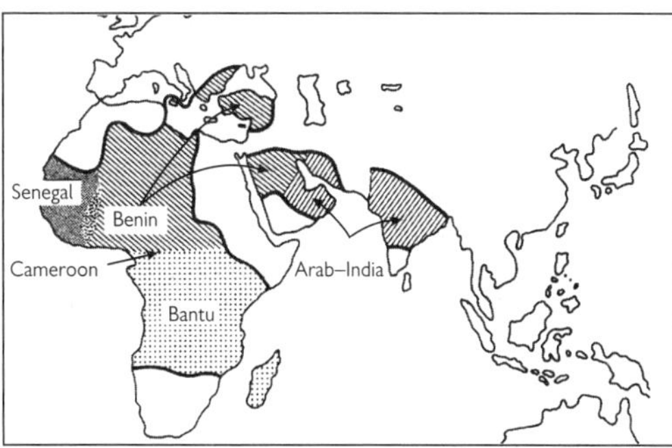

Fig. 11.2 Distribution of haemoglobin S gene and its various haplotypes (Arab-India, Bantu, Benin, Cameroon, Senegal) in the Mediterranean and West Asia.

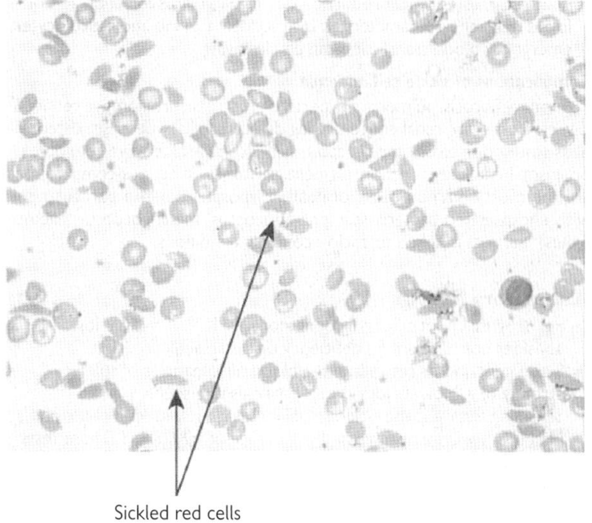

Fig. 11.3 Characteristic sickle-shaped RBCs in peripheral blood film in patient with homozygous sickle cell anaemia. (Reproduced from Provan D, Oxford Handbook of Clinical and Laboratory Investigation 3e (2010), with permission of Oxford University Press.)

The severity of complications depends on a number of factors including the proportion of non-sickle Hb molecules (e.g. HbF) and the ratio of α to β globin chains, which may be modified by concomitant α thalassaemia trait or conditions affecting β-globin chain production.

Types of crises

- *Painful vascular-occlusive:* frequent, precipitated by infections, acidosis, dehydration, or hypoxia. Infarcts often occur in the axial skeleton, lungs, and spleen. Repeated splenic infarction → hyposplenism in adulthood. Crises can involve the CNS (in 7% of patients) and spinal cord.
- *Visceral sequestration:* due to sickling within organs and pooling of blood. Requires emergency transfusion.
- *Chest:* pulmonary infiltrates on CXR, fever, chest pain, tachypnoea, cough, wheeze. There is often concomitant infection, microvascular occlusion, and bronchoconstriction. Chest crises can arise during a painful crisis; patients should be monitored carefully for this complication, which can be fatal.
- *Haemolytic:* ↑ rate of haemolysis with fall in Hb. Usually accompanying a painful crisis. Concomitant G6PD deficiency may worsen haemolysis.
- *Aplastic:* arrested RBC production due to parvovirus infection and/or folate deficiency. Characterized by a sudden ↓ in Hb and reticulocytes; emergency blood transfusion can be life-saving.

Complications of sickle cell anaemia

Pulmonary fibrosis, pulmonary hypertension, stroke, proliferative retinopathy, cardiomegaly, renal concentrating defect, papillary necrosis, osteomyelitis (often due to *Salmonella* spp.), skin ulcers, proliferative retinopathy, priapism, hepatic dysfunction, pigment gallstones. Infectious complications are the most common cause of death. Hyposplenism → a particular risk with encapsulated bacteria (e.g. pneumococcus, meningococcus, haemophilus). Survival is linked to socio-economic conditions.

Laboratory findings

- Hb 6–8g/dL, ↑ reticulocyte count, normal MCV. If is MCV low, consider concomitant Fe deficiency or thalassaemia.
- Sickle cells and target cells in the blood film; features of splenic atrophy (e.g. Howell–Jolly bodies) may also be seen.
- *Screening tests:* e.g. the sickle solubility test (e.g. with dithionate and Na_2HPO^4) will be positive in the presence of >20% HbS. These tests are also positive in sickle cell trait and compound heterozygotes. They are widely available. False –ve results occur in infants <6mths because of the predominance of HbF.
- *Detection of HbS or other Hb variants:* Hb electrophoresis, iso-electric focusing, and HPLC. Some of these tests provide quantification of the abnormal Hb, but are likely to be available only at referral centres. Expect 30–40% HbS with HbAS (≤35% with concomitant α thalassaemia), >80% with HbSS.

Sickle cell disease and pregnancy

- Sickle cell disease → intrauterine growth retardation, pre-eclampsia, pre-term labour, *in utero* foetal death, and ↑ risk of sickle-related complications in the mother.
- Sickle cell trait is not a problem, except UTIs are more common.
- Early access to antenatal care is important to allow monitoring for these complications.
- Folic acid supplements are essential to prevent megaloblastic anaemia and birth defects.
- Delivery should be non-operative where possible. Consider pre-operative exchange transfusion before Caesarian section in complicated pregnancies.
- Test neonate for Hb variants, may need to confirm at 3–6mths.

Sickle cell disease and surgery

The incidence of severe complications is 30–60%, depending on the procedure. Improved outcomes are shown with either top-up or exchange transfusions. Chest physiotherapy is useful. Minor operations can be carried out safely without pre-op transfusion, providing patients are well-hydrated.

Management (Box 11.7)

Painful sickling crises

Acute pain is the most common reason to seek medical attention:

- Exclude other causes of pain.
- *Keep hydrated:* oral, NG, or IV (if other routes have failed).
- Keep the patient warm.
- O_2 therapy is only necessary if hypoxic.
- *Effective pain relief:* can ↓ time spent in hospital; under-treating can → drug-seeking behaviour and a pain-orientated personality.
- Parenteral opiates are often required, but IM route can → abscesses. Monitor response to analgesia; use a pictorial pain scale in children.
- *Oral analgesia:* NSAIDs are good for bone pain. Give with ulcer-protection (e.g. H2-receptor antagonist or PPI) and monitor renal function. Oral opioids are effective.
- *Inhaled NO:* risk of subacute combined degeneration of cord with repeated/prolonged use.

Infections

- Infections are common causes of death in sickle cell anaemia.
- *Treat bacteraemia rapidly:* start antibiotics empirically if febrile and acutely unwell. Greatest mortality from sepsis with encapsulated organisms; cover *S. pneumoniae*, Hib, *N. meningitidis* (e.g. ceftriaxone 2g od). Where microbiological diagnosis is possible, send urine and blood for culture, do LP if features of meningitis, CXR for suspected pneumonia/chest syndrome.
- *Proven/suspected meningitis:* treat with ceftriaxone for 2wks.
- *Acute chest syndrome:* usually triggered by infection. Cover *S. pneumoniae*, Hib, mycoplasma, and *C. pneumoniae* (e.g. ceftriaxone

and erythromycin). Supportive measures, including bronchodilators. Consider exchange transfusion if severe (Box 11.8). Incentive spirometry (use of spirometer to guide deep respirations at regular intervals) can ↓ risk of acute chest syndrome developing from painful crisis involving ribs or back.

- *Osteomyelitis:* confirm organism with cultures, or empirically cover *S. paratyphi*, *E. coli*, and *S. aureus* (e.g. ceftriaxone and ciprofloxacin). Requires at least 6wks of therapy; may require surgery. Monitor closely for recurrence.
- *Malaria:* non-specific cause of fever and associated with mortality in sickle cell anaemia.
- *Good supportive care:* is essential to prevent other complications. Monitor fluid balance carefully to prevent overload; treat pain and hypoxia.

Box 11.7 Maintenance of health in sickle cell disease

- *Screening:* greatest mortality is among children <5yrs so early diagnosis is important. Selective screening (e.g. pregnant women, newborn children born to carriers, relatives of those with the disease) may miss a significant proportion of cases so universal screening is being implemented in some countries.
- *Education:* general health education. Advise to seek medical attention early (especially if high fever), to use clean drinking water and insecticide-treated bed nets to prevent malaria.
- Genetic counselling to identify affected relatives and to plan pregnancy.
- *Avoid factors precipitating crisis:* especially dehydration, hypoxia, infections, cold environments.
- *Folic acid supplements:* 1–5mg/d.
- *Protect against infection:* vaccinate against *S. pneumoniae*, Hib, meningococcus, hepatitis B, influenza. Educate parents/patients about ↓ mortality with prophylactic penicillin (125mg oral bd for children <5yrs, 250mg bd thereafter).
- Advise lifelong anti-malarial prophylaxis in endemic areas.
- *Detection of acute splenic sequestration:* teach parents of young children to palpate the spleen soon after diagnosis and to attend clinic if the child becomes unwell, with an enlarging spleen.
- *Screen for long-term complications:* e.g. annual fundoscopy (for retinopathy) from 15yrs.
- *Hydroxycarbamide:* ↓ frequency of crises, chest syndrome, hospitalisations, and mortality; should be considered for those with painful crises >2–3× per year. It should be avoided around conception and pregnancy.

Box 11.8 Indications for transfusion in sickle cell disease

- ↑ Hb levels above steady state ↑ thrombotic risk. Indications for transfusion include correction of blood loss or ↓ production or sequestration (e.g. post-operatively; during sequestration or aplastic crises; during acute severe illness).
- *Exchange transfusions:* sometimes performed to ↓ HbS%, and thus ↓ risk of vaso-occlusion. Aim for Hb 10g/dL, HCT ≤32%, HbS <30%. Exchange transfusions are beneficial (e.g. to prevent/↓ risk of stroke, during pregnancy in women with a past history of severe complications).

Thalassaemia

α Thalassaemia

α Thalassaemia is a defect or deletion of at least 1 of 4 α-globin genes. α^+ thalassaemia trait is common in Africans and does not cause anaemia. α^0 thalassaemia trait is more common in Asia and Mediterranean region → mild anaemia, ↓ MCV, ↓ MCH; hypochromic, microcytic red cells and target cells. More severe forms of α thalassaemia affect the fetus and neonate because foetal Hb (α2γ2) requires α chains. α thalassaemia is characterized by haemolysis rather than ineffective erythropoiesis.

HbH disease

β chains (HbH) that form inclusions in RBCs; can be detected with specific stains; HbH detected on Hb electrophoresis. HbH very poor at O_2 delivery. HbH levels are 5–30% with Hb 7–10g/dL. Children may have growth retardation and skeletal abnormalities, +/– hepatosplenomegaly. Transfusions are not usually required. Splenectomy may be of benefit.

Hb Bart's hydrops foetalis The fetus lacks all α genes and is stillborn or dies shortly after delivery.

β Thalassaemia

Caused by mutations of the β-globin genes and occurs in people originating from southern Europe, Africa, the Middle East, India, and Southeast Asia. Excess free α-globin chains precipitate as inclusion bodies in RBC precursors, → RBC destruction → ineffective erythropoiesis and ↑ splenic uptake of RBCs. There is compensatory ↑ iron uptake and expansion of erythropoiesis including extramedullary sites. This expansion, together with Fe overload and hypersplenism, → clinical manifestations.

β Thalassaemia minor

Palpable splenomegaly and moderate anaemia during pregnancy. This can → compensatory placental hypertrophy and mild intrauterine growth retardation, but does not cause ↑ perinatal mortality.

Diagnosis Mild anaemia (e.g. Hb 9–11g/dL); blood film shows moderate anisocytosis, microcytosis (MCV<76fL, MCH<26pg), hypochromia with a few target and tear drop cells. Basophilic stippling may occur. Hb electrophoresis shows ↑ HbA2(4–6.5%); HbF may also be ↑. *Note*: Fe deficiency can mask β thalassaemia minor. Test for thalassaemia when patient is Fe replete.

Management Diagnosis avoids future treatment of hypochromic anaemia with Fe, education, and genetic counselling.

β Thalassaemia intermedia

Causes mild to severe anaemia. Generally splenomegaly, bony expansion, and complications of Fe overload are present.

Diagnosis Features intermediate between β thalassaemia major and minor.

General management
Screening of family; active immunization, clean water sources, use of impregnated bed nets to avoid malaria, early attendance at medical facilities if unwell or febrile. Specific measures include: folate 5mg/day for adults; transfusion if severe anaemia or failure to thrive, or to ↓ erythroid expansion (e.g. if skeletal deformity); iron chelation if ferritin >1000micrograms/L even if not regularly transfused; splenectomy if hypersplenism.

β **Thalassaemia major**

- Untreated, most patients die < 5yrs from cardiac failure or infection.
- Failure to thrive at 3–6mths, when the switch from γ to β-chain production should take place; puberty is often delayed.
- Hepatosplenomegaly due to haemolysis, extramedullary haemopoiesis, and later in disease, Fe overload from transfusions. Splenomegaly ↑ blood requirements by ↑ RBC destruction and pooling.
- Bone expansion as a result of intense marrow hyperplasia; → skeletal deformity, including prominent frontal and parietal bones, maxillary enlargement, and flattening of the nasal bridge. There is osteoporosis (↑ fractures) and skull bossing with 'hair-on-end' appearance on X-ray.
- Infections predisposed to infection for a variety of reasons (e.g. defective splenic function). Severe gastroenteritis caused by *Yersinia enterocolitica* is associated with desferrioxamine treatment. Transmission of viral hepatitis is also ↑, probably due to Fe overload and transfusions.
- Iron overload due to transfusion therapy (each 500mL unit of blood contains 250mg of Fe) and ↑ Fe absorption. Fe accumulation → liver damage, failure of growth, delayed or absent puberty, diabetes, hypothyroidism, hypoparathyroidism, and myocardial damage. In the absence of intensive iron chelation, death occurs in the 2nd or 3rd decade, usually from CCF or cardiac arrhythmias. Clinical signs usually appear after >50U (12g of iron), but organ damage and skin pigmentation occur before this.

Diagnosis Severe hypochromic microcytic anaemia with ↑ reticulocyte count. Blood film shows many nucleated RBCs, tear drop and target cells, as well as cells of variable morphology and basophilic stippling. Electrophoresis shows absent HbA; HbF, and HbA2 are ↑.

Management Needs referral to specialist centre. Treat as for thalassaemia intermedia, plus commence ***iron chelation*** (e.g. desferrioxamine by SC infusion) when ferritin >1000micrograms/L, or signs of organ damage.

Start regular transfusions around 6–12mths (of age) when growth chart shows failure to thrive. These help suppress patient's ineffective erythropoiesis, prevent bony deformity and normalize growth. Maintain Hb >9.5g/dL.

- Give HBV vaccination.
- Supplement ***folic acid***.
- ***Splenectomy if hypersplenism***.
- Monitor for complications, e.g. gallstones, CCF, pulmonary hypertension, aplastic crises.

Blood transfusion

Blood transfusion can be life-saving but transfusion-associated risks are high. In countries where supplies of safe blood are scarce, the following may guide the decision to transfuse:

- Anaemic heart failure.
- Hb <5g/dL with symptoms.
- Hb <4g/dL in any situation.
- Acute blood loss → shock or signs of heart failure despite IV fluids.
- Need for emergency major surgery with pre-operative Hb<7g/dL.

Whole blood is used for most transfusions in resource-poor countries.

Ensuring blood safety and supply

Measures to make safe blood available:

- Prevention of unnecessary transfusions.
- Donor screening with a questionnaire designed to exclude those at high risk of transfusion-transmissible infections (e.g. HIV, hepatitis C).
- The use of a panel of voluntary, unpaid donors who have repeatedly tested –ve for transfusion-transmissible infections and who pass a basic medical test (check pulse, BP, screen for anaemia and other major illnesses).
- Standardize procedures for collection, storage, testing, and administration of blood including adequate controls and quality assurance (e.g. two grouping techniques should be used in parallel to prevent fatal ABO-incompatible transfusion reactions).
- Screening all blood for transfusion-transmissible infections, including HIV, hepatitis B, syphilis, hepatitis C, and, if appropriate, trypanosomiasis and malaria.
- Regular training for those involved in transfusion to ensure competency and safety.
- Use of a closed system allowing collection into blood bags with anticoagulant, testing and, if necessary, division, or fractionation of products.
- Appropriate storage in thermostatically controlled fridges with back-up power supplies.
- A labelling system for blood bags, samples, and patient identification as well as a procedure of checks at the bedside to ensure the correct unit is administered to the correct patient.

Administration of blood

Blood should only be removed from the fridge immediately prior to use. When administering a blood transfusion:

- Check the patient details with those of unit of blood to ensure unit has been issued to that patient and is compatible with group of patient.
- Give IV via a blood-giving set with a filter.
- Keep a record of the volume and units given.
- Observe the patient for the first 10min of a transfusion. Check pulse, BP, respiratory rate, temperature at start of transfusion and after 15–30min, and every hour during the transfusion.
- Monitor for signs of fluid overload.

Exchange transfusions

In certain situations, an exchange transfusion is indicated to ↓ the risk of volume overload or to ↓ the concentration of patients' red cells or plasma, e.g. in:

- Heart failure 2° to anaemia.
- Complications of sickle cell disease.
- Haemolytic disease of the newborn.
- Hyperbilirubinaemia in neonates.

Specialist advice should be sought regarding details of volumes and procedures for exchange transfusion.

Transfusion reactions

Severe transfusion reaction

May be due to ABO incompatibility or bacterial contamination of the unit. Heralded by pain at site of cannula, back/chest pain, agitation, dyspnoea, nausea, flushing, or hypotension.

- Stop the transfusion immediately. Do not flush giving set.
- IV access, catheterize patient, and start fluids to ensure diuresis.
- Monitor renal and liver function, clotting parameters, haemoglobinuria.
- Give broad-spectrum antibiotic, e.g. ceftriaxone if possible after taking blood cultures and send donor unit for culture.
- Give bronchodilators if wheezing; give antihistamine and IV hydrocortisone as for allergic reaction.
- Laboratory to re-cross match unit, repeat patient's grouping, and monitor for development of red cell antibodies.

Simple febrile and allergic reactions

If temperature ↑ by >1°C from baseline or the patient develops urticarial rash or itching, stop the transfusion, check vital signs, give paracetamol, and, if the patient remains well after 15min, restart the transfusion at a slower rate.

Delayed transfusion reaction

Usually occurs 5–10d post-transfusion and is due to sensitization to RBCs following previous transfusions or pregnancy.

Clinical features Fever, jaundice, and anaemia. Samples should be taken for grouping, direct Coombs' test, repeat cross-matching, and antibody screening and results compared with a pre-transfusion sample.

Effects of HIV/AIDS

Anaemia

Common in individuals with advanced HIV, usually multifactorial in aetiology and carries worse prognosis. Anaemia of chronic disorders related to OIs and TB is common; HIV itself ↓ erythropoiesis. Thus, anaemia associated with chronic disorders may be far more severe than that seen in HIV– individuals. Bone marrow infiltration by MAC, TB, or other OIs may also contribute (often accompanied by other cytopenias). Malnutrition and malabsorption may → B12, folate and iron deficiency. Avoid inappropriate over-prescription of iron supplementation for HIV-related anaemia, as iron tablets → GI side effects, which may ↓ tolerance of other medication.

Other causes of anaemia in HIV

Medication

AZT (causes anaemia with or without neutropenia), 3TC (pure red cell aplasia, rare), co-trimoxazole (especially at higher doses), amphotericin and rifabutin (marrow suppression), dapsone and primaquine (haemolysis in G6PD deficiency). Drug-induced haemolytic anaemia may also occur.

Infections

Parvovirus B19 can → chronic erythroid hypoplasia in HIV. In endemic areas, malaria should always be considered.

Malignancies and pre-malignant conditions

Lymphoma or Castleman's disease may → bone marrow infiltration or haemolytic anaemia. Gastro-intestinal KS may → GI blood loss.

Immune mediated

Coombs +ve auto-immune haemolytic anaemia, cryglobulinaemias and TTP may all → anaemia.

Thrombocytopenia

The commonest cause is HIV-related ITP. Other causes include drugs (e.g. co-trimoxazole), marrow infiltration (OI, TB, or lymphoma), nutritional (B12 or folate), malaria, and hypersplenism.

Management

Stop/substitute culprit drugs. Bone marrow biopsy if bicytopenia or pancytopenia or if systemic symptoms suggesting OI or lymphoma. ITP is treated with corticosteroids (prednisolone 1mg/kg) and ART initially. HIV-related ITP is an indication for ART.

Neutropenia

May occur related to HIV itself, marrow infiltration (e.g. TB) or drugs (e.g. co-trimoxazole, AZT). Also B12 and folate deficiency.

Coagulopathy

HIV+ individuals have ↑ risk of DVT and pulmonary embolus. This may be related to acquired protein C and S and antithrombin III deficiency and perhaps antiphospholipid antibodies. Thrombosis ↑ during active TB, presumably because of systemic inflammation and immobility.

Acute leukaemias

An excessive proliferation of immature haematopoietic cells → blasts in the peripheral blood. Without treatment, patients with acute leukaemias have a median survival of months. Chemotherapy may be curative. This is not the case with indolent haematological malignancies, which may not require treatment at diagnosis but are incurable with standard chemotherapy.

Diagnosis

Of acute leukaemias relies on analysis of blood and bone marrow samples to establish origin of malignant cells and associated genetic abnormalities.

Treatment

Is with cycles of chemotherapy, and requires urgent transfer to a specialist centre. Normal haematopoietic tissue is also affected by chemotherapy, → anaemia, neutropenia, and thrombocytopenia. Tumour lysis syndrome may occur with 1st cycle and is an emergency (see Box 11.9). Supportive care is essential: RBC and platelet transfusions may be required and there is a significant risk of neutropenic sepsis.

Acute lymphoblastic leukaemia (ALL) has peaks at 2-5yrs and >40yrs. Poor prognostic markers include age <1 or >10yrs and >30yrs; presenting WBC >50 × 10^9/L, and certain cytogenetic abnormalities. Clinical features include bone pain, lymphadenopathy, hepatosplenomegaly, anaemia, haemorrhage, and infections.

Acute myeloblastic leukaemia (AML) has a median age at diagnosis of 70yrs. Clinical features are similar to ALL except that in Africa 10–30% of patients may present with a solid tumour (chloroma), e.g. in the orbit or skin. Gum hypertrophy and DIC can be features. Risk factors include exposure to benzene, radiation, and previous cytotoxic therapy. Poor prognosis is associated with age >55yrs, poor general state of health, and specific cytogenetic abnormalities. Where specialist care is not available, hydroxycarbamide (adult dose 1–2g/d) may temporarily ↓ WBC and symptoms.

Box 11.9 Tumour lysis syndrome

Acute renal failure characterized by ↑ uric acid, ↑ K+, ↑ LDH, ↑ PO_4, ↑ creatinine, ↓ Ca^{2+}. Caused by release of toxic components upon cell death in leukaemia and aggressive NHL. It can occur spontaneously, due to rapid tumour growth or more predictably, upon starting treatment. Occurs more commonly in the elderly, pre-existing renal impairment. Anticipate and prevent: allopurinol 100–200mg tds, aggressive IV hydration to ↑ urine output.

Causes of changes in WBC counts

↑WBC count

Neutrophilia >7.5 × 10^9/L

- Physiological, e.g. pregnancy.
- Acute bacterial infections, e.g. pneumonia, UTI, abscess.
- Tissue damage, inflammation, stress, e.g. burns, pancreatitis, diabetic keto-acidosis.
- Malignant disease.
- Drugs, e.g. steroids.

Basophilia >0.1 × 10^9/L

- Myeloproliferative disorders.
- Allergic reactions.

Lymphocytosis >3.5 × 10^9/L

- Childhood response to infections.
- Certain bacterial infections in adults, e.g. Brucellosis, pertussis.
- Viral and protozoal infections, e.g. CMV, EBV, toxoplasmosis.
- Lymphoproliferative disorders.

Monocytosis >1.0 × 10^9/L

- Rarely, chronic bacterial infection, e.g. TB.
- Chronic myelomonocytic leukaemia.

Eosinophilia >0.5 × 10^9/L

- *Helminth infections:* e.g. hookworm, hydatid disease, schistosomiasis—values >3 × 10^9/L are likely to be due to katayama fever, strongyloidiasis.
- Allergic/skin conditions, e.g. asthma, atopy, drugs, vasculitis, psoriasis; reactive to leukaemia/lymphoma, connective tissue disease.
- Convalescence from viral or other infections, especially in infants.

↓WBC count

Neutropenia <2.0 × 10^9/L

- Acute infection, e.g. dengue, overwhelming sepsis.
- Some chronic infections, e.g. visceral leishmaniasis, miliary TB, AIDS.
- Bone marrow failure or drugs, e.g. chloramphenicol.
- Peripheral consumption, e.g. hypersplenism, Felty's syndrome.
- Miscellaneous, e.g. ethnic, familial, cyclic, chronic, idiopathic.

Lymphopenia <1.5 × 10^9/L

- Very common in many acute infections, e.g. TB, hepatitis, pneumonia.
- Drugs, e.g. corticosteroids.

Lymphoproliferative disorders

Non-Hodgkin's lymphoma

A heterogeneous group of B and T cell tumours. Low-grade lymphomas are incurable and initially run an indolent course even without treatment. High-grade lymphomas are more aggressive but cure is achievable. High-grade NHLs are more common in Asia and Africa and, in Africa, are associated with malaria. Features include: lymphadenopathy, hepatosplenomegaly, ↓ weight, night sweats, pruritus, fever, pancytopenia. Most of these disorders will temporarily respond to corticosteroids if specialist treatment is not available, but beware tumour lysis in bulky high grade disease.

Burkitt's lymphoma (BL)

Highly aggressive NHL and rapidly fatal without treatment. It occurs in malaria-endemic areas, is related to EBV infection, and is the most common childhood cancer in tropical Africa. Commoner in boys, peak incidence 4–7yrs and may be associated with HIV. It classically involves the jaw but can occur in any extra-nodal site. Steroids or a single dose of IV cyclophosphamide may provide temporary control but intensive chemotherapy is needed to achieve a 70% cure rate. Measures to prevent/treat tumour lysis should be taken (see Box 11.9).

Hodgkin's lymphoma (HL)

More common in men, peaking in young adulthood and middle age. There are geographical variations in sub-types; nodular sclerosing HL predominates in published studies, but in developing countries, the mixed cellularity sub-type is more common and linked to EBV exposure. HL usually presents as painless lymphadenopathy and 70–80% of cases are curable with standard radio/chemotherapy.

Chronic lymphocytic leukaemia (CLL)

Characterized by proliferation of mature, dysfunctional lymphocytes → infections or autoimmune haemolytic anaemia. More common in men, median age 60yrs. In temperate regions, the most common form of leukaemia. CLL may present with incidental lymphocytosis (5 to >100 × 10^9/L), lymphadenopathy, hepatosplenomegaly, infections, or bone marrow failure. Treatment consists of chemotherapy (e.g. chlorambucil) or if not available, steroids. Transfusions and antibiotics may be required.

Multiple myeloma (MM)

Plasma cell malignancy infiltrating bone marrow. Incidence is higher in the islands of Pacific, Caribbean, and Africa than in more wealthy countries. Clinical features include bone pain, pathological fractures, osteopenia, ↑ Ca^{2+} (see 📖 Cancer, p. 736), renal failure, and bone marrow failure with anaemia, infection, and bleeding. Definitive treatment → a median survival of 3–5yrs, but where not available, steroids can be used. Supportive treatment includes analgesia, transfusions, and bisphosphonates.

HTLV-1 associated adult T-cell leukaemia/lymphoma (ATL)

HTLV-1 is a retrovirus endemic in parts of the Caribbean, South America, central and southern Africa, southern Japan. It causes ATL with a lifetime risk of 4% in those infected at a young age. HTLV-1 is also associated with chronic neurological conditions.

Transmission

Mainly by sexual contact and breastfeeding in endemic areas. Has also been transmitted by blood transfusion. In Europe and North America it is transmitted through IV drug use.

Clinical features

- *Acute ATL in 2/3 of cases:* high circulating lymphocyte count, lymphadenopathy, hepatosplenomegaly, hypercalcaemia, CNS involvement, skin lesions.
- *Lymphoma type:* clinically like NHL, but with poor prognosis.
- *Chronic ATL:* skin lesions, mild lymphocytosis, protracted course.
- *Smouldering ATL:* low peripheral lymphocyte count, skin lesions, remains stable for many years.

Diagnosis

FBC, WBC (lymphocyte count 30–130 × 10^9/L); blood film shows atypical lymphocytes with convoluted nuclei. HTLV-1 serology is +ve. Elevated serum Ca^{2+} common. CXR may show pulmonary infiltration, osteolytic lesions. Lymph node biopsy or bone marrow biopsy usually diagnostic.

Management Combination chemotherapy for acute or progressive disease.

Myeloproliferative disorders

A group of disorders characterized by proliferation of haemopoietic stem cells. These cells retain their ability to differentiate, resulting in an excess of mature cells of predominantly one lineage. The disorders share systemic symptoms such as malaise, night sweats, fever, and ↓ weight. Often have splenomegaly; gout and pruritus may occur. These disorders are not curable, but may have a long survival if treated. Transformation to acute leukaemia or to marrow fibrosis occurs in a minority.

Polycythaemia

1° Polycythaemia (polycythaemia rubra vera) is characterized by HCT >56% in females, >60% in males, ↑ neutrophils, and/or ↑ platelets, gout, splenomegaly, and, less commonly, thrombosis. 2° causes should be excluded.

Treatment

- Venesection to ↓ HCT to <45%.
- Aspirin (75mg od).
- Hydroxycarbamide for concomitant thrombocytosis or those whose HCT is not controlled by venesection.
- Median survival is >15yrs in younger patients.
- Differential diagnoses include relative polycythaemia (↓ plasma volume, e.g. dehydration) and polycythaemia due to ↑ erythropoietin (e.g. high altitude).

Essential thrombocythaemia

Characterized by platelet count persistently >500 × 10^9/L without an underlying cause (blood loss, iron deficiency, infection, inflammation, hyposplenism, and malignancy). 50% patients are asymptomatic, 25% have splenomegaly and 25% have a history of thrombosis. Platelet function may be abnormal, especially in those with platelets >1000 × 10^9/L. Treatment is with aspirin unless contraindicated. Patients at high risk of thrombosis (e.g. age >60yrs) should also be given hydroxycarbamide to ↓ platelet count to normal range.

Chronic myeloid leukaemia (CML)

Clonal haematopoietic disorder characterized by expansion of mature myeloid cells. It is caused by a chromosomal translocation (Philadelphia chromosome). The median age is 50–60yrs, but can present in childhood. Patients often asymptomatic initially; later, transformation → blast crisis (acute leukaemia) occurs. Continuous treatment with tyrosine kinase inhibitors can → long-term control, but they are costly and regular monitoring is required. The Glivec® International Patient Assistance Program can provide tyrosine kinase inhibitor for free given certain conditions. Otherwise, hydroxycarbamide can be used to ↓ WBC in chronic phase. It is only curable with bone marrow transplantation.

Splenomegaly

Spleen is a major site of antigen presentation and platelet reservoir. Splenic macrophages remove damaged or old RBCs. Spleen enlarges as a result of over-activity of any of these processes.

The high prevalence of chronic infection (especially malaria) as well as haemolytic anaemias in the tropics means that splenomegaly is a common finding. Splenomegaly may → abdominal distension, discomfort, and early satiety. Massive splenomegaly may → pancytopenia.

Hyperreactive malarial splenomegaly (HMS)

Occurs very commonly in areas with high malaria transmission, especially in adults who have taken up residence in the endemic area. HMS is due to polyclonal lymphoid activation because of an abnormal immune response to malaria. HMS is difficult to distinguish from lympho proliferative disorders, hepato splenic schistosomiasis, and visceral leishmaniasis, which may co-exist in the same territory. Once other causes have been excluded (see Box 11.10), HMS is a likely diagnosis. Anti-malaria prophylaxis (e.g. proguanil 100mg/d) for at least 6mths may result in significant ↓ spleen size, supporting the diagnosis.

Splenectomy

Indications for splenectomy include trauma, haemolytic anaemia, immune thrombocytopenic purpura. Post-operatively, there is an ↑↑ risk of sepsis (overwhelming post-splenectomy infection (OPSI)) from encapsulated bacteria, especially *Streptococcus pneumoniae*. Risk of OPSI is ~0.5%/yr, and even with good resources, mortality is ~50%, so prevention is essential. If possible, elective splenectomy should be delayed until age >5yrs because of ↑ susceptibility OPSI. Pneumococcal, meningococcal, and *H. influenza* b vaccinations should preferably be given at >2wks pre-operatively; if splenectomy is unplanned, they should be given >2wks post-operatively; reimmunization for pneumococcus should be repeated every 5yrs. Penicillin V prophylaxis (500mg bd) should be commenced post-op and continued for life. Patients should be educated about the risk of OPSI and seek immediate attention, or start standby broad-spectrum antibiotics, if they develop a fever with fainting or rigors. There is ↑ risk of severe malaria, so long-term malaria prophylaxis (or residence outside a malaria area) should be advised. Immediately post-splenectomy, there is a risk of thrombosis because of transient thrombocytosis, or in the case of haemolytic anaemias, a rise in haematocrit.

Box 11.10 Common causes of splenomegaly

- *Infections:* SBE, brucellosis, typhoid, miliary TB, EBV, CMV, HIV, rubella, hepatitis B, toxoplasmosis, malaria (including HMS*), visceral leishmaniasis*, schistosomiasis*, histoplasmosis, splenic abscess.
- *Malignancies:* lymphoma*, ALL, CLL*, metastatic carcinoma, multiple myeloma, myeloproliferative disorders*.
- *Autoimmune:* SLE, rheumatoid arthritis (Felty's syndrome).
- *Reactive:* autoimmune haemolytic anaemia, haemoglobinopathies*.
- *Congestive:* portal hypertension*, cardiac failure.
- *Other:* sarcoidosis, lipid storage disorders, histiocytosis.

*Can give massive splenomegaly ≥10cm below costal margin.

Causes of DIC in tropical countries

- *Infection:* meningococcal, pneumococcal, staphylococcal, ebola, Marburg, dengue, Lassa fever, malaria (rarely).
- *Malignancy:* disseminated cancer, acute leukaemia.
- *Tissue damage:* burns, fulminant hepatitis, pancreatitis, rhabdomyolysis, fat embolism.
- *Envenoming:* snake bite, *Lonomia* caterpillars (Brazil).
- *Obstetric:* septic abortion, *abruptio placentae*, amniotic fluid embolus, pre-eclampsia/eclampsia, retention of dead fetus.
- *Immune:* ABO-incompatible blood transfusion.
- *Vascular:* vasculitis, malignant hypertension, atrial myxoma.

Disorders of haemostasis

Abnormal bleeding results from disorders of 1° homeostasis (vascular endothelium and platelets) → bleeding into the skin and mucous membranes, or of 2° haemostasis (coagulation and fibrinolytic pathways) → haemorrhage in deep tissues.

Disorders of 1° haemostasis

- Vascular purpura: infections, long-term steroid therapy, and vasculitis. In immunocompromised patients, HSV, VZV, and arboviruses (O'nyong-nyong, chikungunya) can → fatal haemorrhage.
- Defective platelet function: can result from drugs (e.g. NSAIDS, aspirin) and complicate some of the haemorrhagic fevers (e.g. Lassa, dengue, Marburg, ebola), alcoholism, hepatic cirrhosis, uraemia, paraproteinaemias, leukaemias, and myeloproliferative disorders.
- Thrombocytopenia: may result from defective production, ↑ destruction/consumption, and splenic pooling (e.g. malaria, visceral leishmaniasis, HIV).

Onyalai Means 'blood blister' and is a thrombocytopenic disorder of unknown aetiology occuring in central southern Africa.

Clinical features Recurrent haemorrhagic bullae on mucous membranes, epistaxis, hypotension and GI/cerebral haemorrhage. Mortality is 3–10%.

Management Includes blood and platelet transfusion; steroids and IV immunoglobulin have been used to ↑ platelet count.

Management of bleeding due to thrombocytopenia/ defective platelet function

- Treat underlying causes of thrombocytopenia.
- Desmopressin for uraemic platelet dysfunction.
- Tranexamic acid for mucosal bleeding.
- Platelet transfusions, where available, may be necessary for acute bleeding. Their effect only lasts a few days, and they may be ineffective if peripheral consumption is the cause.

Immune thrombocytopenia often occurs after a viral infection in children and remits spontaneously. Adults may have a more protracted course. Remaining FBC and blood film should be normal, unless severe bleeding. Other causes of thrombocytopenia should be excluded (see Box 11.11). Treatment is usually only for bleeding complications in children, or adults at high risk of bleeding: prednisolone (1mg/kg od for at least 4wks) or intravenous immunoglobulin (0.4mg/kg over 5d or 1mg/kg over 2d). Only consider platelet transfusion if severe bleeding complications.

Disorders of 2° haemostasis

Can be congenital, e.g. haemophilia A (factor VIII deficiency), haemophilia B (Christmas disease, factor IX deficiency), and von Willebrand's disease or acquired 2° to malabsorption (→ vitamin K deficiency), liver disease, DIC, and snake envenoming.

Box 11.11 Causes of thrombocytopenia

- ↓ *Production:* Infections (e.g. typhoid, brucellosis, rubella, mumps, hepatitis C, HIV), megaloblastic anaemia, alcoholism, marrow infiltration or failure (e.g. leukaemia, aplastic anaemia, drugs/chemicals).
- ↑ *Peripheral consumption:* Infections (e.g. malaria, visceral leishmaniasis, trypanosomiasis, dengue, and other arboviruses, EBV, CMV, Marburg virus), hypersplenism, pregnancy, chronic hepatic disease, DIC, microangiopathic haemolytic anaemia, ITP, onyalai, acute viral infection, AIDS, drugs (e.g. quinine, penicillin, valproate), lymphomas, CLL.

Congenital disorders of haemostasis

Clinical features

Haemophilia is an X-linked deficiency of factors VIII or IX → prolonged APTT and a spectrum of clinical severity. Boys may present with haemorrhage after surgical interventions, spontaneous bleeding into joints and muscles, which produces crippling arthropathy and deformity of the limbs. Cerebral haemorrhage and spontaneous intra-abdominal or upper respiratory tract bleeding may also occur. Von Willebrand's disease results from a defect in von Willebrand factor and presents with bleeding from mucous membranes because of a defect in platelet function.

Management

General

Requires referral to a specialist. NSAIDS, aspirin, and IM injections should be avoided. Spontaneous musculoskeletal bleeds can be managed with rest, ice, elevation, analgesia, and gentle physiotherapy once the acute symptoms have settled. Tranexamic acid 25mg/kg oral tds can be helpful for mucosal bleeding. Fibrin glue is a helpful adjunct to control intra-operative bleeding. Vaccinate against hepatitis B, screen regularly for other infections especially HCV, HIV if the patient is receiving plasma-based products.

Specific

Recombinant factor replacement very costly, so plasma-derived, on-demand treatment is more common in resource-poor countries. Severe haemophilia A requires factor VIII concentrate and haemophilia B factor IX concentrate. These products should be virally inactivated and freeze-dried, have a defined activity and come from a low-risk donor pool. Cryoprecipitate (haemophilia A), cryosupernatant (haemophilia B) or FFP should only be used as a last resort. Desmopressin (0.3–0.4mg/kg/every 12–24h IV in 50mL 0.9% saline over 20min) is effective in some haemophiliac patients. The World Federation of Haemophilia is an excellent resource: www.wfh.org

Acquired coagulation disorders

Vitamin K is a co-factor for coagulation factors II, VII, IX, and X, and the anticoagulant proteins C and S. These factors are produced in hepatocytes and deficiency of vitamin K, as well as liver failure can → coagulopathy. Vitamin K deficiency results from small bowel fat malabsorption, biliary or pancreatic dysfunction, starvation, or prolonged antibiotic use.

Vitamin K antagonism Warfarin is a competitive inhibitor of vitamin K. Overdose, sepsis, poor vitamin K intake/absorption, or simultaneous administration of potentiating drugs may cause bleeding. For emergency reversal of warfarin, give vitamin K 5–10mg IV and Prothrombin Complex 15mL/kg, where available, or FFP 15mL/kg if not.

Liver disease Bleeding is due to a combination of ↓ clotting factor synthesis, thrombocytopenia, platelet dysfunction, vitamin K deficiency, DIC, and dysfibrinogenaemia and should be treated by IV vitamin K, FFP, and cryoprecipitate if fibrinogen is low.

Disseminated intravascular coagulation

Results from activation of coagulation pathways in the vasculature and a cycle of consumption of coagulation factors and their inhibitors. May be asymptomatic or associated with bleeding, skin purpura, microangiopathic haemolytic anaemia, and arterial or venous thromboses. Depletion of all coagulation factors → prolongation of APTT and PT, ↓ fibrinogen and platelets, and RBC fragmentation on blood film.

Management Treat the underlying condition, careful monitoring, give blood products as required. If there are predominantly thrombotic complications, consider cautious anticoagulation with IV heparin.

Paediatric note: haemorrhagic disease of the newborn (HDN) or vitamin K deficient bleeding (VKDB)

Neonates are vitamin K deficient because of poor placental transfer and ↓ hepatic synthesis. This can cause early bleeding (e.g. intracranial haemorrhage) in the 1st week of life, but bleeding may also occur later. At risk groups include preterm infants and infants of mothers on anti-TB therapy, anticonvulsants, or warfarin. Vitamin K levels are low in breast milk and breastfed infants at ↑ risk of late onset VKDB, at 1–3mths.

VKDB can be prevented with routine prophylaxis of vitamin K. Both oral and IM preparations are available, but IM vitamin K prevents both early and late onset VKDB. For routine prophylaxis at birth, give 1mg vitamin K IM (preterm 400micrograms/kg, max 1mg). Babies at high risk of VKDB should receive prompt IM vitamin K administration after delivery.

Treatment of VKDB is with 1–2mg parenteral vitamin K plus FFP if there are bleeding complications.

Laboratory issues

Most 1° level health centres usually have a light microscope, e.g. for diagnosis of TB and malaria. This enables several important investigations (e.g. WBC and platelet count, RBC morphology, differential WBC%). However, the microscopist should spend <4h/d looking down the microscope to avoid fatigue and poor quality reporting.

The following principles can ↓ errors in tests:

- Use accurate volumes.
- Check date, dilution, and storage of reagents.
- Keep instruments and cuvettes clean and grease/dust free.
- Keep colorimeters away from sunlight.
- Collect capillary or venous blood samples correctly and use appropriate amount of anticoagulant.
- Use correct centrifuge times and speeds.
- Filter stains/diluting mixtures; check for particles and use correctly buffered water.
- Run samples in duplicate.
- Use clean, dry slides.
- Fix slides with water-free methanol when completely dry.
- Consult the standard operating procedures for each test.

Some basic principles of laboratory management

Range of tests

Better to provide a few essential tests to high standards than wide range of poor-quality tests. Test selection should take into account sensitivity and specificity of tests, as well as +ve and –ve predictive values (influenced by disease prevalence in local population), reliability, availability of reagents and consumables, cost, safety, sustainability, and skills of laboratory staff.

Management and operation of equipment

Ensure regular maintenance, availability of manuals, adequate space and light, minimization of dust and heat damage, and reliable supplies of consumables/reagents. Laboratory staff should be appropriately trained and supervised and carry out tests within their skills and knowledge.

Ensure good quality results

Simple ways of promoting confidence in test results include:

- Independent re-analysis of selected slides or samples within one laboratory.
- Regular exchange of samples with neighbouring laboratories.
- Including known samples within a batch of tests to demonstrate that the test is working (e.g. a blood sample known to contain HbS can be included in each batch of sickle-cell screening tests); or use of reference samples.

Standard operating procedures (SOPs)

These are detailed descriptions of laboratory tests designed to prevent errors and ensure consistent results. They must be designed for the local situation, kept up-to-date, and adhered to by all staff. SOPs provide an excellent teaching resource. For each test, they should include:

- The principle of the test and valid reasons for requesting it.
- Details of the specimen required and how it should be collected.
- The equipment and reagents needed, as well as information on how to maintain, procure, and store them.
- The method of the test.
- Quality control measures and sources of error.
- Safety considerations.
- The procedure to be followed in reporting the results (e.g. units to be used).

Chapter 12

Endocrinology and biochemistry

Invited author **Theresa Allain**

Diabetes mellitus

A syndrome caused by the lack, or ↓ effectiveness, of insulin → hyperglycaemia and deranged metabolism. Several forms of DM exist.

Type I DM

An autoimmune disease, with highest prevalence in northern Europe; usually juvenile onset. May be associated with other autoimmune diseases in the patient or family, and environmental factors may also be important in aetiology. Patients always need insulin and are prone to ketoacidosis.

Type II DM

Accounts for >90% of global cases of DM; prevalence is ↑ massively worldwide due to changes in diet and lifestyle accompanying urbanization. Directly associated with ↑ in obesity. Number of cases expected to double by 2025, especially in resource-poor countries. Worldwide DM epidemic is associated with an early age of onset of type II DM, some even presenting in childhood. 20% of type II diabetics eventually need insulin treatment. 'Maturity onset diabetes of the young' has a presentation similar to type II DM.

Malnutrition-related DM

Accounts for 1% of diabetes in a tropical setting. The WHO subdivides this disease into two classes:

- Protein-deficient pancreatic diabetes.
- Fibrocalculous pancreatic diabetes.

Both occur in young patients of low body weight. High doses of insulin are required, but ketoacidosis does not occur. Tropical calcific pancreatitis (see 📖 Persistent diarrhoea and malabsorption, p. 262) may be a cause of fibrocalculous pancreatic DM. Another theory is that consumption of cyanide-containing foods (e.g. cassava/manioc/tapioca, ragi in India, and traditional beers in Africa) on a background of protein-calorie malnutrition → build-up of toxic hydrocyanic acid → direct damage to the pancreas. Conversely, some believe that the malnutrition is a result and not a cause of the DM.

Other types of DM

- Gestational.
- 2° due to:
    - drugs (steroids, thiazide diuretics, ART)
    - pancreatic disease (chronic pancreatitis, tropical calcific pancreatitis, post-surgery)
    - endocrine disease (Cushing's, acromegaly, phaeochromocytoma, thyrotoxicosis).

Clinical presentation of DM

- *Acute:* ketoacidosis, ↓ weight, polyuria, polydipsia. (If blood glucose normal consider hypercalcaemia (📖 Hypercalcaemia, p. 562) and diabetes insipidus (📖 Diabetes insipidus, p. 558, as rarer causes of polyuria and polydipsia).

- *Subacute:* as acute, but occurring over a longer time, plus lethargy, infection (e.g. pruritus vulvae, boils).
- *Chronic:* may present with complications: infection, cataract, microangiopathy (retinopathy, neuropathy, nephropathy) and macroangiopathy (stroke, MI, claudication), foot ulcers.

Diagnosis

- Diagnosis of DM requires demonstration of an ↑ blood glucose level on two separate occasions (if asymptomatic), or on one occasion if symptomatic.
- An ↑ blood glucose level is defined as:
  - *either* a fasting venous plasma glucose level ≥7.0mmol/L
  - *or* a random plasma glucose level ≥11.1mmol/L (Box 12.1).
- Always check urine ketones on diagnosis.
- *The following features favour type I DM*:
  - clinical features—non-fasting ketonuria, short history, ↓↓ weight
  - family history—of type I DM; personal/family history of autoimmune disease
  - age and glucose level are NOT predictive.
- Diagnosis of protein-deficient pancreatic diabetes also requires: onset at <30yrs of age, BMI <19, a history of childhood malnutrition, and the absence of ketoacidosis. Such patients will often require >60U of insulin per day.
- Diagnosis of fibrocalculous pancreatic diabetes: requires recurrent abdominal pain and evidence of pancreatic calculi in the absence of alcoholism, gallstones, or hyperthyroidism.

Impaired fasting glucose

This is defined as a fasting plasma glucose 6.0–7.0mmol/L and is associated with ↑ risk of IHD and progression → diabetes. Monitor fasting glucose annually for progression → DM, and address other risk factors for IHD (e.g. obesity, lipids, smoking, aspirin).

Box 12.1 The oral glucose tolerance test

This should only be used for epidemiological research and diagnosing gestational DM. The patient must be on a normal carbohydrate intake prior to the test.

- Fast the patient overnight.
- Take a fasting plasma glucose sample the following morning.
- Then give 75g oral glucose in 300mL water (children 1.75g/kg, max. 75g) and measure plasma glucose 2h afterwards.

DM is diagnosed if the fasting venous plasma glucose is ≥7.0mmol/L and/or the 2h sample is ≥11.1mmol/L.

Screening for glycosuria is not a cost-effective way of diagnosis in the general population. However, this is an appropriate method of screening for gestational DM. If glycosuria is present, proceed to GTT.

Management of diabetes mellitus

Patient education and motivation are the key to success. Aim of treatment is to restore normoglycaemia and avoid complications. If home monitoring of control not feasible, aim for absence of symptoms of hyper- or hypoglycaemia. Children are more likely to develop ketoacidosis. Glycaemic control important during pregnancy: hyperglycaemia in the 1st trimester → 3-fold ↑ risk of foetal abnormality/birth complications.

Education

Diet and adherence are crucial. Teach monitoring of blood/urine glucose levels. If on insulin or sulfonylureas, advise patient to carry sweets at all times; alert patient/family/colleagues to signs of hypoglycaemia. Diet should avoid rapidly absorbed carbohydrate (e.g. sugar, sweets, fizzy drinks) and other high glycaemic index foods, but include regular meals of complex carbohydrate and foods with low glycaemic index. Avoid long periods of physical activity without food. Explain importance of foot care. Where possible, arrange appointments with dietician and chiropodist. Emphasise regular follow-up.

Conservative management

Treatment should always include a healthy diet: low in fat, sugar, and salt; high in starchy carbohydrate and fibre; with moderate protein; eaten at regular times. Fruit and fruit juice contain a lot of natural sugar. In urban areas, processed foods should be avoided. Obese patients should lose weight. CVS risk factors should be minimized (i.e. smoking, hypertension, lipids, exercise).

Drug therapy

Treatment depends on the type of DM and drug availability. In uncomplicated, newly diagnosed type II DM, try 3-mth trial of diet and exercise. If glycaemic control not adequate by 3mths, start metformin if overweight or a sulfonylurea if slim. Sulfonylureas stimulate insulin secretion and sensitivity and cause hypoglycaemia; tolbutamide (0.5–1.0g bd) is short-acting and preferred. Gliclazide (40–160mg od) and glibenclamide (2.5–15mg od), longer-acting and cause hypoglycaemia in elderly. Metformin (500mg–1g 2–3 × daily with food) does not cause hypoglycaemia, but may cause anorexia, diarrhoea, and rarely, lactic acidosis. It should not be used in patients with renal, heart, or liver failure. The above drugs may be combined. Thiazolidinediones (e.g. pioglitazone) ↓ peripheral insulin resistance. Their maximum hypoglycaemic effect takes 2–3mths to take effect; should not be used as 1st line, but can be used in combination as an alternative to metformin or a sulphonylurea when 2 agents required. Thiazolidinediones should not be combined with insulin. Note that rosiglitazone is not advised – it has lost its European license because of ↑ cardiovascular risk. Pioglitazone can cause hepatitis and increased fracture risk in women.

Combining all 3 oral drug classes not recommended—patients still hyperglycaemic despite 2 oral agents require insulin. Insulin should be used in a non-obese patient on maximal oral treatment who is losing weight.

Oral drugs can be supplemented with daily injection of long-acting insulin; however, it may be simpler (and cheaper) to change completely to insulin. In obese patients who require insulin, adding metformin ↓ weight gain.

Insulin

Soluble insulin (100U/mL) is short-acting, peaking at 2–4h and lasting up to 8h. Medium-acting insulins are suspensions, peaking at 4–6h and lasting up to 16h. Long-acting insulins last up to 32h. Human insulin analogues are available in short-acting, medium, and long-acting forms. They have faster onset, quicker offset, and are associated with less hypoglycaemia than other insulins. Treatment regimes vary, depending upon type of DM, availability of insulins, access to home monitoring, and lifestyle. The typical daily requirement for insulin is 0.5–1.0U/kg/day, (pre-pubertal children 0.6–0.8U/kg/day) in divided doses. Whenever starting insulin in type I or II DM start with 0.5U/kg/d and ↑/↓ the dose at subsequent reviews, usually in 5U/day increments. Type I DM requires insulin action through 24h, whereas insulin-treated type II DM may be controlled with a single injection of medium-acting insulin once or twice/day, or medium acting in the morning, short acting in the evening. For type I DM there are 2 widely used regimes:

- *Two injections/d:* start with 0.5U/kg/d, 2/3 given in morning and 1/3 in evening. Make 1/3 short-acting and 2/3 long-acting. Insulin injections should be given 20min before breakfast and evening meal. Avoiding hypoglycaemia relies on 3 regular meals a day and 2 snacks, one mid-morning and one before bed (Fig. 12.1).
- *Basal bolus:* single injection of long-acting at bedtime (basal) and 3 injections of soluble during the day (bolus) before each meal. Test glucose before each meal and adjust the insulin dose 2U at a time.

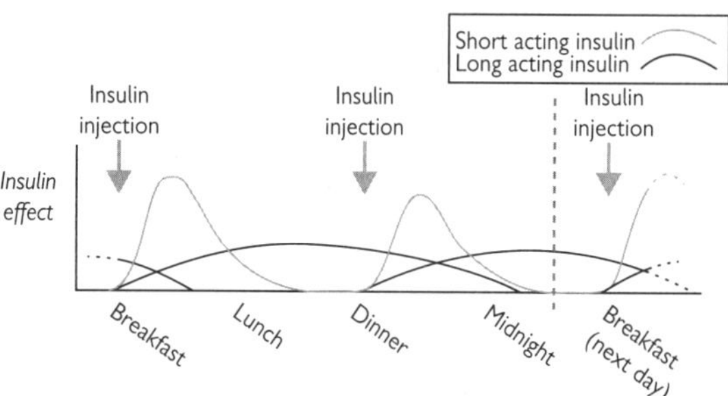

Fig. 12.1 Balancing insulin action and meals. How to monitor and adjust insulin doses with a typical twice-daily regime of short- and long-acting insulin suitable for a type I diabetic. Before breakfast and main evening meal a mixture of short-acting insulin and long-acting insulin is injected. Risk of hypoglycaemia max. at mid-morning and pre-bed, so snacks essential at these times. Check glucose before each meal and at bedtime, and adjust doses accordingly.

Two injections/day involves fewer injections, but is less flexible and means regular meal times and injection times must be adhered to. Basal bolus allows for more flexibility, but requires more injections and is most effective if home blood glucose monitoring can be done.

Diabetic treatment with intercurrent illness

Never stop insulin in type I diabetics, even if they are unable to eat or drink. The stress of illness ↑ insulin requirements. However, oral intake is often ↓ so it is important to monitor blood sugar levels, 4× a day if possible. Drink plenty of water and, if unable to eat, replace meals with frequent, small drinks, e.g. soup, fruit juice or milk. If ↓ calorie intake, ↓ long-acting insulin or biphasic insulin by ~20%. Short-acting insulin may need to be given/altered depending on blood glucose levels (e.g. if blood glucose 11–17mmol/L, give 4 extra units; if 17–28, give 6 extra units; if >28, give 6 extra units and/or consider infusion).

IV insulin regimes

IV insulin may be required in certain circumstances, e.g. diabetic ketoacidosis (DKA, 📖 Diabetic ketoacidosis, p. 548) or acutely unwell patients unable to take/absorb oral hypoglycaemics or whose blood glucose is too unstable to control with regular sc insulin. There is also evidence that careful control of blood glucose with IV insulin may improve the outcome of critical illness including acute coronary syndromes. IV insulin may be given either as a sliding scale or as a glucose-K^+-insulin (GKI) infusion.

Insulin sliding scale infusion

Make 50U of soluble insulin up to 50mL with normal saline (i.e. 1U/mL solution). Measure blood glucose hourly and infuse at a rate according to the blood glucose in Table 12.1. This sliding scale regimen is only a guide—individual scales may vary between institutions, and may need to be adjusted for individual patients.

Give IV fluids through separate vein/IV line: normal saline if blood glucose ≥11mmol/L, 5% glucose when blood glucose <11mmol/L; K^+ according to blood K^+ levels. In DKA, the initial K^+ is often high, but ↓ rapidly after insulin is started. If rapid access to K^+ measurement is not available, give 20mmol K^+/L in the second and subsequent bags of fluid, and then maintenance and replacement K^+ according to blood levels. If IV K^+ is not available use Ringer's lactate instead of saline and oral K^+ supplements.

GKI infusion

Add 15U of soluble insulin to a bag of 500mL 10% glucose with 20mmol K+. Infuse at 100mL/h and check the blood glucose hourly. Make up new bags with altered insulin units as shown in Table 12.2. Unless the blood glucose is quite stable, the GKI regime tends to be more wasteful as new bags need to be made up frequently.

Table 12.1 Blood glucose and insulin infusion

Blood glucose (mmol/L)	Units/h
≤5.0	1
5.1–12.0	3
12.1–20.0	4
>20.0	6

Table 12.2 Blood glucose and insulin in bottles added to bag of 500mL 10% dextrose with 20mmol K^+

Blood glucose (mmol/L)	Insulin in bag (units)
<5	6
5–15	15
>15	25

Diabetic follow-up

Diabetes is an ↑ problem, even in rural areas. Complications of DM can be devastating, but simple measures, e.g. good BP control, effectively ↓ complications. Some complications, such as cataract, can be easily identified and addressed. It is essential to establish locally accessible diabetic clinics in order to:

- Identify and resolve problems with treatment.
- Encourage adherence with treatment and maintain education.
- Encourage ↓ weight.
- Monitor foot care (see 📖 The diabetic foot, p. 654, for diabetic foot management).
- Prevent and monitor development of long-term complications.
- Frequent follow-up and tight control are essential during pregnancy.

Prevention of complications

- Diabetics are at ↑ risk of microvascular and macrovascular complications, including stroke (relative risk, RR 2–3 compared with non-diabetics), MI (RR 2–5), blindness (RR 20), renal failure (RR 25), and limb amputation (RR 40). Although good glycaemic control ↓ complication rates, avoiding hypoglycaemia is even more important.
- Good glycaemic control: assess using the following:
    - *Symptoms*—hyperglycaemia or hypoglycaemic attacks (📖 Hypoglycaemia, p. 550).
    - *Home urine testing*—aim for 0–0.025%
    - *Home glucose records*—aim for 4.5–6.5mmol/L
    - *Glycosylated Hb*—HbA_1c; indicates mean glucose level over the preceding 6wks; aim for 7.5% in type II DM.
- Control of hypertension: good BP control as important at preventing complications as good glycaemic control. Target BP is 130/80mmHg (125/75mmHg if persistent proteinuria).
- IHD risk factor modification: stop smoking, control hyperlipidaemia; aspirin for those with hypertension or vascular disease.

Clinic checklist

Every 6mths check:

- Treatment and glucose control.
- BP.
- Injection sites.
- *Feet:* pulses, numbness, sores, nail care.
- *Both eyes:* check acuity (with glasses if worn, otherwise use pin hole). If acuity ↓, check for cataracts; if no cataracts, maculopathy likely (more common in type II DM). Check fundus for retinopathy—if cotton wool spots or new vessels present, refer for laser treatment, if available.
- *Urine dipstick for albumin:* albuminuria or a ↑ BP may indicate nephropathy. Exclude UTI; check serum creatinine. Albuminuria warrants aggressive treatment of BP (see 📖 Prevention of complications, p. 546).
- If macrovascular disease or nephropathy is present, check lipids.

Diabetic ketoacidosis

Without insulin, glucose is unable to enter cells and the body uses ketones produced in the liver for metabolism. Lack of insulin eventually → hyperglycaemia and a build-up of acidic ketones. This may be precipitated by infection. DKA can occur in type II DM if pancreatic insulin production very low. These patients usually need to be insulin treated.

Clinical features Deterioration is often gradual over several days. There may be hyperventilation (deep Kussmaul breathing, +/– sweet, ketotic breath), vomiting, hyperglycaemia, and coma. May be new diagnosis of diabetes—ask about polyuria, polydipsia and weight loss.

Investigations

FBC, U&Es, bicarbonate, blood gases, infection screen (urine and blood cultures, CXR). Look for ketones in the urine (or in the blood if test available). *Blood glucose may not be very high.* The seriousness of the condition is determined by pH, bicarbonate (HCO_3) levels, and the level of ketones (+/– the underlying precipitant/cause, e.g. infection).

Diagnosis Requires hyperglycaemia (glucose >11.1mmol/L) + acidosis (pH<7.3 or Kussmaul breathing) + ketosis.

Management

- Urgently correct dehydration (may be life-threatening) e.g. normal saline 1–2L/h for the first 2h.
- Give soluble insulin 6U/h IV initially, adjusted according to the sliding scale regimen. If infusion pumps are not available use a GKI regime or IM sliding scale (give soluble insulin 20U IM, then 6U IM/h until blood glucose <10mmol/L, then 3U IM/h). Whichever method is used to control the blood glucose, once the ketones have been cleared from the urine switch to regular sc insulin, using the starting rules above.
- Measure K^+ hourly. Initial K^+ often high , but ↓ rapidly with insulin: if rapid K^+ measurement not available give 20mmol K^+/L in the 2nd and subsequent litres of fluid (unless oliguric, when K^+ may need to be withheld), and then maintenance and replacement K^+ according to blood levels. For management when IV K^+ not available see sliding scale Box 12.2.
- Monitor vital signs and blood glucose every hour.
- When blood glucose concentration falls below 14mmol/L, start a 10% glucose infusion together with a normal saline infusion (two bag system). The rate of glucose infusion can be adjusted to titrate a slow, steady fall in glucose levels without the risk of hypoglycaemia.
- Prevent complications, including aspiration, DVT. Pass NGT to decompress stomach. Be alert to shock, cerebral oedema, and DIC.
- If available give 5000IU heparin sc bd or low molecular weight heparin.
- Giving bicarbonate is unnecessary. Insulin and fluid will correct acidosis provided the underlying cause (e.g. infection) is treated. If there is gross acidosis without ketosis, consider renal failure, aspirin overdose, or lactic acidosis in elderly diabetics or those on ART.
- Identify and manage the precipitant, e.g. poor compliance with treatment, intercurrent illness. Educate to help avoid recurrent DKA.

Box 12.2 Management of DKA in children

❶ Children with DKA are high risk, and can die of cerebral oedema, hypokalaemia or aspiration pneumonia. Always seek senior advice on presentation and follow local guidelines. For more information see: http://www.bsped.org.uk/clinical/docs/DKAGuideline.pdf

- Resuscitate (ABC) if necessary (see inside cover leaf). Give 10mL/kg fluid boluses only if shocked (up to 30mL/kg).
- *Clinical features, diagnosis and investigations:* similar to adults.
- *Consider if child is high risk (may need intensive care):*
  - severe acidosis; pH <7.1 with marked hyperventilation
  - severe dehydration with shock
  - ↓ conscious level (*Note:* risk of aspiration from vomiting)
  - young age (<2yrs).
  - insufficient staffing to allow adequate monitoring.
- *Rehydrate:* calculate fluid requirements over the first 48h as deficit (based on degree of dehydration) plus maintenance. Start fluids 1h before insulin infusion to ↓ risk of cerebral oedema. After 12h may switch from 0.9% to 0.45% saline if Na^+ stable or increasing.
- Insulin infusion is usually started at 0.1U/kg/h:
  - when glucose <14mmol/L add glucose to fluid (e.g. 0.9% saline + 5% glucose); continue insulin to switch off ketogenesis
  - when blood pH is >7.3, blood glucose is <14mmol/L and the fluids contain glucose consider ↓ insulin infusion rate, but no less than 0.05U/kg/h.
- Replace K in all fluids given after initial resuscitation (unless anuric): e.g. 500mL 0.9% saline + 20mmol KCl; adjust according to electrolyte levels where results are available.
- *Monitor closely:* hourly observations including fluid status, GCS, blood glucose, and electrolytes.
- *Resolution of DKA:* change to sc insulin when feels well, able to eat and drink, acidosis resolved blood ketones <1mmol/L or urinary ketones falling. Discontinue insulin infusion 60min (if soluble or long acting insulin) or 10mins (Novorapid® or Humalog®) after the first sc injection to avoid rebound hyperglycaemia.

Hyperglycaemic hyperosmolar non-ketotic coma

Hyperglycaemic hyperosmolar non-ketotic coma (HONK) generally affects older, type II diabetics. Usually a gradual history with intense dehydration and severe hyperglycaemia (>35mmol/L). There is no acidosis or ketosis and the plasma osmolality may be >340mmol/kg. (Plasma osmolality may be estimated as:

$$\text{Osmolality} = 2[Na^+ + K^+] + [\text{urea}] + [\text{glucose}]\text{mmol/L})$$

Treat as for ketoacidosis, but correct the osmolality slowly (over 2–3d) using half normal or normal saline to avoid cerebral oedema after large fluid shifts. DVT is more likely, so use heparin prophylaxis. Seek an underlying cause, e.g. infection, silent MI.

Hypoglycaemia

This is usually due to administration of excess insulin, sulphonylureas, or thiazolidinediones. It presents with altered (often aggressive) behaviour, sweating, tachycardia, and, rarely, seizures and coma of rapid onset. If the patient is unable to take sugar orally, give IV (e.g. 25–50mL of 50% glucose) followed by a saline flush to avoid damaging the vein (may also use larger volumes of 10 or 20% glucose, but larger volumes may be required); improvement should be rapid. This should be followed quickly by feeding with complex carbohydrate. If IV access fails, try glucagon 0.5–1mg IM (0.5mg for children <8yrs old or <25kg) to attempt to promote conversion of hepatic glycogen to glucose (repeated doses of glucagon become less effective as glycogen stores become depleted). If a long-acting insulin or oral agent has been taken, the patient will need monitoring and may require further IV glucose for 48h.

Diabetic nephropathy

Early disease is manifested by microalbuminuria; this may → frank proteinuria (detected by dipstix) and a gradual ↓ renal function, → over 10–15yrs to end-stage renal failure. In type I DM, nephropathy develops ~7–10yrs after onset; in type II it may be present at diagnosis. Retinopathy is usually present in both type I and II diabetics with nephropathy.

Management

- Good glycaemic control: monitor carefully as requirements for insulin and oral hypoglycaemics tend to ↓ in chronic renal failure, due to ↓ renal glucose excretion and ↓ insulin resistance. Avoid glibenclamide (risk of hypoglycaemia) and metformin (risk of lactic acidosis).
- Control BP to ↓ progression of renal damage. Target BP is 125/75. Patients are at high risk of hypertension since salt and fluid loads are less well handled. Fluid-overloaded patient may need high doses of diuretics, unless dialysis is possible.
- ACE inhibitors slow progression of nephropathy, even in normotensive diabetics with microalbuminuria.
- Control hyperlipidaemia.

Nephropathy in the diabetic patient is strongly correlated to the risk of coronary disease and cardiovascular death. Aggressive management of vascular risk factors is also required (smoking/BP/lipids/aspirin). Watch for the abrupt onset of pulmonary oedema or congestive heart failure, which may be the first signs of severe IHD.

Thyroid disease

Thyroid gland may become enlarged either diffusely (goitre) or in single or multiple nodules and, in each case, patient may be euthyroid, hypothyroid, or hyperthyroid. Regulation of thyroid hormones is through hypothalamo-pituitary-thyroid axis (see Fig. 12.2).

Causes of goitre or thyroid nodules

- Physiological: endemic (📖 Iodine deficiency, p. 727) or sporadic (pregnancy/puberty).
- Diffuse, autoimmune: Graves' or Hashimoto's.
- De Quervain's thyroiditis: see Box 12.3.
- Goitrogens: e.g. sulphonylurea drugs, cassava, soya beans.
- Dyshormonogenesis.
- Nodular goitre: single or multi-nodular—euthyroid or thyrotoxic.
- Tumours: benign and malignant.

Hypothyroidism (myxoedema)

Clinical features

Include ↑ weight, lethargy, constipation, dislike of cold, menorrhagia, infertility, dry skin, hoarse voice, depression, dementia, cerebellar ataxia, myopathy, angina, galactorrhoea, and vitiligo. Examination may reveal coarse features, bradycardia, goitre, CCF, non-pitting oedema, ascites, pleural effusion, pericardial effusion, delayed reflexes, loss of the outer third of the eyebrows.

Diagnosis of hypothyroidism ↑ Thyroid-stimulating hormone (TSH), ↓ T_4 (and T_3). FBC may show macrocytic anaemia (check B12/folate) or iron deficiency (menorrhagia); ECG may show bradycardia and/or ischaemia; cholesterol and triglycerides may be ↑. +ve antithyroid antibodies suggest an autoimmune cause.

Management

Levothyroxine 50–150micrograms od, adjusted according to clinical state (aim to keep TSH <5mU/L). In the elderly/those with IHD, begin with 25 micrograms/day and monitor for angina or tachycardia (propranolol may be needed, e.g. 10–40mg 3–4× daily). Usually required lifelong; if de Quervain's thyroiditis is suspected, withdraw levothyroxine after 6mths and monitor. If area is iodine-deficient, use Schiller's iodine (1:30 diluted Lugol's iodine) 2 drops od for 6–12mths.

Myxoedema coma Very rare, with 50% mortality. Often precipitated by infection, MI, CVA, or trauma. Look for hypothermia, hyporeflexia, bradycardia, paralytic ileus, and seizures.

Investigations T_3, T_4, TSH, FBC, U&E (may have hyponatraemia), glucose, cultures, and ABG (hypoxia and hypercapnia).

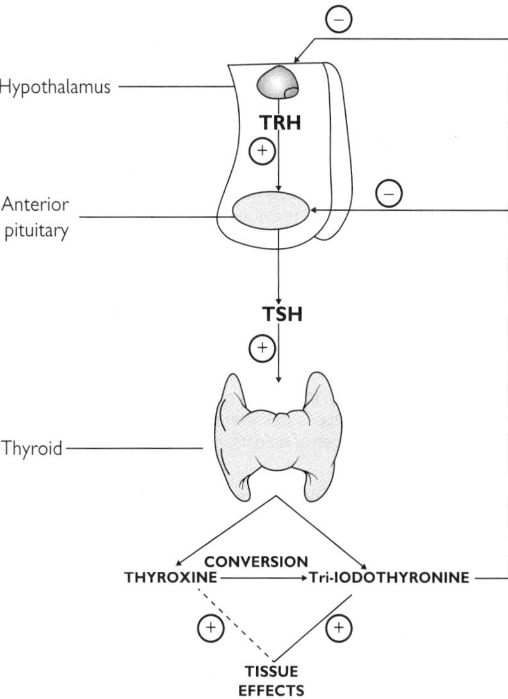

TRH = thyrotropin releasing hormone, TSH = thyroid stimulating hormone

Fig. 12.2 The hypothalamo-pituitary-thyroid axis.

Management

Give O_2 and treat any precipitating cause.

- If available give 5–20micrograms liothyronine by slow IV injection; repeat after 6–12h.
- Give hydrocortisone 100mg tds IV (especially if pituitary failure suspected).
- Pass NGT; unless paralytic ileus, give levothyroxine 300micrograms od.
- Rehydrate with normal saline, avoiding CCF. Hyponatraemia is usually due to water retention so fluid restriction may be necessary.
- Correct hypothermia and hypoglycaemia.
- Monitor for pancreatitis and arrhythmias.
- After 3d, change to usual od levothyroxine dose, orally or per NG.

Compensated/subclinical hypothyroidism

↑ TSH, normal T_3 and T_4, clinically euthyroid. Usually follows treatment for thyrotoxicosis or at an early stage of autoimmune hypothyroidism. Measure thyroid auto-antibodies. Treat with levothyroxine if antibody +ve, hypercholesterolaemia, or subfertility. Otherwise, monitor TFT 6-monthly.

Causes of hypothyroidism

- *Autoimmune hypothyroidism:* usually in women. If goitre present, diagnosis is Hashimoto's thyroiditis; if none, diagnosis is atrophic hypothyroidism. Associated with previous Graves' disease, insulin dependent diabetes mellitus (IDDM), Addison's disease, pernicious anaemia; rarely with thyroid lymphoma.
- Post thyroidectomy or radioiodine treatment.
- *Drug-induced:* anti-thyroid drugs, amiodarone, lithium, iodine.
- *De Quervain's thyroiditis:* see Box 12.3.
- *Iodine deficiency:* (📖 Iodine deficiency, p. 727). Previously widespread (e.g. in Africa). May be endemic, especially in mountain areas, or sporadic (pregnancy/puberty). Iodination programmes have ↓ prevalence, but endemic goitre is still seen in many adults.
- *Dyshormonogenesis:* a number of defects, all autosomal recessive.

Box 12.3 De Quervain's thyroiditis (post-viral thyroiditis)

- Often follows 6wks after a viral infection (e.g. mumps, coxsackie).
- Associated with general malaise. Goitre is tender.
- ↑ Inflammatory markers (WBC, ESR, CRP).
- Can be hypo-, hyper-, or euthyroid.
- Self-limiting illness; usually lasts ~6mths , but may require symptomatic treatment (NSAIDS, prednisolone 30mg od) and occasionally levothyroxine or antithyroid drug treatment in interim.
- 5–25% become hypothyroid months–years later: follow up long term with TFTs.

Abnormal TFTs in non-thyroidal illness

'Sick euthyroid syndrome'

Occurs in severe illness/starvation/fasting. TSH ↓ or normal, T_3 ↓, T_4 ↓ or normal. Patient may be clinically hypothyroid. Does not require treatment; self-corrects when the underlying problem is treated. If abnormalities persist, consider hypopituitarism.

Amiodarone-associated thyroid abnormalities

Abnormal TFTs are common on amiodarone, as well as true thyroid dysfunction. The drug blocks conversion of T_4 to T_3, so may see raised T_4, normal/↓ T_3, and normal/↑ TSH. True thyroid dysfunction more likely if thyroid auto-antibody +ve. Only treat if clinical hypo/hyperthyroidism supported by TFTs.

Hyperthyroidism (thyrotoxicosis)

Clinical features More common in women; ↓ weight, diarrhoea, oligomenorrhoea, tremor, emotional lability, heat intolerance, sweating, itch, fatigue, hair thinning, and proptosis. Examination may reveal tachycardia, AF, fine tremor, eye disease (Box 12.4), goitre/nodule(s), thyroid bruit, myopathy.

Complications Include heart failure, AF, osteoporosis, gynaecomastia.

Diagnosis ↓ TSH, ↑ T_3 and/or ↑ T_4. Nuclear thyroid scanning best way to differentiate toxic nodules and multinodular goitres from Graves' disease (diffuse ↑ uptake) and de Quervain's thyroiditis (↓ uptake). Scan can be done while taking antithyroid drugs. USS, thyroid auto-antibodies, ECG, FBC, U&E also useful. Test the visual fields and acuity.

Management

- Control symptoms with propranolol 10–40mg 3 or 4× daily.
- Start carbimazole 40mg od for 4–6wks (may have to ↑ to 60mg if not achieving control). Propylthiouracil is an alternative. If due to de Quervain's thyroiditis may not need antithyroid drugs. Further treatment then depends on cause of hyperthyroidism.
- *Graves' disease*: either ↓ carbimazole dose according to TFTs and maintain on 5–10mg carbimazole od for 12–18mths before stopping, or 'block and replace'—leave on carbimazole 40–60mg od and once TSH starts to rise add levothyroxine 50–150micrograms od for 18mths. Block and replace is simpler as it does not require regular monitoring of TFTs and may be associated with lower relapse rates. With both regimes ~50% will relapse with thyrotoxicosis, usually in the next 18mths. Toxic nodules/multinodular goitre: use lowest effective dose. Treatment usually lifelong (Box 12.5).
- Tell patient to return if develops a severe sore throat after starting carbamazepine (~0.1% risk of agranulocytosis); check FBC.
- Radioiodine is best treatment for toxic nodule or multinodular goitre. Single treatment should lead to cure with minimal risk of hypothyroidism. Radioiodine can be used for Graves' (usually reserved for relapsed cases); occasionally requires a repeat dose. Post-treatment hypothyroidism is common.
- Surgery is useful for large goitres, but runs similar risks of over- and under-treatment as radioiodine in Graves' disease.
- Patients should be made euthyroid with carbimazole before surgery or radioiodine to avoid thyroid storm.
- In pregnancy, lowest possible dose of antithyroid drug should be used as risk foetal goitre (which may ↑ risk of obstructed labour).

Subclinical hyperthyroidism

↓ TSH, normal T_3 and T_4. Found in multinodular goitre and after treatment for Graves'. Patients are usually clinically euthyroid. Not thought to require treatment , but may be associated with ↑ cardiovascular morbidity and mortality. See Box 12.5 for causes.

Box 12.4 Thyroid eye disease

Thyrotoxic patients may have lid retraction/lid lag due to autonomic overactivity. Patients with autoimmune thyroid disease can develop autoimmune ophthalmopathy, with gritty sore eyes, blurred vision, double vision, eye pain, and/or protrusion. It is worse in smokers.

Box 12.5 Causes of hyperthyroidism

Toxic multinodular goitre Common in areas of iodine deficiency.

Graves' disease Genetic predisposition leads to antibodies to TSH receptors and diffuse goitre. May be ophthalmopathy, pre-tibial myxoedema (oedematous swellings on shins), anaemia, ↑ ESR, ↑ Ca^{2+}, and abnormal LFTs. Associated with other autoimmune diseases in individual or family.

Toxic adenoma Nodule producing T_3/T_4.

Thyroiditis Post-partum or de Quervain's (see Box 12.3).

Others Medication, follicular carcinoma of the thyroid, choriocarcinoma, struma ovarii (ovarian tumour secreting T_3 and T_4).

Addison's disease

Adreno-cortical insufficiency, leading to ↓ gluco- and mineralocorticoids. May occur in disseminated TB, especially during 1st few weeks of rifampicin treatment; or in HIV adrenal disease.

Clinical features Weakness, apathy, anorexia, ↓ weight, abdominal pain, oligomenorrhoea. There may be hyperpigmentation, vitiligo, hypotension (sometimes postural), and sexual dysfunction. Dehydration in crises. Hypoglycaemia.

Investigations Tetracosactide test. Check for hyperkalaemia, hyponatraemia (see 🕮 Hyperkalaemia, p. 562 🕮 Hyponatraemia, p. 560), uraemia, acidosis, hypercalcaemia. Get a CXR (looking for signs of TB) and AXR (adrenal calcification from previous TB).

Management

Treat cause. Replace steroids with oral prednisolone (5mg in morning, 2.5mg at night) or hydrocortisone 2–3× daily with larger dose in morning (e.g. 10mg/5mg/5mg); adjust dose according to symptoms. Warn patient not to stop steroids abruptly. Explain need to ↑ prednisolone dose during intercurrent illnesses. There should be 6-monthly follow-up.

Addisonian crisis Hypotension and shock in a known Addisonian patient or someone on long-term steroids who has omitted their tablets. Often there is preceding infection, trauma, or surgery.

Management

- Take bloods for urgent adrenocorticotrophic hormone (ACTH) and cortisol if available.
- Resuscitate with colloid then crystalloids.
- Give 100mg hydrocortisone IV stat, then every 6–8h.
- Culture blood, urine, and sputum.
- Give a broad-spectrum antibiotic.
- Monitor for hypoglycaemia.
- If stable after 72h, change to oral prednisolone or hydrocortisone regimen as above. (*Note:* hydrocortisone tablets have a high bioavailability; the oral and IV doses of hydrocortisone are similar. 5mg of oral prednisolone is equivalent to 20mg of IV or oral hydrocortisone.)

Cushing's syndrome

Due to chronic glucocorticoid excess. The most common cause is corticosteroid treatment (iatrogenic); important to differentiate this from endogenous over-production of cortisol. Normally, ACTH secreted by the pituitary is regulated by the hypothalamus and stimulates cortisol secretion by the adrenals. Cushing's syndrome may be either ACTH dependent (↑ ACTH drives ↑ cortisol) or ACTH independent (↑ cortisol without ↑ ACTH). Also consider alcoholic pseudo-Cushing's, depression, and ectopic ACTH from, e.g. small cell lung carcinoma.

Clinical features

Moon face, obesity, impaired glucose tolerance, hypertension, hypogonadism, osteoporosis, purple striae, limb wasting and myopathy, hirsutism, thin skin, bruising, peripheral oedema, ↑ infection, poor wound healing, hypokalaemia, psychological change (depression/mania/psychosis). Increased pigmentation if ↑ ACTH.

Diagnosis

First establish if Cushing's syndrome present:

- Overnight dexamethasone (DXM) suppression test is a screening test: give DXM 1mg po at 23.00 hours and take blood for plasma cortisol at 09.00 hours. Normal cortisol <170nmol/L; higher in Cushing's syndrome (*Note:* false high values may be caused by the oral contraceptive pill).
- 24-h urinary free cortisol (>700nmol/24h suggests Cushing's).
- 09.00 hours and midnight cortisols: loss of diurnal variation suggests Cushing's (typically 09.00 hours cortisol 140–700nmol/L, midnight 80–350nmol/L).
- Low-dose DXM suppression test: give DXM 0.5mg 6h for 2d then check 09.00 hours serum cortisol on the 2nd day (should be <50nmol/L). If not suppressed, a diagnosis of Cushing's can be made.

Then identify cause (pituitary/adrenal/ectopic):

- Consider pituitary/adrenal imaging (CT or MRI), CXR (?lung cancer)
- *High-dose DXM suppression test:* as above, but give 2mg DXM 6-hourly for 48h. Pituitary ACTH-driven Cushing's will show some suppression; adrenal or ectopic ACTH will not.

Expert help is required for investigation and management

Will depend on cause. If possible reduce steroid dose (+/– steroid-sparing agent) for iatrogenic Cushing's.

Hyperaldosteronism

Excessive aldosterone production independent of the renin angiotensin system (↑ aldosterone, ↓ renin). Typically, there is ↑ BP, ↓ K^+, alkalosis, and mildly ↑ Na^+. Suspect if K^+ low before treatment of BP or persistent hypokalaemia on thiazides. Most cases are due to adrenocortical adenoma (Conn's syndrome); rarely, adrenal hyperplasia or carcinoma. In 2° hyperaldosteronism (e.g. heart or liver failure, diuretic therapy), aldosterone and renin are both raised. Diagnosis relies on measuring renin and aldosterone levels and requires specialist input. Management may be medical (spironolactone 100–400mg od; glucocorticoids, e.g. dexamethasone 0.75mg in morning, 0.25mg at night), or surgical. Treat 2° disease by treating the cause. Give K^+ replacements.

Hypopituitarism

The pituitary produces ACTH, growth hormone (GH), follicle-stimulating hormone (FSH), luteinizing hormone (LH), TSH, and prolactin. ↓ production of one or more of these is termed hypopituitarism and may be due to: infarction (Sheehan's syndrome post partum haemorrhage or Russell's viper envenoming), cysts, granulomatous disease, abscesses, congenital defects, stroke, basal skull fracture, craniopharyngioma (usually under 20yrs), pituitary adenoma, hypophysectomy, and irradiation. There may be atrophy of breasts, small testes, hair loss, thin skin, hypotension, visual field defects (bitemporal hemianopia, initially of upper quadrants). Investigate with lateral skull X-ray (calcification in pituitary fossa may indicate old granulomatous disease or craniopharyngioma, erosion of sella turcica if pituitary macroadenoma), assessment of visual fields, U&Es, FBC, TFT, testosterone/oestrogen, cortisol, CT head. Endocrine testing requires stimulation tests. A specialist centre is needed for treatment, which involves replacement of hydrocortisone, thyroxine, and oestrogen/testosterone.

Diabetes insipidus

Results from a failure of antidiuretic hormone action either due to lack of production (cranial DI) or renal insensitivity (nephrogenic DI). There is reduced water resorption by the kidney, polyuria, polydipsia. Severe dehydration and ↑ Na^+ will occur if access to water restricted.

Causes

- *Cranial DI:* head injury, metastases, sarcoid, meningitis, surgery.
- *Nephrogenic DI:* ↓ K^+, ↑ Ca^{2+}, drugs (e.g. lithium, amphotericin B, tetracycline), sickle cell disease, renal failure, pyelonephritis, hydronephrosis.

Diagnosis Early morning urine osmolality (if >800mOsmol/L, DI is excluded), U&Es, water deprivation test.

Treatment For cranial DI is desmopressin replacement. For nephrogenic DI, remove underlying cause. May take weeks to recover; thiazides and indometacin 100mg/day may reduce urine output during this time.

Other pituitary syndromes

Acromegaly

- Caused by ↑ GH secretion from a pituitary tumour. (In children → gigantism).
- Clinical features include coarse features, large mandible, tongue, hands/feet, carpal tunnel syndrome, hypertension, muscle weakness, +/– bitemporal hemianopia.

Hyperprolactinaemia

Causes include pituitary adenoma/stalk compression; physiological (pregnancy, stress), drugs (metoclopramide, haloperidol, methyldopa, oestrogens), chronic renal failure, hypothyroidism, sarcoid. Presents with amenorrhoea, infertility, galactorrhoea (women), impotence (men). Treat underlying cause.

In both cases management of pituitary adenoma is often a combination of medical, surgical and radiotherapy, and requires specialist input.

Phaeochromocytoma

A catecholamine-secreting tumour, usually in the adrenal medulla. 10% are extra-adrenal, 10% malignant and 25% multiple. Causes hypertension, cardiomyopathy, weight loss, hyperglycaemia, and crises of fear, palpitations, tremor, and nausea. Check 24-h urinary catecholamine excretion (↑); imaging (e.g. CT/MRI) may aid diagnosis. Management requires specialist input. Cautiously reduce BP with phenoxybenzamine first, then give propranolol to control tachycardia. Phentolamine may be required during crises. Surgery provides the only cure.

Hyponatraemia

Very common. Likely cause depends on fluid status of patient.

↓ Extracellular volume (ECV)

Dehydrated, total body sodium low. Causes include:

- Diarrhoea.
- Vomiting.
- Burns.
- Uncontrolled diabetes.
- Excessive or chronic diuretics.
- Addison's.
- Recovery phase of acute renal failure.

Normal ECV Euvolaemic, total body sodium normal. Causes include:

- Syndrome of inappropriate anti-diuretic hormone (ADH; Box 12.6).
- Over-hydration with hypotonic fluids.
- Severe hypothyroidism.
- Addison's.

↑ ECV Fluid overloaded/oedematous, total body sodium normal. Causes include:

- Nephrotic syndrome.
- Cardiac failure.
- Renal failure.
- Cirrhosis.

Treatment

Directed at the underlying cause. If salt depleted, replace salt and water with ORS, salt tablets (60–80mmol/d, if able to drink) or saline drip +/– K^+. If SIADH fluid restrict (see Box 12.6). *Caution:* if Na^+ corrected too quickly may → central pontine myelinolysis (→ quadriplegia, abnormal eye movements).

Box 12.6 Syndrome of inappropriate ADH

SIADH → water retention and dilutional hyponatraemia

Causes May be secondary to meningitis, pneumonia, TB, cancer, head injury, drugs (e.g. vincristine, carbamazepine, phenothiazines).

Clinical features

- Headache.
- Confusion.
- Nausea.
- Seizures.
- Coma.

Diagnosis Low Na^+, (sometimes low K^+, urea). Plasma osmolality low. Urine osmolality > plasma osmolality. Urinary sodium >30mmol/L.

Treatment Treat the underlying cause.

Fluid restrict 500–1000mL/24h.

Hypernatraemia

Less common. Almost always indicates severe dehydration.

Causes Almost always indicates severe dehydration. Other causes include HONK (📖 Hyperglycaemic hyperosmolar non-ketotic coma, p. 548), anti-diuretic hormone (ADH) deficiency/insensitivity (see 📖 Diabetes insipidus, p. 558 and acute tubular necrosis (ATN)).

Clinical features

- Nausea.
- Vomiting.
- Confusion.
- Fever.
- Seizures.

Diagnosis ↑ plasma osmolality, urine osmolality inappropriately < plasma osmolality.

Treatment Treat underlying cause. Slow rehydration with normal saline.

Hypokalaemia

Causes

Diuretic treatment, IV fluid replacement without K^+, hyperaldosteronism (2°, e.g. liver failure, heart failure; or 1°, e.g. Conn's syndrome). Also consider gastrointestinal losses, e.g. vomiting, diarrhoea, redistribution into cells (insulin+glucose infusion or salbutamol), renal tubular damage, corticosteroid treatment.

Clinical features Usually asymptomatic, but K^+ <2.5mmol/L may → muscle weakness. Very low K^+ can → arrhythmia.

Treatment Treat underlying cause. Adult daily maintenance requirement is 60mmol/24h. Additional K^+ needed if hypokalaemia or ongoing losses. Oral supplements (40–60mmol/day) or fresh fruit, vegetables. If hyperaldosteronism suspected, spironolactone 100–400mg/day (25–50mg/day in heart failure).

Hyperkalaemia

Causes

- Renal failure.
- Spironolactone.
- ACE inhibitors.
- Transfusion of stored blood, acidosis.
- Rhabdomyolysis.
- Addison's.

Clinical features

- Muscle weakness.
- Often asymptomatic.
- Cardiac arrhythmia.

Diagnosis If patient at risk of hyperkalaemia and K^+ result not available check ECG: 'tented' T waves (T wave as tall as the R wave) indicative of hyperkalaemia.

Treatment

Treat the underlying cause/withdraw culprit drugs. In acidosis/DKA K^+ will correct as acidosis/DKA treated (unless concomitant renal failure). In life-threatening hyperkalaemia (K^+ >7.0mmol/L, ECG changes) give 10ml 10% calcium gluconate stat by slow IV injection. Set up insulin+glucose infusion as for GKI regime (*without* the K^+), give salbutamol nebulizers, furosemide, K^+ chelators (e.g. calcium resonium).

Hypercalcaemia

Causes

Malignancy (usually severe); consider:

- Myeloma.
- Lung, breast, or prostate cancer.
- 1° hyperparathyroidism.
- Vitamin D therapy.
- Sarcoidosis.
- TB, thiazide diuretics.
- Thyrotoxicosis.
- Addison's disease.

Clinical features May be asymptomatic or tiredness, malaise, nausea, constipation, ↑ BP, polyuria, dehydration, confusion, vomiting, coma.

Treatment

Treat/remove the underlying cause. If severe symptoms: normal saline 4–6L/24h + furosemide 40mg/L (rehydrates + promotes Ca^{2+} excretion), IV bisphosphonates if available, prednisolone 30–60mg daily (not effective in all cases). If mild and/or suspected hyperparathyroidism encourage good fluid intake, avoid thiazides, consider for parathyroidectomy.

Hypocalcaemia

Causes

- Renal failure.
- Alkalosis (hyperventilation, persistent vomiting).
- Hypoparathyroidism (previous thyroidectomy).
- Vitamin D deficiency.
- Massive transfusion of citrated blood.
- Bisphosphonates.

Clinical features

- Neuromuscular excitability.
- Cramps.
- Tetany.
- Carpopedal spasm (if BP cuff inflated >systolic BP for 3 minutes- Trousseau's sign).
- Twitching of facial muscles if facial nerve tapped (Chvostek's sign).
- Peri-oral numbness.
- Seizures.
- Neuropsychiatric manifestations.
- Psychosis.

Diagnosis

Serum calcium level (should be adjusted for serum albumin level: add/ subtract 0.1mmol/L Ca^{2+} for every 4g/L that albumin is below/above 40g/L, respectively). Check creatinine and phosphate. ECG usually shows long QT.

Treatment

If severe, give 10% calcium gluconate 10mL stat by slow IV injection; then dilute 100mL calcium gluconate 10% in 1L normal saline and infuse at initial rate of 50mL/h, adjusted according to response. Longer term treatment with oral Ca^{2+} supplements. Usually more effective if given with vitamin D (1α-hydroxylated vitamin D required if renal impairment). Monitor for hypercalcaemia.

Acidosis

Causes

- Usually metabolic.
- Renal failure.
- DKA.
- Lactic acidosis (metformin or antiretroviral drugs).
- Severe sepsis.

Clinical features

- Kussmaul respiration.
- +/– Confusion.
- +/– Seizures.
- Plus clinical features of underlying condition.

Diagnosis

↓ HCO_3, ↓ CO_2, may have ↑ K^+, plus biochemical features of underlying cause.

$$\text{Anion gap} = [(Na^+ + K^+) - (Cl^- - HCO_3)].$$

Normal anion gap is <18mmol/L. An ↑ anion gap suggests lactic acidosis, ketoacidosis, renal failure or exogenous acid (e.g. aspirin poisoning). Serum albumin <20g/L gives false low anion gap.

Treatment

Withdrawal of culprit drugs and treatment of underlying cause. For chronic acidosis in patients with chronic renal failure give oral sodium bicarbonate titrated according to symptoms/bicarbonate levels.

Chapter 13

Ophthalmology

Invited author **David Yorston**

Global blindness

WHO estimates that 39 million people worldwide are blind (acuity less than 3/60 in the best eye). 90% of them live in resource-poor countries, and two-thirds are aged ≥50. The number of blind people ↑ every year as world population both increases and ages. However, recent efforts to improve eye care, and to treat cataract and refractive error, have had some success in ↓ global blindness. Another 246 million people have visual impairment (acuity less than 6/18 to 3/60). Cataract is the commonest cause of blindness worldwide, with ~17 million blind people and >100 million eyes needing cataract surgery because of visual impairment. In 1999, ~10 million cataract operations were performed worldwide, but ~30 million cataract operations need to be performed annually if cataract blindness is to be controlled in the next ten years.

With improvements in hygiene and 1° healthcare leading to increased life expectancy, especially in Asia, degenerative conditions, e.g. glaucoma, diabetic retinopathy, and age-related macular degeneration are the fastest growing causes of blindness.

Trachoma and onchocerciasis are responsible for ~5% of all blindness. Both occur in poor communities. Blindness can be prevented through relatively simple, low-cost interventions, including use of antimicrobials. Vitamin A deficiency is major cause of blindness in children in poor communities.

Uncorrected refractive error, especially myopia, is leading cause of visual impairment, especially in Asia. Refraction followed by appropriate spectacle correction will restore sight, but for people living in isolated communities, 'refractionist' and spectacles are often either unavailable or unaffordable. These five diseases (cataract, trachoma, onchocerciasis, vitamin A deficiency, and refractive errors) are all avoidable (preventable or curable) and cause >70% of visual impairment worldwide.

Presenting features of eye disease

Main symptom

- *Visual loss:* cannot see in the distance with one or both eyes. May be rapid or gradual.
- *Red painful eye(s):* eye pain or discomfort, with or without a history of trauma.
- *Inability to read:* ↓ near vision, despite good distance vision. Due to presbyopia > 40yrs.
- *Other symptoms:* include watering eyes, flashing lights.

Examination

- Measure visual acuity (VA) with and without pinhole (Box 13.1).
- Examine the cornea and pupil (Box 13.2) with a torch-light.
- After dilating pupil, examine optic disc and retina with ophthalmoscope.

Box 13.1 Testing visual acuity

All eye patients must have their VA measured. Any opacity of lens or cornea, or damage to central retina or optic nerve, will ↓ VA. Only distance acuity is measured; near vision will always be ↓ in older patients who do not have reading glasses. Distance vision measured at 6m. Each eye is tested individually, using patient's own distance glasses, if they have any.

- Patient stands 6m from chart and covers one eye. Literate patients read out letters, starting at top. Illiterate patients use an 'E' chart, indicating if it is pointing left or right, up or down.
- Each line on chart is labelled with a number. Top line is 60, 2nd is 36, etc. Numbers indicate distance at which that line can be read by a normal eye. 3rd line on chart can normally be read at 24m, so if a patient can only read this line at 6m, the VA is 6/24. 6 identifies distance at which line was read and 24 identifies distance at which that line would be read by normal eye. Normal vision is 6/6. In practice, most people can do most of their normal daily activities with a vision of 6/18.
- If patients cannot see top line at 6m bring them closer. If they can read it at 3m, acuity is 3/60. If they cannot see top line, ask them to count your fingers, see your hand move, or see light. If they have no perception of light, it is probable that eye is permanently blind and no treatment will restore vision.
- Sometimes the VA is ↓ because the patient needs glasses. You can partially overcome a refractive error by using a pinhole: take some dark card and with a hot 21G needle, make a hole in the centre. The patient looks through the hole; if vision improves, the eye has a refractive error.

Box 13.2 Pupil examination

- Seat the patient in a dimly lit room, focused on distant (>3m) object.
- Use a bright light, and test each pupil reaction in turn. Examine reaction of both pupils when one pupil is illuminated.
- Check accommodation response by asking patient to focus on your finger held a few inches in front of their nose. If the patient accommodates, eyes will converge and pupils constrict.
- Observing movement of a darkly pigmented iris against a black pupil in a dim room is difficult. Your examination will be more reliable with magnification.

Visual loss: refractive errors

Usually present with gradual ↓ vision. Five types of refractive errors:

Myopia Short-sightedness, → poor distance vision, but good near vision. Most people with poor distance vision due to refractive errors have myopia. Myopia can be diagnosed as follows:

- The distance vision improves with a pinhole.
- Near vision is good, despite poor distance vision.

Myopia can be corrected with –ve (concave) lenses. In absence of trained refractionist, the following method will usually give an acceptable spectacle correction. If you have trial lenses available, test one eye at a time. Start with –1 lens and gradually ↑ strength by steps of –1, measuring visual acuity with every lens. When ↑ power does not lead to any further improvement, choose minimum power that will give best visual acuity. Repeat process for other eye.

Hypermetropia Long-sightedness, → difficulty with near vision in young people. Hypermetropia uncommon <40yrs, but can be corrected with +ve (convex) lenses.

Astigmatism Different refraction in horizontal and vertical axes of the eye. Can be corrected with cylindrical lenses.

Aphakia Severe hypermetropia due to removal of the lens. Aphakia is becoming less common as most cataract operations include insertion of an intraocular lens. Can be corrected with a +11.0 dioptre lens.

Presbyopia Poor accommodation → difficulty with reading and near vision >40yrs. Can be corrected with reading spectacles that usually have (+ve) strength of between +1.00 and +4.00 dioptres. In patients <50yrs, +1 to +2 is sufficient. Patients >70yrs will require +3 to +4.

Table 13.1 Common causes of poor distance vision

	Causes	Signs and symptoms	Management
Refractive error	Myopia Astigmatism Aphakia (Hypermetropia)	Vision ↑ with pinhole	Spectacles
Cataract	Usually age related Also: Eye injuries Diabetes iritis	White or grey pupil Pupil reacts to light Absent or poor red reflex	Cataract removal if visual acuity is < 6/18, or if lifestyle affected
Corneal opacity	Corneal ulcer Trachoma Vitamin A deficiency Leprosy	White scarring of the cornea in a quiet white eye Pupil difficult to see Absent or ↓ red reflex	Often no treatment Surgery may be considered when both eyes affected
Diseases of optic nerve and retina	Glaucoma Optic atrophy Macular degeneration Diabetic retinopathy Hypertensive retinopathy Retinal detachment	Cornea and lens should be clear Pupil may not react normally to light Specific signs seen with an ophthalmoscope in retina or optic nerve	Management directed at cause

Cataract

Cataracts → gradual, progressive, and painless ↓ VA. Because they progress very slowly, most patients who are blind from cataract never come to an eye clinic, since they accept their blindness as normal for their age. Elimination of cataract blindness requires community involvement to change attitudes and ↓ barriers that block access to eye services. Cataract surgery has a significant impact on poverty. Even one family member with moderate cataract causes a significantly ↓ household income, but income recovers if the affected person has a cataract operation.

Diagnosis

When complete, cataracts can be seen as a white opacity in the pupil, while younger cataracts give a grey-white appearance to the pupil. Examination with an ophthalmoscope, after dilation of the pupil, shows opacity in the red reflex with obscuration of fundus detail due to lens opacity (Box 13.3). The pupil reaction to light is normal in an uncomplicated cataract.

Management

There is currently no way to prevent cataracts forming. The only treatment is surgery to remove the lens and replace it with an artificial intraocular lens. Surgery is usually performed under local anaesthesia. Following surgery, 80–90% of eyes should be able to see 6/18 or better. The patient may then need corrective spectacles to obtain optimal vision.

Box 13.3 Lens examination

Useful tip when studying lens (or other anterior eye structures) is to set your ophthalmoscope to its strongest +ve lens (typically +10 to +30). This allows instrument to focus a few centimetres away. Test by examining your own finger-tip to check distance of focus. By moving in and out you can see cornea, iris, anterior chamber and lens in fairly good detail. This is a low-tech way to inspect eye with good illumination and high magnification.

Corneal opacity

Diagnosis

White opacity on the cornea, which usually prevents clear view of iris and pupil. May follow corneal ulcer, or injury, or it may be caused by trachoma, vitamin A deficiency, or leprosy. Most corneal scars are preventable by 1° prevention strategies (e.g. vitamin A supplements) or by good management of the original condition (e.g. corneal ulcer).

Management

If both eyes have severe visual loss, then a corneal graft or optical iridectomy may improve vision. Specialist care and good follow-up are essential.

Glaucoma

Most glaucoma presents with gradually progressive ↓ peripheral vision due to optic nerve damage. There are no symptoms until VA ↓, which occurs only after most of the optic nerve has been destroyed. Acute glaucoma is uncommon, and presents with a red painful eye (see 📖 Acute glaucoma, p. 581).

Diagnosis

Chronic glaucoma difficult to diagnose. Detecting peripheral visual field loss requires expensive and complex equipment. Measuring intra-ocular pressure (IOP) is simpler, but unreliable, as many patients with ↑ IOP do not have glaucoma. Some patients with glaucoma have normal IOP. More reliable diagnosis is by observing ↑ size of the optic cup. However, this requires expertise.

Management

Consists of reducing IOP with filtration surgery or lifelong eye drops (e.g. timolol 0.25% bd). Treatment prevents progression and preserves sight, but does not improve vision, so patients who are already blind should not be treated.

Macular degeneration

As more people survive into their 8th decade, macular degeneration is becoming a common cause of blindness. Atrophic (or dry) macular degeneration is the commonest type. It causes a gradual, often bilateral ↓ vision in people >70yrs old. Examination of the retina shows atrophy of the central retina. Because it is slowly progressive it usually → visual impairment rather than blindness. At present it is untreatable.

Exudative (or wet) macular degeneration is caused by abnormal new blood vessels that grow out from the choroid under the macula. This usually occurs quite rapidly over a few weeks. The blood vessels leak fluid and bleed. Eventually they are replaced by scar tissue, and the central vision is completely destroyed. This condition is treatable if detected at an early stage (vision 1/60 or better). Patients with recent onset of symptoms, and vision of 1/60 or better, associated with exudates or haemorrhage at the macula should be referred to an eye specialist. Treatment consists of monthly injections of ranibizumab 0.5mg into the vitreous cavity, which was prohibitively expensive. However, bevacizumab 1.25mg, injected into the vitreous every 4wks is as effective, and cheaper.

Diabetic retinopathy

The prevalence of diabetes is increasing globally, and diabetic retinopathy is becoming more common. ~40% of diabetic patients will have some retinopathy; in ~5% it is sufficiently severe to threaten vision. As well as retinopathy, people with diabetes are also at increased risk of cataract.

- Retinopathy is caused by damage to the capillaries in the retina. Capillaries may leak, → oedema and exudates, or they may become blocked, → to ischaemia.
- Commonest cause of visual loss in diabetic retinopathy is *maculopathy*, where macular region of retina (provides central vision) is affected by processes in retinopathy. Oedema is difficult to detect with ophthalmoscope, but hard exudates, lipid deposits in the retina, are easier to see.
- Occlusion of retinal capillaries → ischaemia and hypoxia. Promotes growth of new vessels from surface of retina on posterior vitreous face (proliferative retinopathy). These vessels may bleed, → vitreous haemorrhage, or contract, → traction detachment of the retina.

Diagnosis

In order to detect retinopathy while it is still at an early and easily treatable stage, all diabetic patients should have an annual eye examination, including measurement of VA, and a dilated fundus exam. International classification of diabetic retinopathy gives clear definitions of the different stages and guidelines for referral to an ophthalmologist (see Table 13.2).

Treatment

Laser treatment ↓ risk of loss of vision in maculopathy, but cannot restore sight that has been lost. It can be used to promote regression of new vessels in proliferative retinopathy, to prevent vision loss.

Table 13.2 International classification of diabetic retinopathy

Retinopathy grading	Definition	Action
None	No retinopathy	Re-examine in 12mths
Mild non-proliferative	Microaneurysms only	Re-examine in 12mths
Moderate non-proliferative	More than mild, but less than severe	Re-examine in 6–12mths
Severe non-proliferative	>20 intraretinal hamorrhages in all 4 quadrants. Definite venous beading in >2 quadrants. Intra-retinal microangiopathy in >1 quadrant	Refer to ophthalmologist May need laser treatment
Proliferative	Visible new vessels; vitreous haemorrhage; traction detachment	Refer for urgent laser treatment
Maculopathy grading		
Macular oedema:		
Absent	No exudates or oedema	Re-examine in 12mths
Mild	Exudates in posterior pole, but distant from fovea	Re-examine in 6–12mths
Moderate	Exudates in posterior pole close to fovea	Refer to ophthalmologist for laser treatment
Severe	Exudates in posterior pole involving fovea	Refer to ophthalmologist for laser treatment

Red eye

History and examination

- Ask about any known cause, especially injury.
- Measure the VA.
- Carefully examine eyelids, conjunctiva, cornea, and pupil with a bright torch. Examination will be more reliable if you also use magnification.

Injuries to the eye

Ask about any injury to or foreign body into the eye.

Corneal or conjunctival foreign bodies (FB)

The history is usually straightforward. The FB may be obvious or you may need to evert the upper eyelid to check the conjunctiva for objects scratching the cornea each time the patient blinks.

To remove the FB:

- Lie the patient flat.
- Apply local anaesthetic drops, e.g. lidocaine 4% to the conjunctiva.
- Light the eye with a torch so that the FB is easily visible.
- Loupe magnification is useful.
- Lift off the FB carefully with a sterile needle, or cotton bud.
- Give an antibiotic eye ointment or drops and eye pad for 1d.

Corneal abrasion

This occurs when trauma removes some corneal epithelium. There is sudden severe pain and photophobia. To confirm the diagnosis, apply fluorescein which stains the cornea where there is no epithelium. Treat with an antibiotic eye ointment or drops until the pain has gone and the epithelium is healed, typically in ~24–48 hrs.

Hyphaema

If there is a severe blunt injury (e.g. hit in eye by stone/fist), bleeding may occur inside the eye. A blood level (hyphaema) may be visible between cornea and iris. This will usually resolve over a few days with rest. Avoid aspirin, as this may → further bleeding. If the eye is painful, give acetazolamide 250mg qds for 3–7d to ↓ IOP and topical prednisolone 0.5–1.0% drops qds to ↓ inflammation. If the hyphaema has not resolved after 5d, consult an eye specialist.

Penetrating eye injury

A penetrating injury (involving the full thickness of cornea or sclera) is very serious. Common causes include thorns, and splinters when chopping firewood. Be very careful examining the eye as pressure may aggravate the injury. Gently apply an antibiotic eye drop (not ointment), put an eye pad over the eye, and refer the patient to a specialist immediately. Systemic antibiotics (ciprofloxacin 750mg bd) may ↓ risk of intraocular infection. If immediate referral is not possible, then conservative treatment with antibiotics and an eye pad is probably better than a non-eye surgeon 'having a go'.

Red eye with no injury

If there is no history of eye injury, then consider:

- Conjunctivitis
- Corneal ulcer
- Iritis
- Acute glaucoma

See Table 13.3.

Table 13.3 Common causes of non-traumatic acute red eye

	Acute glaucoma	**Iritis**	**Corneal ulcer**	**Conjunctivitis**
Pain	Severe	Moderate	Moderate to severe	Irritation
Visual loss	Severe	Variable	Variable	None
Redness	Around corneal limbus	Around cornea	Around cornea	Especially in fornices
Cornea	Oedematous and hazy	Keratic precipitates seen with magnification	Opacity on cornea	Normal
Pupil	Half dilated and fixed	Constricted and irregular	Normal	Normal
Special features	↑ IOP	Irregular pupil may be more obvious as the pupil is dilated	Stains with fluorescein	Discharge, often bilateral
Treatment	Acetazolamide 250mg qds to ↓ IOP Surgery usually needed	Dilate pupil and give topical steroids if certain of diagnosis	Topical antimicrobials	Topical antibiotics

Conjunctivitis

Infective conjunctivitis

Infection or inflammation of the conjunctiva is common in the tropics. Important causes and a way of differentiating them are given in Table 13.4.

Diagnosis Irritation of the eye with discomfort, but normal vision. Eye red with ↑ discharge. Severe disease may → swelling of eyelids (chemosis).

Management Give an antibiotic eye ointment or drops, e.g. chloramphenicol 0.5–1%, initially 2-hourly, then qds for 5–7d. Do not pad eye.

Ophthalmia neonatorum

A specific conjunctivitis occurring in the first 4wks of life, usually due to *Neisseria gonorrhoeae* or *Chlamydia trachomatis* (see 📖 Antibiotic therapy of infections in young infants, p. 21). The lids are very swollen and covered with pus. Untreated, gonococcus infection progesses rapidly with complete destruction of the cornea and permanent blindness.

Management

Give appropriate systemic and topical antibiotics which will be effective against local strains of gonorrhoea (see 📖 Gonorrhoea, p. 670). Most cases of ophthalmia neonatorum may be prevented by irrigating eyes of all newborn babies with 2.5% povidone-iodine solution: one drop in each eye immediately after delivery, repeated once within first postnatal day.

Chlamydial conjunctivitis (trachoma)

See 📖 Trachoma, p. 582.

Epidemic haemorrhagic conjunctivitis

Highly contagious viral conjunctivitis usually due to enteroviruses. After 1–2d incubation period, multiple petechial haemorrhages occur. Most patients recover quickly.

Management Give an antimicrobial agent, e.g. povidone-iodine 1.25% 1 eye drop qds, to help ↓ transmission and reassure the patient.

Allergic conjunctivitis

Children and young adults may develop chronic allergic conjunctivitis (vernal conjunctivitis). Severe itching/irritation with a mucus discharge, sometimes with swelling and pigmentation around the cornea.

Management

Treatment with topical steroids is effective, but has serious side-effects. If possible, children with severe disease should be seen and treated by an eye specialist. In milder cases, parents should be reassured that the condition does not lead to loss of sight and is usually self-limiting — children 'grow out of it'. Symptoms may be improved by bathing eyes with cold clean water.

Table 13.4 Common causes of conjunctivitis

Cause	Age	Secretions	Special features	Treatment
Bacterial	Any	Purulent	Red and swollen; purulent discharge	Topical antibiotics for 5d
Ophthalmia neonatorum	First 4wks of life	Purulent	Very red and swollen; purulent discharge	Systemic and topical antibiotics for 10d
Viral	Any	Watery	May have corneal lesions	Symptomatic only
Chlamydial (trachoma)	Usually young children	Mucopurulent	Follicles and papillae on upper lid	Azithromycin 1g tablets or tetracycline ointment for 6 wks
Allergic (vernal)	Children	Stringy mucus	Very itchy, large papillae; infiltrate and pigmentation around cornea	Cromoglicate and possibly steroid eye drops for symptoms

Periocular cellulitis

Cellulitis around eye is commonly divided into pre-septal and post-septal cellulitis depending on whether infection is anterior or posterior to orbital septum (which divides eyelid from orbit). Difference is important:

- *Post-septal (orbital) cellulitis:* an emergency, which → blindness and severe complications (including abscess formation, cavernous sinus thrombosis, optic nerve damage, meningitis). More common in children than in adults.
- *Pre-septal (periocular) cellulitis:* may occur from local superficial infection, spread from sinus infection, or from bacteraemia (this was common with *Haemophilus influenzae* type b in young children, but incidence has ↓ due to Hib immunization). Common pathogens are *Staphylococcus aureus* and Streptococci. It may also be caused by non-typeable *H. influenzae* and, particularly in sinus-associated infection, Gram –ve and anaerobic bacteria. Fungal infection is rare, and more likely to occur with immune deficiencies.

Clinical features

Peri-orbital erythema and tenderness. Orbital cellulitis is suggested by ophthalmoplegia, proptosis, ↓ visual acuity, chemosis or signs of systemic toxicity.

Management

With IV antibiotics (oral treatment might be considered for mild pre-septal cellulitis in a very well patient). Antibiotics should cover likely pathogens, e.g. ceftriaxone 2g IV od (children 50mg/kg IV od) plus metronidazole 400mg tds oral (child 1mth–12yrs 7.5mg/kg tds; max 400mg tds). If available consider CT head for patients requiring parenteral treatment (?sinus infection or complications, e.g. abscess formation), and ear, nose and throat (ENT)/ophthalmology review.

Corneal ulcers

May occur spontaneously or follow corneal abrasion. There are many causes, most frequent are summarized in Table 13.5.

Diagnosis

Usually severe pain, watery discharge, and blurred vision; redness around cornea, which is cloudy, often with localized white or grey opacity, which stains with fluorescein. In severe cases, there may be a fluid level of pus inside eye ('hypopyon'). If ulcer is caused by a bacterium or fungus, organism may be identified by Gram stain and culture of a scraping from edge of ulcer, but this should only be done in an eye clinic.

Management Depends on the cause, and is summarized in Table 13.5.

Snake venom ophthalmia

Spitting elapids have evolved modified fangs that enable snake to eject a spray of intensely irritant venom into eyes of an aggressor, → intense pain, conjunctivitis, corneal erosions (and occasionally anterior uveitis). 2° bacterial infection of corneal erosions may → permanent scarring and blindness.

Management Wash venom from affected eye or mucous membranes with copious amounts of water. Apply topical chloramphenicol or tetracycline ointment. 0.1% adrenaline eye drops relieve the pain.

Table 13.5 Common causes of corneal ulceration

Cause	Predisposing factors	Clinical features	Treatment
Herpes simplex	Fever	Irregular branching ulcer	Aciclovir ointment 5 times daily for 2wks
Bacteria	Trauma	Often severe pain and ↓ vision; +/– hypopyon	Topical and/or sub-conjunctival antibiotics (e.g. ciprofloxacin, ofloxacin, cefuroxime or gentamicin) hourly for 48h then QDS for 5d or until epithelium healed
Fungus	Hot, humid areas, minor trauma	Often severe pain and ↓ vision; +/– hypopyon	Antifungals, e.g. natamycin 5% eye drops hourly for ≥2wks
Vitamin A deficiency	Measles Malnutrition Malabsorption	Dry cornea. Central 'punched out' oval ulcer, often in a quiet eye	Vitamin A 200 000 IU start, then after 1d and 2wks
Exposure	Leprosy Facial burns	Eyelids do not close; lower third oval ulcer	Antibiotic ointment Tape eye closed Tarsorrhaphy

Uveitis

Inflammation of the uvea may involve both anterior uvea (iris and ciliary body) and posterior uvea (choroid). Causes include infections (e.g. leprosy, onchocerciasis, toxoplasmosis, TB, syphilis) and systemic diseases (e.g. certain types of arthritis, sarcoidosis, Behçet's, inflammatory bowel disease). However, most cases, especially of anterior uveitis, have no known cause, and multiple investigations are unnecessary.

Anterior uveitis (iritis, iridocyclitis)

Clinical features

Pain of iritis varies from mild to severe and → photophobia and often some blurring of vision. Blood vessels around margin of cornea (limbus) are dilated. Iris constricts and adheres to front of lens (posterior synechia), making pupil irregular. These synechiae can → 2° glaucoma and cataract. When pupil is dilated, adhesions may be seen before they break, leaving iris pigment on front of lens. Pus collecting in anterior chamber can be seen with a slit lamp microscope.

Management Dilate pupil to break any posterior synechiae (cyclopentolate 1% or atropine 1% 2–3x/d for 2wks); give anti-inflammatory agents to ↓ inflammation (prednisolone 0.5–1.0% drops hourly initially, then gradually ↓ over 4wks).

Posterior uveitis

Clinical features

Presents with visual loss because of involvement of overlying retina and vitreous. Not usually painful, but severe attack may → discomfort. A white inflammatory lesion may be seen in retina. Once inflammation has settled, characteristic scars occur with pigment atrophy and hypertrophy.

Management Requires treatment of cause.

Acute glaucoma

If the IOP ↑ suddenly over a few hours, eye becomes red and very painful with severe loss of vision. Acute glaucoma is unusual in people <50yrs. May occur spontaneously or as a complication of a completely white cataract. Cornea appears hazy and pupil is semi-dilated and does not react to light. IOP is very high, which can → nausea and vomiting. Acute glaucoma may be misleading and can present as a sudden severe headache, or mimic an acute abdomen.

Management Give acetazolamide 500mg stat oral and then 250mg qds oral. Refer to eye specialist, since urgent surgery is usually required.

Trachoma

Trachoma is a chronic conjunctivitis caused by infection with *Chlamydia trachomatis*, serotypes A, B, and C. Inflammation from active infection → scarring of the upper conjunctiva and tarsal plate causing the eyelashes to turn in and scratch the cornea, producing ulceration, scarring, and blindness (see Colour plate 25a–e).

Transmission

Disease occurs especially in poor dry areas of the world, where there is inadequate water supply and poor community sanitation.

The classic trachoma environment can be described as:

- *Dry:* lack of water.
- *Dirty:* lack of sanitation.
- *Discharge:* lack of personal hygiene.

Transmission from child to child, and child to mother occurs through:

- *Flies:* flies go from individual to individual.
- *Fingers:* direct contact with ocular discharge.
- *Family:* within the family, child to child.

Clinical features and diagnosis

See the 5-point WHO grading system in Box 13.4. TF and TI are found mainly in pre-school children; TS, TTr, and CO occur more commonly in women than men, starting at ~15yrs and gradually ↑ in prevalence.

How to examine the eye for trachoma

Use good light (sunlight or strong torch) and ×2–2.5 magnification. Examine each eye separately:

- Look for trichiasis (either inturned lashes or previously removed eyelashes). Push upper lid upwards slightly to expose lid margins.
- Check cornea for opacities.
- Check inside upper eyelid by everting it. Ask patient to look down; gently take hold of eyelashes between thumb and first finger of left hand, and evert upper eyelid using a glass rod or similar instrument in right hand. Steady everted lid with left thumb and examine conjunctiva for follicles, intense inflammation, and scarring.

Management

- Azithromycin 1g oral as single dose (20mg/kg if <45kg) *or*
- For pregnant women, erythromycin 500mg oral bd for 7d *or*
- Tetracycline 1% topical ointment both eyes bd for 6wks.

Studies are still evaluating merits of treatment of whole communities vs. affected individuals. Azithromycin treatment of all children in the community ↓ transmission in adults as well. Where mass distribution of azithromycin has been used, it has been associated with ↓ child mortality. Entropion and trichiasis will require surgery. Although surgery is initially successful, entropion will recur in up to 40% of patients.

Prevention

The acronym SAFE summarizes the strategies for prevention (see Box 13.5). Control requires first identifying a community with blinding disease. This can be done using the grading scheme and a survey of children of 1–10yrs for TF and TI, and women over >15yrs for TT. A prevalence of TF in > 20%, or TT >1%, identifies a community with severe disease.

Box 13.4 WHO's 'SAFE' strategy for the global elimination of trachoma

S Surgery for entropion and trichiasis
A Antibiotics for infectious trachoma
F Facial cleanliness to reduce transmission
E Environmental improvements, e.g. control of disease-spreading flies and access to clean water.

Box 13.5 Trachoma grading

See Colour plate 25. Signs must be clearly seen to be considered present. Grading is important to decide whether mass treatment is warranted.

- *Normal:* normal conjunctiva is pink, smooth, thin, and transparent. Over whole area of tarsal conjunctiva, there are normally large deep-lying blood vessels that run vertically. Dotted line in Colour plate 25a shows the area to be examined.
- *Trachomatous inflammation—follicular (TF):* the presence of >5 follicles in the upper tarsal conjunctiva. Follicles are round swellings that are paler than the surrounding conjunctiva, appearing white, grey, or yellow. Follicles must be >0.5 mm in diameter (see Colour plate 25b).
- *Trachomatous inflammation—intense (TI):* pronounced inflammatory thickening of the tarsal conjunctiva that obscures >50% of the normal deep tarsal vessels. The conjunctiva appears red, rough, and thickened. There are numerous follicles, which may be partially or totally covered by the thickened conjunctiva (see Colour plate 25c).
- *Trachomatous scarring (TS):* scars are easily visible as white lines, bands, or sheets in the tarsal conjunctiva. They are glistening and fibrous in appearance. scarring, especially diffuse fibrosis, may obscure the tarsal blood vessels (see Colour plate 25d).
- *Trachomatous trichiasis (TTr):* eyelash rubs on the eyeball. Evidence of recent removal of inturned eyelashes should also be graded as trichiasis (see Colour plate 25e).
- *Corneal opacity (CO):* easily visible corneal opacity over the pupil. The pupil margin is blurred viewed through the opacity. Such corneal opacities cause significant ↓ VA (worse than 6/18 vision) and, therefore, VA should be measured (see Colour plate 25e).

Xerophthalmia

Xerophthalmia is due to vitamin A deficiency, which may → corneal ulceration and blindness, especially with measles. A medical emergency, as severe vitamin A deficiency has a high mortality (see 📖 Vitamin A deficiency, p. 714). Patients with acute corneal lesions should be referred, whenever possible, to a hospital for treatment of their general condition, as well as their eye disease.

Ocular leprosy

Leprosy (📖 Leprosy, p. 488) can affect eyelids, cornea, or pupils by damaging nerves to eye or by causing iritis.

Eyelids

Nerve damage may occur during a type 1 reaction and cause an inability to close the eye (lagophthalmos), ↑ corneal exposure, ulceration, scarring, and blindness. In the acute stages, systemic treatment of leprosy reaction may restore nerve function.

Management

Protect cornea when patient is asleep by applying ointment and strapping upper eyelid to cheek. If severe and permanent, or if there is corneal ulceration, a tarsorrhaphy will be required to protect cornea. This consists of sewing together lateral third of upper and lower eyelid margins.

Cornea

Ophthalmic nerve damage → corneal anaesthesia. Patient does not blink as much as usual and may be unaware of minor trauma to the cornea, → ulceration, scarring, and blindness.

Management

Prevent by early recognition of problem and educating patient to protect cornea during the day by blinking, and at night with ointment and strapping of eyelid to cheek. If these measures fail, then a permanent lateral tarsorrhaphy is required.

Pupil

There may be acute anterior uveitis with a red painful eye, and small irregular pupil. This may occur as part of an erythema nodosum leprosum reaction. Leprosy also → chronic low-grade anterior uveitis in which the pupil is very small and irregular and will not dilate. Eye is usually white in chronic iritis.

Management

In acute anterior uveitis, pupil should be dilated immediately and patient kept on atropine and topical steroids. In chronic anterior uveitis, it is important to keep pupil dilated and maintain patient on mydriatic eye drops for life.

HIV infection and the eye

Ocular manifestations of HIV infection include:

- Herpes zoster ophthalmicus.
- Squamous cell carcinoma of the conjunctiva.
- CMV retinopathy.

Herpes zoster ophthalmicus

Presents initially with pain over one side of head and face → vesicular rash. Upper eyelids are always involved +/– keratitis and iritis, which can → ↑ IOP. Disease is often blinding in HIV+ individuals with corneal involvement and severe intraocular inflammation. Treatment is with oral aciclovir 800mg 5×/d. Sometimes 1st sign of HIV infection, and all patients should receive counselling and HIV test.

Squamous cell carcinoma of the conjunctiva

Appears as a raised irregular white lesion, usually on temporal conjunctiva, that grows to invade fornices, lids, and cornea. Treatment is by wide surgical excision where possible.

Cytomegalovirus

CMV retinitis is the commonest opportunistic infection of the eye and a major cause of blindness in AIDS patients. Occurs late in the disease (CD4 count <100). Where ART is available, CMV retinitis has become rare. The appearance is one of red haemorrhages and pale necrotic tissue ('cottage cheese and ketchup'). It is bilateral in 50% of cases. It is slowly progressive and can destroy whole retina. Treatment, if available, is with:

- Ganciclovir 5mg/kg IV every 12h for 2–3wks, then 5mg/kg/d *or*
- Foscarnet 60mg/kg IV tds for 2–3wks, then 90–120mg/kg/d.

However, both → severe side-effects and are expensive. Alternatively, ganciclovir can be given by weekly intravitreal injection. This requires much lower doses, with little risk of systemic toxicity, but carries risk of introducing infection (endophthalmitis) and inconvenience of weekly intraocular injections.

Onchocerciasis and the eye

An infection of skin and eye due to filarial worm *Onchocerca volvulus* (see 📖 Onchocerciasis ('river blindness'), p. 630).

Inflammation can affect the:

- *Cornea:* → acute punctate keratitis, which may → sclerosing keratitis and corneal scars.
- *Iris:* → anterior uveitis and posterior synechiae.
- *Choroid and retina:* → chorioretinitis, night blindness, and chorioretinal atrophy (most marked temporal to the macula).
- *Optic nerve:* → optic neuritis and 2° optic atrophy.

No treatment can restore vision that has been lost due to onchocerciasis, but annual treatment with ivermectin prevents eye damage in endemic areas.

Chapter 14

Dermatology

Invited authors **Colette van Hees**
Ben Naafs

Introduction

Skin function and failure

The largest organ of the human body, the skin forms an interface between body and environment. Its main functions are:

- *Barrier against mechanical, thermal, and chemical injury, pathogens and UV-damage:* extensive skin damage, e.g. burns or toxic epidermal necrolysis may be fatal.
- *Sensation:* sense of touch, pain, itch, orientation, temperature, and pressure. Loss of protective sensation may lead to injury or pressure ulcers.
- *Thermoregulation:* control of cutaneous circulation and sweating prevents potentially fatal cooling and overheating.
- *Psychosocial:* healthy skin contributes a 'look good, feel good' factor; skin disease may cause depression, neglect, stigma, and decrease personal and work prospects.

Common problems

Skin disease is among the top three reasons people seek healthcare. The most common problems are:

- Infections and infestations.
- *Absent skin:* burns and ulcers.
- *Sexually-transmitted infections:* affecting skin or mucosae.
- Dermatitis (eczema), psoriasis, and bullous disorders.

Management of skin disease with limited resources

Good skin care may be given using local resources at low cost:

- Take time to examine whole skin to enable pattern recognition. Daylight is proper light for skin examination. Palpate for infiltration and temperature.
- Prevent further damage to diseased skin, both from infection (keep wounds clean and ensure good hygiene) and from trauma. 'Off-loading' the skin is important in preventing pressure ulcers. Well-fitting shoes help prevent foot trauma. Hats provide protection from sun. A blanket may provide warmth, shade, and cover from flies; and injury from fire may be reduced by education and safer cooking devices.
- Preserve and enhance barrier function with locally available moisturisers, such as emulsifying ointment, aqueous cream, and vegetable oils (apply to wet skin). White soft paraffin and mineral oils may cause irritation and 'trap' infectious agents.
- Psychosocial aspects of skin disease may significantly affect quality of life. Skin disfigurement, albinism, leprosy, smell of chronic ulcers or cutaneous manifestations of AIDS may cause stigma and depression. They also fuel a market in ineffective remedies; this and over-usage of cosmetics contribute to the cycle of poverty.

Infections of the skin

For soft tissue infections, see Chapter 15.

Folliculitis

Inflammation of the hair follicle, usually bacterial (*Staphylococcus aureus*), but fungal (*Pityrosporon*) organisms may also be implicated, especially in HIV/AIDS. Treat according to cause with antibiotics or antifungals (imidazole cream bd or itra- or ketoconazole 200mg od for 1–3wks).

Folliculitis keloidalis nuchae

A deep folliculitis of the neck area which is common in African males. It is usually caused by staphylococci → to a chronic fibrosing folliculitis and peri-folliculitis. Keloidal scars are produced in the deeper cutaneous tissue. New papules and pustules occur at the rims of the keloid. The course is very chronic. *Treatment*: doxycycline 100mg od oral for 2wks to several mths. Combine with potent topical steroid e.g. betamethasone cream bd on lesions or intralesional steroids. Full thickness excision of scars left to heal by secondary intention leaves an atrophic scar with no recurrence.

Acne

Blocked sebaceous gland ducts (forming comedones = blackheads and whiteheads), which may progress to inflammatory papules, pustules, and nodules. It commonly occurs on the face and the upper trunk and may be very mild to very severe. In severe acne lesions blend together to form large inflammatory areas with cysts and scar formation. It is very common in puberty, usually regresses in early adulthood, but may persist up to age 30 or lifelong. In dark skin post-inflammatory hyperpigmentation may cause distress. To prevent this, inflammatory acne should be treated at an early stage.

Management

- Stop the use of white soft paraffin, oil, or ointments and greasy cosmetics, which further block sebaceous ducts.
- 'Peeling' of comedones with benzoyl peroxide 5–10% gel adapalene gel or tretinoin 0.01–0.1% cream, lotion or gel; apply at night since both are photosensitizers. An alternative is salicylic acid 1–10% +/−sulphur praecipitatum in a cream, gel or alcoholic solution. Alcoholic solutions remove excess sebum, e.g. dilute methylated spirits with an equal amount of water to give a 35% solution.
- *For pustular/inflammatory lesions:* add topical clindamycin 1% lotion, erythromycin 2% lotion, or use doxycycline 100mg bd until substantial improvement (may be a month or more) followed by 100mg od until acceptable or cleared, which may take many months.

Skin infestations

Arthropod contact or bites are a common cause of itch. Papular urticaria and vasculitic lesions may result in sensitive individuals. Heavy mite or louse infestations may occur in the immunocompromised and the deprived. An itch–scratch cycle contributes to secondary pyoderma. Treatment of household contacts is an essential part of effective management. Bites from gnats, blackfly, and midges are best prevented by thick clothing.

Lice

There are three species of medical importance

- The head louse (*Pediculus capitis*).
- Body louse (*P. humanus*).
- Pubic or crab louse (*Phthirus pubis*).

The body louse is also important as the vector of epidemic typhus (*Rickettsia prowazekii*), relapsing fever (*Borrelia recurrentis*), and trench fever (*Bartonella quintana*).

Transmission is by close personal contact, ↑ by poverty, overcrowding, and poor hygiene. The lice pierce the skin to take a blood meal, injecting saliva and defecating at the same time. A rash occurs due to a hypersensitivity reaction to the saliva. Blue macules <1cm in diameter occur during pubic louse infection probably due to injection of an anticoagulant. Body lice live in the host's clothes, passing onto the skin only to take a blood meal. Head and pubic lice infest the skin directly. Eggs ('nits') are laid and firmly glued to hairs.

Management

For body lice the focus is on laundering clothes. Lice are easily dislodged, but leave eggs in bedding, towels, and clothing. Launder clothes in a very hot wash, then iron the seams; or dust clothes with 1% malathion powder. For head and pubic lice, apply 0.5% malathion liquid on the affected parts, allow to dry naturally, and remove by washing after 12h. (Alternatives to malathion in case of resistance: carbaryl 0.5–1%; permethrin 5%; phenothrin 0.2–0.5%; ivermectin 0.5% lotion).

Scabies (Colour plate 19a–c)

Sarcoptes scabiei is transmitted by close personal contact. The female burrows into the epidermis to lay eggs; burrows can be seen as 0.5–1.5cm long irregular tracks. Sensitization to mite faeces and saliva occurs within a few weeks of 1° infestation. Re-infestation results in almost immediate irritation and, in some cases, a generalized urticaria.

Itchy papules and linear burrows occur in a symmetrical distribution, particularly in the finger webs and on the flexor surface of the wrists (frequent hand washers have fewer lesions on the hands). Other sites commonly include elbows, axillae, genitalia (particularly scrotum), periumbilicus, and breasts. Head infestation is common in infants, but unusual in older age groups. Macules and pustules occur. Scratching results in 2° bacterial infection. Severe, hyperkeratotic ('Norwegian') scabies is seen in immunocompromised (e.g. HIV+) individuals.

Management

Apply permethrin 5% cream, malathion 0.5%, or benzyl benzoate 25% to the body and leave on for 24h before washing off. Malathion and permethrin are applied twice, 1wk apart. Benzyl benzoate is applied on three consecutive days and may require repeated applications to penetrate the crusts. Sulphur 2–10% creams may be used to soften the crusts (also safe in babies). Ivermectin 200micrograms/kg oral stat is an alternative for scabies complicating other skin diseases, for Norwegian scabies, or for communities such as prisons. All clothing worn the previous day, and the day of the treatment, and all bedding, must be washed. Iron the laundry or dry for an hour in a hot dryer. Place any un-washable items into a closed plastic bag for 2wks. The eggs will hatch in ~10d, but mites will die if away from human skin for > 24h. Asymptomatic infection is common, so treat the whole household. *Note:* itching may persist for some days, but does not usually indicate treatment failure.

Trombiculid mites (Chiggers)

Chiggers are the larvae of trombiculid mites, several species of which may cause an itchy dermatitis. The tiny larvae assemble at the tips of grass stems and other foliage and then attach to passing mammals and birds including humans, feeding on the host tissues. Typically, an itchy dermatitis occurs within a few hours of walking through long grass or other vegetation. Application of repellents e.g. diethyltoluamide (DEET) to skin and clothing will help prevent chigger attack.

Ulcers

Ulcers = absence of surface layers of skin. They invite infection and require a greatly enhanced blood supply for repair. Reasons for ↓ healing may be: local (in and around the wound); general ill health; and/or lack of access to care. 2° infection by *Streptococcus pyogenes* or *Staphylococcus aureus* is common. Fig. 14.1 illustrates the causes of ulcers.

Neuropathic (pressure) ulcers

Are due to a prolonged compression of blood supply. They occur in the sick and elderly, and in patients with neurological deficits, e.g. paraplegia, diabetic neuropathy (see 📖 Peripheral neuropathy, p. 486), or leprosy. The latter two may → the 'neuropathic foot'. Pressure ulcers are preventable with frequent off-loading, and by encouraging movement. Skin care with washing and emollients and gentle movement is beneficial since it restores barrier function, ↓ entry points for bacteria and irritants. Supply pressure-relieving footwear. Leprosy may cause neuropathic ulcers and leprosy reactions may rarely ulcerate – see 📖 Leprosy, p. 488. Consider leprosy when 'spontaneous' ulceration appears on hands or feet.

Venous ulcers

Are a consequence of impaired venous emptying, due to damage to venous valves by stasis, trauma or thrombosis. Venous (+/−lymph) stasis occurs, the consequent oedema compromising the skin by depriving it of oxygen and nutrients. Risk factors: obesity, advanced age, and immobility. They occur less commonly in those who frequently sit on the ground in a cross-legged posture or actively use their legs. Arterial ulcers occur due to peripheral vascular disease. Risk factors are those for atherosclerosis: smoking, diabetes, and advanced age.

Sickle cell disease

Contributes to ulceration of the lower leg, especially the ankle, often beginning in early adolescence. The cause is often mild trauma, complicated by obstruction of small blood vessels by the sickling cells.

Tropical ('phagedenic') ulcer

Is a necrotic lesion caused by the synergistic action of anaerobes (*Fusobacteria ulcerans*) and *Treponema vincentii*. It occurs in areas where legs are repeatedly damaged by vegetation. Acacia thorns are notorious. Painful necrotic ulcer develops from a small papule; it mainly affects children and young men, e.g. farmers. After a few weeks, ulcer stops spreading as inflammation reduces and pain diminishes. Some ulcers heal spontaneously leaving a scar; others become chronic and may persist for years. *Noma* is a phagedenic ulcer of mouth.

Anthrax

Inoculation with *Bacillus anthracis* is a result of contact with an infected animal or infected animal material. Itching occurs, followed by a papule with a dark central vesicle after hours to days. Enlargement leads to characteristic necrotic eschar surrounded by a rim of vesicles. Not painful, typically surrounded by extensive non-pitting oedema.

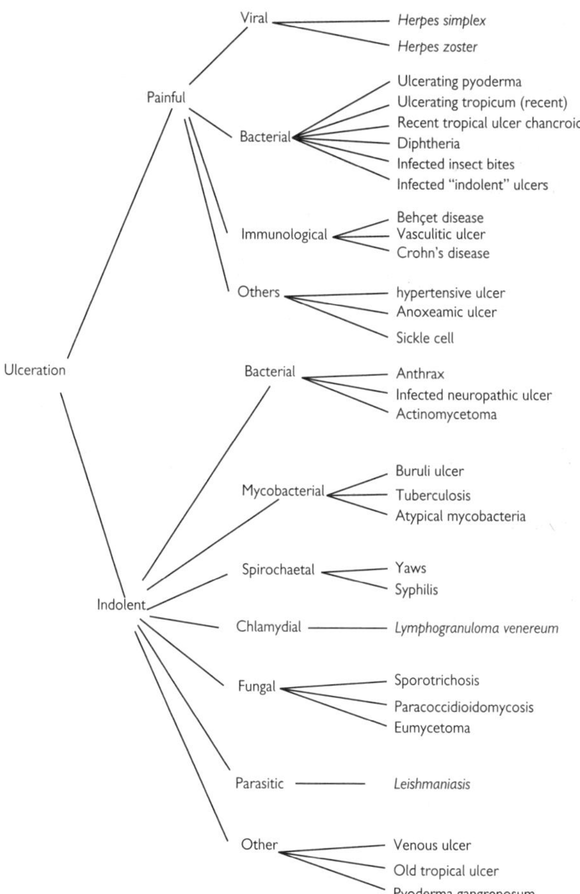

Fig. 14.1 Classification of skin ulcers.

Mycobacterial ulcerating diseases

Buruli ulcer (BU)

Caused by *Mycobacterium ulcerans*, is the 3rd commonest mycobacterial disease (after TB and leprosy) in HIV– individuals (Colour plate 12). It is common in children. BU was first described in Uganda and is endemic in swampy areas in West Africa. BU may be seen elsewhere in the tropics. *M, ulcerans is* inoculated by mild injuries, the bacillus probably residing in muddy water.

A painless papule, plaque or nodule forms, fluctuates after 1–2wks and slowly ulcerates forming an indolent painless ulcer with extensive undermined edges. The patient is not sick and there is no oedema. Mycolactone, a bacterial exotoxin, contributes to necrosis; ulcers may spread rapidly to become very large and disfiguring and 2° infection may occur → sepsis, tetanus, and death. Besides the skin and sc tissue, deeper structures may be involved, e.g. osteomyelitis.

Management

Prevent 2° infection. Until recently, the only effective treatment for BU was wide excision and skin grafting. Recent trials indicate effective treatment (especially in early lesions) with: 8wks rifampicin + 4wks streptomycin + 4wks clarithromycin; or 8wks rifampicin + 8wks clarithromycin. BU may heal spontaneously leaving severe scarring and contractures.

Tuberculosis

Cutaneous TB may cause papules, plaques, warty lesions, cold abscesses, and chronic ulceration, the latter when healing alternates with new ulcerations: lupus vulgaris. Another skin lesion seen in TB is Bazin's disease; panniculitis (sometimes ulcerating) on the calf.

Treatment Standard TB treatment see 📖 Tuberculosis treatment, p. 166).

Other causes of ulcers

These include cutaneous diphtheria, cutaneous leishmaniasis (📖 Cutaneous leishmaniasis, p. 620), sexually-transmitted infections (📖 Sexually-transmitted infections, p. 657), non-venereal treponematoses, actinomycosis, deep mycoses, chronic osteomyelitis, dracunculiasis, trypanosomal chancre, the eschars of rickettsiae, and Behçet's disease.

When an ulcer does not heal *pyoderma gangrenosum* should be considered. This may or may not be associated with IBD, rheumatoid arthritis and myeloproliferative diseases. Small nodular pustules develop into large ulcers at various sites on the body. The pathogenesis of pyoderma gangrenosum is not well understood.

Management of ulcers

Must address the cause; in addition there are some general principles for management of all ulcers.

- Ulcers need covering and should be kept moist. The wound should be carefully cleaned and pus and slough removed. If this is not possible cover the wound with moist (not wet) dressings with saline. As water evaporates saline concentration in dressing increases causing wound secretions and debris to be extracted. Change dressings every 6h till wound is clean. Alternatively clean with 1–6% hydrogen peroxide or dilute sodium hypochlorite solution (≤0.5% available chlorine) at each dressing change.

- Apply clean dressings using short pieces of bandage or well-washed linen. Use dressings with saline or impregnated with honey, coconut oil or white soft paraffin, and cover to prevent evaporation; this will soften crusts and encourage healing. Hydrocolloid dressings may be available in some settings, but may not be suitable in humid climates. Avoid adherent dressings that, when removed, cause pain, bleeding, and take with them any new epidermis growing in the ulcer. Beware evaporation during dressing changes, which may cool ulcer below optimum temperature for cellular repair. Wash and apply emollient on surrounding skin, avoiding maceration of healthy ulcer border with ZnO cream, ointment or paste.
- Blood supply to the ulcer should be optimized by off-loading pressure and encouraging exercise. When the arterial system is healthy, veins and lymph system should be emptied by elevation, compression, and deep breathing exercises. Treat 1° or 2° bacterial infection. Optimize other conditions contributing to poor healing, such as malnutrition.
- Most causes of delayed healing are to be found in the ulcer itself. Foreign bodies, pus, necrotic tissue, and sequestra must be removed and oedema treated. Dead tissue can be excised without pain. Maggots, if available, are a cheap and effective way of debriding an ulcer. Local application of honey or *Aloe barbadensis* (Aloe vera) promotes wound healing, but in general, herbal remedies should be avoided. Large or chronic ulcers may require excision and/or grafting. Pinch or punch grafts can be taken from upper leg or buttocks. They have to be trimmed of the subcutis after being harvested. After they are deposited in a clean ulcer cytokines and chemokines produced by the punch or pinch tissue will promote granulation and vascularization. Often epidermis stays alive and forms a focus of new epithelization. Healthy granulation tissue is generated that can, if needed, be regrafted.
- *Tropical ulcer:* in addition to above measures, antibiotics should be given to eradicate infection, e.g. procaine benzylpenicillin 0.6–1.2g IM daily for 3–7d.
- *Anthrax:* treatment with penicillin.

Rashes

Patient presenting with a skin problem often complains of 'an itchy rash all over the body'. Itch causes severe frustration and should be addressed (Box 14.1). Rashes may be itchy or non-itchy, monomorphic or polymorphic, acute or chronic, symmetrical or asymmetrical, localized, regional or generalized. They may be comprised of macules, papules, plaques, vesicles, pustules, wheals, scales, erosions, or petechiae.

Basis of rashes and topical treatment

- Skin varies in thickness and quantity of hair or sebaceous glands. Rashes affecting only one component of the skin will have a distribution which reflects this component (e.g. hair follicles in folliculitis or dermatomes in shingles).
- In dark skin erythema is not visible, but looks hyperpigmented: palpate to feel inflammation.
- Lesions differ according to depth of inflammation. Near surface it causes vesiculation and scaling, while deep dermal or sc inflammation results in nodule formation.
- Rate of development is determined by type of inflammatory response. Erythema, wheals, and blisters are more acute; white cell infiltration, purpura, and pustules take longer; while ischaemic necrosis and exfoliation are more chronic responses.
- *The distribution of the lesion may be typical:* see Fig. 14.2 and 14.3.
- Endogenous rashes tend to be symmetrical; in contrast, a biting insect produces asymmetric lesions. Unlike rashes of 2° syphilis, site of 1° chancre is not influenced by host symmetry. Fungal infections tend to be asymmetrical, whereas psoriasis is usually exactly symmetrical.
- *Topical treatments:* use cream base for wet and acutely inflamed lesions, an ointment (oily) base for chronic, dry or lichenified lesions. Use topical steroids for short periods of time or intermittently 4d per wk during longer periods. May be diluted with white soft paraffin or vegetable oil.

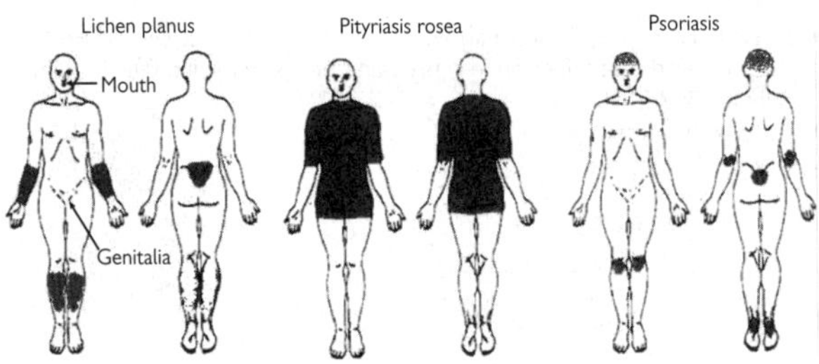

Fig. 14.2 Characteristic distributions of lichen planus, pityriasis rosea, and psoriasis.

Box 14.1 Common rashes (* = itchy)

Maculopapular

Extensive
- Dermatitis*/eczema*
- Body lice*
- 2° syphilis
- Scabies*
- Rubella*
- Measles+/–*
- drug eruption*

Sparse
- Typhoid rose spots
- Gonococcal
- Flea bites*
- Lichen planus
- Pityriasis rosea+/*
- Pityriasis rosea+/*

Hypopigmentation
- Post-inflammatory
- Tinea versicolor
- Vitiligo
- Pityriasis alba
- Pinta
- Post-kala azar dermal leishmaniasis
- Leprosy
- Yaws

Nodules
- Onchocerciasis
- Fungal infections
- Erythema nodosum
- Leprosy
- KS
- Cutaneous leishmaniasis
- Gouty tophi

Plaques/crusts
- Fungal infections
- KS
- Cutaneous leishmaniasis
- Psoriasis
- Trypanosomal chancre
- Crusted scabies
- Impetigo
- Pinta
- Eschar (Rickettsia)

Urticaria*
- Drugs
- Gnathostomiasis
- Strongyloidiasis
- Schistosomiasis (Katayama fever)
- Loiasis

Vesicles
- Chickenpox
- Herpes zoster
- Herpes simplex
- Monkey pox
- Papular urticaria
- Orf
- Vasculitis

Pustules
- Bacterial infection
- Gonococcaemia
- Psoriasis
- Irritant folliculitis

Petechiae
- Meningococcaemia
- Typhus
- Viral haemorrhagic fevers
- Causes of DIC

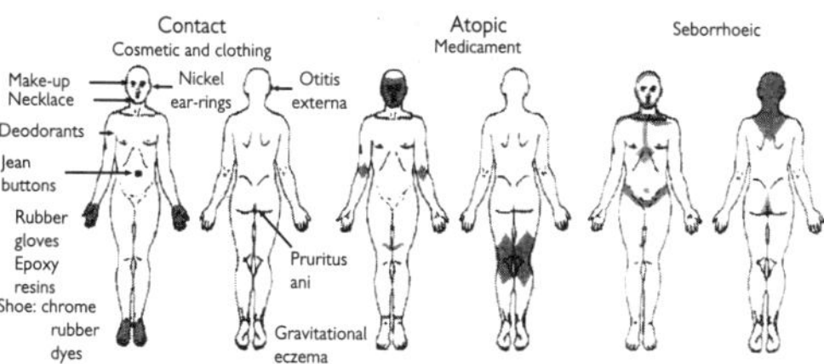

Fig. 14.3 Common patterns of dermatitis/eczema

Dermatitis (eczema)

Inflammatory reaction of the skin that may occur as a (usually asymmetrical) response to an external irritant or as a symmetrical endogenous response to a stimulus (atopic eczema).

Atopic eczema

Atopy is a genetic predisposition to (IgE-mediated) hypersensitivity reactions: asthma, hayfever and atopic eczema. Atopy affects 10–20% of children, usually ≤5yrs and is more common in urban than in rural settings. Whole skin is dry and itchy, lesions are itchy, red, with fine scaling, excoriated and lichenified from scratching and easily superinfected. Deteriorates with dryness, superinfection, heat, sweating, contact with allergens or irritants, and emotional stress. Common in face, elbow and kneefolds, hands, and feet. Differentiate from scabies.

Seborrhoeic eczema

Greasy yellowish scaling and erythema in seborrhoic areas of skin: scalp, eyebrows, nasolabial folds, presternal, axillae and groins. Severe, often superinfected seborrheic eczema is a hallmark of HIV infection.

Irritant contact dermatitis

Common form of dermatitis, generally affecting hands following contact with industrial irritants at work. Also affects feet of barefoot agricultural workers. Skin is dry and breaks easily → deep cracks that may become infected. Previously damaged skin or atopic skin more susceptible to irritants.

Allergic contact dermatitis

Sensitization to an allergen, normally over months or years, results in onset of dermatitis within hours of subsequent exposure to the allergen (e.g. cosmetics, nickel in zips, buttons, stainless steel watches, or jewellery, food, plants, medicines, metals). Irritant dermatitis is a risk factor for allergic contact dermatitis. Patch testing identifies specific allergen: suspected allergens are applied to normal skin, usually on back, and examined at 48 (24h in hot and humid conditions) and 72h for redness, swelling, or vesiculation that identifies an allergen.

Lichen simplex

Usually, a single lichenified (thickened) eczematous patch, which is perpetuated by habitual scratching or rubbing. Common in the neck, groins, shins, lower arms and around the ankles.

Management of dermatitis (eczema)

- Explain chronic, recurrent nature of the disease.
- Eliminate or avoid known irritants or allergens. White soft paraffin may act as an irritant through occlusion.
- Avoid soaps (these dry the skin); wash instead with emollients, e.g. aqueous cream to keep the skin hydrated.
- Moisturize skin daily with emulsifying ointment or aqueous cream, or vegetable oil (e.g. coconut oil).
- Treat acute weeping eczema with creams, chronic lichenified eczema with ointments.
- Apply topical steroids to affected areas 1–2× daily. Use the weakest effective steroid, for short periods of time or intermittently (4d per wk). A weak steroid (e.g. hydrocortisone 1%) can be used on face or in flexures. Avoid strong steroids in children. Strong steroids can be diluted with white soft paraffin or vegetable oil.
- *Seborrhoeic eczema:* add imidazoles and/or sulphur 5–10% and/or salicylic acid 2–5% to a base cream or steroid cream.
- Severe chronic eczema: apply coal tar ointment (2–10%) or paste or strong topical steroids to relieve itch. Covering e.g. with zinc oxide adhesive plaster may be necessary.
- Stop scratching! Instruct and assist with topical treatment and sedating antihistamines at night (not age <2yrs).
- Refractive cases can be relieved by prednisolone and other steroid-sparing immunosuppressive drugs (e.g. azathioprine).
- Treat 2° bacterial infection vigorously: topical povidone iodine or gentian violet, or antibiotics, e.g. cloxacillin or erythromycin.
- Breastfeeding may ↓ risk of atopic eczema. Emphasize for infants with a family history of eczema.

Psoriasis

Psoriasis is a disease of skin, nails an See Box 14.2. ↓ joints. It affects 1–2% western population, ↓ in tropics, ↑ in HIV/AIDS.

- *Classic plaque psoriasis:* sharply demarcated silvery plaques with large scale and +ve candlewax phenomenon (scratch → ↑whiteness). Most common on knees, elbows, lower back and scalp/hairline.
- *Inverse psoriasis:* red, shiny lesions with little scale, often with fissures and maceration in navel, natal cleft, armpits, groins.
- *Guttate psoriasis:* small, poorly defined lesions (often red with little silvery scale) that occur across the whole body; often in youngsters after streptococcal sore throat or vaccination.
- *Palmar/plantar psoriasis:* lesions develop deep cracks and sterile pustules; nails often involved. Differentiate from fungal infection.
- *Generalized pustular psoriasis:* fever, arthropathy, bright red erythema followed by the development of multiple pustules. Can occur after stopping prolonged potent steroid therapy. Resolves spontaneously.

Psoriatic arthritis occurs in ~10% of patients. Five patterns are recognized: a small joint arthritis of hands and feet with distal interphalangeal joint involvement (most common); seronegative rheumatoid-like arthritis; large joint mono- or oligo-arthritis; spondylitis; and arthritis mutilans.

Box 14.2 Management of psoriasis

Chronic condition, partly responsive to agents that ↓ cell turnover and partly responsive to immunosuppressive therapy. Treatment options are:

- *Emollients:* e.g. urea 10% ointment or white soft paraffin restore barrier function and ↓ visibility and dryness. Keratolytics, e.g. salicylic acid 5–10% ointment ↓ thick scale.
- *Strong topical steroids: e.g. betamethasone dipropionate 0.05% or clobetasol propionate 0.5% od for thick lesions, mild steroids, e.g. hydrocortisone 1% or triamcinolone 0.1% in flexures.*
- *Coal tar derivatives (5–10%) and dithranol (0.1–3%): start at a low concentration and gradually ↑; may be combined with UV-exposure.*
- *Severe and/or widespread psoriasis, psoriasis with arthritis:* methotrexate (MTX) 5–20mg once weekly + folic acid 5mg the following day. May be used in HIV+ individuals. TNFalpha inhibitors. In general, systemic corticosteroids should be avoided (rebound).

Pityriasis rosea

Pityriasis rosea is a viral infection of young adults. There may be a flu-like prodromal episode. A single annular erythematous and scaling 'herald patch' appears on trunk or arms, followed within a week by an erythematous and variably pruritic rash of the trunk which typically follows skin lines (Christmas tree pattern). Rash resolves spontaneously in weeks to months. Exclude syphilis.

Lichen planus

Itchy flat-topped, shiny, purplish papules, which may have fine white 'Wickham's' striae' on the surface appear on wrists, lower legs and lower back; lacy white lesions +/– erosions may also occur on the buccal +/– genital mucosa. May resolve spontaneously over months, but mucosal and pretibial hypertrophic lesions last for years. May be very refractive to treatment; 1st choice: strong topical steroids.

Drug eruptions

Drug eruptions may follow both conventional drugs and alternative remedies. Nearly all drugs can cause drug eruptions. Eruptions are usually symmetrical. Exfoliation or vesiculation are rare. They are more common in HIV+ individuals. Drug reactions usually occur >5–10d (up to 3wks) after first exposure, but may occur within days after taking a drug in case of previous exposure.

Exanthems

Are most common, may be maculopapular, urticarial, purpuric (also see 📖 Vasculitis, p. 604). Incidence >1% in penicillins, sulfonamides, NSAIDs, isoniazid, erythromycin, hydantoin derivatives, carbamazepine and others.

Fixed drug eruption

Occurs at same (fixed) site following a particular drug (e.g. sulfonamides, tetracyclines, barbiturates). May blister within a few hours of intake and it leaves an annular pigmented mark.

Management

- Ask the patient about previous reactions to drugs.
- Stop all drugs likely to have caused the reaction.
- Calamine lotion, oral histamines e.g. promethazine, chlorphenamine.
- Prednisolone 30–60mg tapering down fast if reaction is acute/severe.
- *SJS/TEN:* stop any potential drug trigger. Nurse as for extensive burns, attending to fluids, nutrition, and prevention of 2° bacterial infection to prevent high mortality from fluid loss. Steroids may ↓ progression, but later significantly ↑ risk of infection/sepsis through raw skin. Sometimes high dose, short course steroids are given, but only in first days of the disease. IV immunoglobulins (IVIG) may be of benefit. TEN is associated with a high mortality (Box 14.3).
- Never reintroduce drugs that have caused anaphylaxis, TEN, or severe exfoliative dermatitis. In mild cases, restart only essential drugs one by one to identify causative drug.

Box 14.3 Stevens–Johnson syndrome (SJS)

Is a severe form of erythema multiforme (📖 Erythema multiforme, p. 607) complicated by severe blistering of skin and mucosae including the mouth, eyes, and genitalia, and accompanied systemic features such as fever. The target lesions of erythema multiforme may be evident, but in its most severe form, toxic epidermal necrolysis (TEN), causes widespread blistering of the skin. This is associated with a +ve Nikolsky sign, where the top skin layer is rubbed off with light pressure, see Fig. 14.5. Other complications include diarrhoea, anterior uveitis, pneumonia, renal failure, and polyarthritis, A wide variety of triggers may be responsible, including drugs (e.g. sulfonamides; thioacetazone, nevirapine in HIV +ve individuals, allopurinol), streptococcal infections, viral infections (e.g. HSV Orf), malignancy, and some systemic diseases (e.g. SLE).

Vasculitis

Cutaneous vasculitis may occur in isolation or as part of systemic vasculitis. Vessel wall damage may present as urticaria, palpable purpura, ulcers, necrosis, livedo reticularis. Superficial lesions may be vesicular/blistering; deep lesions nodular (e.g. erythema nodosum) and occasionally suppurating. Urticaria occurs more commonly in infants, necrosis more commonly in adults. (*Note:* bruising and non-palpable purpura are more characteristic of platelet deficiency.)

Several mechanisms cause vascular damage, common are:

- *Leucocytoclastic vasculitis:* immune complex deposition → complement activation and neutrophil infiltration and disintegration.
- *Lymphocytic vasculitis:* cell-mediated immune response to, e.g. drugs and infections (viruses, bacteria, rickettsia).

Antigen excess mostly occurs in context of overwhelming acute disease (e.g. streptococcal or meningococcal infection, autoimmune diseases, such as SLE, malignancy) or drugs (including herbal remedies). Circulating noxious agents usually localize to the venular bed; arteriolar damage causes infarcts and embolic phenomena. Arthritis is a common, non-threatening association, classically described in HSP in children (see Box 14.4). Prognosis depends on vital organ involvement. Monitor regularly for haematuria as sign of renal involvement.

Management

- Antibody 'excess' occurs as a physiological mechanism for removal of antigen, and vasculitis frequently resolves spontaneously, particularly in children. Mild renal involvement does not require specific therapy.
- Look for and treat any identifiable cause e.g. infection.
- NSAIDs may help (caution in renal impairment).
- Persistent leg vasculitis benefits from elevation of the limb.
- Consider corticosteroids if multi-organ involvement and fever (caution in severe infections). Azathioprine or cyclosphosphamide may be used in severe disease. Dapsone 50–200mg od in leucocystoclastic vasculitis.

Box 14.4 Henoch-Schönlein purpura

Henoch-Schönlein purpura is the name given to a syndrome of vasculitis (usually manifest as palpable purpura affecting the legs and buttocks), arthralgia, peri-articular oedema, abdominal pain, and glomerulonephritis, most commonly seen in children. It is an immune complex phenomenon, thought to be triggered by a common infection (e.g. viral pharyngitis) in genetically susceptible individuals. Complications include GI bleeding, intussusception, nephritic and/or nephrotic syndrome; rarely protein-losing enteropathy, orchitis, or CNS involvement. The condition is usually self-limiting. Severe renal involvement may require immunosuppressive therapy.

Erythema nodosum

Presents as symmetrical, tender, erythematous nodules on shins or forearms, representing a nodular panniculitis associated with a lymphocytic vasculitis. Some causes are shown in Box 14.5. Investigation is directed at underlying causes. Usual to exclude TB, sarcoid, streptococcal sore throat, leprosy reactions, and inflammatory bowel disease. Treatment is symptomatic (analgesia). Most lesions resolve spontaneously over several days.

Box 14.5 Causes of erythema nodosum

Infections	Streptococci	*Yersinia*
	Tuberculosis	Histoplasmosis
	Chlamydia	Leprosy*
Drugs	Sulphonamides	Aspirin
	Sulphonylureas	Phenytoin
	Oral contraceptive	Dapsone

Sarcoidosis Inflammatory bowel disease

Rarer causes include Behçets disease, rheumatic fever, pregnancy.

* See p. 491 for ENL.

Urticaria

Itchy transient wheals (swelling and flushing of the skin), lasting 30min–24h, although new lesions may continue to develop. May be accompanied by joint pains, stomach aches, and fever.

Causes

Allergens (e.g. food, drugs, helminths) bind IgE → release of inflammatory mediators e.g. histamine in the skin → dermal oedema.

- Immune complex disease and complement activation (e.g. due to antivenom, penicillins, infections).
- Direct effect of histamine releasers in the skin (e.g. drugs such as morphine, shellfish).
- *Urticarial vasculitis:* lesions may be delayed in onset, last many hours to days, and become purpuric.
- *In angioedema:* oedema extends into the subcutaneous tissues. Larger, more solitary lesions lasting 4–48h may occur, and cause dramatic swelling of the eyes, lips, and oropharynx.
- *Chronic urticaria:* recurrent urticaria over >3mths. Causes are very variable. In 80% of cases no cause is found.
- *Papular urticaria:* itchy and persistent papules following damage to epidermis, often by insect bite. Lesions intensely pruritic; may blister.
- *Dermographism:* immediate wheal and flare response to pressure or scratch.

Urticaria may be life-threatening when:

- It is part of an anaphylactic reaction.
- *Angioedema* compromises the airway.
- It is part of a severe systemic disease (e.g. septicaemia, SLE).

Management

Identify and remove/treat stimulus (check for intestinal helminths, trichinosis, onchocerciasis, dracunculiasis, lymphatic filiariasis, strongyloidiasis). Give antihistamine (e.g. chlorphenamine 4mg po 4-hourly; promethazine 10–20mg tds or 25mg bd is more sedative). Steroids may help reduce airway inflammation in angioedema. Treat anaphylaxis as on 📖 Shock, p. 372. Chronic urticaria may require H2 antagonists (cimetidine, ranitidine) or even prednisolone, ciclosporin or dapsone.

Erythema multiforme

As name suggests, lesions of erythema multiforme take a variety of forms, including characteristic 'target lesions'—round, erythematous areas with pale or dusky, and sometimes vesicular centre. Rash is symmetrical and typically involves extensor surfaces and the palms and soles. Recognized triggers are summarized in Box 14.6. It is usually self-limiting.

Box 14.6 Causes of erythema multiforme

Infections	Herpes simplex	Mumps
	Mycoplasma	Streptococci
	Orf	Viral hepatitis
Drugs	Sulphonamides	Aspirin
	Sulphonylureas	Phenytoin
	Tetracyclines	Carbamazepine
	Thiazides	Alopurinol

Connective tissue diseases: e.g. SLE.
Malignancy
Radiotherapy

Blistering disorders

Blistering diseases are common. Clinical signs depend on cause and level of split in the skin (Fig. 14.4). Causes include burns, acute dermatitis from irritants or allergens, infections (e.g. impetigo, fungal infections of the foot), drugs (SJS/TEN see Box 14.3), autoimmune diseases (pemphigus, pemphigoid, dermatitis herpetiformis), genetic disorders (e.g. epidermolysis bullosa, porphyria). Autoimmune blistering disorders may be truly auto immune or triggered by internal malignancies and external factors (infection, drugs).

Pemphigus vulgaris Causes fragile, intra-epidermal blisters in adults. They commonly first appear in the oral and/or genital region before spreading all over the body. The blisters are flaccid (may be more tense in Africans) and enlarge when pressed upon. The roof can easily be rubbed off (Nikolsky sign, Fig. 14.5). Scraping from erosion shows acantholytic (rounded individual epidermal cells) cells (Tzanck test).

Treatment High-dose steroids (prednisolone 60–100mg daily), gradually ↓ as blistering resolves (5mg every 10th day). If new blisters appear ↑ dosage again. Mortality is 20–100%, even when treated.

Pemphigus foliaceus (PF)

Relatively common in rural areas. Endemic type occurs in foci. Very superficial blisters, just beneath the stratum corneum break easily and evolve into well-demarcated scaly, crusted lesions, +/– pustules. (Differential diagnosis: consider impetigo.) Erosions can be painful and extensive, PF may become erythrodermic. Fogo selvagem is an endemic variety of PF in Brazil in which antibodies cross-react with the saliva of a local blackfly. Other endemic variants may have similar aetiologies. PF is not fatal.

Treatment Potent topical steroids or oral dapsone may suffice although often systemic immunosuppressant therapy (prednisolone, methotrexate) is required.

(Bullous) pemphigoid

Sub-epidermal blisters, tense and frequently partially blood-filled, appear on clinically involved itchy erythematous skin and on normal skin. Antibodies are found in a line along the basal membrane, Nikolsky sign is –ve. Pemphigoid is a disease of the elderly. *Treatment*: strong topical steroid cream e.g. clobetasol propionate 0.5% od to bd. More extensive cases respond well to systemic steroids (40–60mg prednisolone); taper dosage ↓ and ↑ guided by the blistering. Erythromycin or doxycycline 100mg bd plus nicotinamide 500mg tid may be effective as a steroid sparing option.

Chronic benign bullous disease of childhood (juvenile dermatitis herpetiformis) Chronic (linear IgA) blistering disease with acute onset in children. Small and large blisters appear predominantly on the lower trunk, genital area and thighs, on the scalp and around the mouth. New blisters form around the old healing blisters forming a 'string of pearls'. (Differential diagnosis: consider impetigo). Dapsone is treatment of choice.

Dermatitis herpetiformis Characterized by intensely itchy rash with papules and vesicles over extensor surfaces. Typical lesions are herpetiform (grouped) arranged vesicles. Coeliac disease often associated, thus incidence ↑ with westernized diets. Treatment with gluten-free diet and dapsone.

Epidermolysis bullosa

An inherited or acquired adhesion weakness at the dermo-epidermal junction causing subepidermal blisters, ranging from mild tot severely multilating and to lethal forms. Inherited forms start early in life. All forms lead to blisters after minimal trauma, which may heal with atrophic or hypertrophic scarring and sometimes milia (small epidermal cysts). Superinfection is common. Malignancies may occur in chronically scarred areas. .

Management Includes trauma prevention, protein rich diet, wound care (e.g. with honey), infection prevention.

Porphyria cutanea tarda

Is a chronic disturbance of porphyrin metabolism, characterized by liver disease (causes include chronic hepatitis C infection and alcohol abuse) and skin lesions. Exposure to sun or trauma induces blistering leading to erosions, crusts, small depressed scars and pigmentation changes. Alcohol or iron intake is a trigger. Sometimes when urine is exposed to light it turns red. *Treatment*: Sun protection, abstain from alcohol, phlebotomy. Low dose chloroquine (e.g. 150mg weekly) may be tried, in higher dose it may exacerbate the disease.

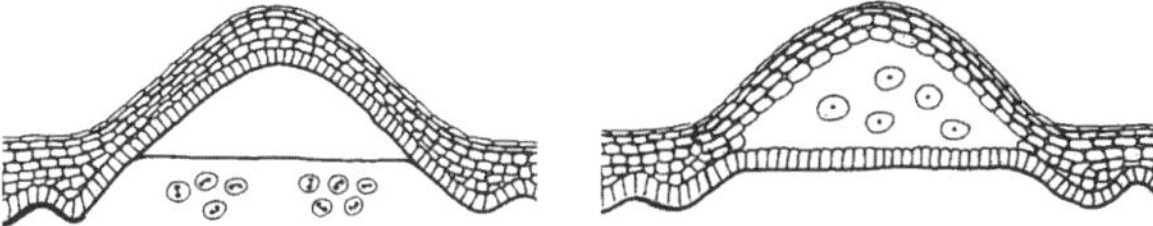

Fig. 14.4 Diagrammatic cross-sections of skin blisters. Left: Pemphigoid, in which blister is thick-roofed. Right: pemphigus, in which the blister is thin-roofed and fragile.

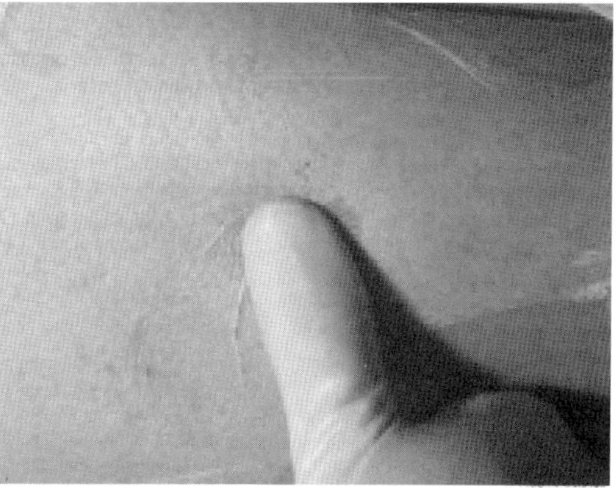

Fig. 14.5 Nikolsky sign – blister roof rubbed off with light pressure

Connective tissue diseases

Seem to be relatively common in tropical areas. Exact epidemiological data are unavailable. In these settings, diagnosis is nearly always clinical.

Lupus erythematosus

An autoimmune disease in which autoantibodies directed against DNA are found and complement is activated → damage to blood vessels, dermal–epidermal junction, and epidermis. Sun may initiate and exacerbate disease in genetically predisposed individuals.

Chronic discoid lupus erythematosus (CDLE)

Lesions occur in sun-exposed areas, e.g. forehead, nose, and cheeks ('butterfly' pattern rash), chest and back, and extensor surfaces of the arms. Scaly with follicular plugging and atrophy with hyperpigmentation and depigmentation. In lighter skins, erythema can be seen. Lesions heal with scarring, and alopecia may follow scalp lesions. CDLE may progress to SLE in 2–20% (📖 Systemic lupus erythematosus, p. 746).

Management Sun protection essential. Strong topical steroids and hydroxychloroquine are standard treatment. Thalidomide, methotrexate, and methylprednisolone pulse therapy are alternatives.

Subacute cutaneous lupus erythematosus (SCLE)

Comprises ~5–10% of all cutaneous lupus erythematosus. Polycyclic erythematous lesions with central depigmentation are seen in the sun-exposed areas. Patients are very sensitive to ultraviolet (UV) exposure, hence, commoner in tropics. Generalized symptoms may be present, most notably tiredness. Very few develop SLE. Lesions heal without scarring.

Treatment Methylprednisolone pulse therapy is effective. Thalidomide may be treatment of choice; chloroquine or methotrexate are usually successful.

Scleroderma

Sclerosis of the skin is seen as a manifestation of morphea, systemic or acrosclerotic, lichen sclerosis and mixed connective tissue disease (MCTD). In rural clinics, diagnosis is only possible on clinical criteria.

Morphea

Circumscribed scleroderma. Dermis is markedly thickened. There may be a single or multiple plaques on the trunk, which progress over 3–5yrs and then stabilize. Treatment is difficult. Potent topical steroids or vitamin D derivatives (e.g. calcipotriene ointment) may be helpful.

Systemic scleroderma

Characterized by atrophy and sclerosus of the skin. Acrosclerosis starts at the extremities and progresses in an ascending fashion. Cutaneous vasculitis may result in ulceration and necrosis of digits leading to claw-like hands. Facial movements become increasingly difficult until the face becomes expressionless. Untreated, the condition progresses slowly , but unremittingly.

Treatment Systemic steroids, methotrexate, cyclophosphamide, chloroquine.

Mixed connective tissue disease

Overlap syndromes occur between rheumatoid arthritis, Sjögren's syndrome, SLE, scleroderma, and polymyositis. Diagnosis is made by clinical features and when possible by laboratory tests. Specific antibodies tests are useful, although none are 100% specific. Patients are typically female and may show features of SLE, systemic sclerosis, dermatomyositis, and polymyositis. Some arthritis or arthralgia is usually present. Fingers may be typically sausage-shaped due to swelling of the joints. There is often a swelling of dorsum of hands. Muscle weakness and pain are common, and sometimes anaemia is present. Raynaud's phenomenon may occur despite a warm climate. Relatively common in East Africa.

Disorders of pigmentation

Skin pigmentation is mainly due to melanin or other endogenous pigments (e.g. haemosiderin, bilirubin). Some common causes of hyper- and hypopigmentation are given in Boxes 14.7 and 14.8.

Hypopigmentation

Melanin is produced by melanocytes and transferred to keratinocytes in melanosomes. Loss of keratinocytes (exfoliation) → hypopigmentation, so skin is often paler following inflammation. When due to mildly dry skin, chapping, or eczema, it is termed *pityriasis alba*. Typically occurs on face and limbs in children.

Treatment Reassure parents that it will clear in time. Apply emollients.

Pityriasis versicolor

Also called *Tinea versicolor*, is due to *Malassezia furfur* and other yeasts, which cause sharply defined confluent slightly scaly patches of hypopigmentation, especially of upper trunk. Often indicates patient has been sweating e.g. TB, HIV; common in humid climate, immunodeficiency.

Treatment Application of selenium sulfide shampoo daily for 1wk, apply lather, and leave in contact for 10min before rinsing; or salicylic acid 5% in 70% alcoholic solution; or fluconazole 400mg as a single dose.

Hypopigmentation due to *tuberculoid leprosy* is more chronic, and scale, if present, is more adherent and does not usually exfoliate easily. These patches will be anaesthetic to cotton wool touch testing.

Vitiligo

Vitiligo is most important cause of depigmentation (distinguish clinically from hypopigmentation). Melanocyte death causes patches of complete depigmentation, often in symmetrical distribution, which may occasionally become generalized. Hair may be affected too (turns white). Affects ~ 2% of the world's population, and can be very upsetting in those with pigmented skin, triggering unjustified fears of contagion and genetic transmission. There may be a personal or family history of associated autoimmune disease (e.g. thyroid, pernicious anaemia, diabetes). Vitiligo severely influences quality of life. Treatment is so unsatisfactory that patients should be protected from spending all their income on a search for cures. Early lesions may respond to potent topical steroids, but the risk of skin atrophy discourages long-term use. Sun exposure may help, although areas of vitiligo will not tan. UVB 311 nm or PUVA (phototherapy in combination with topical or systemic psoralens that sensitize the skin to ultraviolet radiation) may be effective. Camouflage with sweat- and seawater-proof creams is tedious to apply, but safe and effective.

Albinism

Caused by genetic defects in the enzyme tyrosinase, which is required for melanin synthesis. Tyrosinase may be either defective (less severe clinical features) or completely absent. Lack of melanin leads to white skin and hair, with red eyes due to lack of iris pigmentation. Those affected develop potentially fatal squamous cell skin cancers in early adult life. Absence of retinal pigment causes impaired vision, photosensitivity, and nystagmus which disturb schooling. In some communities significant stigma attached to condition. In certain areas (e.g. Tanzania), special programmes exist to educate communities to manage those affected.

Box 14.7 Causes of hyperpigmentation

- Post-inflammatory hyperpigmentation.
- Addison's disease.
- Liver disease, e.g. porphyria cutanea tarda.
- Haemochromatosis.
- Acanthosis nigricans.
- Chloasma (melasma).
- Renal failure.
- Drugs, e.g. amiodarone, clofazimine.
- Naevi.
- Melanoma.
- Congenital, e.g. neurofibromatosis, Peutz–Jeghers syndrome.

Box 14.8 Causes of hypopigmentation

- *Congenital:*
  - albinism
  - phenylketonuria
  - tuberous sclerosis.
- *Acquired:*
  - post-inflammatory hypopigmentation (including onchocerciasis)
  - pityriasis alba
  - pityriasis versicolor
  - tuberculoid leprosy
  - lichen sclerosus et atrophicus
  - drugs (e.g. skin-lightening creams).

Causes of depigmentation

Vitiligo

Skin cancers

Most important risk factor for cutaneous malignancy is sun damage, either long-term exposure to strong sunlight (most skin cancers) or sun burn (melanoma). Melanin protects against sun damage, so albinos and light-skinned individuals have ↑ cancer risk. Seek shade, use sunscreens on sun-exposed parts of body, and wear a hat outdoors. Infants should be protected from sunburn.

Actinic (solar) keratoses

These are pre-malignant, hyperkeratotic, adherent scaly lesions on an erythematous base, which occur post-middle age in light-skinned persons with long-term exposure to the sun. They may develop into squamous cell carcinoma (SCC). Persistent lesions should be destroyed by curettage, cryotherapy, or daily application of topical fluorouracil cream.

Squamous cell carcinoma (SCC)

SCC occurs in sun-exposed areas. May develop from actinic keratoses or at edges of chronic ulcers and areas of inflammation (Marjolin's ulcer). Oral lesions occur in long-term smokers. Usually, a fleshy dry nodule breaks down to form ulcerating lesion with hard raised edges. Systemic metastasis may occur, especially in albinos.

Management Early, radical, local excision.

Basal cell carcinoma (BCC)

Occurs predominantly in sun-exposed areas on the face. Usually slow-growing shiny papule with teleangiectasia which may form a central ulcer with a rolled pearly edge. Usually slow-growing papule grows slowly or breaks centrally to form an ulcer with a rolled 'pearl-coloured' edge. Local infiltration may gradually cause extensive tissue damage and disfigurement, but BCC does not metastasize.

Management Excision, curettage, cauterization, or cryotherapy. Fluorouracil cream or imiquimod cream may be used for superficial lesions or after surgery. Radiotherapy is also effective.

Melanoma

Any pigmented lesion that shows variable pigmentation, changes shape, thickness, or colour, starts to bleed, or ulcerates, should be considered a potential melanoma. Pigmented satellite lesions around a mole also suggest a melanoma. Melanoma frequently originates in moles and is more common in people with many moles, who should be encouraged to examine these regularly and report changes to a doctor. In Africans melanoma commonly occurs on the soles (acrolentiginous melanoma) and may only be recognized following metastasis to lymph nodes or other sites. Original lesion may be quite innocuous.

Management Immediate, wide local excision.

Common cutaneous viral infections

Herpes simplex

HSV-1 and HSV-2 cause mucocutaneous disease, keratitis, encephalitis, and aseptic meningitis. Transmission is by direct contact through mucosal surfaces (oral or genital) or skin abrasions. 1° mucocutaneous disease, including gingivostomatitis, pharyngitis, herpes labialis (cold sores), and genital herpes, may be due to either viral subtype, but *recurrent* oral herpes is most commonly due to HSV-1 and recurrent genital herpes caused by HSV-2. Recurrences are often precipitated by sun exposure, trauma or fever.

After a few days of prodromal burning sensation, erythema appears followed by typically grouped vesicles within 24h. Fever, malaise, and lymphadenopathy are associated with 1° infection. A severe, potentially fatal form with widespread vesiculation particularly affecting face (eczema herpeticum) may occur in patients with atopic eczema. HSV may also trigger erythema multiforme.

Management Treat herpes labialis with zinc oxide ointment or zinc oxide and castor oil. Protect from sunlight. More severe infections: aciclovir (200–400mg 5 × a day) or IV (5–10mg/kg tds) for 5–10d, or valaciclovir 500mg bd or famciclovir 250 tid for 5d, higher doses in the immunesuppressed. Frequent severe recurrences warrant (val-, fam- or) aciclovir prophylaxis.

Varicella zoster virus

This herpes virus (HSV-3) causes chickenpox (varicella) following 1° infection, and shingles (herpes zoster) following reactivation of latent virus in sensory ganglia. Transmission is by respiratory droplet inhalation or contact with vesicular fluid.

Chickenpox is generally a mild infection of children (Box 14.9), but may be severe in neonates, adults (especially in pregnancy), and the immunocompromised. Prodrome of fever, headache, and malaise → an itchy erythematous eruption involving the scalp and face and moving distally to involve trunk. Daily 'crops' of lesions progress from papules to vesicles, pustules, and scabs and all stages may be present at once.

Complications

2° *Staph. aureus* and *Strep. pyogenes* infection is common in children and may cause sepsis or skin scarring; pneumonitis (mainly seen in adults, especially smokers); mild encephalitis (ataxia); thrombocytopenia.

Herpes zoster usually occurs only once, often in the elderly or immunosuppressed, affecting just one sensory ganglion and associated dermatome. Scanty distant vesicles may occur due to haematogenous spread, and rarely disseminated zoster may occur in immunocompromised. Paraesthesia and shooting pains can occur in affected dermatome for several days before appearance of vesicular, erythematous rash and mild fever. Vesicles scab after 3–7d. Zoster (or zoster scars) in patients <40yrs old or in >1 dermatome suggests impaired cell mediated immunity, most commonly due to HIV.

Complications include:

- *Post-herpetic neuralgia:* may be very painful and difficult to treat. Amitriptyline (10–25mg nocte), carbamazepine 600–800mg od or gabapentin 300–900mg od to tds may help.
- *Herpes zoster ophthalmica (of the 1st division of the Vth cranial nerve):* may be complicated by conjunctivitis, keratitis, and periorbital swelling. Delayed healing, multidermatomal zoster, dissemination and complications are more common in HIV-associated herpes zoster.

Management

Antiviral therapy is indicated for herpes zoster and for chickenpox in adolescents, adults, immunocompromised, and patients with complications; it may be considered for chickenpox in high-risk patients, e.g. those with chronic cardiovascular, respiratory, or skin conditions. Treatment should be initiated early, within 72h of onset of the rash and continued for 7d. Give aciclovir 800mg oral 5 × daily or 10mg/kg IV tds in severe infections. Alternatives for herpes zoster are valaciclovir (1g oral tds) or famciclovir (500mg oral tds) for 1wk.

Box 14.9 Chickenpox in children

- Treat symptoms (paracetamol, topical antipruritics, e.g. calamine or phenol-zinc lotion). Add a broad spectrum antibiotic if any indication of local or systemic 2° bacterial infection.
- *In neonates/high-risk groups:* aciclovir may ↓ duration and complications (oral: 200mg qds if age <2yrs; 20mg/kg (max 800mg) qds if ≥2yrs. IV: 10–20mg/kg if age <3mths; 250mg/m^2 if 3mths–12yrs).

Common warts

Warts are caused by many strains of HPV, and affect ~10% of young people at any time. Wart may be nodular, flat, or occasionally filiform (long and slender, e.g. on eyelids). If on sole of foot (plantar wart, verruca) wart is usually painful because pressure forces lesion to form below level of epidermis, and layer of stratum corneum may partly obscure it. Warts of all types may be widespread and persistent in HIV/AIDS.

Treatment Generally regress spontaneously in time; wart paints (e.g. topical salicylic acid 12%–50%), curettage, cryotherapy.

Poxvirus infections

Molluscum contagiosum (Colour plate 16)

Molluscum contagiosum, caused by a poxvirus, produces 0.2–0.4cm smooth 'warts' with central umbilication. It is common in children, in whom spontaneous resolution is the rule. Widespread lesions may occur in HIV/AIDS.

Treatment

Local application of, e.g. phenol or trichloracetic acid spiked into the centre of the lesion; cryotherapy, curettage.

Smallpox

Smallpox was eradicated in 1976, but is a potential agent of bio-terrorism. Control relies on isolation of cases and vaccination of contacts; there is no effective treatment. It carries ~50% mortality.

Monkeypox and tanapox

These poxviruses, closely related to smallpox, cause occasional infections. The rash (1 or 2 lesions in tanapox; many covering the whole body in monkeypox) is preceded by a 2–3d prodromal period with fever and other systemic signs (see Fig. 14.6). Lymphadenopathy occurs in monkeypox, characteristically involving both femoral and inguinal nodes. Unlike chickenpox, lesions are always at same stage and peripheries are involved early. Both infections tend to resolve without treatment. Human–human transmission has been reported within households with monkeypox.

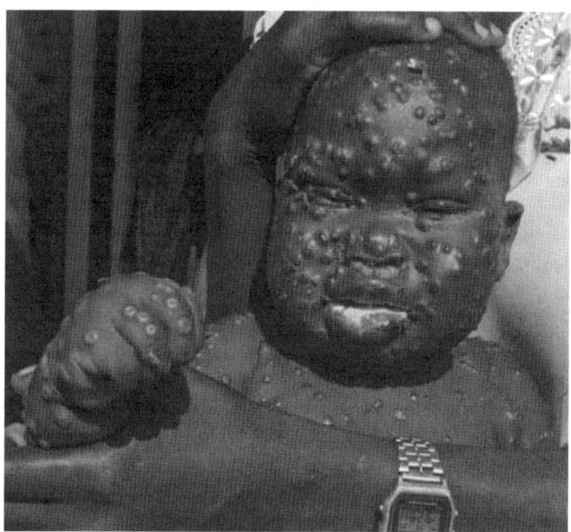

Fig. 14.6 A child in northern Kenya with tanapox. In contrast to chickenpox, these vesicles are umbilicated, less fragile, larger, and occur both centrally and peripherally from the outset. The child made an uneventful recovery. Courtesy of Médecins Sans Frontières.

Cutaneous leishmaniasis

A widespread disease, caused by different species of *Leishmania* parasites manifesting in different ways depending on species and host response. *L. tropica* is anthroponotic; the *L. mexicana* and *L. braziliensis* species complexes (New World) and *L. major* (Old World) are zoonoses of rodents, dogs, or other mammals. Transmission of *Leishmania* promastigotes is by the bite of infected *Phlebotomus* and *Lutzomyia* sandfly vectors, following which the parasite multiplies in skin macrophages, causing local tissue damage (Box 14.10; See 📖 Visceral leishmaniasis (kala-azar), p. 794).

Clinical features

Weeks to months after a bite, a nodule develops at the bite site. This grows slowly (up to 5cm), becomes ulcerated, and is covered by a crust which may drop off to expose a relatively painless ulcer—pain often indicates 2° bacterial infection. The ulcer may be dry or exudative, depending on the species. It heals over months or years, leaving a 'tissue paper' scar. Satellite lesions may occur. 2° infection is uncommon. *L. mexicana* classically causes lesions of the pinna ('chiclero ulcer') that take years to heal, often destroying the pinna.

Less common types

- Mucocutaneous leishmaniasis (MCL) 'Espundia' can occur in New World cutaneous leishmaniasis (CL) and rarely with other species. *L. braziliensis* is the most important cause (also occurs with *L. guyanensis*, *L. panamensis*). 2° mucocutaneous lesions develop months or years after 1° lesion has healed. Starting on the upper lip or nostril edge, MCL eventually destroys the mucosa and cartilage of the nasopharynx, larynx, or lips.
- Disseminated cutaneous leishmaniasis (DCL) is usually caused by *L. mexicana* or *L. aethiopica*: The 1° nodule spreads slowly without ulceration while 2° lesions appear symmetrically on limbs and face. In the immunocompromised, infection continues to spread and responds only transiently to chemotherapy (anergic DCL).
- Recidivans leishmaniasis is usually caused by *L. tropica*, often on the cheek. The lesion heals in the centre , but nodules with scanty parasites persist at the edges for years (see Fig. 14.7).

Diagnosis

This is often clinical in resource-poor settings, supported by identification of Giemsa-stained parasites from microscopy and/or culture from skin smears taken from the edge of active ulcers. PCR, where available may increase sensitivity and allow diagnosis to species level.

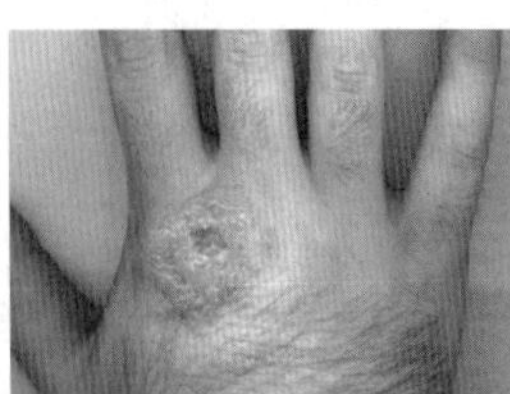

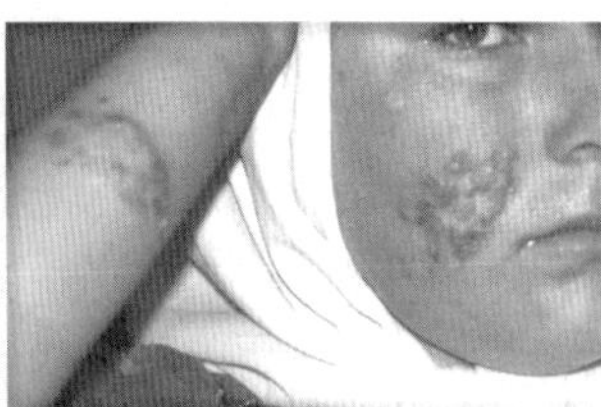

Fig. 14.7 Cutaneous leishmaniasis of the hand due to *L. tropica* (left) and Leishmania recidivans of the face and arm (right).

Box 14.10 Cutaneous leishmaniasis

Local treatments are suitable for Old World CL (*L. tropica* and *L. major*) and *L. mexicana* as there is no risk of these causing later MCL.

- Intra-lesional infiltration of sodium stibogluconate or meglumine antimoniate are widely used: 1mL of undiluted antimonial is injected into the base and edges of lesion Repeat 2–3 × weekly for 2–3wks. If injections are very painful, dilute with lidocaine 2%.
- *Leishmania* are killed at 40–42°C, so heating wound by radiofrequency or heat pads improves healing.
- Cryotherapy is successfully used in Old World CL, either alone or combined with intra-lesional antimonial.
- Topical treatment with paromomycin 15% ointment is effective in *L. major* and *L. mexicana*.

Systemic therapy for Old World CL *L. tropica* and *L. major* only warrant systemic treatment if: Sores too large or badly sited for local therapy.

- Ulcerated or severely inflamed sores, or overlying a joint.
- Disease with lymphatic spread.
- Lesions with involvement of cartilage.

Treatments

- Oral fluconazole 200mg od for 6wks is effective in *L. major* CL.
- Miltefosine or injections of antimonials or amphotericin, see below.

Systemic therapy for New World CL

CL from Central or South America could be caused by *L. braziliensis*. If in doubt, consider all New World CL to be *L. braziliensis*, because differentiation from *L. mexicana* is usually impossible geographically, clinically, or parasitologically unless PCR available. Systemic treatment of *L. braziliensis* CL should prevent subsequent MCL.

Treatments

- 10–20mg/kg/day sodium stibogluconate by IM or slow IV route, or meglumine antimoniate by deep IM for a minimum of 4wks, or until lesion healed.
- Pentamidine isetionate 4mg/kg 1–2 × weekly until lesion no longer visible. For *L. braziliensis guyanensis* 4 doses in 7d (every other day).
- Miltefosine 100mg/d for 28d is successful in many cases.
- MCL responds well to liposomal amphotericin at a dose of 2po mg/kg for at least 20 days (gives similar cure rates as and fewer adverse events than conventional amphotericin).

Treatment of diffuse CL DCL is almost impossible to cure: give sodium stibogluconate or meglumine antimoniate 20mg/kg IM od for several months after clinical improvement; relapse is common.

Lymphoedema (elephantiasis)

Lymphoedema is caused by obstruction to lymph flow → regional accumulation of lymph in the soft tissues. There is ↑ susceptibility to soft tissue infection → further lymphatic damage and a vicious cycle of worsening lymphoedema. In some conditions (particularly lymphatic filariasis), chronic trophic skin changes including hyperkeratosis, nodular fibrosis, and excess adiposity → to the characteristic appearance of elephantiasis of the affected limb or body part.

Causes of lymphoedema include:

- Lymphatic filariasis (see 📖 Lymphatic filariasis, p. 624).
- Malignancy (including lymphatic involvement, radiotherapy, surgery).
- Chronic oedema (e.g. congestive cardiac failure).
- Lymphatic blockage due to TB, leprosy, or KS.
- Podoconiosis (distinguishable from lymphatic filariasis (LF) by its upward ascendance from the foot whereas LF descends from upper leg/genitals).
- Congenital (Milroy's disease).

Management

Involves treating the underlying cause and general measures to promote lymph flow and prevent disease progression and complications (see Box 14.11).

Box 14.11 General measures in management of lymphoedema

Promote lymph flow by ↓ gravitational venous load on the impaired lymphatics and preventing the cycle of inflammation and further lymphatic damage. The following may improve the outcome of lymphoedema by slowing down or halting disease progression. In patients with established severe lymphoedema/elephantiasis, collateral lymphatic channels can re-establish lymph flow if kept free from 2° infection. Prevention/treatment of infection ↓ social stigma associated with foul smelling, chronically infected tissues.

Minimize risk of further lymphatic damage due to inflammation

- Wash the affected part twice daily with soap and water.
- Use emollients (aqueous cream, or local alternatives like vegetable oils or white soft paraffin) to promote skin barrier function.
- Wear shoes; keep nails clean.
- Treat minor wounds or abrasions with topical antiseptics.
- Soak foot in potassium permanganate (1:10,000) solution.
- Ensure early antibiotic treatment of soft tissue infections.

Promote lymph flow in the affected limb

- Exercise.
- Raise affected limb at night.
- Give diuretics to reduce venous load.
- Deep expiratory breathing, e.g. chanting (increases venous return).
- Massage affected limb.
- Compression bandages, stockings or laced boots.

Lymphatic filariasis

Lymphatic filariasis is caused by three geographically distinct (see Fig. 14.8) species of filarial worm, *Wuchereria bancrofti*, *Brugia malayi*, and *B. timori* (Fig. 14.9). The life cycle is shown in Fig. 14.10.

Transmission occurs via bite of mosquito vectors. Infective microfilariae enter host during a blood meal and migrate to lymphatics, particularly around groin and axillae, where they develop into adult worms, which may survive >10yrs. Females grow up to 10cm in length (males ~4cm) and produce microfilaria (~260μm), which enter blood stream. Onward transmission occurs when microfilaria are taken up by several species of mosquitoes during a blood meal. Host pathology is thought to be due to the immune response to adult worms and endosymbiotic *Wolbachia*. Microfilariae are responsible for tropical pulmonary eosinophilia (see 📖 Tropical pulmonary eosinophilia p. 212). In endemic areas, asymptomatic microfilaraemia is common, as are asymptomatic seropositive patients without microfilaraemia.

Acute lymphatic filariasis ('filarial fever')

Usually recurrent, most commonly affects the limbs, spermatic cord/testes (funiculitis/epididymo-orchitis +/–hydrocoele), and breasts, and encompasses two syndromes:

- *Acute filarial lymphangitis (AFL):* caused by death of adult worms leads to a local inflammatory nodule/lymphangitis which spreads distally, accompanied by systemic symptoms including fever, rigors, headache, myalgia, arthralgia +/–delirium.
- *Acute dermatolymphangioadenitis (ADLA):* due to 2° bacterial infection → ascending lymphangitis with associated soft tissue infection/ inflammation (cellulitis) and systemic upset. Lymphatic damage from recurrent attacks → chronic lymphatic filariasis.

Chronic lymphatic filiariasis

Usually occurs as a result of lymphatic damage from recurrent acute attacks, which continue to complicate and exacerbate chronic phase of disease. Clinical features include:

- Hydrocoele, which may be massive and interfere with walking.
- Lymphoedema (elephantiasis) of the legs is common, usually asymmetrical, and starts distally.
- Chyluria and lymphuria are due to rupture into the renal pelvis or bladder of damaged lymphatics draining (i) intestines → fat in urine (chyluria) or (ii) other organs → lymph in urine. Associated haematuria may cause clot retention. Chronic chyluria may cause malabsorption.

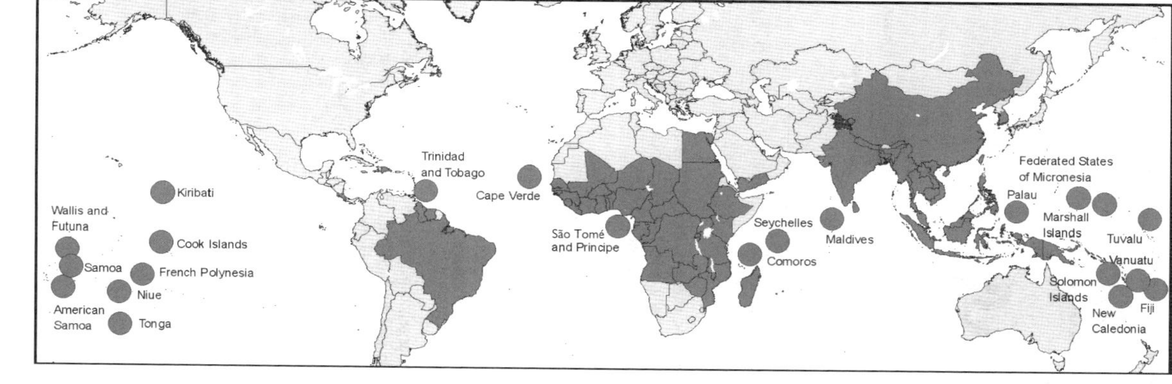

Fig.14.8 Global distribution of lymphatic filariasis which affects 120 million people in 83 countries. (Reproduced from the *Weekly Epidemiological Report*, No. 22, 2006, with permission from the WHO.)

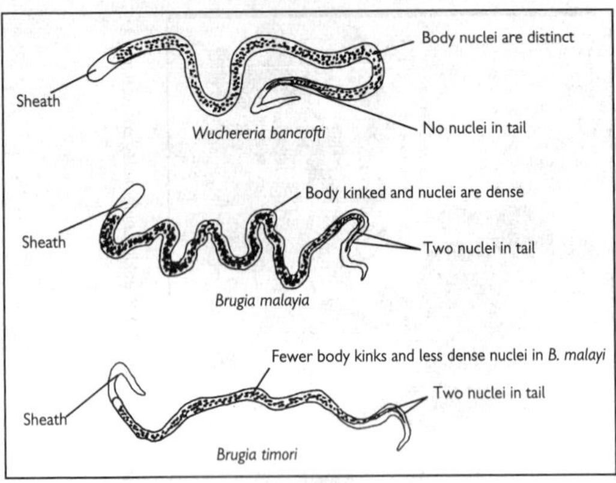

Fig. 14.9 Blood film appearances of the microfilariae lymphatic filariasis.

Other complications

Attributed to lymphatic filariasis, often in the absence of microfilaraemia, include arthritis (especially knee); endomyocardial fibrosis; skin rashes; thrombophlebitis; and nerve palsies.

Microfilarial periodicity

Parasitaemia is periodic, peaking at key biting time of mosquito vector in a particular location. *W. bancrofti* and *B. malayi* usually exhibit nocturnal periodicity (peak parasitaemia around midnight); in the Pacific, *W. bancrofti* exhibits diurnal periodicity (peak about midday). Nocturnal and diurnal *subperiodic* forms also occur with less marked peaks of parasitaemia at night and day respectively.

Diagnosis

In endemic areas is largely clinical and may be overdiagnosed. Parasitological diagnosis relies on isolation of microfilaria from blood; 10mL of blood should be taken during peak parasitaemia into citrated blood bottles (such as used for ESR or prothrombin time). See Table 14.1.

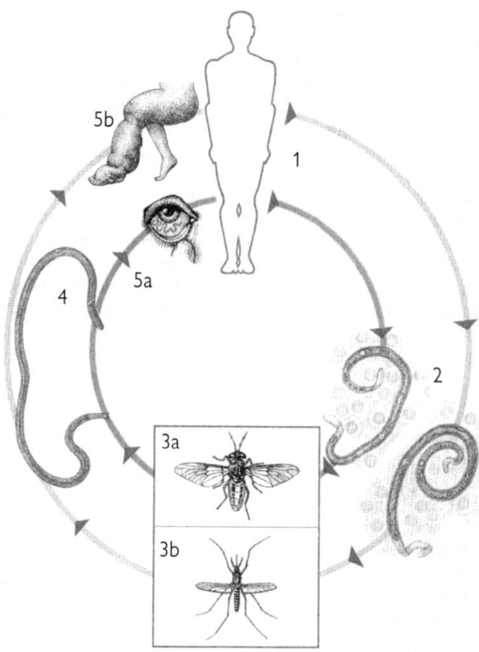

Fig. 14.10 Life cycles of lymphatic filariasis (outer circle) and loaiasis (inner circle). Man is the only host of sexually mature worms (5a, Loa loa, 5b *Wuchereria bancrofti*). Microfilariae (2) appear in the blood periodically - diurnally (loaiasis) and nocturnally (lymphatic filariasis). Microfilariae are taken up during feeding by the intermediate host and vector: day-biting Chrysops flies (3a) or night-biting Culex mosquitoes (3b). In the vector, the microfilariae develop into infective metacyclic forms (4) which infect new human hosts when the vector takes a blood meal.

Adapted from Piekarski, G *Medical, Parasitology in Plates*, 1962, with kind permission of Bayer Pharmaceuticals.

Detection methods

- *Polycarbonate membrane filtration:* this technique is widely used and can detect very low parasitaemias.
  - nucleopore polycarbonate membranes, 25mm diameter, 5-μm pore size, are held in a Millipore Swinnex filter holder, using a rubber gasket to secure the membrane
  - draw up 10–20mL of 1:1 saline diluted blood into a 20-mL syringe
  - connect the syringe to the filter and gently push the blood through the filter membrane
  - repeat until all of the blood has been filtered

- draw up 20mL of saline into the syringe, flush through the filter, repeat using air
- unscrew top of filter and use forceps to transfer to a slide
- add a drop of saline to the membrane and cover with a coverslip. Examine the membrane under the microscope, using a ×10 objective. Examine the slide using the ×10 objective. Active microfilariae can be readily seen and produce a snake-like movement.
- *Saline/saponin method:* add 8mL of 1% saponin in saline to 2mL of blood into a centrifuge tube. Mix by inversion, then allow it to stand at room temperature for 15min to allow the blood to haemolyse. Centrifuge at 2,000rpm for 15min to deposit the microfilariae. Discard the supernatant and use the deposit to make a wet preparation. Stain any microfilariae found using a ×40 objective to note the arrangement of nuclei and presence of a sheath.
- *Simple card tests:* to detect circulating filarial antigens (CFA) are available for *W. bancrofti* , but not *Brugia* species.

Management

- Albendazole 400mg oral bd for 3wks kills adult worms, but is more effective in combination with DEC or ivermectin.
- Albendazole 400mg plus either ivermectin 200μg/kg or DEC 6mg/kg, as a single oral dose repeated annually for 5yrs, is now used for mass drug administration programmes.
- Avoid DEC in *O. volvulus* and Loa loa endemic areas due to risk of Mazzotti reaction.
- Avoid DEC during acute attacks as macrofilaricidal activity +/– release of *Wolbachia* endotoxins may exacerbate symptoms.
- Ivermectin monotherapy only kills microfilaria so needs to be repeated during the lifetime of the adult worms (may be up to >10yrs).
- Doxycycline 100mg oral bd for 6wks (against *Wolbachia*) has been shown to reduce filaraemia and improve lymphoedema.
- Surgical management is required for chronic severe hydrocele. The long-term benefit of surgery for elephantiasis is often limited.
- For general principles of lymphoedema management, see Box 14.12.

Prevention and public health strategies

- *Prevention:* education to reduce vector–human contact; personal protection from mosquito bites; vector control.
- *Mass drug administration:* is promoted by GAELF (Global Alliance to Eliminate Lymphatic Filariasis) for communities with >5% infection prevalence. The whole community is treated once yearly for 5yrs with single-dose albendazole 400mg plus either DEC 6mg/kg or ivermectin 200μg/kg (avoid DEC in Loa loa or *O. volvulus* endemic areas). Addition of DEC to table salt has been used with success.

Table 14.1 Microfilarial periodicity and optimum times to detect microfilariae in blood

Species	Geographic location	Periodicity	Optimum collection time
Wuchereria bancrofti	Tropics/subtropics	Nocturnal	Midnight
Wuchereria bancrofti	Pacific	Diurnal subperiodic	16.00 hours
Brugia malayi	Southeast Asia and Southwest India	Nocturnal	Midnight
Brugia malayi	Indonesia	Nocturnal subperiodic	21.00 hours
Brugia timori	Indonesia	Nocturnal	Midnight
Loa loa	West/Central Africa	Diurnal	13.00 hours
Mansonella perstans	Africa/South America	Non-periodic	Any time
Mansonella ozzardi	Central and South America	Non-periodic	Any time

Box 14.12 *Wolbachia* endosymbionts in human filarial infections

Endosymbiotic *Wolbachia* bacteria (related to *Rickettsia*) live within filarial worms and are now recognized to be important in worm reproduction, development, and pathology. Release from adult worms of *Wolbachia* endotoxins is thought to play a major role in the inflammatory pathology of lymphatic filariasis and onchocerciasis. Early trials of anti-*Wolbachia* chemotherapy with doxycycline have shown significant benefits in both these diseases.

Onchocerciasis ('river blindness')

Onchocerca volvulus occurs in areas with fast-flowing rivers and biting *Similium* blackflies, the parasite's vector. In West African savannah, it was a common cause of blindness until the Onchocerciasis Control Programme ↓ prevalence. Still causes blindness and skin manifestations in other areas.

Clinical features

- Subcutaneous nodules containing adult worms, conspicuous over bony prominences (e.g. iliac crests, ribs, knees, trochanters).
- Cutaneous and eye manifestations due to host inflammatory reactions to dying microfilariae which migrate in the skin (see Box 14.13) and eye.
- Ocular lesions include transient punctate keratitis and potentially blinding conditions, e.g. sclerosing keratitis, iridocyclitis, optic atrophy.

Diagnosis

Confirmed by finding microfilariae in skin snips or the eye. Ask the patient to put their head between their knees for >2min before examining the anterior chamber with a slit-lamp. If skin snip and eye examinations are both –ve, but onchocerciasis is still strongly suspected, perform the Mazzotti test: give DEC 50mg oral; increased pruritus within 24–48h indicates that the patient is infected (Box 14.14).

Management

- Ivermectin 150micrograms/kg oral stat clears microfilariae from skin for 76–79mths. Repeat the dose when patient is symptomatic (typically each 6–12mths) throughout lifespan of adult worms (15–20yrs).
- Doxycycline 100mg oral bd for 4–6wks (against *Wolbachia* endosymbionts) decreases or eliminates microfilariae in skin for 12–18mths and reduces the number of adult worms.

Prevention Ivermectin mass distribution programmes; vector control.

Box 14.13 Forms of dermal onchocerciasis

- *Acute papular onchodermatitis:* small scattered itchy papules, +/– vesicles and pustules, +/– skin oedema, trunk and upper limbs.
- *Chronic papular onchodermatitis:* larger itchy, hyperpigmented, often flat-topped papules +/– hyperpigmentation.
- *Lichenified onchodermatitis:* intensely itchy, hyperpigmented papulo-nodules or plaques, often on the legs, which become confluent.
- *Atrophy:* loss of elasticity with excessive wrinkles particularly on buttocks; inguinal skin forms hanging groins, often filled with enlarged lymph nodes.
- *Depigmentation (leopard skin):* patches of hypo- or depigmentation contrasted with normally pigmented skin around hair follicles.

Box 14.14 Mazzotti reaction

DEC may → severe adverse reactions in *O. voluvulus* infection due to an immune reaction to worm death. Local reactions include skin rashes, exacerbation of eye lesions; severe systemic reactions may occur with fever, myalgia, arthralgia, respiratory distress, and shock. Avoid DEC therapy in onchocerciasis endemic areas.

Loiasis (Loa loa)

Loa loa is transmitted in Central African rainforests by bites of *Chrysops* horse flies. As injected filarial larvae mature, they migrate away from site in the sc layers (producing itching, prickly sensations) or deeper fascial layers (pain, paraesthesia). Transient migratory angioedema,'calabar swellings' of limbs occur at intervals lasting a few hours to days, due to host immune response to migrating adult worms; overlying skin is slightly inflamed (see Fig. 14.11). Worms migrating beneath conjunctiva may be clearly visible for minutes to hours, and produce acute eye irritation.

Diagnosis Clinical or serological; microfilariae can also be found in filtered blood samples collected around mid-day (see Fig. 14.12).

Management

Oral DEC 1mg/kg on day 1; 1mg/kg bd on day 2; 2mg/kg bd on day 3, and 2–3mg/kg tds from day 4–21. Start persons with heavy microfilaraemia at a low dose and give steroid cover for first 2–3d (risk of meningoencephalitis with dying microflaria). Check for mixed infection with *O. volvulus* before using DEC—if present, pre-treat with ivermectin 150micrograms/kg oral stat as there is risk of Mazzotti reaction (see Box 14.14). Doxycycline 100mg bd oral for 4–6wks will produce a more gradual reduction of microfilaraemia by acting on endosymbiotic *Wolbachia* within the worms.

Prevention Avoid vector contact; DEC 300mg oral once weekly may provide effective prophylaxis; vector control.

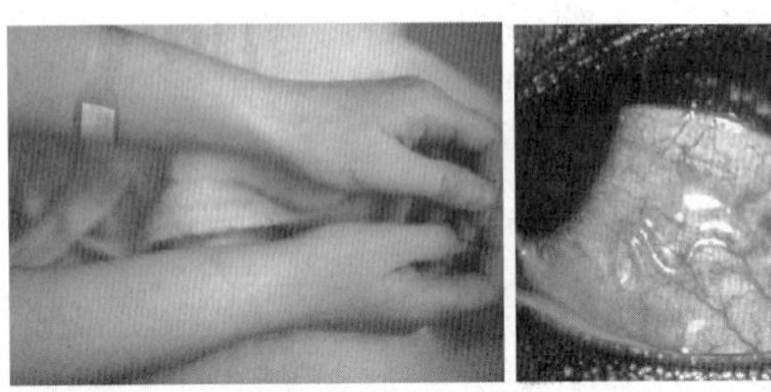

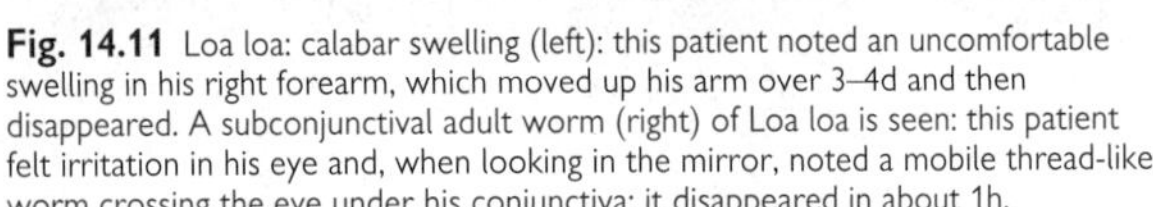

Fig. 14.11 Loa loa: calabar swelling (left): this patient noted an uncomfortable swelling in his right forearm, which moved up his arm over 3–4d and then disappeared. A subconjunctival adult worm (right) of Loa loa is seen: this patient felt irritation in his eye and, when looking in the mirror, noted a mobile thread-like worm crossing the eye under his conjunctiva; it disappeared in about 1h.

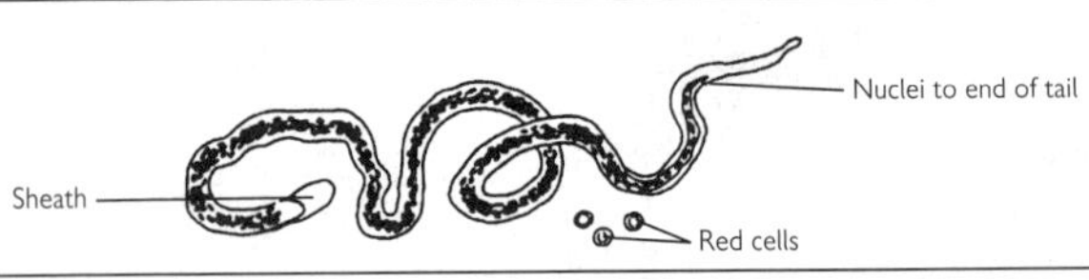

Fig. 14.12 Appearance of Loa loa microfilaria on a blood film.

Dracunculiasis (Guinea worm)

Dracunculus medinensis infection follows ingestion of water containing its copepod crustacean vector (Colour plate 17). Released larvae migrate into body cavities, mature and mate. Months later, adult females (50–100cm long) migrate in sc layers of the skin to extremities, where an ulcer forms and tip of the worm protrudes. In contact with water, larvae worm's uterus prolapses to skin surface to release larvae.

Clinical features

Include systemic hypersensitivity. Protrusion of the gravid female causes a painful blister, which may become 2° infected with bacteria. Some worms migrate to sites, such as brain, joints, or eyes, resulting in cerebral/subdural abscesses, arthritis, or blindness. Diagnosis is clinical in endemic areas in sub-Saharan Africa.

Management

Remove female worms before they blister by identifying them subcutaneously, making a small incision in the skin at their midpoint and pulling the worm out with careful traction and massage along its track. Metronidazole 400mg tds oral check dose for 1wk reduces inflammation and eases the removal. After a blister has burst, analgesics will be needed before the worm can be pulled out. Keep the blister clean and covered.

Prevention

Improve water supply or filter drinking water through cloth to remove crustaceans. The Guinea worm eradication programme has ↓ transmission to scattered foci within affected countries.

Other parasites that invade the skin

Cutaneous (furunculoid) myiasis

This is an infestation of the skin with fly larvae (maggots). *Dermatobia hominis* (the tropical botfly) is endemic in Central and South America. Female flies attach eggs to mosquitoes and other blood-sucking arthropods, which deposit eggs during a blood meal. Warmth from host causes eggs to hatch and larvae penetrate host skin (see Fig. 14.13). In sub-Saharan Africa, female *Cordylobia anthropophaga* (tumbu) flies lay their eggs in shaded soil or clothing hung out to dry (particularly if contaminated by urine); larvae hatch in 2d and penetrate skin. In both cases, as each larva grows subcutaneously, a 'boil'-like lesion with central punctum develops.

Management Removal of the larvae. Occluding punctum with vaseline or fat may allow larva to be grasped as it emerges for O_2. Surgical removal is sometimes required. Treat any 2° bacterial infection.

Prevention Insect repellents, clothing and mosquito nets for *D. hominis*; ironing clothing (including underwear) destroys the eggs of *C. anthropophaga*.

Tungiasis (*Tunga penetrans*, the Jigger Flea)

The 1-mm female pig flea burrows into the skin, usually of the toe webspaces, and grows to about 1cm in 2wks. The female discharges its eggs on the surface and its collapsed carcass is extruded.

Management Careful removal of flea and eggs. Avoid 2° bacterial infection.

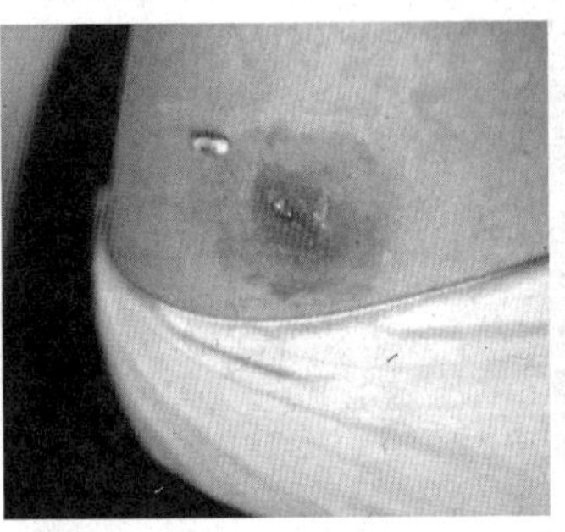

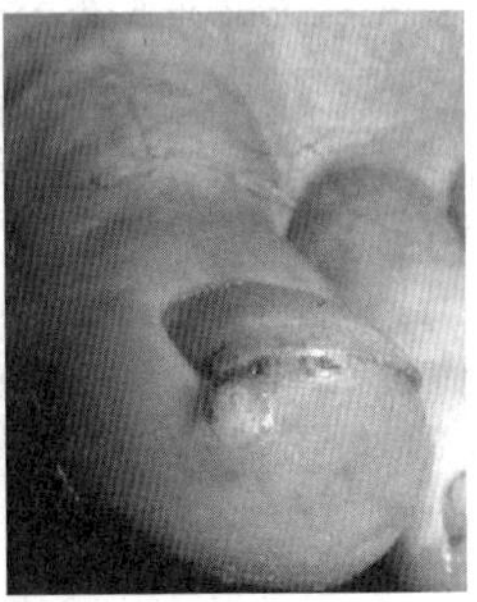

Fig. 14.13 (a) Furunculoid myiasis: this traveller developed a 'boil' on her buttock soon after return from Africa from which the larva of *Cordylobia anthropophaga* (the 'tumbu fly') was extracted. (b) *Tunga penetrans* (the 'Jigger flea'): two lesions are seen at the edge of the toenail.

Cutaneous larva migrans

Infection with filariform larvae of dog and cat hookworms (*Ancylostoma caninum* or *A. braziliense*) for whom humans are accidental hosts (Colour plate 14). Larvae migrate 1–2 cm per day in the skin, leaving an intensely itchy, red irregular track, before they eventually die.

Management Single-dose ivermectin 200 micrograms/kg (12 mg average adukt dose) or albendazole 400mg oral. Thiabendazole 15% cream or 10–15% suspension can also be applied topically. Untreated, the rash will eventually resolve spontaneously.

Larva currens

A cutaneous eruption resulting from autoinfection into the skin (often of the buttocks/perianal area) by *Strongyloides stercoralis* (see 🕮 Diarrhoeal diseases, p. 233). The urticarial wheals are linear and move approx. 1–2cm/h; the abdomen and buttocks are most affected (Colour plate 15).

Podoconiosis

Podoconiosis is a cause of lymphoedema in certain highland areas of East and Central Africa rich in volcanic soils. Microscopic mineral particles penetrate the dermis of the sole of foot and cause chronic lymphatic damage, especially in young adults who habitually walk barefoot. There may be a genetic predisposition.

The non-venereal treponematoses

These disfiguring conditions primarily affect children in communities with poor hygiene. Like syphilis, they have three stages, with a long period of latency before the manifestation 3° disease. Unlike syphilis, the 3° lesions are infective, causing problems for eradication, since it is difficult to identify latent carriers. Transmission is by direct contact; probably through abrasions (spirochaetes cannot penetrate intact skin; see Table 14.2).

Clinical features

Yaws

1° lesion is a papule, which develops into round/oval 2–5cm painless, itchy papilloma. It normally heals in 3–6mths. Weeks to years after this lesion resolves, multiple 2° lesions occur in crops on any part of body and last up to 6mths. They are papules or raspberry-like lesions of various shapes; they may ulcerate and form yellow-brown scabs. Other lesions include dermatitis or hyperkeratosis of palms and soles; local lymphadenopathy; dactylitis; long bone swelling; rarely, osteitis of nasal bones. After latent period, disease reappears with necrotic destruction of skin and bones (gummas). Other clinical features include hyperkeratosis; palatal destruction and 2° infection; saber tibia; bursitis.

Endemic syphilis (bejel)

1° lesion is rarely seen. First lesions are usually painless ulcers of lips and oropharynx. Osteoperiostitis of long bones, condylomata lata, angular stomatitis; rarely a 2° syphilis-like rash; and generalized lymphadenopathy. Late lesions include bone destruction (as in yaws), skin ulcers, and palmar and plantar keratosis.

Pinta

Pinta primarily affects the skin. Satellite lesions surround 1° papule; there is regional painless lymphadenopathy. 2° stage plaques appear within a few months anywhere on the body. 3° disease involves depigmentation and atrophy of the skin.

Diagnosis

Motile spirochaetes can be seen on dark-field microscopy of lesion exudates. There are no serological or morphological features that differentiate syphilis-causing *T. pallidum* from the other treponemes. The precise diagnosis is clinical.

Management A single dose of benzathine penicillin G 0.9g IM (alternatives: erythromycin 250–500mg oral qds or amoxicillin 500mg tds for 15d).

Prevention Identification of active cases, followed by treatment of all contacts. If >10% in community are actively infected, all should receive penicillin.

Table 14.2 Non-venereal treponematoses

	Yaws	**Bejel**	**Pinta**
Organism	*T. pertenue*	*T. pallidum*	*T. carateum*
Age group	15–40	2–10	10–30
Occurrence	Africa	Africa	Latin America
	South America	Middle East	
	Oceania	Asia	
Climate	Warm, humid	Dry, arid	Warm

Chapter 15

Bone, joint, and soft tissue infections

Invited author **Jonathan Underwood**

Infections of skin

Skin infections can be divided into:

- *Pyodermas:* a localized infection where pus is formed within the skin.
- *Spreading infections:* diffuse infection spreading along tissue planes.

Pyodermas

Impetigo

Superficial infection of the epidermis, often at sites of skin damage (e.g. cuts, eczema, chickenpox, scabies, insect bites; Box 15.1). A golden-yellow vesicle quickly bursts to become an area of epidermal loss, which crusts over and enlarges. There may be a little pus under the edges of the lesion. Impetigo is highly contagious: 1° lesion spreads to form satellite lesions elsewhere on the skin (spread by patient's own fingers) leading to infection of contacts. *Staph. aureus* and/or β-haemolytic *Streptococci* (BHS) (e.g. Group A BHS, also known as *Strep, pyogenes*) are most commonly found.

Management

- Topical agents (e.g. mupirocin) if mild.
- Give antibiotics (see Table 15.1) if more extensive/failed topical.
- Apply topical antiseptics (e.g. Gentian violet or chlorhexidine).
- Soak off crusts in saline or weak antiseptic.
- Wash skin daily with soap and water.

Furuncles (boils), carbuncles, and abscesses

Staph. aureus causes abscesses in the dermis or subcutaneous fat. A furuncle (boil, pimple) is pus collecting in a hair follicle or a sebaceous/sweat gland in the skin. Carbuncles are furuncles that have spread deeper (often 2° to patient squeezing or sitting on the furuncle), so multiple points of pus occur. An abscess is a collection of pus at a deeper level—indicated by swelling, erythema, warmth, and fluctuance. Tenderness is common in all skin infections, but pressure on an abscess is very painful.

Management

- Furuncles can often be managed with the application of warm compresses to promote spontaneous discharge.
- Drain pus and remove necrotic tissue and debris
  - abscess cavity should be packed and left to heal by 2° intention
  - do not suture or allow opening to close until interior has healed.
- If the infection spreads in the surrounding soft tissues, give 1–2wks of antibiotics (see Table 15.1). If antibiotics are unavailable or in short supply, drainage and good wound care alone may suffice.

Spreading infections

These are more commonly caused by beta-haemolytic streptococci than by *Staph. aureus*, except when surrounding a staphylococcal abscess.

Erysipelas

Acute, spreading infection in the epidermis, producing a large area of red, shiny, tender skin that is common on the face. The patient is unwell and febrile. The involved area is sharply demarcated from normal skin because the dermo-epidermal junction limits the spread of the inflammatory response. Severe infection → skin blistering; necrotic tissue encourages toxin production so the infection becomes worse if the infection is not treated.

Management: antibiotics (see Table 15.1).

Cellulitis

Acute infection involving the dermis and usually sc fat as well. There is obvious, diffuse swelling and the erythematous area is less clearly demarcated from uninvolved skin than in erysipelas. It commonly involves the lower leg, spreading from breaks in the skin: minor injuries, fungal infection (e.g. athlete's foot), scabies, or insect bites that have been scratched.

Always be aware of an underlying abscess, which may form within cellulitis, especially in the hand. When cellulitis is near the knee or elbow but spares the extremity, consider an underlying prepatellar, pretibial, or olecranon bursitis.

Box 15.1 Soft tissue infections

Insect bites, reduced access to antibiotics, poverty, and malnutrition contribute to a high incidence of soft tissue infections in the tropics. Some conditions, such as pyomyositis (infection of muscle), are particularly common in the tropics compared to temperate zones.

Table 15.1 Causative organisms and antibiotic choices

Condition	Microbiology	Treatment choices	Duration
Superficial infections			
Impetigo Furuncles Abscesses Carbuncles Erysipelas Cellulitis Bursitis	Group A beta-haemolytic streptococci *Staph. aureus* (including MRSA) Group B, C and G beta-haemolytic streptococci	1st flucloxacillin or co-amoxiclav 2nd cephalosporin 3rd clindamycin or erythromycin 4th co-trimoxazole	Until clinical resolution, usually 5–14d
Deep infections			
Acute septic arthritis Osteomyelitis Pyomyositis	*Staph. aureus* (including MRSA) Group A beta-haemolytic streptococci	1st cephalosporin + clindamycin 2nd co-amoxiclav	See individual sections
Necrotizing fasciitis	Mixed aerobes/ anaerobes		

If MRSA suspected add vancomycin.

If diabetic or vascular ulcers present add metronidazole

Usual adult doses

IV route

- Benzylpenicillin 1.2–2.4g IV qds.
- Flucloxacillin 1–2g IV qds.
- Ceftriaxone 2g IV od.
- Cefuroxime 750mg–1.5g IV or IM qds to tds.
- Co-amoxiclav 1.2g IV tds.
- Vancomycin 750mg–1.5g IV bd (depending on weight and renal function).
- Erythromycin 500mg–1g IV qds.

Clindamycin, ciprofloxacin, erythromycin, linezolid and metronidazole are all very well absorbed orally and seldom require IV administration.

Oral route

- Cefuroxime and flucloxacillin have incomplete oral bioavailability, avoid in severe infection.
- Amoxicillin 0.5–1g oral tds (use instead of penicillin, better absorption).
- Cefuroxime 250mg oral bd.
- Ciprofloxacin 500mg oral bd.
- Clindamycin 300–450mg oral qds (active against some strains of MRSA; Box 15.2).
- Co-amoxiclav 625mg oral tds.
- Erythromycin 500mg oral qds.
- Flucloxacillin 500mg–1g oral qds.
- Linezolid 600mg oral bd (active against MRSA).
- Metronidazole 800mg oral initially, then 400–500mg oral tds; or lg tds pr.

Management (see Box 15.3)

Scaling and desquamation are normal after some days of infection; blisters protect the lesion and should be left intact in most cases or incised if they contain pus. Subcutaneous abscesses can develop despite antibiotics. Recurrence is relatively common: if multiple recurrences occur, consider prolonged courses of treatment, long-term prophylaxis, decolonization or standby antibiotics to take at the onset of symptoms.

Bursitis

Bursitis most commonly involves the elbow or the knee, and presents as cellulitis over the joint, or as a red painful swelling. The pathogens are usually BHS or *Staph. aureus*. Although bursitis often restricts the movement of the joint, this is related to the mechanical effects of the swelling and the associated tenderness of the soft tissues, and careful examination can usually distinguish bursitis from the much more serious condition of septic arthritis.

Management (see Box 15.3)

In chronic bursitis, suspect TB, underlying osteomyelitis (erosion of bone detectable on X-ray), or chronic septic arthritis.

Necrotizing fasciitis

Necrotizing fasciitis is a surgical emergency with high mortality. The most common cause is Group A BHS, but other organisms (e.g. mixed aerobe/anaerobe infections following abdominal or perineal wounds) can also cause necrotizing fasciitis.

Infection spreads very rapidly in the loose connective tissue adjacent to the fascial plane → necrosis of subcutaneous tissues and thrombosis of blood vessels that supply the skin or muscle. Infection in deep tissues spreads very fast, and necrosis of the skin ocurs relatively slowly; hence a relatively healthy appearance of the skin is deceptive. At surgery, deeper tissues may be extensively necrotic. As a result, necrotizing fasciitis typically causes severe systemic upset (often with high fever and shock) and pain that seem disproportionate to the local physical signs.

Management (see Box 15.3)

Diagnosis is largely clinical. Imaging (CT or MRI) may confirm the diagnosis in difficult cases but should never delay surgical exploration. Development of fixed tissue staining, ecchymoses, superficial blistering (early in disease, not late as in cellulitis, and on obviously unhealthy skin) makes the diagnosis probable.

Box 15.2 MRSA

Meticillin resistance occurs in clones of *Staph. aureus* that have a mutation in the penicillin binding protein on their surface. Meticillin resistance indicates resistance to all beta lactam antibiotics, including flucloxacillin and co-amoxiclav. MRSA is becoming more common in resource-poor countries and, in particular, in large centres. By 2006, >20% of *Staph. aureus* isolates were MRSA in large urban hospitals in South America, India, Sri Lanka, Kenya, South Africa, Nigeria, and Cameroon, and many other resource-poor countries. In rural settings, the prevalence of MRSA is far lower, but increasing. Thus, whilst flucloxacillin, co-amoxiclav, and cephalosporins are still recommended as 1st line treatment for bone, joint, and soft tissue infections, it should always be borne in mind that poor clinical response may indicate MRSA. In centres in which MRSA is prevalent, empiric treatment for *Staph. aureus* infections is with vancomycin, teicoplanin or linezolid. In most areas, doxycycline has high activity against MRSA, and in many areas chloramphenicol, clindamycin co-trimoxazole and fucidic acid are effective. Rifampicin, although effective against most MRSA strains, is generally restricted for use in TB.

It is important to establish local MRSA rates. Find out where specimens can be sent for culture and sensitivity. Keep updated with the local MRSA antibiotic susceptibilities.

Box 15.3 Management

Cellulitis

- Antibiotics for 1–2wks.
- If cellulitis is 2° to a chronic ulcer, in a diabetic, or follows water contact, broaden the antibiotic cover to include Gram –ve rods and anaerobes (e.g. co-amoxiclav).
- Consider wound debridement and cleaning.
- Drain underlying abscesses (especially in the hand).
- Rest and elevate the limb.

Bursitis

- Antibiotics for 2–3wks.
- Needle aspiration to remove some pus: useful for diagnosis and symptom relief.
- Avoid incision and drainage where possible: the synovial fluid produced in the bursa produces high-volume wound drainage, can delay healing, and sometimes → a synovial fistula.

Necrotizing fasciitis

- Early surgery is mandatory: explore the fascial plane and excise the affected area back to bleeding tissue.
- Repeated surgery is often necessary.
- *Broad-spectrum antibiotics:* high-dose penicillin plus gentamicin plus metronidazole is a good 1st choice. Where available, add clindamycin (anti-toxin effect, beneficial in animal models of necrotizing fasciitis). Duration of treatment should be guided by clinical response. Adjust antibiotics when cultures are available from surgical samples.
- *Intensive care support and reconstructive surgery:* without these, prognosis is poor.

Infections of muscle

Pyomyositis

Also called 'tropical pyomyositis', it is a 1° bacterial infection of skeletal muscle that is common throughout the tropics and subtropics, particularly in young men.

Clinical features

There are three characteristic phases:

- *Invasive phase:* affected muscle is painful, hard, and woody on palpation. Patient may have little systemic illness; this phase may last for days–months. Condition is difficult to diagnose, and can sometimes be mistaken for a tumour.
- *Suppurative phase:* muscle liquefies → IM abscess, with very tender swollen muscle. US shows IM collections; for psoas abscess, CT or MRI scanning may be necessary. (*Note:* psoas abscess is also a complication of lumbar spinal infections and does not represent 'pure' pyomyositis.) Gram stain and culture of aspirated pus usually reveals *Staph. aureus* (rarely β haemolytic streptococcus (BHS)).
- *Systemic phase:* sepsis, bacteraemia and progression to metastatic infection can occur.

Management

- Antibiotics for >3wks.
- Drain abscesses surgically or percutaneously.

The overall prognosis is generally good.

Gas gangrene

A rapidly progressive, life-threatening and necrotizing infection within muscle, characterized by severe systemic illness, muscle pain, and crepitus due to gas formation. Gas gangrene is generally caused by *Clostridium perfringens*, which produces toxins that → muscle necrosis. The infection is acquired through environmental (particularly soil) contamination of deep wounds involving muscle.

Management

- Emergency surgical exploration and debridement of dead tissue is needed, often with excision of massive areas of muscle (for trunk wounds) and early amputation (for limb infection).
- The systemic effect of the toxins is invariably fatal without successful treatment.
- High-dose penicillin with clindamycin if available is important, but unlikely to be effective without surgery.

Prevention Through good wound care/wound debridement.

Septic tenosynovitis

Infections of the tendon sheath occur predominantly in the hand and the traumatized foot (including the chronically ulcerated).

Aetiology

As well as common bacteria, tenosynovitis in the non-traumatized hand can be caused by atypical mycobacteria such *as M. marinum*, *M. chelonae*, and *M. kansasii*, and environmental fungi such as *Sporothrix schenckii*. If related to trauma or ulceration, a wide range of organisms may be involved. It can also occur 2° to disseminated gonococcal infection, sepsis with other bacteria, or *M. tuberculosis*.

Clinical features Swelling of one or more fingers, palm, or dorsum of the hand. Swelling in the foot can be minimal if fluid drains via an ulcer.

Diagnosis Can be clinical, confirmed by surgery, or made with ultrasound or MRI.

Management

- *Generally requires drainage of the involved tendon sheath:* to control the infection and to prevent adhesions and long-term stiffness.
- *Tendons heal slowly if exposed:* soft tissue or skin cover is important.
- See Table 15.1 for antibiotics: for pyogenic infections, treat for 2–4wks; for mycobacterial or fungal infections, use standard courses for the pathogen.

Septic arthritis

Bacteria infect the joint by haematogenous spread or direct inoculation (trauma, ulceration or iatrogenic). Bacterial multiplication in the joint → acute inflammation → destruction of articular cartilage and resorption of exposed bone, → deformity, chronic osteomyelitis, and joint fusion. Bacteraemia and septicaemia may occur. If pus tracks and discharges externally, a sinus is formed.

Clinical features

Although most cases of acute or chronic infection involve a single joint, multiple joint involvement occurs in 5–10% of cases (Box 15.4).

- *Acute septic arthritis:* fever, pain, and loss of function. The joint is highly irritable; the patient resists both active and passive movement. Usually, the joint is obviously swollen, warm, and tender to touch, with little or no erythema unless accompanied by bursitis or cellulitis (Box 15.5).
- *Chronic septic arthritis:* swollen and painful joint, but little systemic illness. There may be obvious deformity or crepitus from gross joint destruction (Box 15.6).

Complications

Without timely and effective treatment, joint destruction ensues. There may be osteomyelitis, septicaemia, and, in young child, growth plate disturbances → deformity or ↓ limb length. Complications are much more likely if treatment is delayed.

Diagnosis

- *Blood tests:* FBC, CRP, and ESR demonstrate inflammation, but lack specificity.
- *Cultures:* aspiration of synovial fluid is essential for diagnosis. Microscopy shows neutrophils and can exclude crystals (gout, pseudogout), bacteria may be seen on Gram stain and cultures are often +ve if antibiotics have not been previously given. Blood cultures are +ve in ~50% so should be taken in all cases of suspected septic arthritis.
- *Radiology:* plain X-rays determine extent of joint damage but only if infection present for >10d. CT and MRI reveal the extent of bone and soft tissue infection and are useful in joints that are difficult to examine (e.g. hips). Radiological changes, especially MRI changes, lag behind clinical recovery.

Management

- Drainage of the joint should be performed urgently by aspiration (may be required daily) or arthroscopic washout. Open drainage may be needed when repeated drainage has failed or for hip joints. There is no place for continuous irrigation of the joint: this carries the risk of introducing antibiotic-resistant bacteria (e.g. *Pseudomonas*). Removal of the prosthesis is often required in prosthetic joint infections.
- Chronic septic arthritis usually requires surgery.
- Antibiotic choice should be guided by the initial Gram stain and subsequent culture and sensitivity results. Treatment is at least 3wks

(ideally parenterally). Shorter durations of therapy can be used for gonococcal arthritis. In joints with extensive pre-existing arthritis and exposed bone, or in compromised hosts (rheumatoid arthritis is a good example of both), treat for longer.

Box 15.4 Causes of bone and joint infections

- Skin infections can seed via the bloodstream → septic arthritis and acute osteomyelitis.
- If ineffectively treated, these acute conditions become chronic (e.g. when surgery is unavailable and prolonged courses of antibiotics are unaffordable).
- Commonly caused by injuries on roads and in factories, armed conflict, and landmine injuries.
- Some 1° infections of bone and joint are more common in the tropics: TB, brucellosis, melioidosis, histoplasmosis, and blastomycosis.

Box 15.5 Organisms causing acute septic arthritis

- *Staph. aureus:* most common in all age groups and all countries. Flucoxacillin 1st choice (MSSA). Vancomycin for MRSA.
- *Haemophilus influenzae:* in populations without access to HiB vaccine. Ceftriaxone 1st choice in serious infections.
- *Beta-haemolytic streptococci of all groups (including Group B in pregnancy, neonates, and diabetics):* penicillin 1st choice.
- *Enterobacteriaciae (e.g. E. coli):* in neonates and elderly. Ceftriaxone or co-amoxiclav 1st choice.
- *N. gonorrhoeae:* in sexually active individuals. Ceftriaxone 1st choice.

Box 15.6 Organisms causing chronic septic arthritis

The same organisms as acute septic arthritis, plus:

- *M. tuberculosis.*
- *Brucella.*
- Occasionally fungi (e.g. *Sporothrix schenckii*).

Osteomyelitis

Infection of the bone → progressive bone destruction and sequestrum formation. Acute or chronic, it may be caused by haematogenous or contiguous spread of microorganisms or by direct inoculation. Organisms causing acute osteomyelitis are largely the same as those causing acute septic arthritis.

Clinical features

- *Acute osteomyelitis:* fever, localized bone pain, and loss of limb function. Osteomyelitis can → septic arthritis, especially in young children.
- *Chronic osteomyelitis:* chronic drainage from wound or sinus tract, pain, flares of intercurrent acute infection, impaired function, and/or chronic ill health. Visible or palpable bone in a wound makes osteomyelitis highly likely. An orthopaedic implant or an open fracture with a chronically draining wound is almost certainly infected.

Diagnosis

- *Blood tests:* WBC may be normal, but ESR and CRP are often raised. Anaemia is common in chronic infection.
- *X-rays:* become abnormal after ~10d, as involved the bone is demineralized (lytic areas), attempts to heal (periosteal reaction), and–in parts–dies (sclerotic areas). Changes evolve over a few weeks; the process is aggressive. There may be evidence of loosening of metalware.
- *Other imaging:* US can show abscesses adjacent to bone and delineates sinus tracts. Bone scans are sensitive but not specific, CT and MRI are superior. CT is useful for assessing bony union, bone destruction and sequestrum. MRI detects marrow oedema, cortical breaches, sinus tracts, and soft tissue collections, but is less useful in patients with extensive metalware or recent surgery.
- *Cultures:* blood cultures may be +ve in ~50% and may obviate the need for more invasive tests. Bone biopsy, obtained radiologically or surgically, ideally before antibiotics are started, is useful to identify the causative organism(s). Sinus tract swabs are of dubious value unless they demonstrate *Staph. aureus.*

Management

Goal of treatment is to eradicate infection and restore/preserve function. Usually achieved by a combination of surgical debridement, removal of foreign bodies if present and antibiotic therapy.

- *For acute osteomyelitis:* give antibiotics (see Table 15.1) for >6wks. Use IV, then consider oral route. Evaluate need for surgery.
- *For chronic osteomyelitis:* evaluate need for surgery, patient's general fitness, and goals of treatment.

Control of intermittent flares Especially if flares infrequent and respond to antibiotics. Monitor for progression of bone involvement.

Suppression with long-term antibiotics If surgery impossible for technical reasons, unaffordable, or worse than disease. Long-term antibiotics can → drying of sinuses, ↑ in general health, and ↓ pain.

Surgical exploration, debridement, and excision with subsequent antibiotics. Aim to remove all dead bone, ensuring the skeleton is stable and soft tissue covers the bone at the end of surgery. Dead space inside debrided bone can be filled with muscle, cancellous bone graft (usually delayed until infection is arrested), or antibiotic-laden carriers. Antibiotics added to acrylic bone cement will generate very high local levels. With expert surgery, >90% of cases can be arrested. However, even without surgery or antibiotics, spontaneous long-term arrest can occur if sequestra discharge spontaneously. Many patients can live with their bone infection for long periods; in some situations, this may be the best that can be achieved.

Spinal infections

Common causes are *Staph. aureus*, *Brucella* spp., and TB. Initial blood-borne seeding to disc space is followed by involvement of adjacent vertebral bodies. Paraspinal muscles may also become involved, with collections (e.g. psoas abscesses). Retropulsion of disc and inflammatory tissue, or spinal epidural abscess, may compress the spinal cord → paralysis.

Clinical features Unusually severe back pain, especially at night; sudden paraparesis on a background of back pain and/or fever.

Diagnosis

Plain X-rays may show irregularity and destruction of end-plates adjoining the infected disc space (which becomes ↓ in height). MRI is the investigation of choice. CXR or sputum examination may provide evidence of TB; the organism may be cultured from blood, aspirate of paraspinal or disc space abscesses, or guided biopsy of the disc.

Management

- Antibiotics (see Table 15.1). Treat pyogenic infections of the spine for 6–12wks.
- Surgery is reserved for cases with acute spinal epidural abscess, persistent pain, mechanical instability, recurrent infection with abscess formation, or cord compression.
- Steroid therapy may be useful as an adjunct to ↓ oedema in spinal TB with neurological involvement.
- Patients with spinal TB infection may recover neurologically on anti-TB medication, even if presenting with paralysis.

The diabetic foot

The dramatic worldwide ↑ in type II diabetes → ↑ in patients with foot complications. These arise from diabetic peripheral neuropathy, with or without ischaemia, plus impaired systemic resistance to infection. A foot ulcer precedes most amputations in diabetics; most patients undergoing amputation for non-traumatic causes are diabetic. Good long-term glycaemic control is important.

- Motor neuropathy → ↑ curvature and height of the arch of the foot, → hyperextension and subluxation at MP joints → clawing at the IP joints → pressure on metatarsal heads, heel and clawed toes, the tips of toes, and over the PIP joints.
- These deformities co-exist with a sensory neuropathy, which means that patient does not perceive pain until too late (or not at all).
- Patient may also sustain penetrating injuries or burns without knowing.
- Autonomic neuropathy → dry, fissured skin, which is more susceptible to injury and infection.
- There is also ↓ white cell function.
- Peripheral vascular disease, if present, further ↓ healing of ulcers.

Diabetic foot infections are frequently polymicrobial. The extent of infection determines the likely pathogens.

- Superficial infections (inc infected ulcers and cellulitis) are commonly caused by *Staph. aureus* (including MRSA) and BHS.
- Deeper ulcers often involve Gram –ve bacteria (including *Pseudomonas* sp.) in addition to the above.
- Extensive local infection, gangrene or necrosis with systemic upset usually indicates anaerobic involvement in addition to the above.

Clinical features

Soft tissue infection and loss, draining sinuses with exposed bone, sometimes necrotizing fasciitis or septicaemia. Purulent drainage suggests infection, as does erythema, swelling, pain (which often occurs to some extent, despite neuropathy), and systemic symptoms.

Diagnosis

Blood tests may show ↑ WBC, CRP, ESR, glucose, and creatinine. Plain foot X-rays may show gas in the soft tissues, bone destruction, and/or changes consistent with infection or diabetic osteopathy. Serial X-rays may show progressive changes over weeks. MRI is imaging modality of choice in indeterminate cases.

Management

- Assess fever, cardiovascular stability, hydration, and diabetic control.
- Examine sensation, peripheral perfusion (Buerger's test, palpation of pulses, and Doppler assessment including ankle-brachial pressure indices), and presence of cellulitis, necrosis, swelling, or crepitus.
- Debride the ulcer to determine its extent. If possible, probe with a sterile metal probe: palpable bone suggests underlying osteomyelitis. Other features that make osteomyelitis probable are: ulcer size >2 × 2cm, ulcer depth >3mm, ulcer duration >2wks or an ESR >70mm/h.
- See Table 15.1 for antibiotics.

Durations

- 72h for amputation through healthy tissue.
- 1–2wks for amputation through infected soft tissue, without residual infected bone.
- 4wks for amputation or surgery through ischaemic or severely infected soft tissues, including deep tissue involvement (e.g. tendon sheaths).
- 4–6wks for osteomyelitis, fully resected, with restoration of soft tissue cover.
- 6–12wks for osteomyelitis with residual infected or dead bone.

Prompt surgery is essential for significant soft tissue necrosis, crepitus, gangrene, necrotizing fasciitis, abscess drainage, or bone and joint involvement.

Vascular surgical input if ischaemic; may be able to avoid amputation.

Prevention

Diabetic foot ulcers often recur without special attention to foot care and footwear. Appropriate long-term care, with off-loading of pressure points, is also essential to obtain 1° healing of ulcers, even if not infected. Improve glycaemic control, daily foot inspection, stop smoking, and control BP.

Fungal skin infections

Cutaneous infections

Dermatophytoses (tinea)

Common skin infections caused by fungi, particularly *Trichophyton* and *Microsporum* spp. (see Box 15.8).

- Cause scaling or maceration between toes (tinea pedis).
- Itchy, scaly, red rash with definite edges in the groin area (tinea cruris).
- Annular lesions with raised edges (often itchy) anywhere on the body (tinea corporis).
- Scaling and itching of the scalp with loss of hair (tinea capitis).
- Treat with local application of Whitfield's ointment (benzoic acid compound) or clotrimazole for 2–4wks.
- For severe cases and nail involvement, use 4–6wks of griseofulvin 10mg/kg oral (alternatives: terbinafine or itraconazole).

Pityriasis versicolor

A superficial, hypopigmented, macular rash normally of the upper body. If extensive, can indicate a cause of chronic sweating (e.g. TB or HIV). Treatment with 2% selenium sulfide shampoo—apply lather and leave in contact for 10min before rinsing; or fluconazole 400mg as a single dose. (see 🕮 Dermatology, p. 587).

Superficial candidiasis

In addition to vaginal and oral infection, *C. albicans* can infect moist folds of skin (groin, under breasts, nappy area of baby) producing a very red rash and skin damage. Treat with topical nystatin or clotrimazole and keep dry.

Subcutaneous infections

Mycetoma (Madura foot)

Chronic infection of sc tissue (see Fig. 15.1), bone, and skin that is due to environmental organisms, either fungi (eumycetes, producing eumycetomas) or bacteria (actinomycetes or *Nocardia* spp., producing actinomycetomas), probably introduced into deep tissue by a thorn. The infecting organisms grow very slowly, typically forming 'grains' that are macroscopic colonies of fungi or bacteria. Mycetomas commonly occur on the foot or leg, but may occur anywhere. Start as area of hard swelling; infection eventually spreads from sc tissues to invade and destroy bone. Considerable swelling and usually multiple sinus tract formation, through which grains may discharge, but pain is rarely severe.

Diagnosis On X-ray, underlying bone is expanded, eroded, and ultimately destroyed. There is some local lymphatic involvement. The cause needs to be determined by microscopy of the sinus discharge.

Management Fungal mycetomas rarely respond to systemic antifungals and frequently require amputation. Actinomycetomas may respond to streptomycin or rifampicin for 2–3mths plus co-trimoxazole for many months until there is clinical improvement.

Sporotrichosis: Sporothrix schenckii
Inoculated into the skin at sites of minor trauma. It may present as a single ulcer or nodule. In the lymphangitic form, the fungus spreads down the lymphatics, forming nodules at intervals which may then ulcerate through to the skin. Chronic lesions may look like psoriasis or a granuloma.

Treatment Saturated aqueous solution of potassium iodide mixed with milk, 0.5–1mL oral tds, increased in small increments to 3–6mL tds, until 1mth after clinical resolution. (*Alternative:* itraconazole 100–200mg oral od.)

Box 15.8 Skin signs of systemic fungal infection
Systemic mycoses, such as histoplasmosis, blastomycosis, coccidioidomycosis, paracoccidioidomycosis, and other fungal infections in immunocompromised individuals, often show skin signs. Such signs include purpura, ulcers, slow spreading verrucous plaques, nodules, papules, pustules, and abscesses.

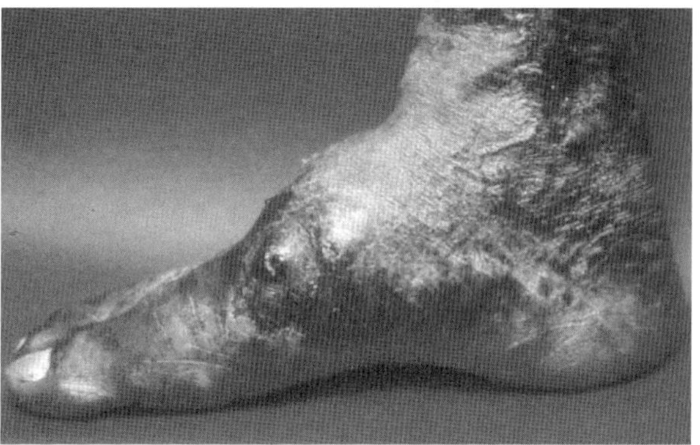

Fig. 15.1 Madura foot: fungal mycetoma caused by *Fusarium* species.

Chapter 16

Sexually-transmitted infections

Invited author **Henrietta Williams**

Why are sexually-transmitted infections important?

STIs have short- and long-term health consequences, with a significant impact on health of both individual and population. These include:

- *Acute problems:* urethral/vaginal discharge, pain, fever.
- *Chronic problems:* pelvic pain, infertility, tubal pregnancy, malignancy, miscarriages, perinatal infection, neurological and cardiovascular disease.

In addition:

- Psychological health and well-being may be affected by stigma.
- Prevalence is ↑ among the most vulnerable and marginalized groups in society that, combined with the stigma, → difficulties in accessing healthcare.
- Many STI also ↑ risk of HIV transmission.

Understanding the health consequences of STI for individuals and society is critical to the implementation of effective control policies. Recent understanding of the role of male circumcision in ↓ HIV transmission means it is also now important for future public health initiatives.

Epidemiology and control of sexually-transmitted infections

The May and Anderson equation encapsulates important factors in the epidemiology of STI. This states that:

$$R_0 = BCD,$$

where: R_0 is the number of 2° cases resulting from an infected individual in a susceptible community; B is the probability of an infection being transmitted per sexual activity; C is the rate of change of sexual partners; D is the average duration of infectiousness

Factors influencing these variables are listed in Box 16.1. The success of public health interventions for control of STI depends on reaching certain 'core groups' in the community in which ↑ STI prevalence is usually associated with frequent changes of partner and unsafe sexual practices. Such groups may include commercial sex workers (CSW), men who have sex with men (MSM), and sexually active adolescents.

Challenges and opportunities in control of STI

The model in Box 16.1 is effective for bacterial STI such as gonorrhoea, syphilis, and chancroid. Viral STIs (e.g. HSV, HPV) have additional challenges. Lack of curative treatment and poor accessibility to suppressive treatment → symptomatic or asymptomatic viral shedding and ongoing transmission. HSV-2 is often a commoner cause than chancroid of genital ulceration, even in countries with high rates of ulcerative STI.

There are new preventative measures.

Vaccines

Recently developed HPV vaccines can ⇊ HPV related disease, including cervical cancer and genital warts, if dissemination and uptake of vaccine is successful (📖 Immunization, p. 893).

Box 16.1 Variables influencing the reproductive rate (R_0) of an STI

Variable	Factors impacting these variables
Probability of an STI being transmitted (B)	• Condom usage • Sexual practices, e.g. 'dry sex' • Treatment of other STI • Circumcision • Suppressive treatment, e.g. HSV
Rate of change of sexual partners (C)	• Safer sexual behaviour patterns • ↓ partner change (especially concurrent partners) • Delayed initiation of sexual intercourse
Average duration of infectiousness (D)	• Education and awareness of STI • Availability and access to diagnostic and treatment services • Availability and access to syndromic treatment • Screening of high risk individuals

Male circumcision

↓ Transmission of HIV from women to men by ~60%. In countries where heterosexual HIV transmission predominates, HIV prevalence rates are high, with low background rates of male circumcision. If circumcision can be carried out safely, it is being actively promoted to ↓ HIV transmission. Information available at: http://www.who.int/hiv/topics/malecircumcision/en/index.html

Syndromic management of sexually-transmitted infections

Rapid, definitive diagnosis and treatment of STI, together with partner notification, effectively ↓ further transmission and reinfection. Rapid diagnostic tests are becoming increasingly available worldwide, and should be used when possible. Where this is not available, STI services focus on syndromic management, using treatment algorithms to cure common causes of defined clinical syndromes. HCWs are trained to identify these syndromes by easily recognizable symptoms and signs.

Syndromic management is only aimed at symptomatic patients. Treatment reflects local antibiotic resistance patterns. To ↑ compliance, directly observed single dose treatment is used whenever possible. Syndromic management also includes partner notification and sexual health promotion.

Advantages of syndromic management

- Prompt and rapid treatment at the point of presentation.
- Does not need expensive or sophisticated laboratory resources.
- Does not need highly trained laboratory staff.
- Involves local trained HCWs.

This chapter outlines the management of the following STI syndromes based on WHO guidelines:

- Urethral discharge.
- Vaginal discharge.
- Genital ulcer disease.
- Inguinal buboes.
- Scrotal swelling.
- Lower abdominal pain in women.
- Neonatal conjunctivitis.

See: http://www.who.int/hiv/pub/sti/pub6/en/

Urethral discharge in men Urethritis is diagnosed if urethral discharge or an inflamed meatus is seen on examination (see Colour plate 31), or dried discharge is seen on the penis.

Clinical features

Most common presentation is urethral discharge and dysuria. In men with no definite signs of urethritis the urethra can be 'milked' to detect the presence of a discharge.

Cause

- *Most common pathogens: Neisseria gonorrhoeae, Chlamydia trachomatis*
- *Less common pathogens:* genital mycoplasmas (*Mycoplasma genitalium, Ureaplasma urealyticum*), *Trichomonas*, HSV, and *Adenovirus*.
- In ~50% of cases, no causal pathogen can be identified.
- *Sexual behaviour may predict aetiology:* e.g. HSV and *Adenovirus* are common causes of urethritis in those practising insertive oral sex.

Diagnosis
If laboratory services are available, a sample of discharge can be swabbed for culture and air-dried on a glass slide for microscopy . Gram –ve intracellular diplococci suggest *N. gonorrhoeae*. Presence of >5 pus cells in a Gram smear has traditionally been used to confirm the presence of urethritis, but this may not be sufficiently sensitive.

Management
- Treatment of the index case.
- Partner notification.
- Treatment of contacts.

If gonorrhoea cannot be reliably excluded by laboratory tests, treatment should be for both gonorrhoea and *Chlamydia* (📖 Chlamydial infections, p. 672), ideally with single dose treatment to aid compliance. The index patient should return if symptoms persist for >7d. Persistence suggests failure of treatment or reinfection. If reinfections unlikely, refer for laboratory investigations to identify less common causative pathogens; if no laboratory investigations are available treat for trichomoniasis.

Recommended treatment regimens Therapy for uncomplicated gonorrhoea (📖 Gonorrhoea, p. 670) plus therapy for uncomplicated *Chlamydia* (📖 Chlamydial infections, p. 672).

Alternative regimen if tetracyclines are contraindicated/not tolerated Therapy for uncomplicated gonorrhoea (📖 Gonorrhoea, p. 670) plus erythromycin 500mg oral qds for 7d.

Vaginal discharge

The usefulness of vaginal discharge as a symptom in syndromic management of STI is uncertain. Personal and cultural factors influence the subjective interpretation of vaginal discharge so it does not always reliably indicate cervical infection. Vaginal speculum examination is used to confirm the presence of discharge and to view the cervix when feasible.

Clinical features
Abnormal vaginal discharge is usually caused by vaginitis or vaginosis; cervicitis (often caused by an STI) is also common and cannot be reliably distinguished from symptoms alone. Cervical mucus or pus, presence of cervical erosions, cervical friability and intermenstrual or post-coital bleeding are more frequent in cervicitis, but do not exclude vaginitis or vaginosis. Risk assessment (📖 Management, p. 662) takes account of local STI prevalence, as well as local sexual behaviour patterns.

Causes
Commonly bacterial vaginosis, candidiasis, trichomoniasis; also cervical infection caused by *Chlamydia* sp. and *Neisseria gonorrhoeae*. These cervical infections are frequently asymptomatic. Non-infective causes of vaginal discharge usually present with a less acute history and include malignancy, foreign body, atopic vulvovaginitis, and cervical ectropion.

Diagnosis

History of the discharge and associated symptoms, as well as a risk assessment (📖 Management, p. 662). If microscopy is available, a Gram stain for *N. gonorrhoeae* from the cervix and a wet preparation for *Trichomonas* from the vagina are helpful.

Management

All women are treated for vaginitis and those women with ≥1 risk factors below for STI are also treated for common causes of cervicitis:

- <21yrs.
- Unmarried.
- >1 sexual partner in < 3mths.
- New partner in <3mths.
- Current partner with an STI.

Treatment

- *Cervicitis:* therapy for uncomplicated gonorrhoea (📖 Gonorrhoea, p. 670) and *Chlamydia* (📖 Chlamydial infections, p. 672).
- *Vaginitis:* therapy for bacterial vaginosis (📖 Bacterial vaginosis, p. 677) and *Trichomonas vaginalis* (📖 Trichomoniasis, p. 676), and, if indicated, for *Candida albicans* (📖 Candida vaginitis, p. 680).

Lower abdominal pain

Endometritis, salpingitis, and pelvic inflammatory disease (PID) resulting from STI can present with lower abdominal pain (LAP) in sexually active women. PID may also occur in the absence of STI; in these cases the aetiology is often polymicrobial and may result from inadvertent introduction of flora from the lower genital tract, e.g. during a gynaecological procedure.

Causes

Of PID include *Chlamydia* and gonorrhoea and, less commonly, genital mycoplasmas. Non-sexually transmitted pathogens responsible for PID include *Actinomyces*, TB, anaerobes, and *Mobiluncus*.

Diagnosis

In addition to LAP, PID commonly presents with fever, vaginal discharge, deep dyspareunia, menstrual disturbance, and less commonly nausea and vomiting. Signs include fever, lower abdominal tenderness, vaginal discharge, uterine tenderness, including pain with movement of the cervix (cervical excitation), and adnexal tenderness and/or adnexal masses. Clinical examination has low diagnostic sensitivity and specificity for PID and no reliable non-invasive investigations exist. Low threshold for treatment is advocated because delayed treatment increases risk of long-term sequelae.

Management

Admit to hospital if severely unwell, for surgical emergencies (e.g. ectopic pregnancy, appendicitis), during pregnancy, if a pelvic abscess cannot be excluded, or if outpatient treatment has failed. PID often has polymicrobial aetiology so treatment should be broad spectrum, but must also target commoner identifiable known bacterial causes.

Treatment

Outpatient treatment

Stat treatment for gonorrhoea (📖 Gonorrhoea, p. 670), plus doxycycline 100mg bd (or tetracycline 500mg qds) plus metronidazole 400mg bd for 14d. Avoid alcohol with metronidazole and avoid tetracyclines in pregnancy.

Inpatient treatment

- Ceftriaxone 2g IV daily for 7d, plus doxycycline 100mg oral/IV bd (or tetracycline 500mg oral qds) and metronidazole 400–500mg bd oral/IV (or chloramphenicol 500mg oral/IV qds) for 14d *or*
- Clindamycin 900mg IV tds plus gentamicin 1.5mg/kg tds or substitute single dose regimen
- Ciprofloxacin 500mg oral bd plus doxycycline 100mg oral/IV bd (or tetracycline 500mg oral qds) and metronidazole 400–500mg oral/IV bd (or chloramphenicol 500mg oral/IV qds).

For inpatient regimens IV treatment needs to be continued for 2d after severe symptoms improving and then treat for a further 14d with doxycycline 100mg oral bd or tetracycline 500mg oral qds.

If an IUD is present and PID is mild, it is reasonable to leave IUD in situ, if the patient is monitored for improvement. If IUD is to be removed, usually recommended >48h of antibiotics. Alternative contraception will be needed.

Scrotal swelling

Testicular torsion

Should always be excluded in patients with a painful swollen scrotum. In acute torsion there is usually severe pain, which is worse when walking and is not relieved by supporting testicle. Often associated nausea and vomiting. Testicle may be red and swollen. Urgent surgical exploration is needed as the testicle will not survive for >6h with compromised blood supply.

Epididymitis

Is one of the commonest causes of scrotal swelling. In young, sexually-active men this is usually due to an STI and often associated with testicular infection/inflammation epididymo-orchitis.

Infective causes of epididymitis or epididymo-orchitis may be either STIs or non-STIs. In men >35yrs (and in children and adolescents prior to sexual debut), non-sexually transmitted pathogens are more common. Associated urethral discharge strongly indicates an STI.

- *STIs: Chlamydia* and gonorrhoea.
- *Non-STIs: E. coli, Klebsiella* spp., or *Pseudomonas aeruginosa*. TB and *Brucella* infection may also need to be considered. Other less common causes include *M. leprae* reactions, syphilis, *Candida albicans, Streptococcus pneumoniae* and *Haemophilus influenzae* type b. Mumps can also cause an orchitis.

Non-infectious causes of scrotal swelling (less common) include malignancy and trauma.

Management

Treatment for *Chlamydia* and gonorrhoea if suspected, and supportive care: bed rest, support of the testicle and pain relief. NSAIDs are helpful for pain.

Recommended treatment regimens

- *If likely STI:* treat as for uncomplicated gonorrhoea (📖 Gonorrhoea, p. 670) plus treatment of *Chlamydia* with 14d doxycycline 100mg bd (📖 Chlamydial infections, p. 672).
- *If not likely to be STI:* treat coliform organisms with ciprofloxacin 500mg bd for 10d. If severe infection *then* cefuroxime 1.5g tds IV + gentamicin for 3–5d can be used.

Genital ulcer

Causes

Genital ulcer disease often has multiple aetiologies. Commonest cause in a particular area is influenced by local prevalence of STIs and HIV. Ulceration caused by syphilis, lymphogranuloma venereum (LGV), granuloma inguinale, chancroid and HSV cannot be accurately distinguished clinically. HSV-2 is commoner than previously realized, even in areas where other causes of genital ulceration are common. Unusual or atypical presentations are common in HIV+ patients. 2° bacterial infection of genital ulcers is common.

Diagnosis

Offer serological testing for syphilis and HIV. Swab ulcer and test for HSV (if available) and *Treponema pallidum*, either by dark ground microscopy or other method if available. Chancroid and donovanosis may be considered depending on local prevalence. Microscopy with Giemsa staining may help in diagnosing donovanosis and culture can be used to diagnose chancroid. In some places a multiplex PCR is available for genital ulcer diagnosis (includes syphilis, HSV, chancroid and donovanosis).

Management

Counselling includes advice on period for infectivity of HIV and syphilis, and natural history of HSV and its transmission. Treatment depends on local causes, and should cover syphilis and HSV. Treatment for LGV, granuloma inguinale and chancroid depends on local prevalence rates. Advise patient to return for review if lesion not healed <7d. Individuals with HSV/HIV co-infection often have persistent multiple lesions and are at ↑ risk of transmitting HIV. HIV –ve patients with genital HSV are more susceptible to contracting HIV infection.

Recommended treatment

- Therapy for syphilis (📖 Syphilis, p. 666) *plus*
- Therapy for HSV if available (📖 Genital herpes, p. 678) *plus*
- Therapy for chancroid (📖 Chancroid, p. 674) *or*
- Therapy for granuloma inguinale (📖 Granuloma inguinale (donovanosis), p. 675) *or*
- Therapy for LGV (📖 Lymphogranuloma venereum, p. 672).

Inguinal buboes

Inguinal buboes are localized enlarged lymph nodes in the groin that are tender and sometimes fluctuant. LGV and chancroid are the most common causes. They are rarely the only signs of an STI and chancroid in particular is usually associated with a genital ulcer.

Recommended treatment

Ciprofloxacin 500mg oral bd for 3d plus *either* doxycycline 100mg oral bd *or* erythromycin 500mg oral qds for 14d.

Treatment may need to be continued beyond 14d. Fluctuant lymph nodes can be aspirated through skin, but should not be incised or drained as this can delay healing. Biopsy for diagnosis if treatment fails.

Neonatal conjunctivitis

Causes

Neonatal conjunctivitis can be caused by *Neisseria gonorrhoeae*, *Chlamydia*, *Staphylococcus aureus*, *Streptococcus pneumoniae* and *Haemophilus* spp. *N. gonorrhoeae* is the most important and often commonest cause—without appropriate treatment it can → blindness.

Diagnosis A red swollen sticky eye occurs 2–5d after delivery in gonococcal conjunctivitis and at 5–12d in chlamydial conjunctivitis.

Management

- Should cover both gonorrhoea and *Chlamydia*.
- *Treatment of gonococcal neonatal conjunctivitis:* ceftriaxone 50mg/kg (max 125mg) IM stat.
- *Treatment of chlamydial neonatal conjunctivitis:* erythromycin syrup 50mg/kg oral daily in 4 divided doses for 14d *or* trimethoprin 40mg with sulfamethoxazole 200mg oral bd for 14d.

Prevention

Neonatal gonococcal conjunctivitis can be prevented by washing carefully at the time of birth and applying 1% silver nitrate solution or 1% tetracycline ointment to eyes. Recommended for all babies born to mothers at high risk of gonorrhoea. Provides little protection from *Chlamydia*, which may also be present.

Syphilis

A worldwide disease caused by the spirochaete *Treponema pallidum*. The disease can be divided into four stages:

- Local 1° infection.
- Dissemination, associated with 2° syphilis.
- A latent period during which infectivity is low (relapses into 2° syphilis may occur during the 1st 4yrs after contact—early latent period).
- Late syphilis (> 2yrs duration), which occurs after many years with widespread gumma formation (granulomatous lesions with a necrotic centre and surrounding obliterative endarteritis) and long-term damage to the cardiovascular and CNS.

Transmission

Commonly through abraded skin at sites of sexual contact with infected persons. Other modes include congenital transmission (→ severe disease in the infant) and infection by blood transfusion.

Clinical features

1° syphilis

9–90d after infection a 1° genital ulcer or chancre forms. This is typically solitary, 'punched out', indurated, and painless, with a clear exudate. Atypical lesions occur and there may be multiple ulcers in HIV+ individuals. Lesions, which are highly infectious, resolve over a few weeks. There is painless regional lymphadenopathy.

2° syphilis

Coincides with the greatest number of treponemes in the body and blood, 1–6mths after contact. Specific features include:

- A transient, variable (but not vesicular) rash, particularly on trunk, soles, and palms. Not itchy.
- In warm, moist areas where two skin surfaces are in contact (e.g. perineum), papules enlarge and coalesce to form highly infectious plaques called condylamata lata.
- Silver-grey lesions with red periphery on mucosal surfaces called mucous patches (e.g. snail track ulcers in the mouth).

There is also:

- Low-grade fever.
- Malaise.
- Generalized lymphadenopathy.
- Arthralgia.
- Occasionally, focal involvement of eyes, meninges, parotid glands, or viscera (kidney, liver, GI tract).
- 2° syphilis symptoms generally resolve spontaneously <12mths.

Late syphilis

Areas of local gummatous tissue destruction in skin, bones, liver, and spleen are most common. Other cardiovascular and CNS manifestations include:

- Ascending aortic aneurysm +/– aortic regurgitation.

- Coronary artery stenosis.
- Chronic meningitis → cranial nerve damage, hemiparesis, seizures.
- CNS parenchymal disease (general paralysis of the insane, GPI)—psychoses, dementia, hyperactive reflexes, tremor, speech, and pupillary disturbances (Argyll–Robertson pupils).
- *Tabes dorsalis:* shooting pains in limbs, peripheral neuropathy, ataxia, Charcot's joints, +ve Romberg's sign.

Diagnosis of syphilis

- *Dark field microscopy:* of ulcer exudate for motile spirochaetes.
- *PCR and fluorescence staining of exudates:* increasingly available, which may be more appropriate for oral/GI specimens because of potential confusion with commensal spirochaetes on dark field microscopy.
- *Serology:* either treponeme-specific (fluorescent *Treponema* antibody (FTA), *Treponema pallidum* haemagglutination assay (TPHA)) for exposure, or non-specific (VDRL, rapid plasma regain (RPR)) for active disease and screening. An enzyme immunoassay (EIA) to detect anti-treponemal IgG and IgM is also available: IgM usually detectable towards the end of 2nd week, and IgG in 4–5th week of 1° infection.
- *CSF examination:* should be performed in any patient with neurological symptoms or signs. It remains controversial as to when asymptomatic patients need CSF examination. Recommendations include late latent (> 2yrs) syphilis with an RPR > 32, HIV+ individuals with latent syphilis and patients with inadequate serological response to treatment. CNS can be involved in any stage of syphilis.
- *HIV testing:* should be offered to all patients with syphilis since dual infection is common, and affects assessment and management.

Management

Early syphilis (stages 1 and 2 or latent syphilis of <2 y duration)

- Either benzathine benzylpenicillin 2.4 million units IM stat (usually given as two injections into separate sites because of the large volume).
- *Or* procaine benzylpenicillin 600 000 units IM od for 10d.

For penicillin-allergic patients alternatives include:

- Either tetracycline 500mg oral qds for 14d.
- Or doxycycline 100mg oral bd for 14d.
- Or erythromycin 500mg oral qds for 14d for penicillin allergic *pregnant* patients.

Patients should be followed-up at 3, 6, and 12mths to assess treatment and possible reinfection.

Late syphilis (not neurosyphilis; includes latent syphilis of >2 y or indeterminate duration)

- Either benzathine benzylpenicillin 2.4 million units IM (given as two injections into separate sites) once weekly for 3wks.
- Or procaine benzylpenicillin 600 000 units IM od for 17d.

For penicillin-allergic patients, alternatives include the following (however penicillin is preferred therapy and should be given whenever possible):

- Either tetracycline 500mg oral qds (probably better) for 30d.
- Or doxycycline 100mg oral bd, for 30d.
- Or erythromycin 500mg oral qds for 30d.

Neurosyphilis

- Either aqueous benzylpenicillin 2–4 million units IV every 4h for 14d.
- Or procaine benzylpenicillin 1.8–2.4 million units IM od plus probenecid 500mg oral qds for 17d: ensure patient compliance with this outpatient regimen.

For penicillin-allergic patients, alternatives include:

- Either tetracycline 500mg oral qds for 30d.
- Or doxycycline 200mg oral bd for 28d.

Consult a neurologist if possible and follow-up carefully.

Management of syphilis in pregnancy

Pregnant women with syphilis should be treated with penicillin whenever possible. Pregnant women who are allergic to penicillin, but whose allergy is not manifested by anaphylaxis, may be given ceftriaxone 1g od for 10d. Alternatives include erythromycin 500mg oral qds for 14d (early syphilis) or 30d (other forms of syphilis). *Note:* effectiveness of erythromycin is highly questionable, particularly for neurosyphilis, and many failures have been reported. Tetracyclines are contraindicated in pregnancy. The baby should be evaluated and treated soon after birth.

Congenital syphilis

Transplacental infection may occur during any stage of syphilis, but is most likely during the early stages (and if untreated results in premature delivery or perinatal death in 40–50% of infections). Untreated late maternal infection ↑ perinatal mortality by 10 and 10% of children will be born with congenital syphilis.

Neonatal features of congenital syphilis include rhinitis, a diffuse maculopapular, desquamative rash involving palms and soles (may be vesicular/bullous), hepatosplenomegaly, lymphadenopathy, generalized osteochondritis/periostitis, CNS involvement, anaemia, jaundice, and thrombocytopenia, although any organ may be affected and some newborns are asymptomatic. Death may occur, e.g. due to pneumonia, liver failure, pulmonary haemorrhage, or hypopituitarism.

In those children who survive the neonatal period, infection normally becomes latent, but there may be characteristic chronic signs and sequelae involving the bones (frontal bossing, saddle nose, protruding mandible, short maxilla, saber tibia), joints (recurrent arthropathy and effusions), teeth (peg-shaped upper incisors—'Hutchinson's teeth'), eyes (interstitial keratitis), and neurological system (neurosyphilis, deafness).

Diagnosis

Diagnosis is often clinical, supported by routine bloods, X-rays (look for raised periosteum on plain X-rays of the long bones), VDRL/RPR on blood and CSF, +/– specific serology and/or PCR if available. Test the mother. Treatment is cheap and safe, so all children born to infected mothers should be treated empirically, even if mother received treatment during pregnancy.

Management

Early congenital syphilis (≤2yrs) and infants with abnormal CSF:

- Either aqueous benzylpenicillin 100 000–150 000U/kg/d administered as 50 000U/kg IV bd for the first 7d of life and then tds for a total of 10d.
- Or procaine benzylpenicillin, 50 000U/kg IM od for 10d.

Congenital syphilis of ≥2yrs;

- Aqueous benzylpenicillin, 200 000–300 000IU/kg/day, administered as 50 000IU/kg IV/IM every 4–6h for 10–14d.

Penicillin allergic patients:

Penicillin is the treatment of choice in infants with congenital syphilis and alternatives should only be considered if there is a significant allergy to this antibiotic. An alternative (after the first month of life) is:

- Erythromycin 7.5–12.5mg/kg oral qds for 30d.

Gonorrhoea

Gonorrhoea results from infection with the Gram –ve diplococcus *Neisseria gonorrhoeae*. 1° infection through sexual contact usually involves the mucosal surfaces of the urethra, cervix, rectum, and oropharynx (see Colour plate 31).

Without early effective treatment, both local and disseminated complications occur. Recent decades have seen the rise in strains resistant to penicillin, tetracycline, doxycycline, and other antibiotics. Conjunctival infection of neonates during vaginal delivery may cause blindness if not treated early.

Clinical features

In *men*, urethral discharge and dysuria occur 2–5d after infection. Discharge is initially mucoid, but becomes profuse and purulent (in contrast to non-gonococcal urethritis). Local complications include acute epididymitis, prostatitis, peri-urethral abscess, and urethral stricture.

In *women*, infection produces signs of cervicitis (+/– urethritis) after ~10d with vaginal discharge, dysuria, intermenstrual bleeding or post-coital bleeding. However, unlike men, many women are asymptomatic. Local complications include PID and peri-hepatitis. Frequency and urgency are uncommon symptoms in both men and women.

Haematogenous dissemination is a rare complication in untreated patients, which may → meningitis, endocarditis, osteomyelitis, sepsis, or acute destructive monoarthritis. Reactive polyarthropathy and papular/pustular dermatitis are recognized complications.

Diagnosis

Gram –ve intracellular diplococci in smears from the urethra in men (>90%) and endocervix in women (less reliable); culture. In some settings, PCR testing for gonorrhoea is available. This may be more sensitive but in low prevalence populations the +ve predictive value of a test may be correspondingly low.

Management

Resistance to penicillin, tetracyclines, and fluoroquinolones is ↑ worldwide. In addition ↓ sensitivity to ceftriaxone has been reported. Many national guidelines now recommend dual therapy for treatment of gonorrhoea to ↓ the ability of the gonococcus to become resistant to ceftriaxone (widely used therapy). Local patterns of resistance must be considered when treating gonorrhoea and test of cure should be performed 1wk after treatment (especially important for asymptomatic infections). See Box 16.2 for recommended regimens. Unless facilities available to exclude chlamydial infection, patients should also be treated for *Chlamydia*, since they are often co-infected. Treat sexual partners at the same time.

Box 16.2 Recommended regimes for gonorrhoea

In uncomplicated genital and anal infection

Ceftriaxone 500mg IM stat plus 1g azithromycin oral stat.

Other regimens depend on local resistance patterns. Always use the locally recommended regimen.

Options include:

- Azithromycin 2g oral single dose ***or***
- Spectinomycin 2g IM single dose.
- Ciprofloxacin 500mg oral stat (not during pregnancy) only recommended now if susceptibilities known before treatment–widespread resistance is documented, especially in Asia.

In disseminated infection

- Ceftriaxone 1g IV/IM od for 7d ***or***
- Spectinomycin 2g IM bd for 7d.
- Treatment can be oral after 48h if response is good, e.g. cefixime 400mg bd oral, or ciprofloxacin 500mg bd oral.
- Extend treatment to 14d in meningitis, and 28d in endocarditis.

Gonococcal conjunctivitis in adults is highly contagious. Manage with barrier nursing, frequent saline irrigation and antibiotics: ceftriaxone 1g IM single dose (or ceftriaxone 500mg od IM for 3d) plus 1g azithromycin oral stat.

If penicillin allergy:

- Azithromycin 2g oral stat, plus doxycycline 100mg bd oral for 1wk, plus ciprofloxacin 250mg od oral for 3d.
- Spectinomycin 2g IM od for 3d.

Neonatal gonococcal conjunctivitis (📖 Conjunctivitis p. 22, 📖 Neonatal conjunctivitis, p. 665)

- Ceftriaxone 50mg/kg (max 125mg) IM stat.
- Neonatal patients should be reviewed at 48h.

Chlamydial infections

Chlamydia trachomatis is an obligate intracellular bacterium. *Chlamydia* serovars D-K are the most common STI in resource-rich regions. They occur worldwide, frequently co-exist with gonorrhoea, and are the most common cause of non-gonococcal urethritis (NGU) in men. These serovars cause infection of the urethra, endocervix, or rectum, and may → upper genital tract infection in women and cause epididymo-orchitis in men. Less commonly these serovars cause conjunctivitis, arthritis and perihepatitis.

Other serovars include:

- Serovars L1–L3, which cause lymphogranuloma venereum.
- Serovars A–C, which are not sexually transmitted, but are an important cause of blindness worldwide due to trachoma (see 🕮 Trachoma, p. 582).

Uncomplicated urethritis/endocervicitis/proctitis

Clinical features Infections in women are often subclinical or asymptomatic.

Diagnosis

Screening asymptomatic women at risk of infection should ↓ complications. Diagnostic tests that detect *Chlamydia* DNA in urine (= do not require cervical or urethral swabs) are widely available and reliable for diagnosis of asymptomatic individuals. These tests have now replaced culture and other testing techniques in many parts of the world, especially for screening purposes.

Management

Single dose treatment (directly observed where possible) for uncomplicated genito-urinary infection (azithromycin 1g) is the preferred option in most situations. This eliminates need for a test of cure as compliance is not an issue; effectiveness is excellent with cure rates ~90%, and resistance is not documented.

Complicated chlamydial infections

Clinical features Complications in men include epididymitis and epididymo-orchitis and (in MSM) chronic proctitis. Infections in women may → cervicitis, salpingitis, and endometritis. They are a major cause of female infertility worldwide.

Management Standard treatment is doxycycline 100mg oral bd for 2wks +/– azithromycin 1g oral stat (see under syndromic management).

Lymphogranuloma venereum

LGV is a chronic STI caused by the L1, 2, and 3 serovars. Although LGV has long been endemic in many parts of the world a recent epidemic has been seen amongst MSM in Europe and other resource-rich countries. Most of these men have also been infected with HIV.

Clinical features

1° lesion is a painless genital ulcer (rarely visible in women) that heals in a few days. After a latent period (days to months), acute, fluctuant inguinal lymphadenopathy (buboes) develop. Buboes may spread locally and ulcerate → sinuses/fistulae. Chronic blockage of lymphatic drainage → genital lymphoedema, often quite severe in women.

Diagnosis

This is by enzyme-linked immunosorbant assay, DNA probe, direct fluorescent antibody test or culture of bubo aspirate. Complement fixation testing is helpful if there is a ≥4-fold rise in titre or a single titre of >1:64; a –ve antibody test rules out the diagnosis. Specific serovars responsible for LGV can be identified in some laboratories which may help with diagnosis.

Management

Doxycycline, erythromycin or tetracycline for 2wks, see Box 16.3. In LGV fluctuant lymph nodes should be aspirated through healthy skin. Incision and drainage or excision of nodes will delay healing and is contraindicated (late sequelae such as stricture/fistula, however, may require surgical intervention). Partner notification and treatment for all sexually transmitted infections is important.

Box 16.3 Antibiotic regimens for chlamydial infection

Uncomplicated anogenital infection

- Doxycycline 100mg oral bd for 7d **or**
- Azithromycin 1g oral stat.
- *Alternatives:* amoxicillin 500mg oral tds for 7d, **or** erythromycin 500mg oral qds for 7d, **or** ofloxacin 300mg oral bd for 7d, **or** tetracycline 500mg oral qds for 7d.

Uncomplicated anogenital infection during pregnancy Erythromycin (base/ethylsuccinate) 500mg oral qds for 7d **or** amoxicillin 500mg oral tds for 7d.

LGV

- Doxycycline 100mg oral bd for 14d **or**
- Erythromycin 500mg oral qds for 14d.
- *Alternative:* tetracycline 500mg oral qds for 14d).

Neonatal chlamydial conjunctivitis

- Erythromycin syrup 50mg/kg per day in 4 divided doses for 14d.
- *Alternative:* co-trimoxazole 240mg oral bd for 14d.

Chancroid

An acute STI caused by *Haemophilus ducreyi* characterized by painful necrotizing ulceration and painful bubo formation; highly infectious and a common cause of genital ulcers in Africa and Southeast Asia. Chancroid is much more common in males, suggesting a female carrier state.

Clinical features

- 3–7d post-infection, painful papules form, which rapidly develop into soft ulcers with undermined, ragged edges.
- Ulcers are haemorrhagic and sticky (often secondarily infected); if multiple they may become confluent; they occur at sites of trauma during intercourse (extra-genital ulcers are rare).
- 7–14d later inguinal nodes may become involved: painful, matted, and tethered to erythematous skin → bubo. A discharging sinus may develop, in time becoming a spreading ulcer. Lesions heal slowly and commonly relapse.

Diagnosis

- Clean ulcer with saline, then remove material from the undermined edge; or aspirate pus from bubo.
- *Gram stain smear: H. ducreyi* are Gram –ve rods (fine, short, round-ended) sometimes seen in 'shoal-of-fish' or 'railroad track' formation.
- *Culture is difficult:* PCR, immunofluorescence and serology may be available for diagnosis in some laboratories.
- *Without treatment:* infectivity may continue for several months, but with appropriate antibiotic therapy (see Box 16.3) lesions often heal in 1–2wks. As with all STIs, intercourse should be avoided until lesions have completely healed.

Management

- Erythromycin 500mg oral qds for 7d.
- *Alternatives:* ciprofloxacin 500mg oral bd for 3d, ***or*** azithromycin 1g oral stat, ***or*** ceftriaxone 250mg IM stat).

Single dose treatments have higher failure rates than longer courses of antibiotics, so erythromycin is treatment of choice. With HIV co-infection treatment is less effective. Co-infection syphilis and HSV may occur.

Granuloma inguinale (donovanosis)

Calymmatobacterium granulomatis causes chronic, destructive ulceration of genitals and surrounding tissues. Males are more frequently infected than females. It is not easily transmitted; patients' sexual partners are often uninfected.

Clinical features

- 1–6wks following infection a painless indurated papule forms, which slowly develops into a 'beefy' granulomatous ulcer with characteristic rolled edges. Lesion is elevated, well defined, and bleeds easily with trauma.
- Usual sites are anogenital region, thighs, and perineum; rarely vaginal (or rectal) lesions may present with PV (or PR) bleeding. Healing is uncommon without treatment; 2° infection can follow → painful, destructive lesions, and may → SCC.
- Inguinal nodes are not involved unless there is 2° infection.
- Sc granulomas form, which may be mistaken for enlarged lymph nodes (hence, the name 'pseudo-bubo'). They may also become an abscess, discharging via a sinus, or an infected ulcer.
- Lymphoedematous enlargement of genitalia may occur during healing.

Diagnosis

- Crush a piece of granulation tissue from the active edge of the lesion between 2 slides, air dry, and stain with Giemsa or Gram stains.
- Look for large mononuclear cells filled with Donovan bodies (intracytoplasmic Gram –ve rods that look like closed safety pins due to bipolar staining).
- Culture is difficult; PCR and serology are available in some facilities.

Management

Treatment should be for at least 3wks or until all the lesions have epithelialized.

- Azithromycin 1g oral stat then 500mg od.
- Doxycycline 100mg oral bd.
- *Alternatives:* erythromycin 500mg oral qds, ***or*** tetracycline 500mg oral qds, ***or*** co-trimoxazole 960mg oral bd.

Trichomoniasis

Clinical features

~50% of women with *Trichomonas vaginalis* infection are asymptomatic. Infection in men usually asymptomatic, but may cause symptoms of urethritis. Vaginitis due to *Trichomonas vaginalis* can produce an irritating, pruritic (rarely foul smelling) discharge 5–28d post-infection, +/– dyspareunia. Urethral infection may cause dysuria. The vaginal discharge is often copious, sometimes yellow or green, and pools in the posterior fornix. The vagina and cervix become inflamed; colposcopic examination reveals cervical haemorrhages in ~50% of symptomatic cases—'strawberry cervix' (this can also be seen by the naked eye during speculum examination in ~5% of women with trichomoniasis).

Diagnosis

In women this is by wet preparation microscopy of vaginal discharge for motile *Trichomonas vaginalis* (sensitivity 40–80%). Culture of vaginal discharge has a sensitivity of ~80%. Cervical smears often identify *Trichomonas*, but this is not a reliable method of diagnosis as there is a significant risk of both false –ves and false +ves.

Diagnosis in men is not easy. *Trichomonas* can produce urethritis in men, but urethral swabs, urethral smears, and first catch urine specimen are not sensitive in making a diagnosis. Often *Trichomonas* infection in men is only suspected and treated once other causes of urethritis have been excluded.

In some settings, PCR for trichomonas is available and sensitivity by PCR > culture.

Management of trichomoniasis

- Metronidazole 400–500mg oral bd for 7d.
- *Alternatives:* efficacy less certain; metronidazole 2g oral stat or tinidazole 2g oral stat.
- All sexual partners should be notified and treated.
- Patients should return after 7d if symptoms persist. Failure can be due to resistance or reinfection. Patients often respond well to retreatment with the 7-d regimen.
- Refractory infections should be treated with metronidazole 2g oral od plus 500mg applied intravaginally each night for 3–7d.

Pregnancy

Treatment with metronidazole in all trimesters of pregnancy is appropriate, but avoid higher stat doses. Trichomonas in pregnancy can be treated with 5–7d course of metronidazole 400–500mg oral bd. There is evidence that trichomonas can be harmful in pregnancy, but there are no recommendations to screen for trichomonas in asymptomatic pregnant women as case detection and treatment has not been shown to improve outcomes.

Bacterial vaginosis

Bacterial vaginosis (BV) is a common cause of vaginal discharge (Colour plate 32).

Characterized by:

- ↓ In hydrogen peroxide-producing lactobacilli.
- ↑ In other bacteria in greater amounts than normally present in the vagina and include *Gardnerella vaginalis*, *Mycoplasma hominis*, *Bacteroides*, *Mobiluncus*, peptostreptococci, and a newly-identified bacterium *Atopobium vaginae*.

Clinical features

Most women complain of an offensive whitish discharge that tends to recur and may often seem worse after intercourse. There are usually no associated symptoms of vaginitis (itch or irritation). BV in non-pregnant women is associated with postpartum endometritis and surgical procedures, e.g. hysterectomy, termination of pregnancy. In pregnancy, it can be associated with chorioamnionitis and amniotic fluid infection, ↑ rates of miscarriage (all stages of pregnancy), premature rupture of membranes, low birth weight and preterm birth. BV increases susceptibility to and transmissibility of HIV.

Diagnosis

This is by microscopy and culture plays no part. Amsel's criteria for diagnosis suggest 3 of 4 of the following need to be present for diagnosis:

- White homogenous vaginal discharge.
- Vaginal pH >4.5.
- Clue cells (>20% vaginal epithelial cells stippled with bacteria).
- A fishy smell on addition of KOH to a sample of vaginal discharge.

Management

- Metronidazole 400mg oral bd for 7d. A single dose of metronidazole 2g is an alternative if adherence is likely to be poor.
- Clindamycin cream 2% intravaginally bd for 7d can be used as an alternative.
- Partners are not routinely treated as it is a polymicrobial condition and not technically an STI.

Women often suffer from recurrence; >50% of women will have a recurrence < 1yr. The trigger for ↓ in hydrogen peroxide-producing lactobacilli in the vagina is not understood. Optimal management of recurrent BV is unclear: 14d of metronidazole plus intravaginal clindamycin 2%, followed by monthly 2g doses of metronidazole may be of benefit. Pregnant women who are symptomatic should be treated. It is unclear whether treating asymptomatic pregnant women improves pregnancy outcomes.

Genital herpes

Most genital herpes (see Colour plate 34) is caused by HSV-2, although there are ↑ number of 1° HSV-1 genital herpes infections.

- Recurrent genital ulcers are due to reactivation of the latent virus from the dorsal root ganglia, and occur more frequently with HSV-2 than HSV-1 infection.
- Asymptomatic shedding is common and is an important cause of transmission: most infections are transmitted by people unaware they are infected.
- HSV ↑ likelihood of transmitting HIV and susceptibility to HIV.
- Persistence of HSV ulceration and frequent recurrences are common in HIV+ individuals, and acute episodes are often prolonged, atypical and severe.

Transmission Occurs by direct contact with infected genital secretions. After an incubation period of 2–7d, local infection and inflammation → multiple vesicular lesions that rapidly ulcerate.

Clinical features

The ulcers are greyish and extremely painful; they occur on the penis in men and the vagina, cervix, vulva, and perineum in women, often accompanied by a vaginal discharge. The ulcers may be present in the anus (usually in MSM). 1° infection is accompanied by fever, malaise, and inguinal lymphadenopathy; vulval oedema and urinary retention may occur. Extragenital involvement occurs in up to 20% of cases. Encephalitis is a recognized complication of genital herpes. Non-primary initial infection (e.g. HSV-2 infection with pre-existing antibodies to HSV-1) is often less severe.

Diagnosis of genital herpes

Swabs from the lesion can be tested by PCR (highly sensitive), culture, or direct immunofluorescence. Reliable Western blot type-specific serological tests are available and so serological testing may be useful, e.g. for discordant couples, as part of preconception counselling.

Management

- Analgesia and salt baths may help ↓ discomfort and pain associated with 1° infections.
- *In those with a first clinical episode (take a careful history):* aciclovir 200mg oral 5 × daily for 5d, or valaciclovir 1g oral bd for 5d ↓ formation of new lesions, duration of pain, time required for healing, and viral shedding, but probably not the rate of future recurrence. Treatment should be started as soon as possible.
- *Recurrences:* can be managed with either episodic treatment or suppressive treatment. Episodic treatment is aciclovir 200mg oral 5 × daily for 5d (*alternatives:* valaciclovir 500mg bd or famciclovir 125mg bd, for 5d). Patient-initiated high dose, short-course antivirals are also effective and safe: aciclovir 800mg tds for 2d, famciclovir 1g bd for 1d or valaciclovir 500mg bd for 3d. Treatment should be started as soon as early symptoms of recurrence are recognized, hence these regimens are given in advance to patients to treat themselves.
- *Suppressive treatment:* usually considered if >6 episodes/yr. Regimens include aciclovir 400mg bd, famciclovir 250mg bd, or valaciclovir 500mg od. These regimens should ↓ recurrences by ~80%. If patients suffer from >10 episodes/yr valaciclovir 1g od is often used. Recurrences become less common with ↑ duration, so try stopping antivirals after 1yr so that recurrence rates can be reassessed. Minimum continuous dose that will suppress recurrence should be determined empirically.
- *Decreasing transmission:* Condoms can ↓ transmission; long-term suppressive treatment with valaciclovir also appears to ↓ transmission. Lubrication with water-based lubricants is also advisable as trauma to the genitals can → recurrence.

Candida vaginitis

Candida vaginitis is not an STI. Occurs due to overgrowth of the commensal vaginal yeast, *Candida albicans* (and less commonly other *Candida* spp.). Antibiotic therapy, pregnancy, and immunosuppression all predispose to symptomatic candidiasis.

Clinical features

Commonly there is vulvitis, as well as vaginitis and intense vulval pruritus and erythema are characteristic. Discharge is thick, curd-like, and white (rarely it may only be scanty), and microscopy shows Gram +ve budding yeasts +/– hyphae; visualization of the yeasts is made easier by the addition of 10% KOH to clear the epithelial cells.

Recurrent vulvo-vaginal candidiasis is defined as >4 episodes of microbiologically proven *Candida* infection in a 12mths period; affects 5–8% of women in their reproductive life. The majority of women have no demonstrable risk factors and it may be due to a cell-mediated immunodeficiency at the vaginal mucosal level.

Men can suffer from candida balano-prostitis, but this is not as a result of transmission between partners, and treatment of partners is not generally helpful unless the male partner is symptomatic.

Management

- Miconazole or clotrimazole 200mg intravaginally od for 3d ***or***
- Clotrimazole 500mg intravaginally stat ***or***
- Fluconazole 150mg oral stat.
- *Alternative:* nystatin 100 000IU intravaginally od for 14d, will treat all species of *Candida*.
- Women with recurrent vulvo-vaginal candidiasis can be treated with a 2-wk induction course of clotrimazole followed by weekly maintenance treatment with clotrimazole 500mg as a pessary for 3–6mths. Alternatively fluconazole 150mg oral can be given every 72h for 3 doses, then maintenance dose of 150mg oral once every week for up to 6mths.

Occasionally candida vaginitis may be caused by a strain of *Candida albicans* resistant to routine treatment, or to less common *Candida* spp., such as *C. glabrata* or *C. krusei*. Standard treatments should initially be used as *Candida glabrata* may, e.g. be present as a commensal and not responsible for symptoms. Symptoms may be due to other *Candida* spp. or even genital pain syndromes. Nystatin 100 000IU intravaginally od for 14d is effective against all species of *Candida*. Extended and higher dose 1st line treatments should also be considered for persistent symptoms, as well as boric acid pessaries, used intravaginally for 14d (if available). These are highly toxic, especially if taken orally, but can also be absorbed from skin and mucous membranes causing toxicity, and this should be discussed with patients.

Human papillomavirus and genital warts

Epidemiology

Genital warts are caused by infection with human papilloma virus (HPV) transmitted by skin to skin contact (see Colour plate 33). There are >100 serotypes of HPV, of which 35 preferentially infect the anogenital area. Serotypes 6 and 11 are typically responsible for warts and rarely insert themselves into the host genome. Infection with these types has no malignant potential.

Oncogenic types (16, 18, 31, 33, 35 and 45) may integrate with the host genome and can eventually → cervical squamous cell carcinoma if infection is persistent and other cofactors are also present. These oncogenic types do not cause genital warts.

Genital wart virus infection is common and prevalence rates amongst sexually-active populations may be as high as 50%. Many HPV infections are subclinical, with evidence of infection histologically or on colposcopy. HPV typing on clinical specimens is available in some countries.

Management of genital warts

Genital warts are a cosmetic problem and, although natural history is for them to resolve spontaneously, treatment is often requested. Treatment options include the following (application of topical treatments can often be done by patient themselves):

- Cryotherapy with liquid nitrogen.
- Surgical excision.
- Laser treatment.
- Podophyllotoxin cream (0.5%) or liquid (an anti-mitotic) can be applied to accessible warts bd in cycles of 3d/wk for max 4wks. Local irritation is a common side effect.
- Imiquimod 5% cream is a topical treatment that induces production of local cytokines and is associated with ↓ recurrence rate compared with other treatments. It should be applied ×1 daily, 3 × per week max 16wks.
- Cervical warts are best treated by cryotherapy after colposcopic examination. Warts can be resistant to treatment and cause problematic recurrences in pregnancy and in HIV+ individuals.
- Infection with oncogenic type HPV → squamous intraepithelial lesions is best identified, treated and followed up by colposcopy and regular cervical smears.

Prevention

Vaccines against HPV serotypes 16 and 18 (two of the commonest causes of cervical squamous cell carcinoma) have excellent efficacy in preventing the 'pre-cancerous' stage cervical intraepithelial neoplasia. One of the vaccines also targets serotypes 6 and 11 (together responsible for most genital warts) (📖 Immunization, p. 893).

Human papillomavirus and genital warts

Chapter 17
Nutrition

Invited author **James A. Berkley**

Malnutrition, health and survival

Why does malnutrition occur?

- Poverty, infant feeding practices, food insecurity, infections, chronic intestinal inflammation, and lack of care are the main direct causes.
- Underlying factors include global food prices, trade tariffs, ↓ political commitment, political instability, civil unrest, disasters, climate, geography, agricultural factors (e.g. soil characteristics, and factors affecting animal husbandry).
- Seasonal availability of cereals, fruit, or vegetables affect dietary intake.
- Cultural preferences include gender inequality, early weaning, lack of exclusive breastfeeding, ↓ birth intervals, and large family size.
- ↓ Breastfeeding because of fears of HIV transmission contribute to malnutrition.
- Inadequate care by sick parents, and orphanhood.
- Certain cereals may limit bioavailability of micronutrients.
- Infection ↓ appetite, intake and absorption, ↑ nutrient requirements, and ↑ urinary and intestinal losses.
- This results in a vicious cycle of infection and malnutrition. Infections → malnutrition, especially persistent diarrhoea, pertussis, measles, intestinal parasites, TB, and HIV/AIDS.

Effects of malnutrition on health and survival

- Immunity: malnutrition kills by ↑ susceptibility to infections. Malnutrition contributes to ~45% deaths among children by ↓ barrier functions of skin, gut and respiratory mucosa, ↓ systemic immunity, and slowing tissue repair after infection. Vitamin A and Zn deficiency are important.
- Growth and development: dietary and genetic factors affect growth. Better diet before the age of 2yrs → lifelong improvements.
- Organ function: severe malnutrition → profound physiological and metabolic disturbances, with failure of normal homeostatic mechanisms (📖 Measuring nutritional status, p. 686). Nutritional deficiencies affect the eye (vitamin A), thyroid gland (iodine), brain (Fe, essential fatty acids), respiratory and intestinal epithelia (vitamin A and Zn), and ovaries (anorexia).
- Pregnancy outcomes: maternal malnutrition affects maternal health, intrauterine development, ↓ birth weight, lactation, and infant/child health.
- Foetal programming: intrauterine malnutrition, ↑ risk of cardiovascular diseases, hypertension, diabetes, and stroke in adulthood.

What are the main aspects of treatment?

- Immediately treat life-threatening complications.
- Re-establish physiology and metabolism (stabilization).
- Treat infections.
- Promote growth and repair.

Malnutrition with medical complications should be treated in a hospital or inpatient feeding centre. Uncomplicated moderate acute malnutrition (MAM) or severe acute malnutrition (SAM) may be treated in an outpatient or community setting with ready to use therapeutic food (RUTF).

See Box 17.1 for a summary. Also see http://www.thelancet.com/series/maternal-and-child-nutrition and http://www.cmamforum.org

Box 17.1 Key points in malnutrition

- Most cases of severe malnutrition occur in children <5yrs. In older children or adults, suspect an underlying infection (e.g. HIV, TB) or malignancy.
- Complicated SAM has a high mortality because immunity, metabolism and physiology are dysfunctional, → ↓ appetite, malabsorption, and failure of homeostasis.
- Children and adults with kwashiorkor have severe physiological disturbances and high mortality.
- Assessment and management requires the same rigour of management as severe microbial or metabolic illness. These often co-exist.
- Infections may not demonstrate the usual clinical signs. Children may develop overwhelming sepsis quite suddenly after apparently making progress.
- Medical treatment differs from that for non-malnourished individuals.
- Initially, in complicated SAM, cautious feeding aims to re-start metabolic processes and improve absorption by carefully replacing energy and micronutrients without overloading a fragile system.
- RUTF enables effective management of uncomplicated SAM in the community.
- Children and adults with MAM are also at ↑ risk of death in community and in hospital.
- Modern programmes integrate management of SAM and MAM.
- The HIV epidemic has had a profound impact on presentation and outcomes of malnutrition.
- After rehabilitation has started, children and adults may return to homes with continuing poor diet and a high burden of exposure to infections before fully recovering immunity.
- Poverty and social exclusion are often underlying factors. Your patient may not be able to afford fare to come for follow-up or buy drugs that have been prescribed.
- Role of health professionals in advocacy for prevention of malnutrition is vital.
- Obesity is also an increasing problem in resource-poor countries. Over- and under-nutrition may co-exist in the same household.

Measuring nutritional status

Anthropometry (body measurement) quantifies malnutrition according to international standards. In children, measurement of mid-upper arm circumference (MUAC) is increasingly used, and the most simple to undertake (see Fig. 17.1). Weight and height measurements are more traditional, but require more equipment. They can be useful to detect wasting and stunting (see Tables 17.1 and 17.2), as well as for individual monitoring over time, e.g. growth velocity.

Weight and height

- *Weight for height (W/H):* weight relative to standard weight for a child of the same height. W/H indicates acute malnutrition. <2yrs, measure length (lying), rather than height (W/L). Low W/H = *wasting*, and indicates acute malnutrition.
- *Height for age (H/A):* height relative to the standard height for a child of the same age. Low H/A = *stunting* and indicates chronic malnutrition. Wasting and stunting may occur together.
- *Weight for age (W/A):* weight relative to the standard weight for a child of the same age. Low W/A = *underweight*. W/A does not distinguish acute from chronic malnutrition since a tall thin child may be the same weight as a short fat child of the same age. W/A is thus not used for diagnosis of acute malnutrition, but plotted over time, W/A is a useful marker of progress (see Fig. 17.2).

W/A, H/A, and W/H are expressed as *Z* scores, e.g. if weight is 2SD below mean weight of normal children of same age, *Z* score is –2 (📖 Table 17.1, p. 688); or it can be expressed as centiles.

Mid upper arm circumference

MUAC is measured using a tape or marked plastic strip around the left upper arm. Between ages 6mths–5yrs MUAC increases slowly, so simple cut-off values may be used for nutritional assessment. MUAC <115mm is equivalent to a W/H *Z* score of –3 (i.e. SAM). MUAC <125mm is equivalent to a W/H *Z* score of –2 (i.e. MAM). MUAC is much quicker and easier than calculating W/H, especially in sick patients. MUAC is a good predictor of mortality. There is no need to use both MUAC and W/H.

Body mass index (BMI)

BMI assesses under-nutrition or obesity among non-pregnant adults. Normal values vary with age in childhood and BMI is affected by individual variation in build and muscle bulk, so should be interpreted with this in mind. BMI = weight/(height)^2.

'Visible severe wasting' (VSW)

VSW = muscle wasting in buttocks, loss of sc fat, or prominence of bones, e.g. ribs/spine/pelvis. VSW is very insensitive, identifying mostly very severe cases of SAM. It is better to use MUAC.

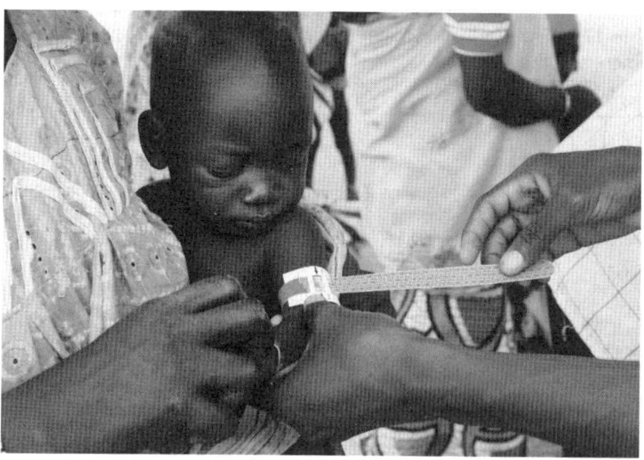

Fig. 17.1 Measuring MUAC of a young child in Niger. The tape has three colours, red indicating severe acute malnutrition, yellow indicating moderate acute malnutrition and green indicating normal nutritional status.

Reproduced with permission of David di Lorenzo, Medecins Sans Frontieres—Switzerland.

Table 17.1 Thresholds for malnutrition in children, adults, pregnant women, and the elderly

Age group	Severe	Moderate	At risk
MUAC			
Infants <6mths	–		
Children 6mths–5yrs	<115mm	115–124mm	125–135mm
Children 5–18yrs	–		
Adults*	<160mm	160–185mm	–
Elderly*	<160mm	160–175mm	–
Pregnant/lactating women*	<185mm	185–210mm	210–230mm

*Decisions to admit may also be influenced by recent weight loss or chronic illness e.g. HIV.

Age group	Severe	Moderate	At risk
*W/H Z score***			
Infants <6mths	<–3	–3 to –2	–2 to –1
Children 6mths–5yrs	<–3	–3 to –2	–2 to –1
Children 5–18yrs	<–3	–3 to –2	–2 to –1
Adults	–		
Elderly	-		
Pregnant/lact. women	-		

**See WHO charts and tables at: http://www.who.int/childgrowth/standards/en/

Age group	Severe	Moderate	At risk
BMI			
Children 0–18yrs	Varies with age**		
Adults***	<16	16–17	17–18.5
Pregnant/lactating women	–		
Elderly	–		

*** In adults, BMI >25 is overweight and BMI >30 is obese.

Kwashiorkor	Kwashiorkor = severe malnutrition at any age

Reference growth standards and growth charts

Table 17.2 Example W/L reference tables for boys and girls 0–2yrs

Weight-for-length GIRLS Birth to 2 years (Z-scores)					**Weight-for-length BOYS Birth to 2 years (Z-scores)**				
cm	**−3 SD**	**−2 SD**	**−1 SD**	**Median**	**cm**	**−3 SD**	**−2 SD**	**−1 SD**	**Median**
60.0	4.5	4.9	5.4	5.9	60.0	4.7	5.1	5.5	6.0
60.5	4.6	5.0	5.5	6.0	60.5	4.8	5.2	5.6	6.1
61.0	4.7	5.1	5.6	6.1	61.0	4.9	5.3	5.8	6.3
61.5	4.8	5.2	5.7	6.3	61.5	5.0	5.4	5.9	6.4
62.0	4.9	5.3	5.8	6.4	62.0	5.1	5.6	6.0	6.5
62.5	5.0	5.4	5.9	6.5	62.5	5.2	5.7	6.1	6.7
63.0	5.1	5.5	6.0	6.6	63.0	5.3	5.8	6.2	6.8
63.5	5.2	5.6	6.2	6.7	63.5	5.4	5.9	6.4	6.9
64.0	5.3	5.7	6.3	6.9	64.0	5.5	6.0	6.5	7.0
64.5	5.4	5.8	6.4	7.0	64.5	5.6	6.1	6.6	7.1
65.0	5.5	5.9	6.5	7.1	65.0	5.7	6.2	6.7	7.3
65.5	5.5	6.0	6.6	7.2	65.5	5.8	6.3	6.8	7.4
66.0	5.6	6.1	6.7	7.3	66.0	5.9	6.4	6.9	7.5
66.5	5.7	6.2	6.8	7.4	66.5	6.0	6.5	7.0	7.6
67.0	5.8	6.3	6.9	7.5	67.0	6.1	6.6	7.1	7.7
67.5	5.9	6.4	7.0	7.6	67.5	6.2	6.7	7.2	7.9
68.0	6.0	6.5	7.1	7.7	68.0	6.3	6.8	7.3	8.0
68.5	6.1	6.6	7.2	7.9	68.5	6.4	6.9	7.5	8.1
69.0	6.1	6.7	7.3	8.0	69.0	6.5	7.0	7.6	8.2
69.5	6.2	6.8	7.4	8.1	69.5	6.6	7.1	7.7	8.3
70.0	6.3	6.9	7.5	8.2	70.0	6.6	7.2	7.8	8.4
70.5	6.4	6.9	7.6	8.3	70.5	6.7	7.3	7.9	8.5
71.0	6.5	7.0	7.7	8.4	71.0	6.8	7.4	8.0	8.6
71.5	6.5	7.1	7.7	8.5	71.5	6.9	7.5	8.1	8.8
72.0	6.6	7.2	7.8	8.6	72.0	7.0	7.6	8.2	8.9
72.5	6.7	7.3	7.9	8.7	72.5	7.1	7.6	8.3	9.0
73.0	6.8	7.4	8.0	8.8	73.0	7.2	7.7	8.4	9.1
73.5	6.9	7.4	8.1	8.9	73.5	7.2	7.8	8.5	9.2
74.0	6.9	7.5	8.2	9.0	74.0	7.3	7.9	8.6	9.3
74.5	7.0	7.6	8.3	9.1	74.5	7.4	8.0	8.7	9.4
75.0	7.1	7.7	8.4	9.1	75.0	7.5	8.1	8.8	9.5

Full tables are found at: http://www.who.int/childgrowth/standards/en/

Pathophysiological consequences of severe malnutrition

- *Energy:* ↓ energy intake, malabsorption, ↓ liver glycogen stores and gluconeogenesis → ↑ susceptibility to hypoglycaemia and hypothermia.
- *Gut:* achlorhydria, ↓ gut motility, bacterial overgrowth, villous atrophy, and gut enzyme deficiencies impair digestion and absorption.
- *Liver:* ↓ protein synthesis (e.g. albumin, transferrin) and ↓ detoxification. Abnormal metabolites of amino acids and drugs are produced. ↑ production of acute phase proteins (e.g. CRP, ferritin).
- *Renal function:* may ↓ with inability to excrete Na+ and phosphate.
- *Whole body Na+ ↑ and K+ ↓:* Na^+/K^+ ATPase pumps are impaired, electrolytes are not normally distributed across cell membranes.
- *Muscle wasting and diarrhoea:* → K^+, Zn^{2+}, Ca^{2+}, Mg^{2+}, Cu^{2+} deficiency.
- *Red cell mass ↓, liberating Fe:* unbound Fe, free radicals, and anti-oxidant deficiency → infections, inflammation, and cell membrane dysfunction.

Immunity

- Surface and mucosal barriers are impaired → pathogen/antigen entry.
- Skin excoriation → local sepsis and septicaemia.
- Gut inflammation and damage → bacterial translocation (bacteraemia).
- *Cellular immunity:* thymic atrophy, ↓ cellular immunity, ↓ neutrophil function.
- *Humoral immunity:* SAM has little effect on antibody production following immunization. Secretory IgA is ↓.

Kwashiorkor (oedematous malnutrition)

- First described by Dr Cecily Williams in Ghana, in 1935, among children weaned from the breast onto a maize-based diet.
- Unclear why some children develop kwashiorkor and others not (see Box 17.2 for clinical features of kwashiorkor and marasmus).
- Dietary deficiencies of energy, protein, and micronutrients are common to both kwashiorkor and marasmus.
- Oedema of kwashiorkor improves on a low protein initial diet.
- Anti-oxidant deficiencies have been postulated as cause of kwashiorkor. However, multiple anti-oxidant supplements do not affect subsequent incidence of kwashiorkor.
- Kwashiorkor may be related to enteropathy.

Pathophysiology of micronutrient deficiencies

- ↓ Intake of micronutrients → depletion of body stores → specific clinical signs in severe cases: xerophthalmia (Vitamin A), pellagra (niacin), scurvy (Vitamin C), anaemia (iron/folate/Vitamin B12), rickets (Vitamin D/calcium), clotting abnormalities (Vitamin K) and goitre (iodine).
- ↓ Intake of protein, essential amino acids and minerals → ↓ growth rate or ↓ weight, usually without specific signs of deficiency.

Box 17.2 Comparisons of clinical features of marasmus and kwashiorkor

Clinical features of marasmus

- *Wasting:* low MUAC or W/H Z score.
- *Emaciated:* thin, flaccid skin ('little old man' appearance), grossly ↓ fat and muscle tissue; prominent spine, ribs, pelvis.
- *Behaviour:* alert and irritable.
- Distended abdomen due to weakened abdominal muscles and gas from small bowel bacterial overgrowth.

Clinical features of kwashiorkor

- Low or normal MUAC or W/H Z score.
- *Oedema:* bilateral pitting limb oedema; periorbital oedema. May be generalized.
- *Skin changes:* desquamation, often in the flexures and perineum.
- *Hair changes:* dry, thin hair which may become depigmented appearing brown, yellowy-red, or white.
- Hepatomegaly is common.
- *Behaviour:* miserable, lethargic, and apathetic with sad facies.

These may occur together: marasmic–kwashiorkor.

Clinical assessment of nutrition

History and physical examination

Look for complications, physiological dysfunction, infections, signs of specific nutrient deficiencies, underlying illness, feeding patterns and modifiable risk factors.

History

Concurrent illness/symptoms

- Current or recent illness (diarrhoea, malaria, lower respiratory tract infection (LRTI), etc.).
- Duration, frequency, and nature of vomiting or diarrhoea.
- Behaviour and activity changes (crying, irritable, apathy, anorexia).
- *Hydration:* recent sinking of eyes, time when urine was last passed.

Feeding history

- Food and fluids taken in past few days? Thirst? Appetite?
- *Breastfeeding history:* how long for? Mixed or exclusive BF? Is child breastfeeding now? Age of introduction of complementary feeds?
- Usual diet before current illness, lack of food in household or quality of food, recent change in diet.

Growth history

- Birth weight; prematurity; whether a twin.
- Review growth chart.

Other medical history

- HIV/AIDS status of child or mother.
- Development milestones reached (e.g. sitting unsupported 9mths, standing unsupported for 1–2s at 12mths).
- Immunization and Vitamin A doses up to date? (📖 Immunization, p. 893).

Family history

- Deaths of siblings or parent.
- Is the mother ill or malnourished?
- TB contact?

Physical examination

- General appearance, behaviour, mood (apathy, irritability), level of consciousness, facial appearance, signs of kwashiorkor/marasmus (see Fig 17.2).
- Fever or other signs of infection.
- Pallor.
- Enlarged or tender liver, jaundice; abdominal distension, tenderness.
- *Skin changes:* desquamation, oedema, rash (e.g. post measles), exfoliation, fungal infection, cancrum oris.
- Signs of cerebral palsy or congenital syndrome (e.g. Down's syndrome).
- Appetite test (see Box 17.3).

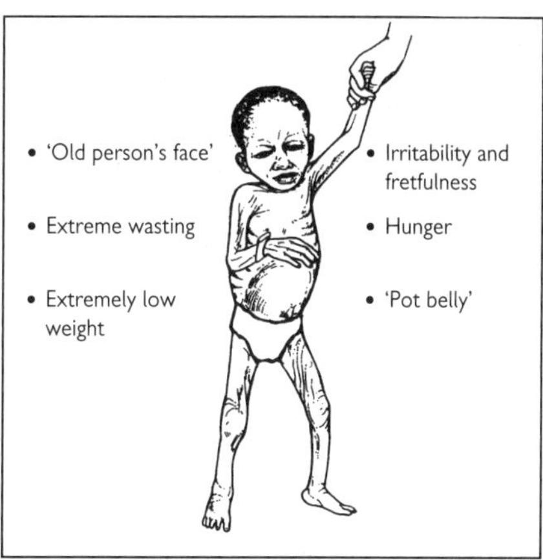

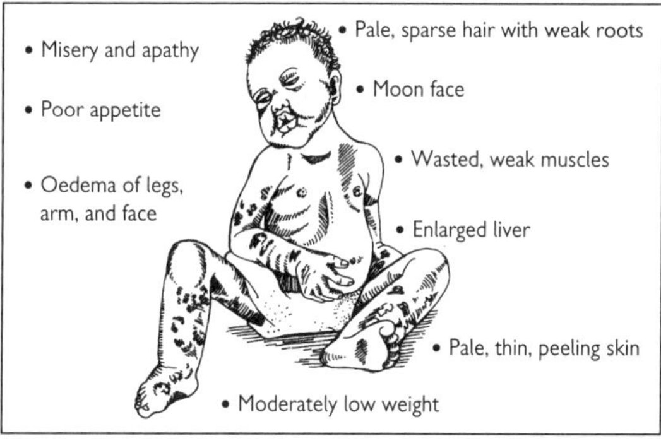

Fig. 17.2 Signs of marasmus (top) and kwashiorkor (bottom).

Complicated or uncomplicated malnutrition?

Complicated malnutrition indicates severe physiological or metabolic changes, or infection. The child must be treated as an in-patient until stabilized. Uncomplicated malnutrition may be treated in the community.

Children with uncomplicated malnutrition:

- Are alert with no respiratory distress, shock, hypoglycaemia, hypothermia, severe diarrhoea, dehydration, convulsions or severe oedema
- *And* have no other reason for admission to hospital (e.g. pneumonia)
- *And* pass an appetite test (see Box 17.3).

Children with *complicated malnutrition* fail one or more of these criteria.

Laboratory evaluation

The following can be used, but are rarely available. Some altered by inflammation:

- *Serum proteins:* e.g. albumin, transferrin.
- *Micronutrients:* e.g. Vitamin A, Zn, Vitamin B12, Vitamin D, Ca, folate, ferritin.
- *Red cell enzymes:* e.g. glutathione reductase.
- *Urinary micronutrients:* e.g. iodine.

Management plan

This depends on whether the child has complicated or uncomplicated malnutrition, and MAM or SAM. Use the algorithm in Fig. 17.3 to classify the malnutrition and decide on type of treatment.

Box 17.3 Appetite test

Appetite is a good marker of metabolic disturbance, and whether a malnourished child needs to be admitted.

- In a quiet area, explain to the mother/carer the purpose of the test.
- The caregiver washes her hands, with soap and water.
- The caregiver either offers the RUTF (see Box 17.1) from the packet, or puts a small amount on her finger and gives it to the child.
- If child refuses, caregiver continues to encourage child. Child must not be forced to take the RUTF.
- Child might refuse to eat the RUTF because of the strange environment—in this case the carer should take the child to a quiet place and gently encourage them.
- Offer plenty of water to drink from a cup while he/she is taking RUTF.
- The mother must be happy that child is eating RUTF and clinic worker should actually see child eat the RUTF.
- The child should be able to eat about a quarter of a 92-g sachet.
- Any child not eating RUTF has failed and should be admitted.

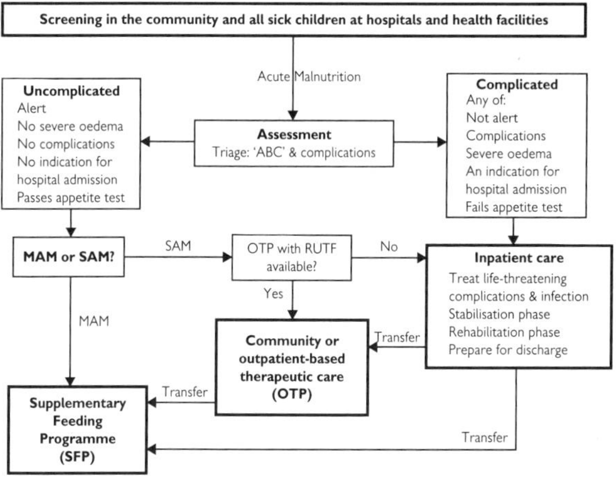

Fig. 17.3 Algorithm for categorization and management of children with malnutrition.

Medical management within inpatient therapeutic nutrition programmes

Manage life-threatening complications

See Chapter 1 on management of airway, breathing, circulation (ABC) and shock in severe acute malnutrition (📖 Emergency management of the sick child—ABC, p. 8). Infection, dehydration, hypothermia, hypoglycaemia, severe anaemia, and electrolyte abnormalities are common complications. See for management of hypoglycaemia 📖 Hypoglycaemia, p. 548. Other complications are discussed below.

Hypothermia

Defined as rectal temp <35.5°C, it is associated with infection and/or hypoglycaemia. It is a dangerous prognostic sign. Change wet nappies and bedding, ensure child does not get cold during washing. Provide blankets/lamps/heaters especially at night. Encourage 'kangaroo' technique: mother lies supine with child on her chest, covered by her clothes and blankets. Cover child's head with a cap to ↓ heat loss.

Severe anaemia Transfuse if Hb<4g/dL; or 4–6g/dL with respiratory distress. If not shocked, give 10mL/kg body weight of whole blood, slowly over 3h. If shocked, you should not be reading here yet – see 📖 Management of shock in children with severe acute malnutrition, p. 12.

Dehydration

❗ IV fluid resuscitation is controversial and may result in potentially dangerous under- or over-hydration. Use oral rehydration fluids designed for severely malnourished children (ReSoMal) unless there is established shock (📖 WHO defined shock, p. 7 and Management of shock in children with severe acute malnutrition, p. 12).

Dehydration may be difficult to assess as sunken eyes and ↓ skin turgor may be due to acute malnutrition. Assessment is best made on the basis of history or observed fluid losses. Use ReSoMal, rather than standard oral rehydration solution (📖 p. 738): give 5mL/kg orally/NG every 30min for the first 2h; aim to give 70–100mL/kg over 12h. ReSoMal can be given with F-75. Once rehydrated, continue F-75 and replace volumes lost in stool. Once rehydrated, continue F-75 and replace volumes lost in stool. Continue breastfeeding wherever possible. Reserve IV fluids for children in shock, or maintenance only in those not tolerating oral/NG fluids (with monitoring as described above). Useful signs of rehydration include return of tears, moist mouth, less sunken eyes and fontanelle, and improved skin turgor. Daily weight is a guide to changes in hydration status.

Infection

Bacterial sepsis

A common cause of death in severely malnourished children. Signs of infection may be absent, so give all children with complicated SAM broad-spectrum antibiotics:

- Ampicillin (50mg/kg 6-hourly IM/IV) plus gentamicin (7.5mg/kg IM/IV daily) or ceftriaxone (50mg/kg daily by IV injection over 2–4min) for 7d for complicated SAM.

- Metronidazole (7.5mg/kg 8-hourly for 7d) may be added if suspected protozoal (e.g. amoebiasis) or anaerobic infection.
- If receiving co-trimoxazole prophylaxis for HIV, this should continue.

Other infections

- Blood film/rapid diagnostic test for malaria on admission (📖 Malaria, p. 33).
- UTIs are common in malnourished children. Do a urine dipstick test and if possible, culture (📖 Urinary tract infection, p. 414).
- All severely malnourished children should have a DTC for HIV performed by the clinician at admission.
- After stabilization give a single dose of albendazole 400mg oral to children >24mths; (children 12–23mths, 200mg) to treat helminth infection.
- Screen for other infections as clinically indicated, consider if available chest X-ray; LP; blood cultures; consider TB.

Diarrhoea

Is common; may be due to infection, osmotic load of the food, lactose intolerance, or premature transfer to the next feeding phase. Cohort patients and wash hands to avoid spread.

- If severe diarrhoea, go back to F-75 or a non-milk-based feed. If possible, test stool for reducing substances (= lactose malabsorption; stool pH usually <5.5). Check volumes of feeds are correct—large boluses may → diarrhoea.
- Severely malnourished children with HIV may have *Cryptosporidium* or other intestinal parasites—do microscopy if possible.
- Treat dysentery with antibiotics according to local protocols.
- Diarrhoea can be due to systemic infection (e.g. sepsis).
- Zn is already included in therapeutic feeds, no extra Zn is required.

Tuberculosis

Severely malnourished children have ↑ TB risk, but clinical features are non-specific and microbiological diagnosis rarely possible. Consider TB in children who do not respond quickly to standard nutritional and medical treatment, and in those with a history of household TB contact (see 📖 Tuberculosis, p. 151). Cohort patients with TB to avoid nosocomial transmission. Investigations for TB include fine needle aspiration of cervical glands, sputum induction (nebulized hypertonic saline) or gastric washings (📖 Tuberculosis, p. 151).

Electrolyte abnormalities

Hyponatraemia may be present, but does not reflect a deficiency in total body Na^+; avoid giving too much Na^+. Hypokalaemia is common, especially with diarrhoea, and contributes to cardiac arrhythmias. Hypomagnesaemia may contribute to cardiac arrhythmias and muscle twitching. Phosphate levels are often low. K^+, Mg^{2+}, and other electrolytes are contained in therapeutic feeds. ReSoMal and recommended IV fluids contain less Na^+ and more K^+ than ORS and fluids used for well-nourished children.

Inpatient therapeutic nutrition programme

The principles are similar for all ages and for both marasmus and kwashiorkor. Combine therapeutic nutritional treatment with intensive medical care (see 📖 Medical management within inpatient therapeutic nutrition programmes, p. 696). Management of infants <6mths is covered on 📖 Severe malnutrition in infants <6 months old, p. 708. Nutritional treatment may be divided into stabilization, transition, and rehabilitation phases.

Stabilization phase

Establish low protein, fat and energy feeds (F-75) with just enough micronutrients to restart metabolic and physiological processes. This also allows oedema to begin to clear (Box 17.4).

- Give 130mL/kg F-75 daily, divided into 3-hourly feeds (see Table 17.3).
- Continue feeding at night to prevent hypoglycaemia.
- If unable to take sufficient feed orally, give via NGT. Offer each feed by mouth and give remainder via NGT. NGT may be removed when child takes most of daily diet orally.
- Weigh child each morning before feed; assess oedema daily.
- Monitor vital signs at least twice a day.
- Give folic acid 5mg on admission.
- Sufficient vitamin A is contained in the recommended therapeutic feeds and unless there are signs of deficiency or measles, additional vitamin A is not required.
- If signs of vitamin A deficiency or measles, (see 📖 Vitamin A deficiency, p. 714), give on days 1, 2, and 14.
- All other micronutrients are contained in *commercial* F-75.
- Iron should not be given in the stabilization phase as it is pro-inflammatory, pro-oxidant and can promote infection (e.g. *Salmonella*).

Transition phase

Once appetite returns, oedema starts to clear and medical complications are treated (usually after ~3–7d), child may enter transition phase in which dietary intake ↑ under close monitoring. Problems can occur with ↑ dietary Na^+, fluid, osmolality, and amino acids. Key components of transition phase:

- Switch to same amount of F-100 therapeutic milk.
- Continue to feed regularly (e.g. 8 feeds in 24h).
- Gradually ↑ successive feeds by 10mL until refusal.
- Monitor vital signs at least twice a day.
- Weigh and assess oedema daily.
- Once tolerating feeds, provided improving and not losing weight → rehabilitation phase.

***Note:* oedematous children lose weight before starting to gain.**

❗ Failure to lose oedema or gain weight: is almost always because of inadequate intake of feeds or infection.

Box 17.4 Therapeutic and supplementary feeding products

Milk-based products

F-75 and F100 are specially formulated milks, available commercially or locally prepared (see 📖 Recipes and formulas, p. 712). F-75 (75kcal and 0.9g protein/100mL) is used for cautious feeding in the stabilization phase to restart metabolic processes, ↓oedema and regain appetite. F100 (100kcal and 2.9g protein/100mL) is for catch up growth in the transition and rehabilitation phase. F-75 and F100 contain a balance of protein, energy, fats and commercial (but not all local) preparations contain micronutrients. They do not contain additional iron. Because of a short shelf life they are not suitable for use at home. Commercial F-75 and F100 contain maltodextrin instead of sugar, which ↓ osmolarity and ↓ risk of osmotic diarrhoea.

Ready to use therapeutic food

RUTF is a paste based on peanuts, or cereals/legumes that is lipid, protein, energy, and micronutrient-rich. RUTFs are very palatable, with a nutritional composition similar to F100 (including extra K^+). RUTF is resistant to microbial contamination (unopened, it can be stored safely at ambient tropical conditions for many months), has lower osmolarity than F100 and micronutrients (e.g. vitamin A) are preserved. Typically, a 92-g sachet = 500kcal.

RUTF can be eaten from the packet and needs no cooking. Encourage breastfeeding and adequate water intake; other foods should not be encouraged until weight has been restored. RUTF can be used at home for uncomplicated SAM or interchangeably with F100 in hospital. Give plenty of drinking water with RUTF. There is no RUTF equivalent of F-75 and RUTF is unsuitable for the stabilization phase of complicated SAM.

RUTF can be produced locally, but commercial formulations are usually widely available, often supported by NGOs or UNICEF. Commercial RUTF contains maltodextrin instead of sugar, which ↓ osmolarity. Local production requires a properly formulated vitamin and mineral mix, which must be bought. Aflatoxin contamination can be a risk. Mechanical mixing is required. Instructions are available on the WHO website: http://www.who.int/nutrition/topics/backgroundpapers_Local_production.pdf

Supplementary feeds

Supplementary feeds used to treat MAM in supplementary feeding programmes (SFP). They typically include micronutrient fortified, blended cereals and pulses as dry rations and vegetable oil. Local food habits may be important in determining appropriate rations. Ready to use supplementary food is also available, and specially designed for nutritional requirements in MAM.

Rehabilitation phase

When ↑ appetite, ↓oedema and medical complications are stable, child may enter the rehabilitation phase, which aims to promote rapid growth. See Table 17.4.

- Gradually ↑ to >200mL/kg/d F100 (=200kcal/kg/d).
- 5 feeds/d are usually needed.
- RUTF and F100 are interchangeable: 20g RUTF = 100mL F100.
- Give iron 3mg/kg/d, except when using RUTF, which contains 11.5mg iron per sachet.
- Record the dietary intake.
- Give albendazole as described 📖 Medical management within inpatient therapeutic nutrition programmes, p. 697.
- Check temperature and general condition daily.
- Check weight and oedema 3 × per week.
- Encourage play therapy and physical activity to promote speech and motor development.
- Promote breastfeeding.

Preparing for discharge from inpatient care

Discharge should be planned in advance with the mother/carer. Refer to an outpatient therapeutic nutrition programme (OTP) or a supplementary feeding programme (SFP), if now moderately malnourished. Key issues during this phase include:

- Stable children may be discharged to OTP, even if they still meet criteria for SAM. However, they must pass an appetite test with RUTF (see 📖 Appetite test, p. 695).
- Discharge to SFP means being completely stable, and eating well.
- Provide nutrition and health education, cooking demonstrations.
- Support increasing household food security.
- Support families with serious social problems.
- Encourage regular visits to under-5s clinics, immunization, and regular vitamin A prophylaxis (3 × per year).
- Vaccinate all children aged 9mths–15yrs against measles, unless proof of previous vaccination. Children immunized <9mths should be re-vaccinated as their previous immune response may be inadequate.

Follow-up

- Follow-up should ideally be through an established OTP or SFP.
- If no OTP/SFP is available, therapeutic feeding should continue until the WHZ is >–2 or MUAC >12.5cm and oedema has resolved for at least 2wks. See child after 1wk then every 2wks to check weight gain (after nutritional recovery child should grow at 1–2g/kg body weight/d). Check for dietary/medical reasons for poor weight gain.
- Ensure child is integrated into clinic or community-based programme for monitoring progress of 'at risk' children, and can be referred back in case of problems.

❗ ***Deterioration… → ABC, complications → stabilization phase.***

Table 17.3 Amounts of F-75 required for stabilization phase

Weight (kg)	2-hourly feed	3-hourly feed	4-hourly feed	Weight (kg)	2-hourly feed	3-hourly feed	4-hourly feed
2.0	20	30	45	6.2	70	100	135
2.2	25	35	50	6.4	70	105	140
2.4	25	40	50	6.6	75	110	145
2.6	30	45	55	6.8	75	110	150
2.8	30	45	60	7.0	70	115	155
3.0	35	50	65	7.2	80	120	160
3.2	35	55	70	7.4	80	120	160
3.4	35	55	75	7.6	85	125	165
3.6	30	60	80	7.8	85	130	170
3.8	40	60	85	8.0	90	130	175
4.1	45	65	80	8.2	90	135	180
4.2	45	70	90	8.4	90	140	185
4.4	55	70	95	8.6	95	140	190
4.6	50	75	100	8.8	95	145	195
4.8	55	80	105	9.0	100	145	200
5.0	55	80	110	9.2	100	150	200
5.2	55	85	115	9.4	105	155	205
5.4	60	90	120	9.6	105	155	200
5.6	60	90	125	9.8	110	160	215
5.8	65	95	130	10.0	110	160	220
6.0	65	100	130				

Table 17.4 Amounts of RUTF required for rehabilitation phase

Weight (kg)	92-g sachets/d	92-g sachets/wk
3.5 – 3.9	1.5	11
4.0 – 5.4	2	14
5.5 – 6.9	2.5	18
7.0 – 8.4	3	21
8.5 – 9.4	3.5	25
9.5 – 10.4	4	28
0.5 – 11.9	4.5	32
≥12	5	35

Outpatient therapeutic nutrition programme

The aim of an OTP is to conduct screening, identify the severity of malnutrition and plan a treatment regimen. For uncomplicated SAM, provide medicines and therapeutic feeds, and advise patients/carers.

Treat infection (often subclinical)

- Treat all children with SAM for infection whether they have clinical signs or not. For uncomplicated SAM, give amoxycillin oral for 5d. If the child is on co-trimoxazole prophylaxis, this should continue.
- Give a single dose of albendazole (doses see 📖 Medical management within inpatient therapeutic nutrition programmes, p. 697).
- Test for HIV and refer to comprehensive care services if HIV+.
- Diagnose and treat malaria and UTIs, URTIs, skin infections etc.
- Ensure child is up to date with immunizations.
- Give vitamin A (doses see 📖 Vitamin A deficiency, p. 174) if signs of deficiency on days 1, 2 and 14.
- Additional iron and folate are not needed, they are in RUTF.
- Follow up the child weekly until adequate weight gain is achieved.

Outpatient RUTF programme

The aim of this programme is to manage children with SAM at home provided they can eat adequate amounts of RUTF.

Give sufficient RUTF till the next visit:

- Follow up every 2wks until weight gain satisfactory (e.g. >5g/kg/d).
- Advise carer to give up to 100kcal/kg body weight/d (using teaspoon equivalents of RUTF) until oedema has resolved.
- If no oedema, or once oedema resolved, give 150–220kcal/kg body weight/d.
- RUTF of 200kcal/kg body weight/d can → a daily weight gain of up to 20g/kg body weight.
- Advise carer of need to feed frequently, to keep child warm (especially at night), and to come back to clinic if child develops an infection or refuses RUTF.
- RUTF is sometimes shared with other children. If intake of RUTF falls to 100–150kcal/kg body weight, daily weight gain to falls to ~5–10g/kg body weight/d. Give cereal/legume (e.g. corn-soy blend) supplement to the family to ensure other children in the family do not eat RUTF intended for the index child.
- Give plenty of drinking water with RUTF.

Give nutritional guidance to improve dietary intake

- Advise on need to give extra food in convalescent phase of an illness and how to ↑ the protein and micronutrient content of traditional diet if possible.
- Advise on access to local programmes which ↑ food security (using local community development programme and/or a local programme of food supplements).
- Provide a 'take home' ration of food to provide protein, energy and micronutrients in a form which is palatable and can be stored safely without refrigeration (e.g. nutritional pastes).
- Discharge to SFP when appropriate (MAM).
- For kwashiorkor, therapeutic feeding should continue until oedema has resolved for >2wks.

Supplementary feeding programmes

The aim of an SFP is to conduct screening; identify severity of malnutrition; and plan a treatment regimen (refer to paediatric ward, OTP, SFP, or home). For MAM, provide supplementary feeds, identify and advise patients/carers. MAM ↑ risks of infections and development of SAM.

Food rations

Include cereals, pulses, legumes, oil, sugar and micronutrients, e.g. corn-soy blend (see 📖 Outpatient RUTF programme, p. 702). In some areas, ready to use supplementary foods (RUSF) may be available. RUSF is similar to RUTF, but designed for MAM and to be used alongside other foods.

Medical treatment

- Albendazole (📖 Medical management within inpatient therapeutic nutrition programmes, p. 697), unless already given.
- Iron and folate as per national recommendations.
- Measles immunization unless proof of previous immunization.
- Children immunized <9mths should be re-immunized.

Nutrition counselling

Mother or carer should be advised on giving healthy diet using locally available foods. Work with nutritionist to make chart of foods available, rather than trying to 'educate' mothers about carbohydrates, fats, protein, etc.

Discharge criteria

- *Children age 6–59mths:* MUAC >12.5cm.
- *Children of any age:* W/H >–2 Z scores.
- *Adults:* MUAC >18.5cm, or if pregnant or HIV+, MUAC >23cm.

HIV/AIDS and malnutrition

Among severely malnourished children in sub-Saharan Africa, the prevalence of HIV approaches 15% in community treatment programmes, and 60% in complicated SAM. Almost all severely malnourished HIV+ children have low CD4 counts and need ART. CD4 counts are not low in severely malnourished children without HIV.

All severely malnourished children should be tested for HIV because selective testing increases fear and stigma. A +ve test in child reveals that mother is also HIV+. The benefits of making the diagnosis include appropriate treatment of OIs, co-trimoxazole prophylaxis, ART, improving mothers' health, advice on infant feeding, and prevention of future mother-to-child transmission (see 🕮 HIV/AIDS, p. 69).

Specific issues in HIV+ children:

- Poor dietary intake due to weakness, painful oral lesions (e.g. candidiasis), anorexia due to fever/infections, and sickness of a parent or guardian (often also HIV+) → limited care and food provision.
- Malabsorption and chronic diarrhoea due to intestinal parasites (e.g. *Cryptosporidium*) → nutrient losses from the intestine.
- ↑ Energy expenditure due to intercurrent infections.
- Severe weight loss and growth faltering are common.
- Micronutrient deficiencies (including vitamin A, Zn) are common.
- Anaemia is common in HIV+ children, usually result of chronic inflammation, rather than micronutrient deficiency. Iron supplements may be harmful in HIV due to the ↑ in oxidative stress and HIV viral load.

Management

- Give co-trimoxazole prophylaxis (🕮 HIV/AIDS, p. 69).
- Give stabilization therapy (see 🕮 p. 698).
- During rehabilitation, aim at 220kcal/kg/d.
- Manage diarrhoea energetically. Persistent diarrhoea due to *Cryptosporidium* may not improve until ART is started.
- Treat infections and OIs vigorously (🕮 Symptomatic HIV infection, p. 84).
- Refer to an ART clinic; measure CD4 count if possible.
- Optimum time to start ART is unknown. Because of metabolic effects of ART, children should ideally have stabilized, appetite returned and oedema resolved, then start without further delay.
- Failure to gain weight is common in HIV. Investigate co-morbidities including TB and intestinal parasites, and consider early ART.
- Prevent mother-to-child transmission — see 🕮 HIV/AIDS, p. 69.
- Provide health care for the mother and/or carer, including HIV testing +/– CD4 count to assess need for ART. A healthy mother/carer is crucial to the child's recovery.

See Box 17.5 for summary of nutrition in people with HIV/AIDS.

During follow-up: Ensure nutrition during OIs. Ensure best possible food and drinking water hygiene.

Outcome: HIV roughly doubles the case fatality of SAM. Weight gain is often slower and may not increase until ART is started.

Box 17.5 Nutrition in people with HIV/AIDS

Good nutrition is essential, in order to maintain immune competence and strength and minimize the impact of infections. HIV/AIDS patients (even when asymptomatic) need ↑ food intake:

- At least the RDA of vitamins A, B, C, E, folic acid; and minerals (e.g. selenium, Zn).
- Even more during recovery from an infection.

Nutritional education should start once a person is identified as HIV+. Focus on how to meet ↑ dietary needs and prevent OIs and improve hygiene. Support the entire family, including food security, hygiene, and psychosocial care of the HIV+ individual.

To optimize intake

Eat small, frequent meals; make food softer. Include body-building food (legumes, cereal, animal products), protective foods (fruits and vegetables, fortified food), and energy foods (sugar, starch and fat, staple foods).

Problems

- *Nausea and vomiting*: eat frequent small meals and avoid fatty food.
- *Mouth sores:* avoid hot and spicy foods; eat soft, mashed or liquid food.
- *Anorexia:* eat frequent small meals. Time ART to minimize impact of GI side-effects (e.g. nausea) on meals.

Breast feeding and HIV/AIDS

- HIV+ mothers are usually worried about transmission during breastfeeding. Mixed breast/replacement feeding has greater HIV transmission than exclusive breastfeeding or replacement feeding.
- Many mothers end up mixed feeding because they cannot afford to sustain replacement feeding.
- Exclusive breastfeeding has lower risks of inadequate intake and infection (contamination).
- Cow's milk is especially hazardous. Although recipes for modification for infant use are available, these are impractical for poor mothers.
- Clinical trials of prophylactic ART given to the mother or child reduces transmission to ~2% during breastfeeding, with few maternal side effects. Where ART prophylaxis to mother or breastfeeding is available this is preferable to replacement or mixed feeding (see 🕮 Prevention of mother to child transmission, p. 144).
- WHO recommends exclusive breastfeeding up to 6mths and partial breastfeeding continue to at least 12mths, with maternal ART or infant nevirapine until 1wk after breastfeeding ceases to prevent transmission.
- Replacement feeding should not be used unless it is acceptable, feasible, affordable, sustainable and safe—in resource-poor countries these criteria are *very rarely* met.

Severe malnutrition in infants <6 months old

Feeding problems, including sickness or absence of the mother, insufficient breastmilk (stress, war, drought), inappropriate alternative infant feeding (unsafe bottle feeding, use of cow's milk, early introduction of complementary (weaning) foods) and inappropriate attempts to avoid breastmilk transmission of HIV, may cause SAM and illness in infants. Diagnosis of SAM <6mths is based on:

- W/L <–3 *Z* scores *or*
- Bilateral oedema of kwashiorkor *or*
- Weight loss and too weak to suckle effectively.

Breastfeeding

Breastfeeding ↑ immunity, is hygienic, clean, and cheap, and there is usually a good supply, although mothers need support. Artificial feeding risks contamination (teats, bottles, milk left standing too long, unclean water) and dilution (cost, sharing with siblings). This can → malnutrition through inadequate intake, wrong concentration, and repeated episodes of diarrhoea.

During insecurity, anxiety, and migration, breastmilk might be ↓. Mothers often think they produce less breastmilk because they are themselves malnourished. Milk *quantity* is usually only reduced once maternal energy intake is <1600kcal/d. Breastmilk *quality* (especially of micronutrients) is quickly affected by the mother's diet. A mother's complaint that she does not have enough milk should be properly investigated. When the milk production is reported to be ↓ or stopped, breastfeeding should be encouraged, and mother supported with nutritious food. Only if there is no other option should artificial feeding be used and then mother (or caretaker) must be trained in using the milk safely.

Medical treatment

Severely malnourished young infants require similar medical treatment regimes to older infants and children with severe malnutrition:

- Antibiotics—(📖 Medical management within inpatient therapeutic nutrition programmes, p. 696).
- Vitamin A (50 000IU) if they will not receive a therapeutic feeding product.
- Folic acid 2.5mg on admission.
- *Note:* commercial F100 already contains iron.
- Ensure that the mother has her illnesses diagnosed and treated. Maternal depression affects infant feeding and growth. Test infant for HIV and counsel mother appropriately.

Nutritional treatment

Aim to re-establish breastfeeding whilst treating infant. There is no stabilization phase unless infant has kwashiorkor.

- Supplement breastmilk with diluted F100 (see 📖 Recipes and formulas for management of malnourished children, p. 712) 130mL/kg/d. Kwashiorkor, use F-75 (130mL/kg/d) until oedema is resolving then use diluted F100. *Breastfeed as often as possible.*

- *Use a supplementary suckling technique to continue to stimulate breastmilk production:* http://www.docstoc.com/docs/48486395/UNICEF-IMAM-Publication-pdf-National-Guideline-for-malnutrition
- *When infant is gaining weight at 20g/kg/d, gradually ↓ diluted F100 until the infant is gaining weight on breastmilk alone.*

If no prospect of breastfeeding

Start with diluted F100 (or F-75 if kwashiorkor) 160mL/kg/d. When stable and tolerating, gradually ↑ diluted F100 up to 320mL/kg/d. Once gaining weight for 3 consecutive days, very gradually replace diluted F100 with 'normal' breastmilk substitute. ↑ From 120kcal/kg/d (normal intake) to 150kcal/kg/d for extra growth until recovered.

Monitoring

Monitor weight gain daily. If an infant loses weight for 3 consecutive days, check the amount of food offered is not enough (breastmilk plus therapeutic milk), re-screen for infections or medical causes of poor feeding. Address social problems.

Discharge

The following conditions should be met before discharge:

- Clinically well; no infections.
- Weight gain ≥100–125g/wk without therapeutic milk supplementation for 7d (min 5g/kg/d, target 10g/kg/d).
- *Breastfed infants:* active suckling; established breastmilk production.
- *Non-breastfed infants:* supply of breastmilk substitutes must be ensured, and the caretaker should understand hygienic preparation and the dangers of artificial feeding.

Complications of severe malnutrition in infants

- *Hypothermia:* a major cause of mortality in malnourished infants. Keep infants warm—skin-to-skin contact (kangaroo position); provide blankets and caps.
- *Dehydration:* use ReSoMal.
- *Anaemia:* iron is only given as treatment for anaemia, not as routine therapy. Give iron 2mg/kg tds (preferably in a suspension) for >3mths, but only start after 14d of nutritional treatment. If Hb <5 g/dl, consider blood transfusion (see Severe anaemia, p. 696).
- *Candidiasis:* is frequent in newborns—treat with nystatin.

Pregnancy

Nutritional counselling

There is no strong evidence that nutritional advice to ↑ energy and protein intake during pregnancy → better outcome for infants or mothers.

Energy/protein supplementation

Trials have reported ↓ in small for gestational age (SGA), ↓ stillbirths and possibly ↓ neonatal deaths. There is no effect on prematurity or on long term nutritional status in mothers or infants, or improved neuro-cognitive development.

Iron and folic acid

In pregnancy ↓ risk of maternal anaemia, maternal mortality and stillbirth. Give iron 60mg and folic acid 400µg daily.

Multiple micronutrient supplementation

Widely used in wealthy communities during pregnancy. However, in developing countries has very little benefit over iron and folate alone. Multiple micronutrient supplementation cannot be universally recommended.

- Energy/protein supplementation during pregnancy is justified in malnourished women as part of an SFP. Advise non-acutely malnourished pregnant women on a healthy, balanced diet rather than any specific regime.
- Avoid vitamin A, except for overt vitamin A deficiency (see 📖 Vitamin A deficiency, p. 714).
- Cut-off values used for MUAC to diagnose SAM and MAM are higher than for non-pregnant adults (see 📖 Malnutrition, health and survival, p. 684).

Breastfeeding: key issues promoted by WHO/UNICEF

- Early discontinuation of breastfeeding is associated with ↑ risk of death. Give infants no food and drink other than breastmilk, unless medically indicated = exclusive breastfeeding up to 6mths.
- Train healthcare staff and have a written breastfeeding policy.
- Inform all pregnant women about benefits of breastfeeding.
- Help mothers initiate breastfeeding within a half-hour of birth.
- Show mothers how to breastfeed and how to maintain lactation even if they may be separated from their infants.
- *Promote 'rooming in'*: mothers and infants should remain together 24h/d wherever possible. Encourage breastfeeding on demand.
- Do not give artificial teats or pacifiers (also called dummies or soothers) to breastfeeding infants.
- Foster establishment of breastfeeding support groups.

Nutrition in emergencies

Emergencies are typically due to famine, natural disasters, epidemics, armed conflict, and population displacement (refugees), and are exacerbated by poverty, long-term food insecurity, weak infrastructure, and endemic diseases, e.g. HIV or kala-azar (see 📖 Health emergencies in humanitarian crises, p. 913). Acute malnutrition (SAM and MAM) are common in emergencies and outbreaks of micronutrient deficiencies occur where diet is restricted. High rates of malnutrition and mortality occur during emergencies.

Current strategies are broad-based including

- Nutritional surveillance, baseline data and early warning systems.
- National programmes on food security and training in nutrition in emergencies.
- Standardized, rapid nutrition assessments (e.g. MUAC).
- Food distribution including general foodstuffs, food for work, and school-based programmes.
- Targeted therapeutic and supplementary feeding with RUTF or blended dry rations with micronutrients as described below.
- Provision of other aspects of healthcare.
- Promotion of breastfeeding.
- Non-food interventions, e.g. livelihood generation, agricultural improvement.
- Coordination between humanitarian agencies, health providers, social welfare institutions and government, and occasionally military authorities.

A set of resources can be found at: http://www.unscn.org/en/resource_portal/index.php?themes=203

Recipes and formulas for management of malnourished children

Electrolyte/mineral solution (EMS)

This is used in the preparation of starter (F-75) and catch up (F-100) feeding formula and ReSoMal (low Na^+ oral rehydration solution (ORS), see recipe for ReSoMal http://www.who.int/chd/publications/referral_care/app3/app3.htm#a3.1). Sachets containing these formulas are manufactured, but if not available, prepare by dissolving the ingredients in Table 17.5 in cool, boiled water made up to 2500mL solution.

Store EMS in sterilized bottles in the fridge to retard deterioration. Discard if turns cloudy and make fresh each month.

Commercial mineral and vitamin mix may be available; this is preferable as it contains all necessary micronutrients.

Nutritional rehabilitation formulas F-75 and F-100

Ready-made sachets of F-75 and F-100 are widely available, but where these are not, they can be prepared using the following ingredients by mixing the milk, sugar, oil, and electrolyte mineral solution (EMS or commercial mineral and vitamin mix) into a paste, and then slowly adding warm, boiled water to make up to 1000mL. If available, use an electric blender or hand whisk (see Tables 17.6 and 17.7).

Commercial packets of F-75 starter formula have lower osmolality because maltodextrins replace sugar, and already contain the required micronutrients.

Alternative milk ingredients

- If only whole dried milk (WDM) available, an alternative to F-75 may be prepared using 35g WDM, 100g sugar, 20g oil, 20mL EMS, and water up to 1000mL. Similarly, to prepare an alternative to F-100, use 110g WDM, 50g sugar, 30g oil, 20mL EMS, and water up to 1000mL.
- If only fresh cow's milk available, another alternative to F-75 may be prepared using 300mL milk, 100g sugar, 20g oil, 20mL EMS, and water up to 1000mL. Similarly, to prepare an alternative to F-100, use 880mL milk, 75g sugar, 20mg oil, 20mL EMS, and water up to 1000mL. The use of fresh cow's milk carries ↑ risk of microbial contamination.

Diluted F-100 (infants only)

This is a 75% dilution of F-100 used for severely malnourished infants (see Severe malnutrition in infants <6 months old, p. 708). It is made by adding 350mL water to 1L of prepared F-100. It supplies 75kcal/100mL, 10kcal % protein, 50kcal % fat, and is isotonic with a medium Na^+ concentration.

Diluted F-100 is used because infants <6mths cannot handle the renal solute load of full strength F-100.

Table 17.5 Electrolyte/mineral solution (EMS)

EMS ingredients	amount (g)	mol/20mL
Potassium chloride: KCl	224	24mmol
Tripotassium citrate	81	2mmol
Magnesium chloride: $MgCl_2$, $6H_20$	76	3mmol
Zinc acetate: Zn acetate, $2H_20$	8.2	300μmol
Copper sulphate: $CuS0_4$, $5H_20$	1.4	45μmol
Water make up to	2500mL	

If possible, add selenium (28mg of sodium selenate, $NaSe0_4.10H_20$) and iodine (0.012g KI/2500mL).

Table 17.6 Nutritional rehabilitation formulas

Ingredients	F-75	F-100
Dried skimmed milk (g)	25	80
Sugar (g)	100	50
Vegetable oil (g)	27	60
Electrolyte/mineral solution (mL)*	20	20
Water: make up to (mL)	1000	1000

*Commercial mineral and vitamin mix is often available, use one 'red' scoop (6.35mg) per 2000mL of F-75 or F-100 instead of EMS.

Table 17.7 Nutritional contents of F-75 and F-100

Contents per 100mL	F-75	F-100
Energy (kcal)	75	100
Protein (g)	0.9	2.9
Lactose (g)	1.3	4.2
K^+ (mmol)	4.0	6.3
Na^+ (mmol)	0.6	1.9
Mg (mmol)	0.43	0.73
Zinc (mg)	2.0	2.3
Copper (mg)	0.25	0.25
% energy from protein	5	12
% energy from fat	32	53
Osmolality (mOsm/L)	413	41

Vitamin A deficiency

In resource-poor regions, >80% vitamin A is derived from dietary carotenoids found in breastmilk, dark green vegetables, and yellow and orange fruits. Margarine and meat (especially liver) are also sources. Vitamin A deficiency → ↑ morbidity and mortality among children and is a preventable cause of blindness from xerophthalmia. Xerophthalmia is classified as follows:

- *Night blindness (XN):* individual bumps into objects in poor lighting.
- *Conjunctival xerosis (X1a):* dry conjunctiva has glazed appearance.
- *Bitot's spots (X1b):* white foamy spots on conjunctival surface, commonly at the corneoscleral junction on the temporal side (see Fig. 17.4).
- *Corneal xerosis (X2):* dry cornea, associated with the onset of visual impairment. Most common in children aged 2–4yrs.
- *Corneal ulceration (X3a):* often worse in measles; central corneal ulceration may profoundly affect vision.
- *Keratomalacia (X3b):* severe destruction of the eye with blindness; occurs especially in severe malnutrition precipitated by measles.
- *Corneal scarring (XS):* follows healing after vitamin A replacement, often with permanent visual impairment.

Treatment

For xerophthalmia, severe malnutrition, measles, and pneumonia/diarrhoea in HIV-infected children:

- Give 3 doses of oral vitamin A at days 1 and 2, and in week 3 as per Box 17.6.
- For xerophthalmia, also give topical antibiotic eye ointment (e.g. tetracycline 1% or chloramphenicol 1%) for 10d.
- If cornea is involved, close the eye and gently cover with an eye pad.

Pregnancy

Vitamin A is teratogenic and high doses are contraindicated in pregnancy. However, a pregnant woman with xeropthalmia should receive vitamin A 5000–10 000IU oral od for ≥4wks.

Public health note: prevention of vitamin A deficiency

- ↑ *Dietary vitamin A:* carotenoids in breastmilk, spinach, carrots, sweet potatoes, mangos, papaya, milk, eggs, red palm oil, liver, fish liver oils.
- Prophylactic supplementation (200 000IU) given 2–3 × per year to children aged 6mths–5yrs in endemic deficiency areas.

Box 17.6 Curative doses for vitamin A deficiency

- 0–6mths: 50 000IU*.
- 6–12mths: 100 000IU*.
- >1yr (including adults): 200 000IU*.
- Vitamin A deficiency in pregnant women: 10 000IU**.

* Give 3 doses of oral vitamin A (days 1 and 2, and in week 3).

** Give daily dose for >4wks, but see notes above.

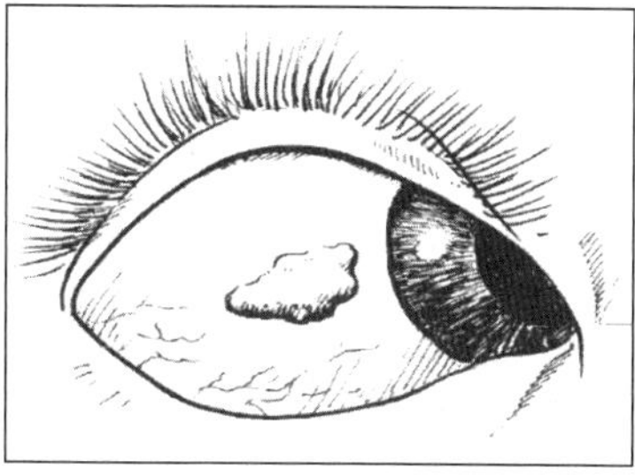

Fig. 17.4 Bitot's spot, xeropthalmia and conjunctival xerosis.

Reproduced from World Health Organization, *Pocket Book of Hospital Care for Children* (2005), with permission of WHO.

Vitamin B1 (thiamine) deficiency: beriberi

Thiamine is widely available, but deficiency may occur when cereals, e.g. rice, are highly milled. Deficiency may also complicate alcoholism and nitrofurazone therapy for trypanosomiasis. (📖 African trypanosomiasis, p. 782; 📖 American trypanosomiasis, p. 788).

Clinical syndromes

- *Dry beriberi:* peripheral sensory and motor neuropathy: gradual onset of distal limb weakness and wasting with 'glove and stocking' sensory loss; foot drop and calf wasting common. Affected muscles may show oedema and painful contraction when hit. Reflexes and joint position sense are ↓ or lost; ataxia +/– incontinence may develop in the later stages. Death occurs due to generalized and diaphragmatic paralysis.
- *Wet beriberi:* high-output cardiac failure. Typically, peripheries are warm with a bounding pulse, due to peripheral vasodilation. In acute, fulminant beriberi, peripheries become cold due to poor cardiac output. Death occurs due to CCF.
- *Infantile beriberi:* occurs in infants breastfed from a thiamine-deficient mother and is an important cause of infant mortality in parts of Asia. Irritability and oedema typically occur aged 2–3mths and may be confused with kwashiorkor; progressive heart failure occurs (+/– convulsions due to CNS involvement) and death is due to cardio-respiratory failure.
- *Wernicke's encephalopathy:* classically complicates thiamine deficiency in chronic alcohol abuse, but may also be precipitated by infections or by administration of carbohydrate (including IV glucose) before thiamine replacement. Clinical features: confusion, ataxia, nystagmus, and ophthalmoplegia due to haemorrhagic degeneration in the midbrain and mamillary bodies. Korsakoff's psychosis may also occur with confusion, confabulation, and loss of short-term memory. This is reversible with thiamine replacement, unlike the other clinical features.

Diagnosis

Usually clinical. CXR shows cardiolmegaly and pulmonary oedema in cardiac beriberi. Plasma pyruvate and lactate are ↑, red cell transketolase levels are low. Thiamine deficiency may be confirmed *in vitro* by ↑ activation of red cell transketolase after addition of thiamine.

Management

- *Acute fulminant beriberi:* thiamine 50–100mg IV tds until acute symptoms improve followed by 10–25mg/d oral.
- *Chronic beriberi:* thiamine 10–25mg/d oral for ≥6wks. Pain in limbs is relieved rapidly; peripheral neuropathy may take months to years to resolve.
- *Infantile beriberi:* thiamine 25–50mg given IV slowly followed by 10mg IM daily for 1wk; then 3–5mg/d orally for 6wks. Treat mother with thiamine 10mg/day oral for 7d, then 3–5mg/d for 6wks.

Vitamin B2 (riboflavin) deficiency

Riboflavin is found in meat, vegetables, milk, and wholemeal flour. Overt deficiency is uncommon. Some drugs, e.g. phenothiazines and tricyclic antidepressants interact with riboflavin.

Clinical features

Angular cheilosis/stomatitis, sore red lips, atrophic glossitis. There may be plugging of sebaceous glands, giving a roughened appearance to the skin, and scrotal dermatitis. Anaemia occurs because riboflavin deficiency → poor iron absorption.

Management Riboflavin up to 30mg oral od. Usually rapidly cured.

Vitamin B3 (niacin) deficiency: pellagra

Niacin and its precursor tryptophan are found in meat, fish, nuts, fruits, and vegetables. Deficiency → pellagra, which is common in communities where maize or sorghum are the staple, as bioavailability of niacin in maize is low, and ↑ leucine levels in sorghum ↓ nicotinic acid and tryptophan metabolism; deficiency may be prevented by dietary tryptophan, e.g. in beans. Pellagra also occurs in malabsorption, isoniazid therapy, alcoholism; it may contribute to diarrhoea, depression, and skin disorders in HIV/AIDS.

Clinical features

The classical triad is of dermatitis, diarrhoea, and dementia.

- *Skin:* a photosensitive, sunburn-like rash at sun-exposed sites; there may be a collar-like ring around the neck (Casal's necklace). Lesions are sensitive/inflamed, later becoming scaly and desquamate. Atrophic patches of skin remain between the fingers; the nails become brittle and atrophic.
- *Gastrointestinal:* gingival swelling +/– bleeding; raw, fissured tongue; dysphagia; villous atrophy and malabsorption; diarrhoea and nausea.
- *Neurological:* insomnia, anxiety, depression, memory loss, photophobia; mania or psychosis (which may be permanent); pyramidal and extra-pyramidal signs; frontal reflexes. Confusion can precede death. Peripheral and cranial neuropathies also occur.
- *Eyes:* conjunctival oedema, corneal dystrophy, and lens opacities extending from the periphery to the centre.

Management Treatment with nicotinamide 500mg daily until complete recovery (at least 3–4wks).

Prevention In confirmed outbreaks, consider vitamin B complex supplements for the entire population as a short-term measure.

Vitamin B6 (pyridoxine) deficiency

Clinical signs of deficiency are rare, except as peripheral neuropathy during isoniazid therapy, and pyridoxine antagonists, e.g. pyrazinamide and cycloserine may → sideroblastic anaemia. Dietary sources include meat and vegetables.

Management

Pyridoxine 50–150mg/d oral in divided doses is widely used, but little evidence for efficacy. Doses up to 400mg/d may be partially effective in idiopathic and hereditary sideroblastic anaemia. Give pyridoxine 10mg/d during isoniazid therapy and to malnourished alcoholics.

Toxicity Peripheral neuropathy is reported following prolonged high-dose pyridoxine. Improvement is limited even after stopping treatment.

Vitamin B12 deficiency

Vitamin B12 is available in animal products including liver, fish, meat, eggs, and dairy products, but not in vegetables. Absorption depends on intrinsic factor from the stomach binding vitamin B12 to facilitate uptake in the terminal ileum. Deficiency may be due to poor dietary intake (e.g. vegans), atrophic gastritis (pernicious anaemia), previous gastrectomy, and terminal ileal disease.

Clinical features

- *General:* angular cheilosis, glossitis; hyperpigmentation of the hands and feet is noted in some populations.
- *Macrocytic anaemia:* see 📖 Macrocytic anaemias, p. 504.
- *Subacute combined degeneration of the cord:* dorsal column and corticospinal tract degeneration → sensory and both upper and lower motor neuron signs, classically with extensor plantars but absent knee and ankle reflexes, +/– ataxia due to ↓ proprioception; pain and temperature sensation are preserved as spinothalamic tracts are not involved. May be precipitated by administration of high doses of folate to patients with combined B12 and folate deficiency.
- *Other neurological sequelae:* peripheral neuropathy, optic atrophy, dementia, neuropsychiatric symptoms, neurodevelopmental delay.

Diagnosis Low serum B12; macrocytosis; anaemia; low WBC and platelets (📖 Causes of anaemia due to ↓ RBC production, p. 495). Tests for pernicious anaemia: parietal cell/intrinsic factor antibodies, Schilling test.

Management

Hydroxocobalamin 1mg IM 3× per week for 2wks to replenish body stores, then 1mg IM every 3mths (often needed for life); if neurological involvement, give 1mg on alternate days until no further improvement, then 1mg every 2mths.

Folate deficiency

Leafy green vegetables (e.g. spinach), fruits (like citrus fruits and juices), and dried beans and peas are all natural sources of folate. Folate is heat labile and water soluble so is lost in prolonged cooking or boiling. Deficiency occurs in malabsorption, in pregnancy or haemolysis, and in patients on anti-folate drugs, e.g. methotrexate or trimethoprim.

Clinical features

Blood changes are similar to vitamin B12 deficiency (📖 Vitamin B12 deficiency, p. 718), but without neurological sequelae. Deficiency in pregnancy ↑ risk of neural tube defects; intrauterine growth retardation, premature delivery, low birth weight.

Diagnosis ↓ RBC folate; macrocytic anaemia (📖 Macrocytic anaemias, p. 504).

Management Treat deficiency with folic acid 5mg oral od. Folate is increasingly being added to flour as part of national government policies.

Vitamin C deficiency: scurvy

Vitamin C (ascorbic acid) is essential to collagen formation, ↑ iron absorption, maintaining healthy epithelial tissues, e.g. mouth and skin, and promoting wound healing. Found in fresh citrus fruit and potatoes but easily destroyed by overcooking. Deficiency occurs when fruit and vegetables are scarce, in the elderly, and in young children (who have ↑ requirements).

Clinical features

- *General:* weight loss, stiffness, weakness, swollen painful large joints.
- *Skin:* dry skin, hyperkeratosis of hair follicles, 'corkscrew hairs', bruising, perifolicular petechial haemorrhages, poor wound healing.
- *Mouth:* gingivitis, bleeding gums, dental caries, loss of teeth.
- *Anaemia:* microcytic anaemia due to iron deficiency, and/or megaloblastic anaemia as vitamin C is required for folate metabolism.

Treatment Oral ascorbic acid, in divided doses per day for 2wks (infants <1mth 50mg/d; 1mth–4yrs, 125–250mg/d; 4–12yrs, 250–500mg/d; adults 500mg/d).

Prevention

- Avoid overcooking vegetables; eat citrus fruit, mangos and guavas. If necessary, supplement with tablets (children and adults 25–75mg/d).
- Avoid artificial feeds without fortified vitamin C.

Paediatric note: scurvy in infants

Infantile scurvy typically presents at 6–12mths in premature or artificially fed infants. Erupting teeth → bleeding of the gums. Sub-periosteal haemorrhages → limb pain and swelling, especially in the long bones, e.g. distal femur and proximal tibia; costochondral beading may also be palpable (scorbutic rosary). Occasionally, there is bloody diarrhoea. There may be a microcytic and/or megaloblastic anaemia. Plain X-rays of the long bones show epiphyseal changes and ground glass appearance of the shafts.

Vitamin D deficiency: rickets/ osteomalacia

Vitamin D regulates calcium homeostasis by controlling intestinal absorption and renal excretion of Ca^{2+}, and mobilizing Ca^{2+} from bone. Vitamin D is also important in cell signalling, gene expression, platelet aggregation, and host immunity (e.g. TB). The best food source of vitamin D is oily fish, although most vitamin D3 is formed in the skin by UV light. Deficiency may be due to dietary insufficiency, malabsorption or lack of UV exposure, which is exacerbated by skin-covering and lack of outdoor play. It may also be due to liver disease, renal failure, or anticonvulsant therapy (↑ vitamin D metabolism 2° to enzyme induction). Deficiency → rickets in children and osteomalacia in adults.

Clinical features

- Rickets is due to disordered bone mineralization at the growth plates of growing children, usually <2yrs. Features include:
  - irritability, hypotonia, painful wrists, and tender legs (which may be bowed once the child starts standing)
  - swollen costo-chondral junctions ('rachitic rosary'), pigeon chest, indrawing of the lower ribs (Harrison sulcus), spinal deformities, bossing of the skull and craniotabes
  - hypocalcaemia may → tetany and jaw, tongue or laryngeal spasm
  - neurodevelopmental delay also occurs
  - presentation ∴ depends on age.
- Osteomalacia occurs in adults, often in women or in the elderly. It presents with aching muscles and bones (pelvis, ribs, femora), pathological fractures, proximal myopathy (waddling gait).
- Vitamin D deficiency is associated with susceptibility to TB and pneumonia.

Diagnosis

Is clinical, aided by the following investigations:

- *X-rays:* cupping and fraying of the metaphyses with widening of the epiphyses in rickets; osteopenia, Looser's zones (partial fractures without bony displacement e.g. of lateral scapular border, femur, or pelvis), biconcave deformity of the vertebrae. (See Fig. 17.5).
- *Bloods:* low plasma 25-hydroxy vitamin D. Only in severe deficiency is there ↓ serum Ca^{2+}, ↓PO_4^-, ↑ ALP.
- *Bone scanning:* shows characteristic changes.

Management

- *Oral ergocalciferol (vitamin D2):* the RDA for adults is 400–800 units.
- *Deficiency should be corrected with a few days of high dose replacement:* adults 40 000U, children <6mths 3000U; 6mths–12yrs 6000U; 12–18yrs 10 000U daily.
- A single IM dose of 150 000–300 000IU of vitamin D2 in oil will protect for >6mths. Unless there is plenty of calcium in the diet or water, give calcium 500mg oral od for the first 15d of treatment. Specialist regimens are required if vitamin D deficiency is due to renal disease or malabsorption.

Paediatric note: calcium deficiency and rickets

- Rickets may occur as a result of calcium deficiency and/or of vitamin D deficiency, e.g. in African children fed a maize diet low in calcium.
- Vitamin D deficiency may occur in infancy, due to maternal deficiency and low sunlight exposure.
- Calcium deficiency usually occurs later e.g. bow legs.

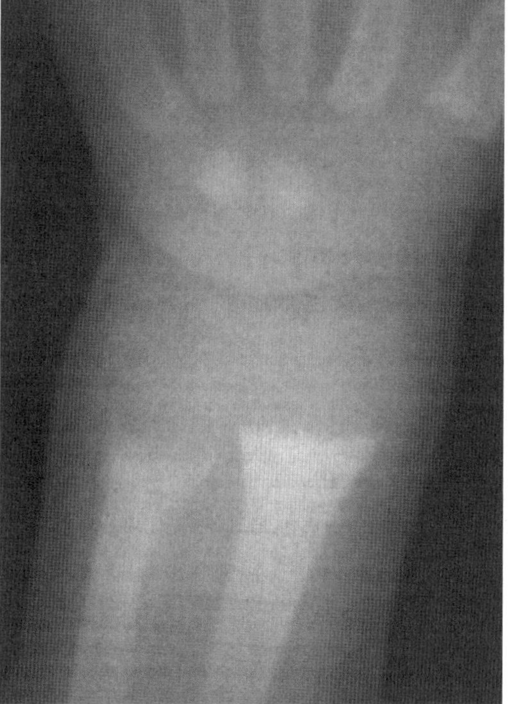

Fig. 17.5 Wrist X-ray of a 15-mth child with rickets showing cupping and fraying of the distal ends of the radius and ulna.

Vitamin E (alpha-tocopherol) deficiency

Vitamin E deficiency develops in patients with fat malabsorption (e.g. cholestatic liver disease) and in patients with congenital abetalipoproteinaemia. Premature infants often have inadequate vitamin E stores → haemolytic anaemia.

Clinical features Haemolytic anaemia, ataxia, and peripheral neuropathy.

Diagnosis Plasma vitamin E (alpha-tocopherol) level.

Treatment

Few patients need treatment. Treat deficiency with vitamin E in neonates (10mg/kg oral od) and children (1mth–18yrs 2–10mg/kg oral od, up to 20mg/kg has been used). Children with a β-lipoproteinaemia (neonate 100mg/kg oral od, child 1mth–18yrs, 50–100mg/kg oral od). Children with cholestasis or severe liver disease treat (neonate 10mg/kg oral od; child 1mth–12yrs, initially 100mg oral od adjusted according to response; up to 200mg/kg od may be required; child 12–18yrs, initially 200mg oral od, adjusted according to response; up to 200mg/kg oral od may be required).

Vitamin K deficiency

Vitamin K is essential for production of clotting factors II, VII, IX, and X, proteins C and S, and for bone growth. It is found in leafy green vegetables and is produced by intestinal bacteria. Deficiency occurs in poorly fed neonates and adults with malabsorption, and → bleeding tendency with ↑ prothrombin time. Neonates have low body stores, especially those born prematurely, and deficiency causes 'haemorrhagic disease of the newborn.' This can be prevented with vitamin K (see 📖 Paediatric note: haemorrhagic disease of the newborn (HDN), p. 532 for details).

Treatment For vitamin K deficiency associated haemorrhage, give vitamin K (1mth–18yrs: 250–300micrograms/kg IV stat, up to a maximum of 10mg; in adults 5–10mg IV) Dietary advice suffices in most non-bleeding cases.

Iodine deficiency

Iodine is essential for thyroid hormone synthesis, brain development and function. Deficiency is usually due to low levels in soil and water, especially in mountainous areas (e.g. Nepal and Bolivia) and low-lying areas where flooding has washed iodine out of the soil (e.g. Bangladesh). Limited iodine availability can be worsened by eating brassicas, cassava, or soya beans. Deficiency → goitre +/– hypothyroidism; it is the commonest cause of preventable mental retardation ('cretinism') worldwide.

Clinical features

- *Goitre:* ↑ TSH from the pituitary → thyroid enlargement. Large goitres may → dysphagia and hoarseness (recurrent laryngeal nerve compression). Patients may be euthyroid (most commonly) or hypothyroid. Not associated with ↑ risk of malignancy.
- *Endemic (neurologic) cretinism:* mental retardation, speech and hearing deficits, strabismus, spastic diplegia, and a characteristic apathetic facies with thickened features. May occur as a result of maternal hypothyroidism in any population, even in absence of iodine deficiency.
- *Hypothyroidism:* clinical features are described on 🕮 Thyroid disease, p. 550. Severe hypothyroidism → 'myxoedematous cretinism', with short stature, ataxia, and mental retardation without hearing deficit.

Diagnosis Is clinical, supported by ↑ TSH +/– ↓T_4; urinary iodine measures of dietary iodine intake.

Treatment

- Iodized oil as a single dose repeated after 1–2yrs (see Public health note).
- Lugol's iodine (often kept for sterilization) may also be given as 1 drop every 30d, or 1 teaspoon daily of a solution containing 1 drop of Lugol's iodine in 30mL of water.
- Surgery may be required for massive goitre.

Public health note: prevention of iodine deficiency

Visible goitre in >10% of the population indicates severe iodine deficiency and mass prevention should be undertaken with IM injections of iodized oil or oral iodine. Iodine should also be given to pregnant women in endemic areas to prevent congenital hypothyroidism.

- *Iodized salt:* satisfactory iodization of salt can be tested using simple colour change kits based on starch/iodine interaction colours.
- *Iodized poppy seed oil (IPSO):* can be used in endemic areas where salt is not iodized: women should take IPSO 400mg as a single dose, preferably before conception; children should receive 100mg <12mths, 200mg aged 1–5yrs, 400mg aged 5–18yrs. In areas where intestinal parasites are endemic, give albendazole to ensure absorption. The dose lasts for up to 2yrs.
- Over-replacement in endemic areas may → thyrotoxicosis.

Other micronutrients

Zinc

Zinc has antioxidant properties and is essential to several proteins and enzymes, including those regulating gene expression. Body stores are minimal so deficiency occurs quickly, especially in catabolic states or if intestinal losses are high. Zn is found in meat and fish; bioavailability from cereals is often poor because phytate binds Zn. Deficiency occurs in severe malnutrition (especially oedematous malnutrition) and low birth weight infants.

Clinical features

Failure to thrive, recurrent infections, persistent diarrhoea, scaly lesions (probably due to local *Candida*) on the feet and buttocks, stunting, developmental delay. The classical rash of acrodermatitis enteropathica is rare, usually due to a congenital disorder of Zn malabsorption. Plasma Zn is often ↓ in individuals but single measurements are unreliable as they ↓ in acute infection.

Treatment Zinc 10mg/day ↓ frequency/severity of respiratory infections and diarrhoeal disease, including in HIV+ individuals, and improves wound healing. A 2-wk course of zinc given for diarrhoea ↓ mortality in the following 6mths.

Copper

Cu is important for several enzymes with antioxidant properties and for development of collagen. Cu is widely available in shellfish, liver, kidney, nuts, and wholegrain cereals. Deficiency is uncommon and → osteoporosis and leukopenia with ↑ risk of infection. Cu deficiency may be precipitated by high Zn doses → impaired Cu absorption. Menke's disease is a rare cause due to defective Cu metabolism. Dietary excess (+/– genetic predisposition) is implicated in Indian childhood cirrhosis (📖 Indian childhood cirrhosis, p. 333).

Treatment Copper should be included in the electrolyte/mineral mix for treatment of severe malnutrition.

Selenium

Several enzymatic processes require Se. Dietary sources include cereals, meat, and nuts. Deficiency occurs where cereals are grown in low Se soils → ↓ antioxidant activity. This may → to coronary artery disease. Se stimulates immunity and has been advised in nutritional support for HIV.

Clinical features Se deficiency → cardiomyopathy in China where soils are deficient in Se.

Treatment and prevention Se should be included in the electrolyte/mineral mix for treatment of severe malnutrition (see 📖 p. 708). Fertilizers help mitigate the effect of low Se levels in the soil.

Iron Iron deficiency is a common cause of anaemia (see 📖 Iron-deficiency anaemia, p. 500).

Fluoride

Fluoride is essential for mineralization of bones and teeth, and is present in the majority of foods and drinking water. Deficiency contributes to dental caries. Excess dietary fluoride may occur where the drinking water is very high in fluoride (e.g. Rift Valley in East Africa, the Punjab) causing clinical fluorosis.

Clinical features

Signs of deficiency include dental caries and softening of long bones with deformity. Conversely, fluorosis is characterized by excess fluoride deposition in teeth and bones, with chalky discolouration of teeth enamel, spinal rigidity, restricted joint movement, ectopic mineralization of tendons, ligaments, and occasionally muscles, ↑ bone density.

Prevention Add fluoride to drinking water at source where fluoride levels low. Where fluorosis is endemic and fluoride levels in water are high, advise on alternative drinking water sources.

Obesity

The terms overweight and obese are interchangeable. People become obese because they take in more calories than they consume in metabolism and work. There is ↑ evidence for differences between individuals in appetite, fat metabolism, and metabolic responses to a meal. There is a global epidemic of obesity. Changes in dietary intake in recent years have been associated with ↓ physical activity. Obesity tended in the past to be a disease of the prosperous and urbanization, but the present epidemic of obesity affects the poor who buy cheaper, high-energy foods. Obesity may also result from programming occurring when intrauterine malnutrition, or malnutrition in the first 2yrs of life, has been present. Obesity ↑ risk of coronary heart disease, stroke, hypertension, type II diabetes, gallstones and other digestive disorders, back problems, arthritis of the knees and hips, accidents, fractures, and fatigue.

Diagnosis

BMI >25kg/m^2 indicates probable obesity; >30 definite obesity in adults. Children should be assessed with charts and table of W/H or BMI. Children are obese if they are >+2 Z scores (>97th centile) for W/H (see 📖 Measuring nutritional status, p. 686).

Management

Weight loss difficult:

- Eat foods containing more fibre and less fat or sugar. Instead of high-energy snacks, eat fruit or maize cobs. Avoid sweets, chips, crisps, and cakes; ↓ alcohol.
- Exercise for >20min/d at a level sufficient to raise the pulse and respiratory rates.
- Be realistic and offer encouragement, not scorn.
- Advise stopping smoking to ↓ cardiovascular risk.
- Avoid drugs that suppress appetite and metabolism: evidence for these is lacking.

Metabolic syndrome

Central (abdominal) obesity leads to insulin resistance, and to the production by adipocytes of cytokines implicated in endothelial dysfunction, dyslipidaemia, hypertension, vascular inflammation, and thereby atherosclerotic cardiovascular disease. The term 'metabolic syndrome' has been given to the co-association of central (abdominal) obesity, hyperglycaemia, dyslipidaemia and hypertension, which together identify people at high risk for developing type 2 diabetes and cardiovascular disease. Its prevalence is increasing in both the industrialized and developing world. Other associations include fatty liver disease, chronic kidney disease, polycystic ovary syndrome, obstructive sleep apnoea syndrome, gout, and an increased risk of dementia.

Management involves aggressive lifestyle modification focussed on weight reduction and increased exercise, in addition to treatment of cardiovascular risk factors that are not controlled by lifestyle modification alone.

Chapter 18

Multi-system diseases and infections

Invited authors

Charles M. Stein
Chris Parry
John Frean
David Warrell
Yupin Suputtamongkol
Kevin Griffith
Sharon Peacock
Robert Spencer
François Chappuis
Tania C Araujo-Jorge
Erwan Piriou
Sam Nightingale
Tom Solomon
Cecilia Chung

Differential diagnosis of fevers

Fever is a common presentation of infections (and, less commonly, inflammatory conditions or malignancy; Box 18.1).

Fever pattern does not reliably distinguish bacterial, viral, parasitic, fungal, or non-infectious causes of fever. Distinctive patterns of fever and pulse rate, (e.g. a step-wise increase in fever and relative bradycardia previously described as typical of typhoid) are now seldom emphasized. In fever from whatever cause, body temperature tends to rise in the late afternoon/evening and fall during the night. This → a sensation of being cold in the afternoon/evening and night sweats. Fever is often intermittent; it may be absent in the morning, or if anti-pyretics (e.g. paracetamol) have been taken. Patients on steroids may have little or no fever.

- Rigors (chills or shivering, often uncontrollable and lasting for >20min) are always highly significant, and generally indicate malaria or bacterial sepsis, and occasionally severe viral infection (e.g. dengue, Lassa fever). TB (except miliary TB), kala-azar, and other chronic infections do not generally cause rigors, and nor do mild viral infections (e.g. EBV or respiratory viruses), malignancy, or connective tissue diseases.
- Drenching sweats especially at night are highly significant, but can occur in any cause of fever.
- Patients with prolonged fever will invariably lose weight due to ↓ appetite.

History and examination

During a detailed history and complete physical examination, consider:

- Where is site of infection?
- Which are likely infecting organisms?
- Is this presentation unusual? Has it become more common recently? Might an epidemic be occurring?
- Is the patient immunocompromised? If so, consider the differential diagnoses for both immunocompetent and immunocompromised individuals.
- Serious infections, such as meningococcal sepsis and malaria may have 'false localizing' symptoms and signs such as headache, breathlessness, vomiting, or diarrhoea.
- In the presence of localizing features, investigations are targeted towards the presumed cause. Specimens (blood, urine, CSF, etc.) for microscopy and culture, if available, are most useful.
- Treatment with antibiotics can be started based on a clinical diagnosis and the likely infecting organisms. Consult local guidelines for choosing antibiotics, if available.
- Be aware of risk factors (such as HIV+, or malnutrition) putting a patient at higher risk of both severe infection and death.

Box 18.1 Common infections with localizing features

• Pneumonia	Breathlessness, cough, sputum, pleurisy
• Pulmonary TB	Prolonged cough, haemoptysis
• UTI	Urinary frequency, dysuria, haematuria, loin pain
• Gastroenteritis	Vomiting and watery diarrhoea
• Infective enteritis	Watery diarrhoea, central abdominal pain
• Colitis/dysentery	Diarrhoea with blood and mucus, lower abdominal pain, tenesmus
• Cellulitis	Red, hot skin
• Septic arthritis	Painful, swollen joint
• Osteomyelitis	Bone pain
• Meningitis	Headache, confusion, neck stiffness
• Streptococcal, EBV, or diphtheria infection	Sore throat, exudate over tonsils/pharynx
• TB lymphadenitis	Prominent cervical lymphadenopathy

Fever without localizing features

Challenging clinical problem; the following are helpful in determining likely cause:

- Blood smears for microscopy for malaria.
- FBC, to include total and differential WBC and platelet count.
- Blood culture (where available).

The importance of malaria

In many tropical areas, malaria is a common and important cause of fever and should be considered and excluded. Patients generally have evening fevers, so may be afebrile in a morning clinic. In endemic areas, low-grade parasitaemia without symptoms is common in adults and older children (due the development of partial immunity to malaria). Thus, the finding of low-grade parasitaemia (or a +ve RDT) in an individual with fever does not prove that the fever is caused by malaria—always consider differential diagnoses. Febrile patients with no visible malaria parasites (or a –ve RDT) should not normally be treated for malaria. Exceptions may include severely ill children or adults, who are unlikely to have acquired any immunity, who may need to be treated whilst awaiting malaria blood films (or RDTs) repeated daily × 3d to be sure they are –ve (time of day does not matter, do not wait for a fever spike), whilst treatment is given. Undertake repeat testing in other patients with persistent, unexplained fever to ensure they do not have malaria.

Note: that artemisinins can rapidly ↓ parasite counts so consider this if prior treatment has been given at another health facility.

Blood counts in a patient with fever (See Tables 18.1and 18.2) WBC and platelet count may give useful clues to the cause, although this must be considered in the context of careful clinical assessment of the patient.

Treatment of fever of unknown cause

Quite commonly, a +ve diagnosis cannot be made after the initial clinical assessment and tests. The management then depends on:

- Judgement of the most likely diagnoses.
- How severely ill patient is.
- Resources.

Patients who you judge to be (or at risk of becoming) seriously unwell should be given 'best guess' empirical antimicrobial therapy, using local guidelines if they exist. Admission to hospital, if possible, is best course if worried about patient's condition. In time, diagnosis is likely to become apparent, particularly if patient is regularly reassessed.

Persistent fever despite antimicrobial therapy

- Antimicrobials chosen do not treat the infecting organism.
- Infecting organism is resistant to chosen antimicrobials.
- Inadequate drug concentration at site of infection; think about compliance, dose, absorption, drug penetration into special sites (e.g. CSF, collections/abscesses).
- Non-infectious causes.

Table 18.1 If total WBC ↑, look at the differential WBC count

Differential white cell count	Common or important causes
Neutrophilia	Bacterial infections (sepsis, focal infection, deep-seated abscess, leptospirosis, borreliosis) Amoebic liver abscess
Lymphocytosis	Infectious mononucleosis (EBV), pertussis, brucellosis
Eosinophilia	Invasive worm infections (e.g. acute schistosomiasis)

Table 18.2 If total WBC normal or low, look at the platelet count

Platelet count	Common or important causes
Normal	Viral infections (including the prodrome of acute viral hepatitis), typhoid, rickettsial infection
Low	Malaria, dengue and other viral infections, HIV Bacterial infections (especially Gram–ve)

Sepsis

Bacterial infections are the most common cause of sepsis, but other serious infections (e.g. falciparum malaria, Lassa fever) can → an identical clinical syndrome. Some non-infectious insults can also → identical clinical syndrome (e.g. pancreatitis, chemical toxins, burns). Sepsis may also occur at the same time as other infections, such as malaria.

Sepsis syndromes

Systemic inflammatory response syndrome (SIRS)

- Recognized clinically as the presence of two or more of:
  - temperature > 38.3°C or < 36.0°C
  - heart rate > 90bpm
  - respiratory rate (RespR) > 20bpm
- Hypotension (adults: systolic BP <90mmHg).
- WBC >12 or <4, or >10% immature forms.

Sepsis SIRS plus confirmed or strongly suspected infection.

Severe sepsis

Sepsis and at least one of:

- Hypoperfusion, area of mottled skin, or capillary filling >3s.
- Urine output < 0.5mL/kg for at least an hour.
- Lactate > 2mmol/L.
- Confusion.
- Platelet count <100 000cells/mL; DIC.
- Hypoxia, acute lung injury or acute respiratory distress syndrome.
- Cardiac dysfunction.
- Renal impairment.
- Hepatic impairment.
- Coagulopathy.
- ↑ Or ↓ blood glucose in non-diabetic.

Septic shock Severe sepsis with hypotension despite adequate fluid resuscitation.

Management

The cornerstones of treatment are IV fluid resuscitation and antimicrobial therapy. Antimicrobial therapy empirical treatment ('best guess') should be started immediately (after blood cultures, if available).

In severely ill patients, a wide range of supportive measures (e.g. vasopressor therapy, mechanical ventilation, haemofiltration, IV hydrocortisone) may be indicated if available.

Despite intensive treatment, mortality from sepsis remains high; overall ~20–30% in sepsis, rising to ~50% in adult patients with severe sepsis or shock, and >80% in patients with multi-organ failure.

Cancer

Cancer is an increasingly important cause of mortality in resource-poor countries. The global burden of cancer is likely to double by 2020, and most of the ↑ will come from resource-poor countries. Populations are expanding and ageing, tobacco consumption increasing and diets are westernized. ~ 60% of global cancer occurs in resource-poor countries.

There is wide geographical variation in the prevalence of some cancers. Lung cancer is the most common cancer worldwide, followed by stomach, liver, colon and rectum, oesophagus, and breast. Breast cancer is the most common fatal cancer in women.

Cancer requires early intervention for therapy to be effective. Bearing this in mind, basic rules include:

- Suspect cancer in any unexplained illness, particularly in the elderly.
- An attempt should be made to get a histological or cytological diagnosis as soon as feasible.
- Once diagnosed, patients should start a planned regimen of treatment within days, not weeks. Tumours grow exponentially and there is no room for delay.

Signs and symptoms common to many forms of cancer

- *Pain*: due to direct effect of tumour (e.g. infiltration of nerves or compression), or metastatic spread to the bones. Any patient with unexplained persistent pain should be suspected of having malignant disease. Treatment may also cause pain.
- *Weight loss*: due to involvement of GI tract (obstruction, metastatic liver involvement), anorexia, or general cachexia due to a catabolic state. This may be exacerbated by treatment.
- *Tumour mass*: enables early diagnosis by biopsy, preferably by fine needle aspiration.
- *Fever*: while normally caused by superimposed infection, fever may itself be a feature of cancers e.g. lymphomas, renal CA, and tumours metastasizing to the liver. Frequently occurs as drenching night sweats without rigors.
- *Anaemia:* normocytic normochromic (sometimes hypochromic) due to bleeding, malabsorption, or anaemia of chronic disease.
- *Hypercalcaemia:* due to widespread metastases to the skeleton or, more commonly, to paraneoplastic syndromes.

Paraneoplastic syndromes

These occur relatively commonly and are due to tumour-derived cytokines or hormones or to a tumour-induced immune response cross-reacting with normal tissue. The range includes endocrine, neurological, dermatological, musculoskeletal, and haematological syndromes. Paraneoplastic symptoms often improve on therapy. Most neurological problems are due to metastases, and most endocrine problems due to endocrine tumours themselves, not paraneoplastic syndromes.

WHO performance status

This is useful for grading the status of cancer patients and determining prognosis.

- **0** Able to carry out normal activity without restriction
- **1** Restricted in physically strenuous activity, but walking about and able to carry out light work
- **2** Walking about and capable of self-care, but unable to carry out any work; up and about >50% of waking hours
- **3** Capable of self-care; confined to bed or chair >50% of waking hours
- **4** Completely disabled; cannot carry out self-care; totally confined to bed or chair

Important complications of some tumours

- Spinal cord/cauda equina compression†
- Cerebral metastases and ↑ intracranial pressure†
- Carcinomatous meningitis → to headache and ↑ intracranial pressure
- Pleural and pericardial effusions

† *Management* requires immediate administration of dexamethasone 8mg bd IV. Neurological symptoms should settle quickly. Delay in the treatment of spinal cord compression will result in paraplegia.

Further reading

Website: http://www.inctr.org/about/develop.shtml

General rules of cancer management

Whenever you see a patient with cancer, consider the following points:

Could the patient have neutropenia?

Infection in a neutropenic patient often presents suddenly with sepsis, but without localizing features, and cultures are usually –ve. Neutropenia commonly occurs if the patient has had chemotherapy. Bacterial flora from the mouth, digestive tract, respiratory tract, or skin are usually responsible, and indwelling lines and catheters may be the source. Any cancer patient who is feeling 'run down' and especially with a fever must have their WBC checked immediately and not be sent home. Such patients can deteriorate quickly and be dead within hours.

Could the patient have hypercalcaemia?

Unlike 1° parathyroid disease, the onset is rapid and there are none of the classical 'stones, bones, or groans'. Instead, clinical features include: polyuria, thirst, confusion, fatigue, coma. Treatment of hypercalcaemia → a marked improvement in the patient's condition (Box 18.2).

Is patient's pain controlled?

Use morphine, it is a very effective drug. The following regimen is useful:

- Give morphine 10mg 4-hourly at 07.00, 11.00, hours, etc., until 23.00, at which point give a double dose so that 03.00 dose can be missed out, offering the chance of a good night's sleep.
- If pain breaks through, give an extra dose of morphine 10mg (even if the next 4-hourly dose is only 10min away), continuing other doses as normal.
- As more breakthrough doses are required, ↑ regular 4-hourly dose (e.g. to 20mg).
- If using long-acting morphine (e.g. MST® 80mg bd), take total daily dose (160mg) and divide by 6 doses to give size of the IV morphine dose to use for breakthroughs—here 160/6 = ~25mg).

Could the patient have early cord compression?

Ask:

- Can you walk?
- When was the last time you walked?
- Have you been incontinent of urine and/or faeces?
- Do a neurological exam including anal tone and sacral sensation, and check for a palpable bladder.
- Missing spinal cord compression may → patient spending their last few weeks or months in a miserable paraplegic state.

Box 18.2 Hypercalcaemia

- Rehydrate with 0.9% saline IV (e.g. 4–6L in 24h depending on hydration status).
- Once rehydrated consider forced saline diuresis: continue 0.9% saline infusion and give e.g. furosemide 40mg bd oral/IV.
- Consider single bisphosphonate infusion (e.g. pamidronate) to ↓ Ca^{2+} over 2–3d (max effect at 1wk). Dose varies according to serum Ca^{2+} level (see Table 18.3).
- Steroids may help in some conditions e.g. sarcoidosis, malignancy.
- If possible treat the underlying cause.

Table 18.3 Treating hypercalcaemia

Corrected Ca^{2+}	Disodium pamidronate dose
<3mmol/L	15–30mg
3–3.5mmol/L	30–60mg
3.5–4.0mmol/L	60–90mg
>4.0mmol/L	90mg

Management of acute pain in hospital

- Effective relief can be achieved with oral non-opioid and NSAIDs. Ibuprofen 400mg is very effective and is associated with fewer gastrointestinal bleeds than some other NSAIDs. Also effective are paracetamol 1g and paracetamol combined with codeine.
- Initial management of moderate pain, e.g. in post-surgical patients, should ideally be an oral NSAID, such as ibuprofen, supplemented if necessary with paracetamol. In the elderly, paracetamol may be preferred, although it is less effective. There is no evidence that parenteral is more beneficial than oral administration.
- Opioids are the 1st choice treatment for severe acute pain. Additional, often smaller doses can be given if the patient is still in pain and you are sure that all the previous dose has been delivered and absorbed. Repeat doses can be given 5min after IV injection, 1h after IM or sc injection, and 90min after an oral dose. The route of administration can be changed to achieve faster control if there is no response to the repeated dose.
- Titrate opioids against degree of pain relief. Inadequate pain control results from too little drug, too long dosing intervals, too little attention being paid to the patient, or too much reliance on rigid regimens.
- Morphine is the most appropriate opioid and it is popular amongst pain specialists. Its analgesia lasts a reliable 4h and is easier to titrate than opioids with a longer half-life. Set up a 4-hourly regimen which prevents the occurrence of pain (see above).
- As the pain ↓, the patient can be switched to ibuprofen and paracetamol. Supplementation of morphine with an NSAID allows the morphine dose to be reduced.
- See Fig. 18.1.

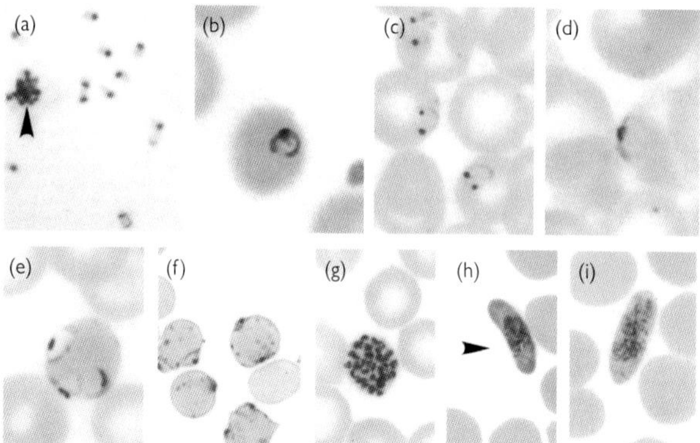

Plate 1 *Plasmodium falciparum*. (a) Thick film showing ring trophozoites + schizont (arrow); and thin films showing: ring trophozoites [(b) to (f)]—note the single and double chromatin dots, multiply infected erythrocytes, accolé form (d) and Maurer's clefts (f); schizont (g); macrogametocyte (h); and microgametocyte (i). Reproduced from WHO Bench Aids for the Diagnosis of Malaria Infections, 2nd ed.

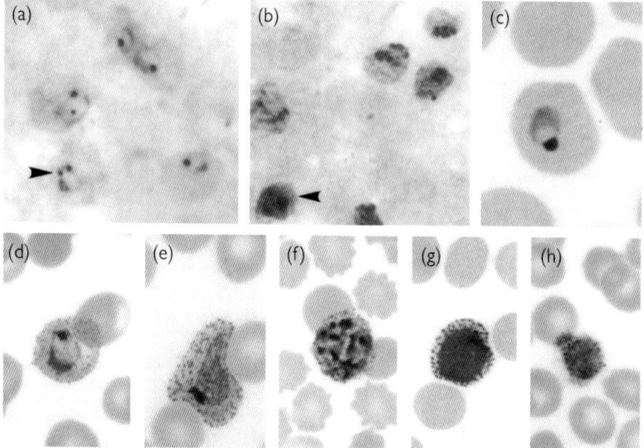

Plate 2 *Plasmodium vivax*. Thick films (a) and (b) showing ring forms; and thin films showing: ring trophozoites of varying size and shape [(c) to (e)], schizont (f), microgametocyte (g), and macrogametocyte (h). Note Schüffner's dots seen as stippling in the surface of the erythrocyte. Reproduced from WHO Bench Aids for the Diagnosis of Malaria Infections, 2nd ed.

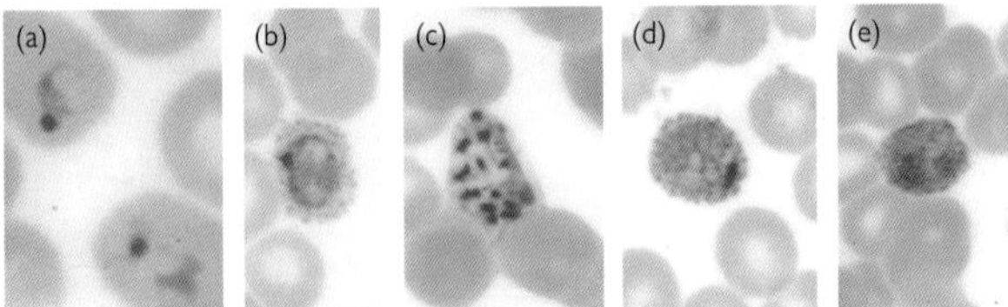

Plate 3 *Plasmodium ovale*. (a) and (b) Thin films showing trophozoites; (c) schizont; (d) microgametocyte and; (e) macrogametocyte. Reproduced from WHO Bench Aids for the Diagnosis of Malaria Infections, 2nd ed.

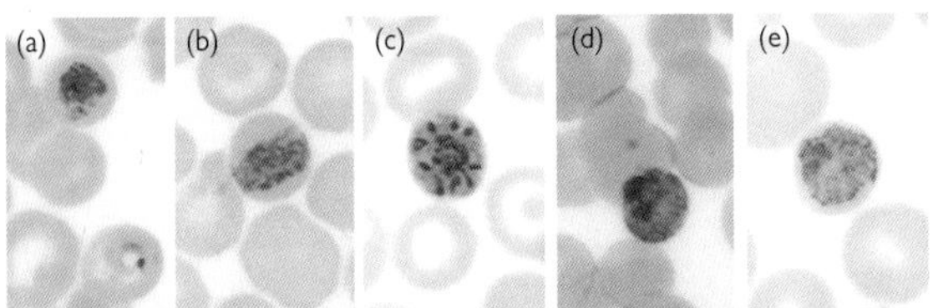

Plate 4 *Plasmodium malariae*. (a) Thin films showing trophozoites, including (b) band form; (c) schizont; (d) microgametocyte and; (e) macrogametocyte. Reproduced from WHO Bench Aids for the Diagnosis of Malaria Infections, 2nd ed.

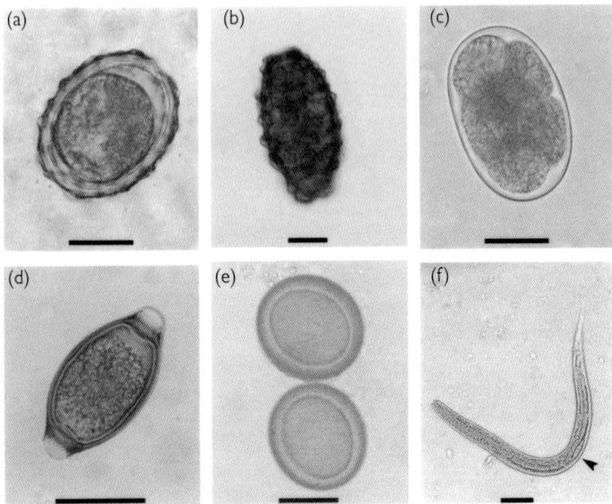

Plate 5 Faecal parasites 1. (a) Ascaris egg (fertile); (b) Ascaris egg (infertile); (c) Hookworm egg; (d) Trichuris egg; (e) Taenia eggs; (f) Rhabtidiform larva of *Strongyloides stercoralis*. [Scale: bar = 25 μm]. Reproduced from WHO Bench Aids for the Diagnosis of Faecal Parasites.

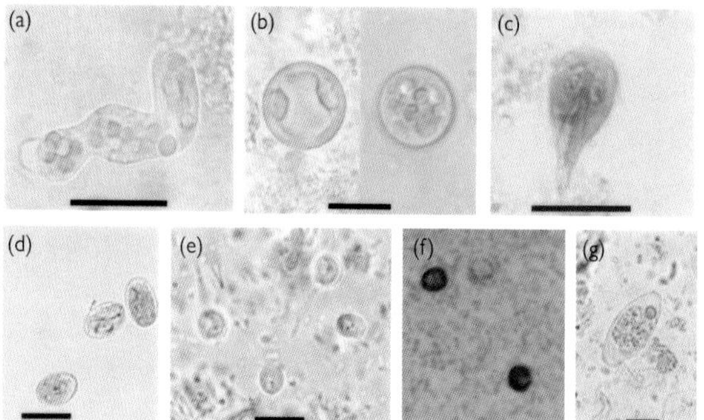

Plate 6 Faecal parasites 2. (a) *Entamoeba histolytica* trophozoite (note phagocytosed erythrocytes); (b) *E. histolytica* cysts; (c) *Giardia lamblia* trophozoite; (d) *G. lamblia* cysts; (e) *Cryptosporidium parvum* oocysts (wet prep); (f) *Cryptosporidium parvum* oocysts (Ziehl–Neelsen stain); (g) *Isospora belli* cyst. [Scale: bar = 10 μm]. Reproduced from WHO Bench Aids for the Diagnosis of Faecal Parasites.

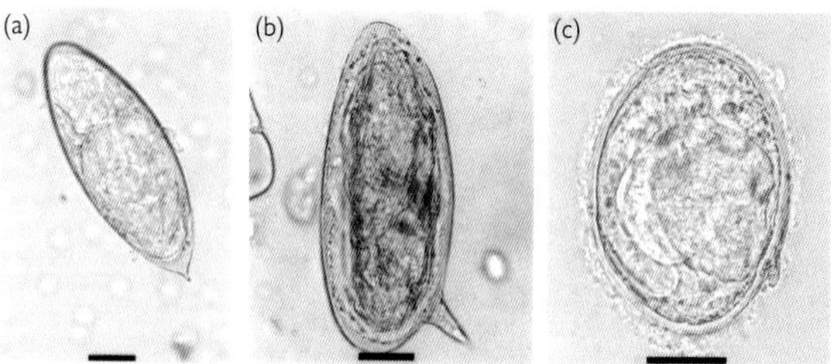

Plate 7 Schistosomiasis eggs. (a) *S. haematobium* (in urine); (b) *S. mansoni* (in stool); (c) *S. japonicum* (in stool). [Scale: bar = 25 μm]. Reproduced from WHO Bench Aids for the Diagnosis of Faecal Parasites.

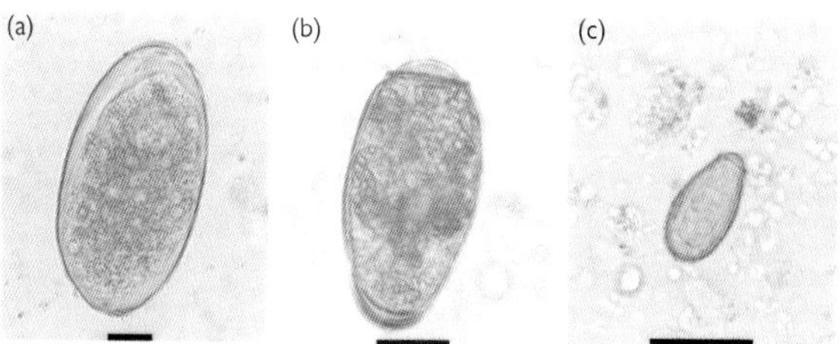

Plate 8 Other trematodes. (a) *Fasciola hepatica* egg; (b) *Paragonimus westermani* egg; (c) *Clonorchis sinensis* egg. [Scale: bar = 25 μm]. Reproduced from WHO Bench Aids for the Diagnosis of Faecal Parasites.

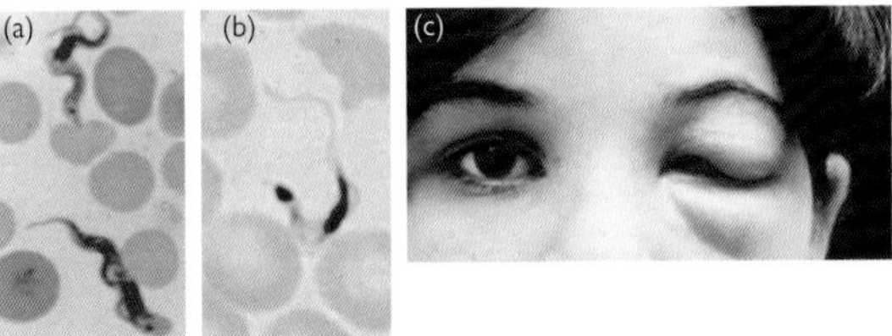

Plate 9 Trypanosomes. (a) *Trypanosoma b. rhodesiense* (Giemsa); (b) *Trypanosoma cruzi* (Leishman stain); (c) Romaña's sign (unilateral oedema and conjunctivitis at the portal of entry in acute Chagas' disease). (c) Reproduced from WHO/TDR Image library http://www.who.int/tdr/tropical_diseases/databases/imagelib.pl?imageid=9305157

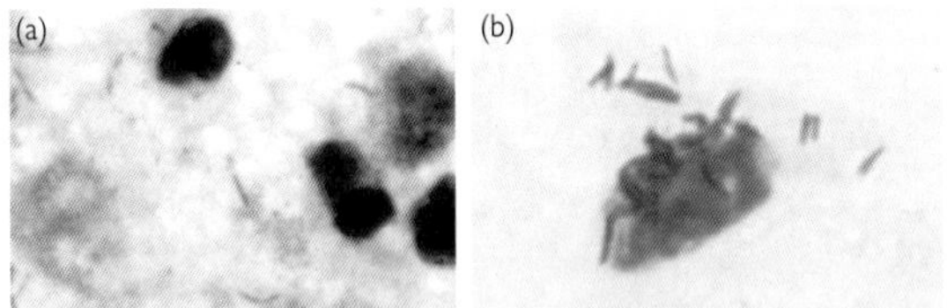

Plate 10 Mycobacteria. (a) *M. tuberculosis* in sputum smear; (b) *M. leprae* in skin smear—note acid-fast bacilli in and around macrophage (both Ziehl–Neelson stain). Oxford Handbook of Tropical Medicine 2e.

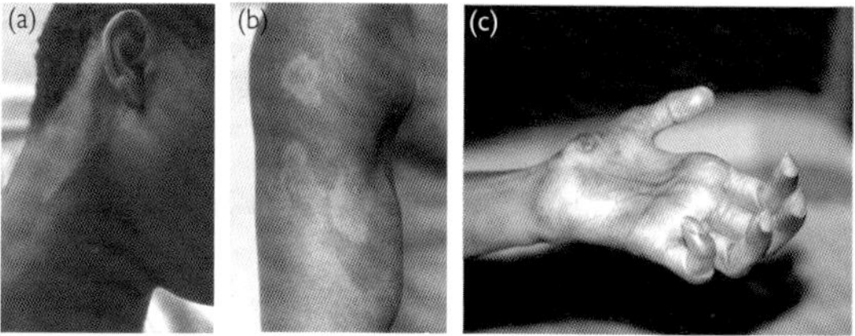

Plate 11 Leprosy. (a) Thickened greater auricular nerve; and (b) hypopigmentation in tuberculoid leprosy; (c) typical deformity and neuropathic ulcer in lepromatus leprosy. (a) Courtesy of Robert Davidson; (b) Courtesy of Anthony Bryceson; (c) Reproduced from WHO http://medicine.plosjournals.org/perlserv/?request=slideshow&type=figure&doi=10.1371/journal.pmed.0020341&id=41756

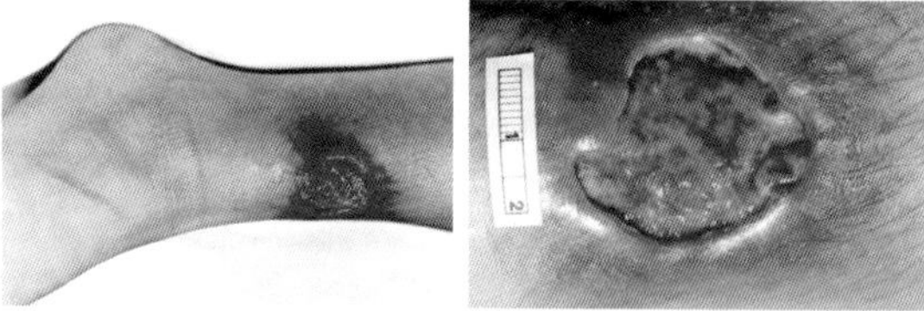

Plate 12 Buruli ulcer. Note the undermined edges of the ulcer. Reproduced from PLoS (http://medicine.plosjournals.org/perlserv?request=slideshow&type=figure&doi=10.1371/journal.pmed.0020108&id=25784)

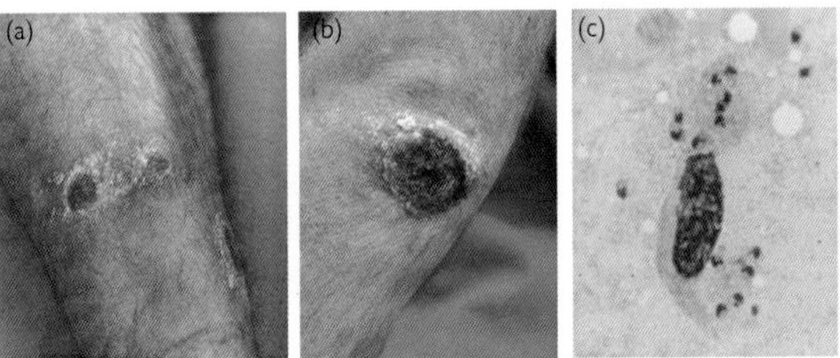

Plate 13 Leishmaniasis. (a) Leg and (b) elbow with cutaneous leishmaniasis from Belize due to *Leishmania braziliensis*; (c) *Leishmania* amastigotes in slit skin smear. Courtesy of Rob Davidson.

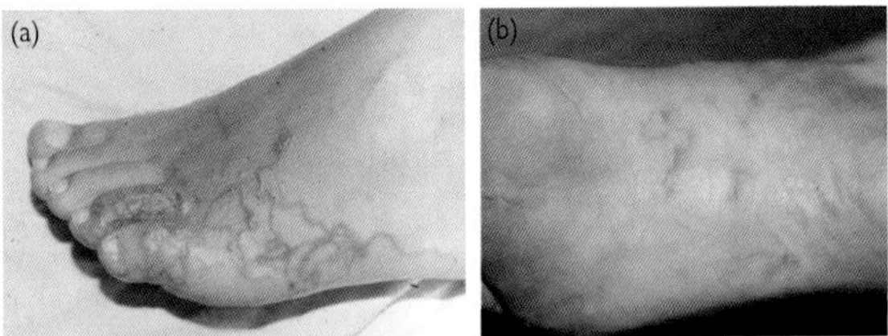

Plate 14 Cutaneous larva migrans. (a) Courtesy of Anthony Bryceson; (b) Courtesy of Terence Ryan.

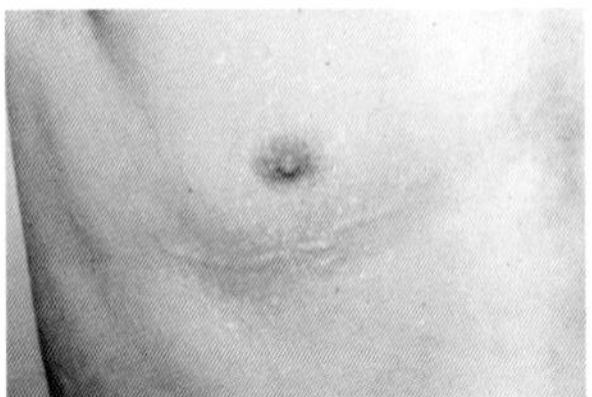

Plate 15 Larva currens. Courtesy of Anthony Bryceson.

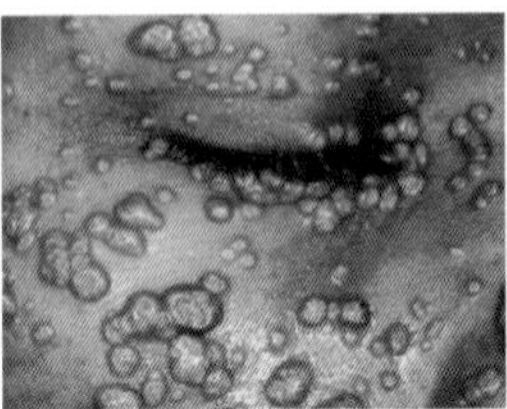

Plate 16 Molluscum contagiosum. Reproduced from Cotell SL, Roholt NS. Images in clinical medicine. *Molluscum contagiosum in a patient with the acquired immunodeficiency syndrome*. N Engl J Med. 1998;338:888, with permission.

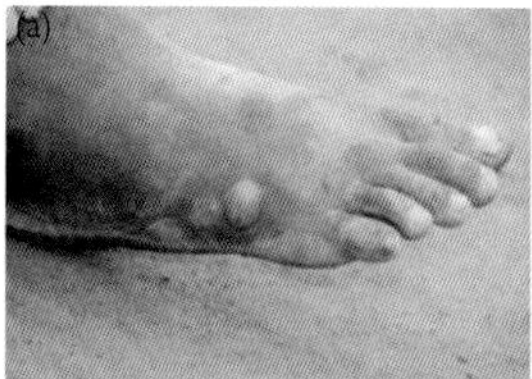
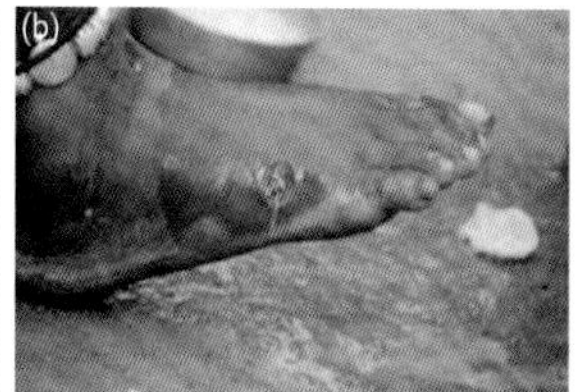

Plate 17 Dracunculiasis. The female guinea worm induces a painful blister (a), through which she protrudes (b) to lay her eggs when water is poured over the site. Reproduced from CDC ☞ www.dpd.cdc.gov/dpdx/HTML/ImageLibrary/Dracunculiasis_il.htm

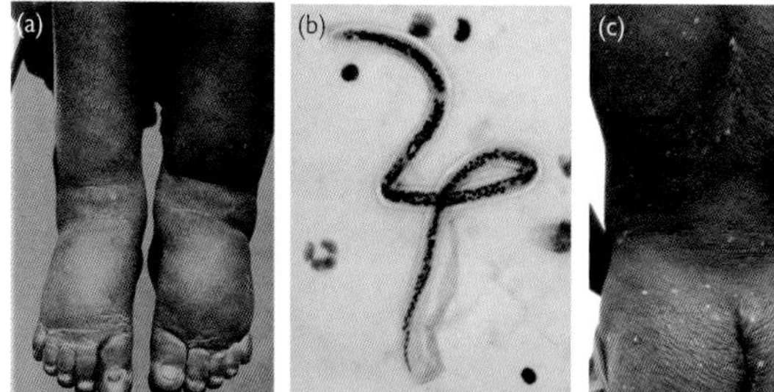

Plate 18 Filaria. (a) Lymphoedema (elephantiasis), due to (b) *Wuchereria bancrofti* (blood smear, haematoxylin); (c) onchocerciasis—chronic papular onchodermatitis. (a) and (c) Courtesy of Anthony Bryceson. (b) Reproduced from CDC ☞ http://www.dpd.cdc.gov/dpdx/HTML/ImageLibrary/Filariasis_il.htm

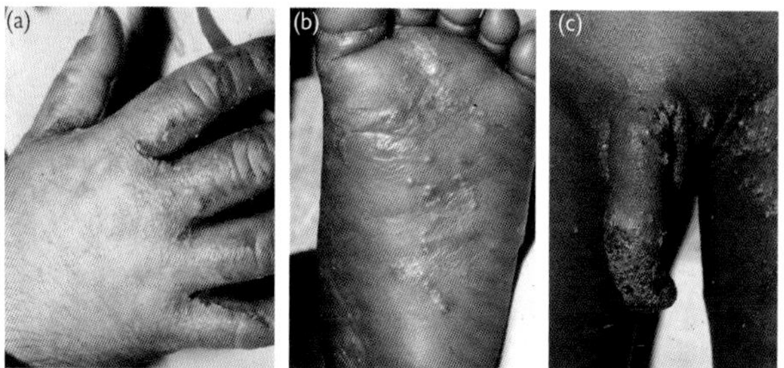

Plate 19 Scabies. (a) Hand (note predilection for web spaces), (b) foot, (c) groin. Reproduced from TALC Bench Aids for Dermatology, with permission.

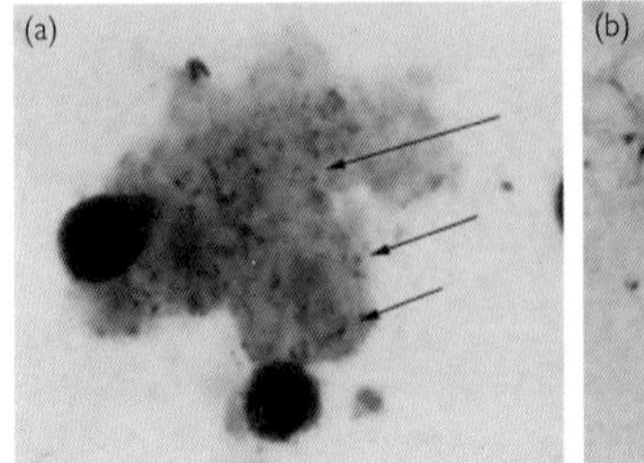

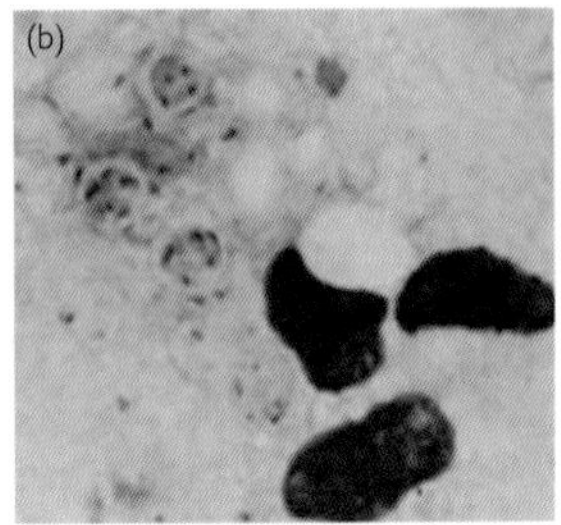

Plate 20 Pneumocystis pneumonia (PCP). (a) *Pneumocystis jirovecii* trophozoites in bronchoalveolar lavage (BAL) from patient with HIV (Giemsa). The trophozoites are small (1–5 μm), and only their nuclei, stained purple, are visible (arrows). (b) 3 *Pneumocystis jirovecii* cysts in BAL (Giemsa stain). The rounded cysts (4–7 μm) contain 6 to 8 intracystic bodies, whose nuclei are stained by Giemsa; the walls of the cysts are not stained; note the presence of several smaller, isolated trophozoites. Reproduced from CDC ℛ http://www.dpd.cdc.gov/dpdx/HTML/ImageLibrary/Pneumocystis_il.htm

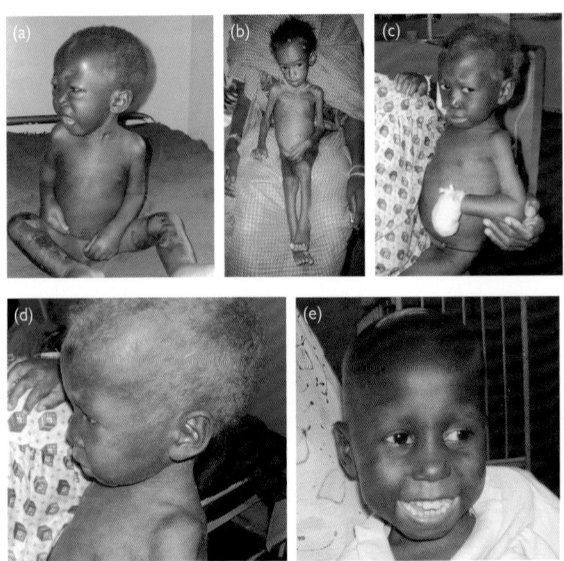

Plate 21 Malnutrition. (a) kwashiorkor—miserable affect, periorbital and limb oedema, protuberant belly, skin and hair changes; (b) marasmus—severe wasting; (c) & (d) marasmus-kwashiorkor—wasting, hair changes, and early skin changes in axilla and groin; (e) is the same child one month later after nutritional rehabilitation. (a), (c) – (e) Andrew Brent; (b) Rob Davidson.

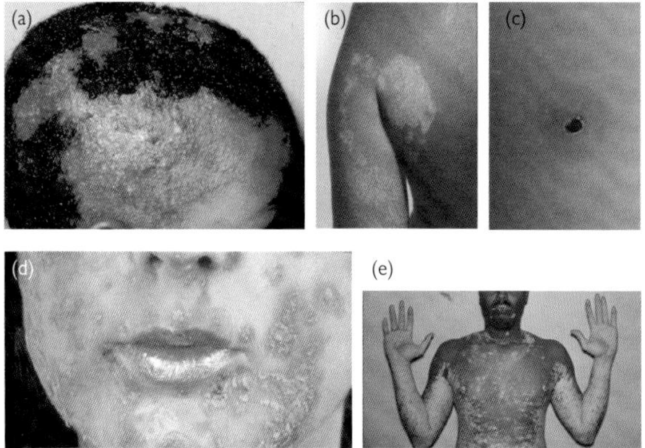

Plate 22 Miscellaneous dermatology. (a) Tinea capitis; (b) tinea corporis; (c) Rickettsial eschar (African tick bite fever); (d) impetigo; (e) vitiligo. (a) TALC Bench Aids for Dermatology; (b), (d), (e) Terence Ryan; (c) Andrew Brent.

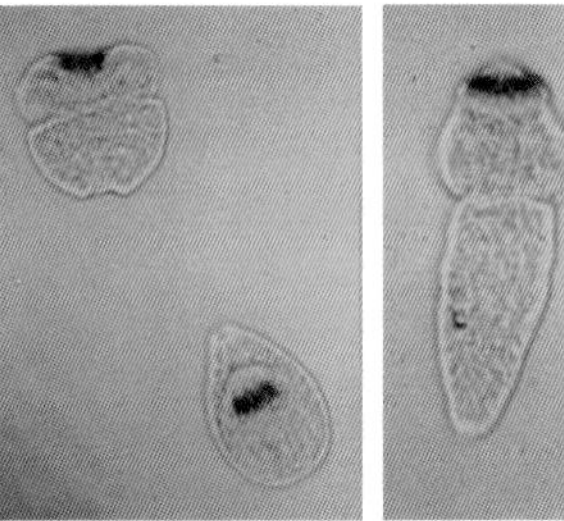

Plate 23 Hydatid sand. *Echinococcus granulosus* protoscolices in hydatid cyst fluid. Reproduced from CDC 🖱 http://www.dpd.cdc.gov/dpdx/HTML/ImageLibrary/Echinococcosis_il.htm

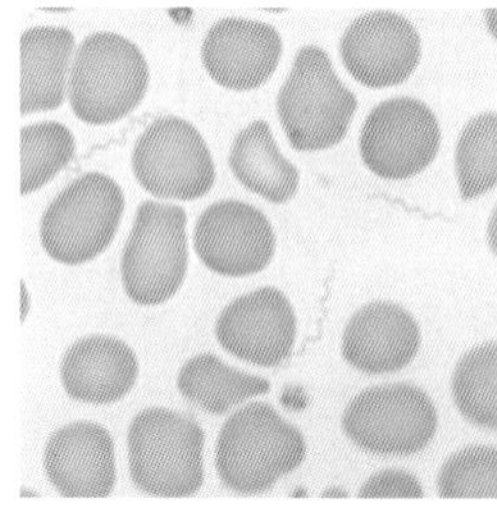

Plate 24 *Borrelia recurrentis* spirochaetes in blood film. Reproduced from 🖱 http://library.med.utah.edu/WebPath/COW/COW077.html

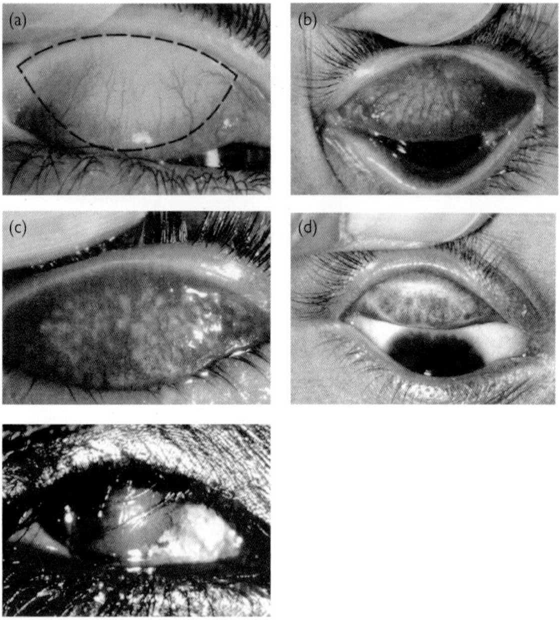

Plate 25 Trachoma. (a) Normal tarsal conjunctiva (area to be examined outlined by dotted line); (b) follicular trachomatous inflammation (>5 follicles in the upper tarsal conjunctiva); (c) intense trachomatous inflammation (inflammatory thickening partially obscures numerous follicles; (d) trachomatous scarring (white bands or sheets in the tarsal conjunctiva); (e) trachomatous trichiasis and corneal opacity (eyelashes rub on cornea which eventually clouds).

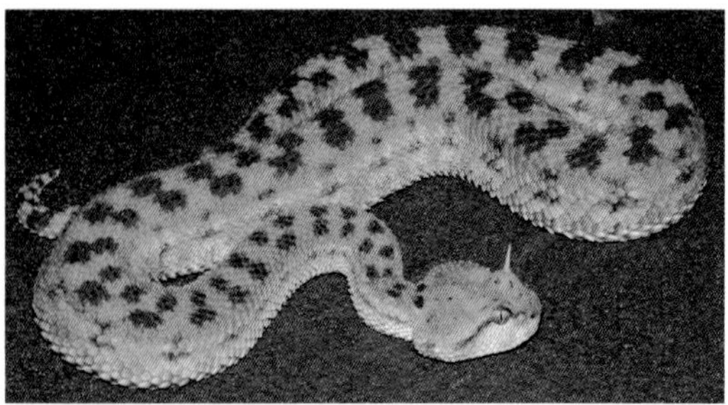

Plate 26 Saharan horned viper (*Cerastes cerastes*) specimen from Egypt. The commonest cause of venomous snake-bite throughout the Sahel region and some Middle Eastern countries. Not all specimens have the supra-ocular horns. Venom causes local swelling, blood clotting disorders, and acute kidney injury. Picture courtesy of Prof David Warrell.

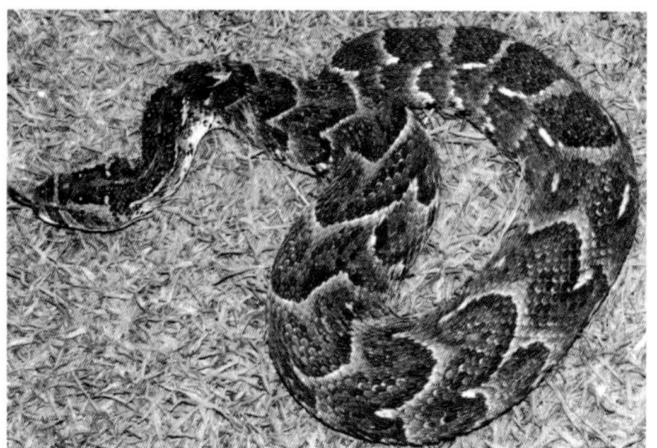

Plate 27 Puff adder (*Bitis arietans*) specimen from Babile, Ethiopia. The commonest cause of venomous snake-bite throughout the savannah region of Africa. Distinguished by the 'U' or 'V' markings down its back. Causes shock and severe local envenoming often leading to necrosis. Picture courtesy of Prof David Warrell.

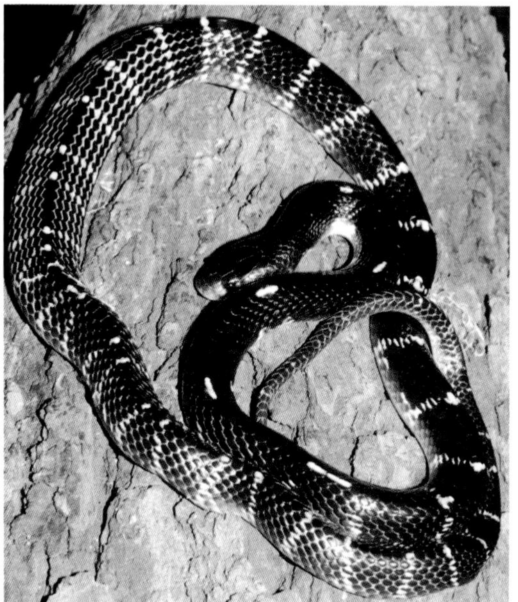

Plate 28 Common krait (*Bungarus caeruleus*) specimen from Pune, India. One of the commonest causes of fatal snake-bites throughout South Asia. Black with a white belly and paired narrow dorsal white bands. It bites people who are sleeping on the floor of their dwellings, causing severe abdominal pain and descending paralysis. Picture courtesy of Prof David Warrell.

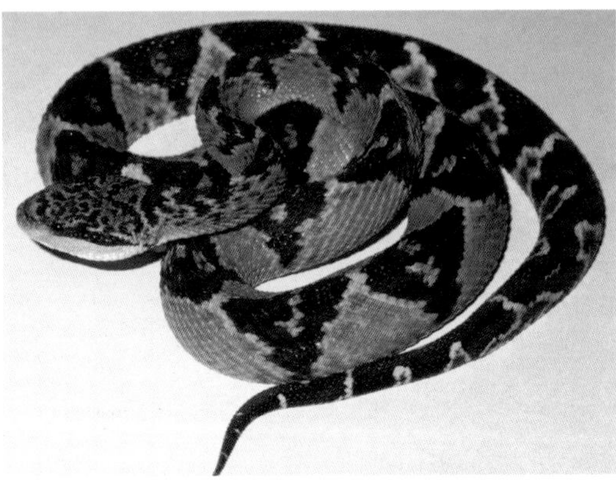

Plate 29 Bushmaster (*Lachesis muta rhombeatus*) specimen from Alagoas, Brazil. The Western hemisphere's longest venomous snake, growing up to 3.5 m in length. Its rough skin is likened to a pineapple or jack fruit. Its venom causes shock, myocardial damage, gastrointestinal symptoms, and blood clotting disorders. Picture courtesy of Prof David Warrell.

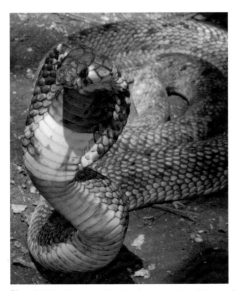

Plate 30 Egyptian cobra (*Naja haje*) specimen from Watamu, Kenya: Cleopatra's 'asp'. It occurs in many colour varieties and is favoured by snake charmers throughout Africa, some of whom it has killed. Its venom causes descending paralysis. Picture courtesy of Prof David Warrell.

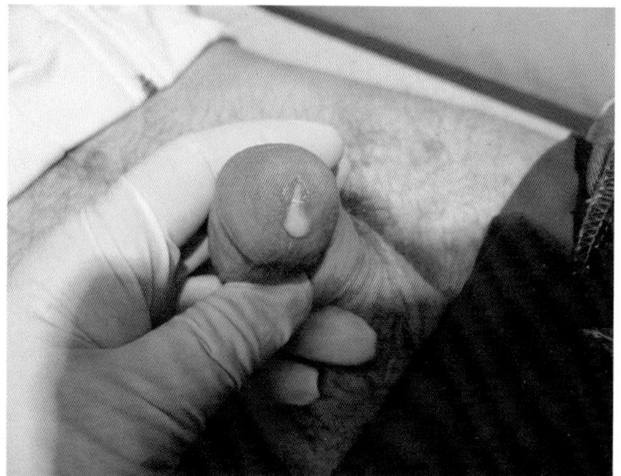

Plate 31 Gonorrhoea causing urethral discharge. Picture courtesy of Melbourne Sexual Health Centre (www.mshc.org.au), Alfred Health, Melbourne, Australia, reference ☞ http://stiatlas.org/

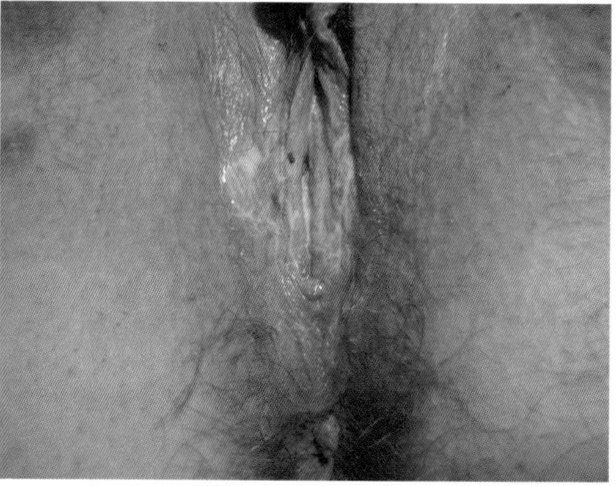

Plate 32 Vaginal discharge (BV). Picture courtesy of Melbourne Sexual Health Centre (www.mshc.org.au), Alfred Health, Melbourne, Australia, reference ☞ http://stiatlas.org/

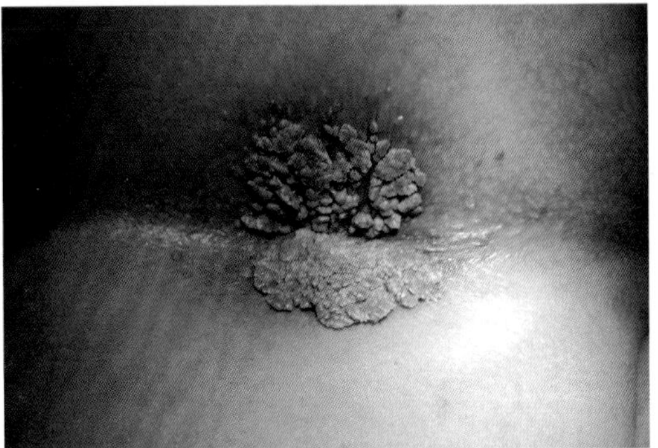

Plate 33 Genital warts. Picture courtesy of Melbourne Sexual Health Centre (www.mshc.org.au), Alfred Health, Melbourne, Australia, reference ☞ http://stiatlas.org/

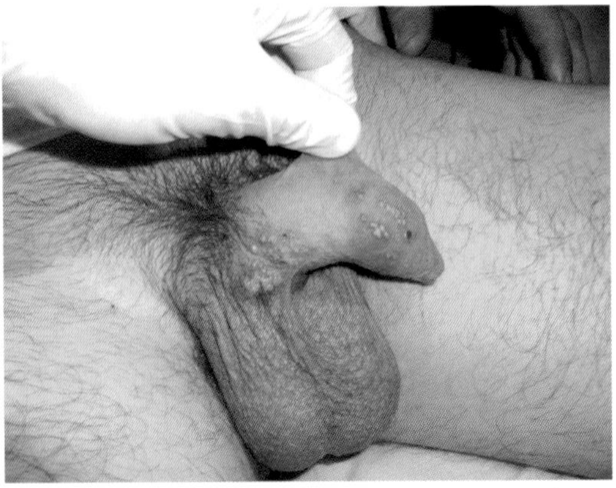

Plate 34 HSV. Picture courtesy of Melbourne Sexual Health Centre (www.mshc.org.au), Alfred Health, Melbourne, Australia, reference ☞ http://stiatlas.org/

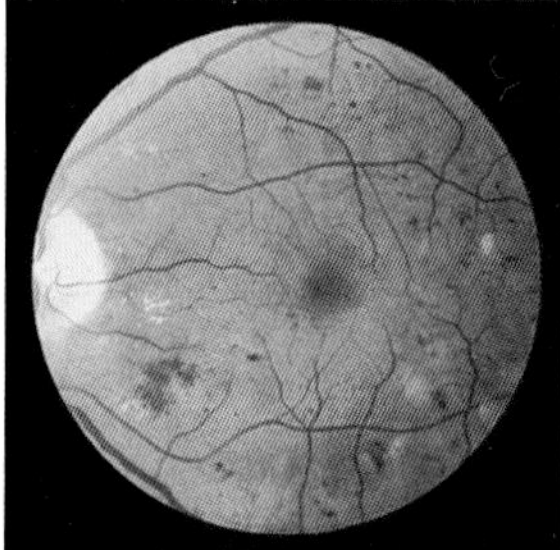

Plate 35 Diabetic, background retinopathy. The hallmarks of background retinal changes are red dots (either microaneurysms or small haemorrhages) and blots (larger haemorrhages) together with glinting hard exudates which are no closer than one disc diameter from the central fovea and vision is normal. Reproduced from Warrell, D, et al, Oxford Textbook of Medicine 5e (2010), with permission from Oxford University Press.

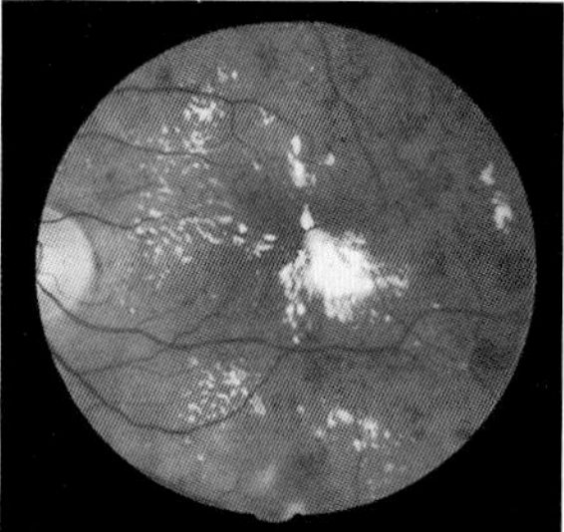

Plate 36 Diabetic, maculopathy. Hard exudate, containing lipid and protein which has leaked from damaged retinal capillaries, has congregated at the fovea. Central vision is irretrievably impaired. Diabetes may present in this way, especially in the elderly. Reproduced from Warrell, D, et al, Oxford Textbook of Medicine 5e (2010), with permission from Oxford University Press.

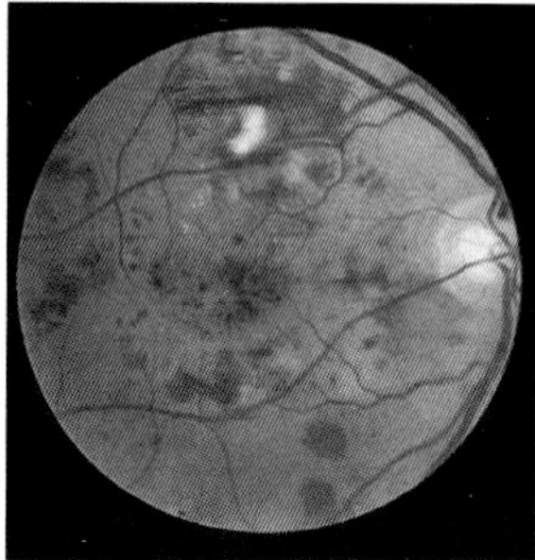

Plate 37 Diabetic, ischaemic retinopathy. Capillary ischaemia creates multiple cotton wool spots—microinfarcts within the nerve fibre layer. Other features are dilatation of retinal veins and multiple blot haemorrhages. Frank proliferation of new vessels is almost inevitable and the retinal changes must be carefully observed. Reproduced from Warrell, D, et al, Oxford Textbook of Medicine 5e (2010), with permission from Oxford University Press.

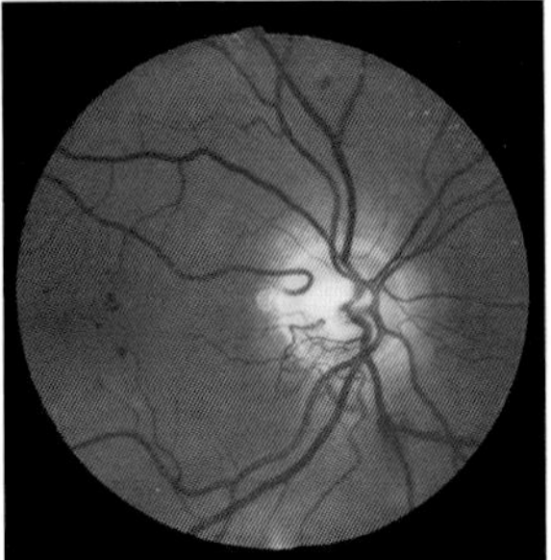

Plate 38 Diabetic, proliferative retinopathy. New vessels have formed on the inferior part of the optic disc. They are fine, looping, and aimless. There may be others in the peripheral retina. If the vessels bleed, vision will become acutely obscured by 'floaters'. Reproduced from Warrell, D, et al, Oxford Textbook of Medicine 5e (2010), with permission from Oxford University Press.

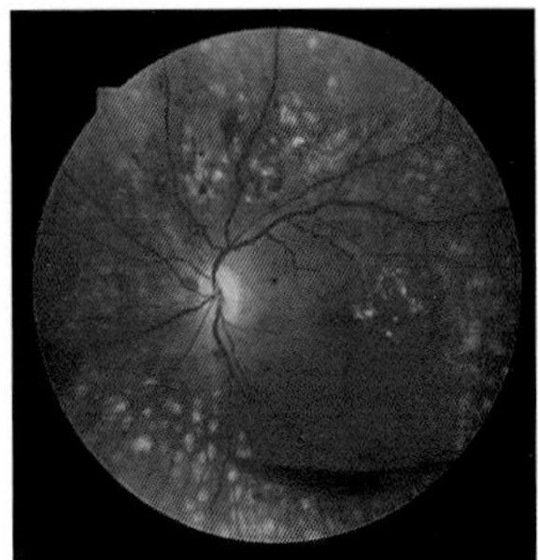

Plate 39 Diabetic, preretinal haemorrhage and laser scars. Neovascular fronds may bleed in front of the retina or into the vitreous, obscuring vision acutely. Here blood has sedimented into a characteristic 'boat' shape and multiple laser scars have been placed outside the major vascular arcades. There are haemorrhages and hard exudate temporal to the fovea. Reproduced from Warrell, D, et al, Oxford Textbook of Medicine 5e (2010), with permission from Oxford University Press.

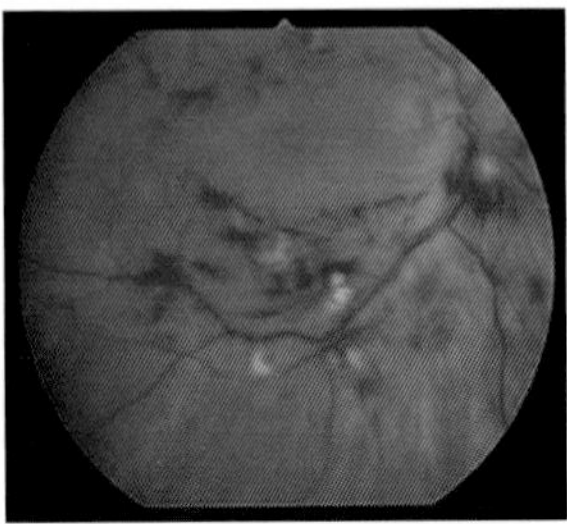

Plate 40 Hypertension, accelerated. Multiple flame shaped haemorrhages, microinfarcts, and swelling of the optic disc margin are characteristic features of accelerated hypertension. Vision may be normal, yet the changes dictate immediate treatment to reduce blood pressure. The diastolic level is usually greater than 110 mmHg and proteinuria is to be expected. Reproduced from Warrell, D, et al, Oxford Textbook of Medicine 5e (2010), with permission from Oxford University Press.

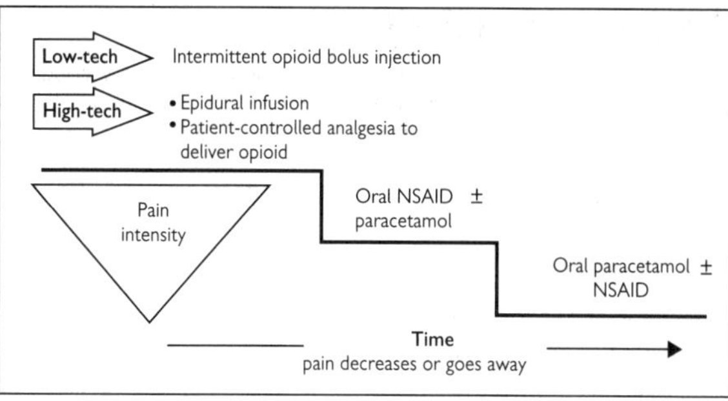

Fig. 18.1 Overview of the management of acute severe pain.

Rheumatoid arthritis

Rheumatoid arthritis (RA) is a chronic, systemic inflammatory condition of unknown cause that primarily involves joints. It is associated with disability, accelerated atherosclerosis, and ↑ mortality. Lack of treatment and poor response to treatment → permanent joint destruction and deformity. Onset usually in the 3rd to 5th decade and RA affects women 2–3 × more frequently than men.

Clinical features

Symptoms Joint pain, swelling, and morning stiffness.

Clinical signs Usually chronic symmetrical joint swelling (often proximal interphalangeal (PIPs), metacarpophalangeal (MCP)s, metatarsophalangeal (MTPs), wrists, knees; affects the cervical but not the lumbar spine.

Extra-articular disease

Anaemia of chronic disease, subcutaneous nodules (usually extensor), fatigue, pleuropericarditis, myocarditis, lymphadenopathy, nerve entrapment (e.g. carpal tunnel syndrome), mononeuritis multiplex, splenomegaly, episcleritis, scleritis, Sjögrens syndrome, interstitial lung disease, vasculitis, and coronary artery disease.

Complications

Patients with longstanding RhA and poor disease control may → irreversible joint damage and deformity, ↓ functional capacity and atlanto-axial instability. Premature death is mainly attributed to atherosclerosis and infection.

Diagnosis

By history and physical examination. There is no definitive test (see Box 18.3). The American College of Rheumatology (ACR) and the European League Against Rheumatism (EULAR) have proposed new classification criteria for patients with at least 1 joint with definite clinical synovitis not better explained by other disease (see Box 18.4).

X-rays Affected joints may show typical changes (soft tissue swelling, symmetric joint space narrowing, bone erosions, and deformities).

Immunology

Rheumatoid factor (RhF) is +ve in ~80% (false +ve in 5% of healthy people, more often in old age, chronic infections, liver disease, fibrotic lung disease, and other rheumatic diseases). Anti-citrullinated peptide antibodies (ACPA) and RhF have similar sensitivity, but ACPA are more specific (95%).

Management

- *Non-pharmacologic:* patient education, aerobic and resistance exercise, physical and occupational therapy, stop smoking.
- *Pharmacologic:* disease-modifying anti-rheumatic drugs (DMARDs) are critical to prevent permanent damage. They should be prescribed as early as possible and are often needed lifelong. Monitoring for drug

toxicity is needed (see Table 18.4). DMARDs are used alone or in combination for disease control. Most widely used are methotrexate, sulfasalazine, and antimalarials = chloroquine and hydroxychloroquine. A common combination is methotrexate + sulfasalazine + hydroxychloroquine. Other DMARDs include leflunomide and biologic agents. Biological agents include anti-TNF drugs (infliximab, etanercept, adalimumab, golimumab, or certolizumab pegol), anti-CD-20 (rituximab), CTLA-4 Ig (abatacept), and anti IL-6 (tocilizumab). The anti-IL-1 agent (anakinra) is not as efficacious. All are extremely expensive. Rarely used DMARDs include: gold salts, minocycline, penicillamine, ciclosporin and azathioprine.

- *Oral NSAIDs:* ↓ pain and swelling; they only provide symptomatic relief and do not affect outcome, and if used, should always be used with DMARDs.
- *Corticosteroids:* can be used orally in low-doses (equivalent to <7.5mg of prednisolone/d) or as intra-articular injections. If steroids are used, it should be in low doses, in combination with a DMARD, and with a plan to slowly taper to lowest dose of steroid required.
- *Surgery:* for deformity and complications.

Contraindications to drugs for RhA

- *NSAIDs:* GI bleed, peptic ulcer; if past history of GI bleed or ulcer and NSAID required combine with a proton pump inhibitor (PPI) e.g. omeprazole.
- *Methotrexate:* pregnancy, elevated creatinine, alcohol use, liver disease, abnormal LFTs, HIV, HBV, HCV.
- *Sulfasalazine:* allergy to sulfas, G6PD deficiency.

Box 18.3 Differential diagnosis of RhA

- Acute viral polyarthritis: caused by hepatitis, rubella.
- *Parvovirus:* self-limited (weeks); history of rash IgM viral antibodies.
- Connective tissue diseases: symmetric polyarthritis without joint deformities. Look for other multi-systemic features (e.g. SLE).
- *Septic arthritis:* usually acute monoarthritis. Immediate joint aspirate (for Gram and stain, crystals, culture) and antibiotics are required to prevent permanent joint damage.
- *Fibromyalgia:* diffuse pain without inflammation. Insomnia and fatigue are common features.
- *Reactive arthritis:* asymmetric oligoarthritis, sausage digits. Look for urethritis, conjunctivitis, and history of enteric infection.
- *Gout/pseudogout:* acute attacks. In gout, monoarthritis of the 1st MTP is common. Definitive diagnosis made by finding crystals in synovial fluid.
- Osteoarthritis (see 🕮 Osteoarthritis, p. 745).
- Paraneoplastic syndromes.
- HIV-associated arthritis.

Box 18.4 2010 ACR/EULAR classification criteria for RhA

A score of ≥6/10 is diagnostic of RhA.

- Number and site of involved joints:
  - 2–10 large joints = 1 point
  - 1–3 small joints = 2 points
  - 4–10 small joints = 3 points.
  - >10 joints (at least one small joint) = 5 points
- Serological abnormality (RhF or ACPA):
  - low +ve RhF or ACPA = 2 points
  - high +ve RhF or ACPA = 3 points.
- *Elevated acute phase reactant:* abnormal CRP or abnormal ESR = 1 point.
- Symptom duration ≥6wks = 1 point.

Table 18.4 Monitoring of drugs commonly used to treat RhA

Drug (usual doses)	Monitoring
NSAIDs	FBC +/– yearly LFT and creatinine
Methotrexate (15–25mg once a week)	FBC, LFT, albumin, creatinine at 2–4wks then every 8wks
Chloroquine (150mg [base] od*)	Fundoscopy and visual fields every 12mths
Hydroxychloroquine (400mg od)	Fundoscopy and visual fields every 12mths
Sulfasalazine (max 3g od)	FBC 2–4-weekly for 3mths, then 3-monthly

*Note: chloroquine base 150mg = chloroquine sulphate 200mg = chloroquine phosphate 250mg

Osteoarthritis

Osteoarthritis (OA) is a chronic, non-inflammatory arthropathy that can be idiopathic or 2° to trauma or other conditions.

Symptoms

Non-inflammatory joint pain (see Box 18.5). The knees, hips, and distal interphalangeal (DIPs) are most commonly affected. If unusual joints are involved (elbows, ankles, MCPs) look for 2° causes: previous trauma, haemochromatosis, Wilson's disease, or reconsider diagnosis (could be RA).

Clinical signs Bony swelling, crepitus.

Diagnosis By history and physical exam.

X-ray findings Non-uniform joint space narrowing, osteophytes, and juxta-articular osteosclerosis.

Management

- *Non-pharmacological:* patient education (↓ weight if obese, exercise to strengthen muscles around affected joint), physical and occupational therapy.
- *Analgesia:* paracetamol +/– NSAID.
- Intra-articular hyaluronans.
- Intra-articular glucocorticoids.
- Topical NSAIDs.
- Surgery including prosthetic joint replacement.

Box 18.5 Characteristics of joint pain and type of arthritis

Inflammatory, e.g. RA	*Non-inflammatory, e.g. OA*
• Pain ↓ with activity.	• Pain ↑ by activity.
• Worse in the morning.	• Worse at night.
• Morning stiffness >60 minutes.	• Morning stiffness <30 minutes.
• Systemic features: sometimes.	• Systemic features: absent.
• Soft swelling (effusion).	• Hard swelling ('bony').
• Sometimes erythema.	• No erythema.
• Sometimes warmth.	• No warmth.

Systemic lupus erythematosus

Multisystem chronic inflammatory disease, characterized by facial rash, photosensitivity, alopecia, nephritis, serositis, non-erosive arthritis, CNS involvement, vasculitis, and fever. Aetiology unknown. Women affected 10× more often than men; peak incidence 15–40yrs of age. Causes of death include infections and disease activity in early phases of the disease, and atherosclerosis in the long-term (see 🕮 Dermatology, p. 610, for details on cutaneous lupus erythematosus).

Clinical features

- *General:* fever, fatigue, ↓ weight, Raynaud's phenomenon.
- *Joints:* arthralgia/arthritis (similar to RA, but usually non-erosive).
- *Skin:* photosensitive rash, purpura, alopecia, livedo reticularis, mouth ulcers.
- *Renal:* nephritic or nephrotic syndrome; renal failure.
- *Neurological:* cognitive defects, psychosis, seizures.
- *Serositis:* pleural and pericardial effusion.
- *Pulmonary:* pneumonitis, fibrosis, bronchiolitis.
- *Cardiovascular:* hypertension, pericarditis, sterile (Libman–Sacks) endocarditis.
- *Blood:* normocytic anaemia, haemolysis (Coombs +ve), leukopenia, thrombocytopenia.
- *Thrombosis and miscarriage:* may be part of the antiphospholipid antibody syndrome.

Laboratory tests

Several auto-antibodies that react with the cell nucleus are a feature of SLE. Anti-nuclear antibodies (ANA) are +ve in > 98% of patients. However, ANA are not specific; patients with other rheumatic conditions or chronic diseases, and 5% of normal subjects can have +ve ANA. Anti-double-stranded DNA and particularly anti-Smith (anti-Sm) antibodies are more specific but less sensitive. Other autoantibodies sometimes present are anti-Ro, anti-La, anti-RNP. Patients can have low complement levels.

Diagnosis

American College of Rheumatology classification criteria for SLE are given in Box 18.6.

Management of SLE

- *Education:* avoid sun, sunscreen, hat, long sleeves, stop smoking, prevent atherosclerotic disease.
- *NSAIDS:* useful for musculoskeletal symptoms and serositis.
- *Antimalarials (chloroquine/hydroxychloroquine):* effective for skin and musculoskeletal symptoms; prevent renal and CNS flares, ↓ risk of thrombosis.
- *Systemic corticosteroids:* prednisolone <0.5mg/kg for moderate disease; higher doses (1mg/kg) for severe or life-threatening disease, e.g. renal disease, pneumonitis, severe cytopenias, or CNS lupus. Consider high-dose IV methylprednisolone 1g boluses for severely ill patients.

Box 18.6 American College of Rheumatology classification criteria

Four or more required to fulfil criteria to diagnose SLE:
- Malar rash.
- Discoid rash.
- Photosensitivity.
- Oral ulcers.
- Arthritis.
- Serositis.
- *Renal involvement:* proteinuria (>0.5g/d) or cellular casts.
- *Neurological disorders:* seizures or psychosis.
- *Haematological disorders:* haemolytic anaemia, leukopenia, lymphopenia or thrombocytopenia.
- *Immunological disorders:* anti-DNA, anti-Sm, or antiphospholipid antibodies (lupus anticoagulant, IgG or IgM anticardiolipins or false +ve serological test for syphilis).
- Anti-nuclear antibody.

- Corticosteroids should be tapered early according to response; combine with steroid-sparing agents to minimize steroid side-effects.
- *Cyclophosphamide:* for severe SLE including proliferative lupus nephritis, vasculitis, CNS involvement, and alveolar haemorrhage.
- *Mycophenolate mofetil:* for lupus nephritis; may be as effective as cyclophosphamide with less adverse events.
- *Azathioprine:* as a steroid-sparing agent.
- *Methotrexate or leflunomide:* for arthritis.
- *Others:* chlorambucil, ciclosporin, and expensive biologics that deplete B-cells: rituximab (anti-CD20 antibody) and belimumab (antibody that binds to soluble B-lymphocyte stimulator).
- *Anticoagulation:* for the antiphospholipid syndrome.
- *Manage co-morbidities:* such as hypertension, diabetes, osteoporosis, and heart disease.

Markers of poor prognosis in patients with SLE

- Diffuse proliferative renal disease.
- Hypertension.
- Male sex.
- Lower socio-economic and education status.
- Black and Hispanic ethnicity.
- Antiphospholipid antibodies.
- Disease activity involving multiple organs.
- Renal failure.

Further reading

Useful website http://www.hopkins-arthritis.org/

Typhoid and paratyphoid fevers

These conditions, also called enteric fever, follow infection with *Salmonella* spp. (*S. enterica typhi* [typhoid]; *S. enterica paratyphi* types A, B, and occasionally C [paratyphoid]). Endemic and important causes of morbidity across developing world. Typhoid and paratyphoid A are most severe; paratyphoid B mildest, with type C falling somewhere in between.

Early antibiotic treatment

Essential to prevent complications and ↓ mortality. Start treatment empirically if clinical suspicion strong. Following ingestion, bacteria survive gastric acid barrier, then penetrate through wall of ileum, probably through M-cells, and pass to mesenteric lymph nodes. After 1° multiplication in mesenteric lymph nodes, bacteria then infect cells of the reticulo-endothelial system where further multiplication occurs, → 2° bacteraemia, infection of multiple organs, and clinical illness. If untreated, ≥10% die from overwhelming toxaemia or 2° organ involvement, particularly encephalopathy, toxic myocarditis, or GI haemorrhage and/or perforation and peritonitis.

For infection control, note that short-term post-typhoid convalescent faecal carriage and chronic asymptomatic gall bladder infection is common. Carriers have highly infectious stools.

Transmission

Via ingestion of food or water contaminated by infected faeces (or occasionally, infected urine). Gastric acid is protective so any condition/drug that ↓ acid production (e.g. proton pump inhibitors) will ↑ susceptibility to infection.

Clinical features

Incubation period is 10–20d; untreated illness typically lasts 4wks (may be longer in severe infections and shorter in mild cases).

- *1st week:* non-specific symptoms—malaise, headache, rising remitting fever with mild cough, constipation or mild diarrhoea, vomiting and abdominal pain.
- *2nd week:* patient becomes 'toxic' and apathetic; often mentally dull (e.g. slow response to questions) or occasionally psychotic (e.g. an agitated, febrile patient admitted to psychiatric ward); sustained high temperature with relative bradycardia; rose spots (2–4-mm pink papules on central torso, fading on pressure) may transiently occur; distended abdomen; hepatomegaly and/or splenomegaly.
- *3rd week:* ↑ toxicity with persistent high temperature; patient becomes delirious and weak with feeble pulse, tachypnoea +/– basal crepitations, profuse 'pea soup' diarrhoea. Look and listen for abdominal distension and bowel sounds. Neurological complications may occur (may rarely be the presenting complaint). If death occurs it is usually during weeks 2, 3, or 4.
- *4th week:* if patient survives, fever, mental state, and abdominal distension gradually improve. Intestinal haemorrhage, perforation, and peritonitis may occur at any time, most commonly in weeks 2–4.

Diagnosis

By culture of bone marrow (~75% culture +ve) or blood (~50% culture +ve). There are ~10× more bacteria/mL of bone marrow than per mL blood. A +ve stool culture, or rectal swab culture, may indicate acute infection but could also represent carriage with the acute illness having another cause. The Widal test is a serological test that measures antibodies against the causative bacteria. It has poor sensitivity and specificity (giving many false +ve and false –ve results) and is not recommended for diagnosis.

Management

- *Give antibiotics:* see Box 18.7.
- *Give dexamethasone:* 3mg/kg IV stat, then 1mg/kg qds for 2d to patients with shock or ↓ consciousness. May ↓ mortality.
- Toxic patients must be observed carefully for signs of GI haemorrhage (treat conservatively and with blood transfusion if significant blood loss) or peritonitis (treat with surgery).

Relapse

5–10% of treated patients relapse after treatment and initial recovery, even if organism is sensitive to antibiotic used. Relapses tend to occur within 1 month of end of treatment. Relapses are generally milder and shorter than 1° illness, but may be equally severe; 2nd and 3rd relapses have been reported, ∴ arrange follow-up if possible. Co-infection with schistosomes may result in chronic or recurrent fever, since bacteria survive within adult worms, protected from antibiotics.

Prevention

Good sanitation and clean water are most important preventative measures. Two vaccines are currently available (📖 Immunization, p. 893).

- Live attenuated oral vaccine (Ty21a) requires 3 doses over 5d with a booster every 5yrs. Not recommended for children <6yrs.
- Purified Vi antigen vaccine, given as a single dose IM; boosters every 3yrs. Not recommended for children <2yrs.

In development are: a modified conjugate Vi vaccine; a single dose attenuated oral vaccine; vaccines for paratyphoid; vaccines for very young children.

Box 18.7 Treatment of typhoid

Initial choice of antibiotics varies due to local resistance. In most areas of the Americas 1st and 2nd line antimicrobials can be used. In many areas of Asia and Africa, infection with MDR strains (resistant to the 1st line antibiotics chloramphenicol, amoxicillin, co-trimoxazole) is common. Infections also occur, particularly in Asia, with ↓ susceptibility to fluoroquinolones (nalidixic acid resistance) or full resistance to fluoroquinolones.

1st line antimicrobials

- Chloramphenicol 1g oral qds for 14–21d.
- Amoxicillin 500mg oral tds for 14d.
- Co-trimoxazole 960mg oral bd for 14d.

MDR strains that remain nalidixic acid susceptible

- Ciprofloxacin 500–750mg oral bd for 7–10d.
- Ofloxacin 400mg oral bd for 7–10d.
- Ceftriaxone 50–80mg/kg IV od for 10–14d.
- Azithromycin 500mg oral od for 7d (not in severe disease).

MDR strains that are nalidixic acid (or fluoroquinolone) resistant

- Ceftriaxone 50–80mg/kg IV od for 10–14d.
- Azithromycin 500mg oral od for 7d (not in severe disease).

In severe disease

- Add dexamethasone 3mg/kg IV stat, then 1mg/kg qds for 2d.
- Dosages for each antibiotic drug can be increased 1.5× initially and given IV.

Public health note

- Typhoid fever vaccination may be offered to travellers, including those visiting friends and relatives, to destinations where risk of typhoid fever is high, especially if staying in endemic areas >1 month or visiting locations where antimicrobial resistant *S. typhi* common.
- Immunization of school-age and/or pre-school children recommended by WHO in areas where typhoid fever has been shown to be a significant public health problem, particularly where antimicrobial resistant *S. typhi* common.
- Whether this should be school- or community-based depends on - age-specific disease incidence, subgroups at particular risk and school enrolment rates.

Rickettsioses

Rickettsioses are zoonoses caused by small intracellular Gram –ve bacilli. Ticks, fleas, or mites act as vectors and/or reservoirs; the commonest is African tick bite fever.

Spotted fever group

Usually transmitted by the bite of ixodid (hard) ticks. Dogs, rodents, and other animals are reservoirs. After 3–14d (usually 5–7d) incubation, fever, headache, muscle pain, rash, local lymphadenopathy, and an inoculation eschar (small ulcer with black centre and red areola) typically develop.

- *Rocky Mountain spotted fever (Rickettsia rickettsii, USA):* frequently severe, with mortality 13–25% in untreated cases. There is no eschar.
- *Boutonneuse fever or Mediterranean spotted fever (Rickettsia conorii, Africa, India, Europe, and the Middle East):* usually less severe, but occasional fatal cases occur, especially in elderly or when treatment has been delayed.
- *Rickettsialpox (Rickettsia akari):* transmitted by mites in eastern USA and former Soviet Union. Rash vesicular. May be confused with chickenpox.
- *African tick bite fever:* most common. More fully described in 📖 African tick bite fever, p. 756; Table 18.5.
- *Flea-borne spotted fever/cat flea typhus (Rickettsia felis):* recently-recognized illness with clinical picture similar to spotted fever group. Transmitted by cat flea.
- *Other types:* Queensland tick typhus, and North Asian tick fever.

Typhus group

Epidemic (louse-borne) typhus fever (Rickettsia prowazekii)

Rickettsia prowazekii is transmitted between humans by the human body louse in cold, unhygienic conditions, particularly during war and famine (see Fig. 18.2). The disease is endemic in mountainous areas in eastern Africa, Mexico, Central and South America, and Asia.

- Rickettsiae are excreted in faeces of infected lice and inoculated into abrasions or bite wound by scratching.
- After 1–2wks incubation, abrupt onset of fever, headache, prostration, myalgia, conjunctival injection, rales. No eschar. Macular rash appears on days 5–6. Fatality ranges from 10–40% (untreated) and with age.
- Brill–Zinsser disease is a milder recrudescent disease, which may occur years later in those who have not been adequately treated.
- In the eastern USA, flying squirrels have been the source of occasional human infections that tend to be milder than classical typhus.

Endemic (flea-borne) typhus fever (Rickettsia typhi)

Transmitted from rats → humans by fleas. Found worldwide, especially in warm, humid climates, where rats and humans co-exist. Rickettsiae transmitted via flea faeces by scratching itchy fleabites. Illness similar to louse-borne typhus, but milder.

Scrub typhus

Scrub typhus (*Orientia tsutsugamushi*) transmitted by the bite of trombiculid mites living in sharply delimited rural and suburban areas ('mite islands') in Central, East, and Southeast Asia, and northern Australia.

- Punched-out eschar develops in ~50% after 6–21d followed by severe acute febrile illness resembling typhus. Deafness and pneumonitis are common. Case fatality varies with infecting strain and ↑ age.
- Unlike other rickettsial illnesses, repeat infections may occur, since immunity does not cross-protect against heterologous strains.

Diagnosis and management of rickettsial infection

Diagnosis

Often clinical in right epidemiological setting, if typical triad of fever, rash, and eschar are present. Can be verified by serology (ideally, immunofluorescence; classical Weil–Felix test is now obsolete); PCR on blood or skin biopsy, or isolation of rickettsiae in cell culture from such samples early in infection, are possible, but not widely available.

Management

Give antibiotics (in severe cases, drugs can be given IV):

- Doxycycline 100mg oral bd or 200mg od for 7–10d is standard therapy for rickettsial infections. In some situations (e.g. louse-borne typhus) a single 200mg dose is sufficient.
- Alternative: chloramphenicol 500mg oral qid for 7–10d.
- Quinolones are effective in boutonneuse fever, but like macrolides, are not recommended for moderate or severe spotted fever infections. They are not effective in scrub typhus.

Paediatric note

Doxycycline favoured for treatment of moderate to severe rickettsial infections in children. Milder infections (e.g. Mediterranean spotted fever) can be treated with newer macrolides, e.g. azithromycin 10mg/kg/day for 3d. Also suggested for treatment of rickettsial infections in pregnant women.

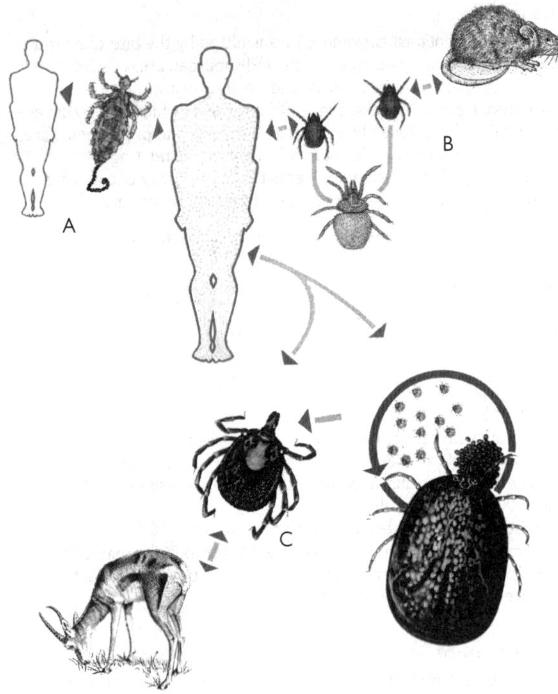

Fig. 18.2 Life cycles of rickettsial infections.

A: *Epidemic (louse-borne) typhus.* Body louse, *Pediculus humanus* feeds on patient infected with *R. prowazekii*; new host is infected when louse faeces are inoculated into skin.

B: *Scrub typhus:* larvae of *trombiculid* mites are infected with *Orientia tsutsugamushi* from feeding on infected animal or trans-ovarially; man accidentally infected when bitten.

C: *African tick-bite fever:* infection with *R. africae* is prevalent in many animal species and sustained in *Amblyomma* ticks trans-ovarially and -stadially; man accidentally infected when bitten.

African tick bite fever

Epidemiology

- Seroprevalence is 70% or higher among adults living in endemic areas in southern Africa. Whereas reports on African tick bite fever in indigenous populations are scarce, the number of reported cases in travellers from Europe and elsewhere has recently ↑ significantly.
- Vectors ixodid *Amblyomma* ticks, mainly *A. variegatum* (the tropical bont tick) and *A. hebraeum* (southern African bont tick; see Fig. 18.4). Infection in ticks is maintained at very high levels (30% to >70%) by

Table 18.5 Signs and symptoms in African tick bite fever

Characteristic		Frequency (%)
Fever		59–100
Headache		62–83
Myalgia		63–87
	Neck muscle myalgia	81
Inoculation eschar		53–100
	Multiple eschars	21–54
Regional lymphadenitis		43–100
Cutaneous rash		15–46
	Maculopapular rash	15–26
	Vesicular rash	0–21
Aphthous stomatitis		11

trans-ovarial transmission (from adult female → offspring) and trans-stadial transmission (from larva → nymph → adult). Ticks aggressive, actively seek mammalian hosts, crawling up the legs before attaching to thin, moist skin especially in folds behind knees, groin, and buttocks.

- Patient has typically walked in long grass, e.g. in game reserve, within 10d preceding onset. Rainy season is time of greatest tick abundance.

Clinical features

- Most patients present with abrupt onset of fever, nausea, fatigue, headache, and myalgia.
- Of note is a prominent neck muscle myalgia with subjective neck stiffness.
- Inoculation eschar is present in most cases but may be overlooked, particularly on dark skin, in hair, or in the anogenital region. Sometimes, non-typical eschars mimicking acne are seen. (see Fig. 18.3).
- Rash typically maculopapular erythema, becoming confluent in areas, with regional lymphadenopathy draining the site of eschar. Rash may be absent or there may occasionally be scattered vesicles. Reactive arthritis occasionally occurs.

Diagnosis In first 10d of illness, ↑ CRP and moderate lymphopenia seen in most cases; ↑ liver enzymes occur in 40% and ↑ platelets in 20%. Diagnosis can be confirmed in most cases by +ve rickettsial serology, but usually only after the acute illness. Serology lacks sensitivity and specificity for *R. africae*.

Treatment Give doxycycline 100mg oral bd for 7d or until 48h without fever; most cases improve in 48h. *Alternatives for pregnant women and young children*—azithromycin. In severe cases, start with doxycycline for a few doses then change to azithromycin. Erythromycin has high failure rate.

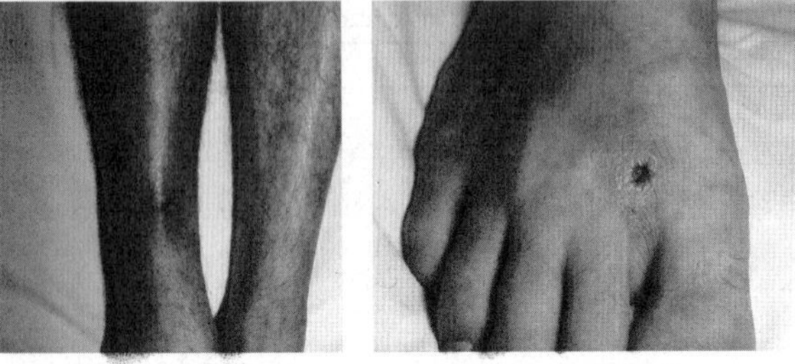

Fig. 18.3 Eschars at the site of vector bites resulting in rickettsial infections. Left: eschar on shin, with surrounding halo of erythema and macular rash in patient with African tick bite fever (*R. africae*). Right: eschar of scrub typhus (*Orientia tsutsugamushi*) without a rash.

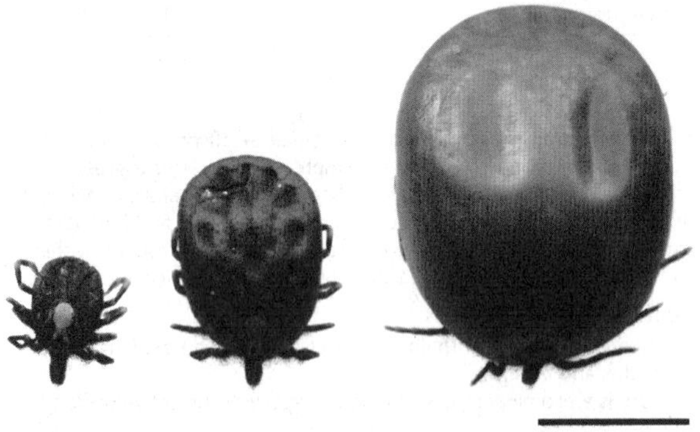

Fig. 18.4 *Amblyomma hebraeum* (vector of African tick bite fever): females at different feeding stages: unfed, partially fed, and fully engorged. (Picture courtesy Alex Smith, University of Alberta, Canada.)

Bartonella

Bartonellas are intracellular bacteria with tropism for red cells and endothelial cells. Clinical features overlap for some species, as below.

- *B. quintana* is transmitted by the human body louse amongst the homeless, those living in crowded, unhygienic conditions, and during war. It causes *trench fever*, chronic bacteraemia, and endocarditis in the immunocompetent, and *bacillary angiomatosis* (BA) in the immunocompromised.
- *B. henselae* is transmitted amongst cats by the cat flea and to humans by cat scratch or bite. It causes *cat scratch disease* (uncommonly, bacteraemia and endocarditis in immunocompetent persons) as well as BA and *peliosis hepatis* in the immunocompromised.
- *B. bacilliformis* is unlike other bartonellas in being transmitted by sandflies in the Andes; it causes *Oroya fever* (especially in tourists and transient workers) and *verruga peruana* (especially amongst natives of the Peruvian Andes). See Box 18.8 for notes.
- Other, unusual species are occasionally associated with *endocarditis* (*B. elizabethae*, *B. vinsonii*) or *cat scratch disease* (*B. clarridgeiae*).

Clinical features

- *Trench fever:* presents with acute onset fever ('5-day fever'), headache, dizziness and shin pain. Most cases are self-limiting, but the course in some patients may be prolonged, and relapsing in others. A minority develops chronic infection (attacks of fever, chronic bacteraemia, endocarditis).
- *Cat scratch disease:* usually presents as a tender, self-limiting (2–3mths) regional lymphadenopathy without fever. Complications are rare (retinitis, encephalopathy, visceral forms).
- *Bacillary angiomatosis and peliosis hepatis:* due to vascular proliferative lesions, respectively, in the skin or liver/spleen, but can involve any organ. Typically occur in immunocompromised (HIV) patients. Skin lesions are nodules or papules which may be red to purple, may ulcerate, or bleed (see Fig. 18.5).
- *Endocarditis* mainly affects middle-aged patients, presenting with fever, emboli, and occasionally glomerulonephritis. Previously normal or damaged valves may be infected.

Diagnosis

- *Serology:* extensive cross-reactions between *B. henselae* and *B. quintana*.
- PCR of lymph node aspirate, tissue biopsy, or blood.
- Culture from blood is possible, but technically difficult.
- For cat scratch disease and bacillary angiomatosis, organisms can be seen in tissue sections stained with Warthin–Starry silver stain (but not Gram or ZN stains).

Management

- *Trench fever:* doxycycline 200mg po od for 4wks plus gentamicin 3mg/kg IV od for the first 2wks.

- *Cat scratch disease:* no therapy unless extensive or complicated: azithromycin 500mg po on day 1 then 250mg po on days 2–5.
- *Bacillary angiomatosis and peliosis hepatis:* azithromycin 250mg po od or erythromycin 500mg po qds for 2–3mths or doxycycline.

Box 18.8 *Bartonella bacilliformis:* Oroya fever and verruga peruana

Clinical features

- *Oroya fever:* has a variable incubation period (~ 2mths) and is characterized by fever and severe anaemia, and in some cases, multiple organ failure. Death is frequently caused by opportunistic bacterial (especially salmonellosis and *Staphylococcus aureus*), protozoal, or viral infections.
- *Verruga peruana:* may follow Oroya fever or occur independently; the classical presentation is that of recurrent crops of erythematous papules, nodules, or angioma-like skin lesions, caused by vascular endothelial proliferation. The verrucae dry up and slough, leaving no scars. Usually relatively benign, lesions may bleed or become secondarily infected.

Diagnosis

- History of travel and possible exposure is important.
- Serology; PCR of blood, in reference laboratories.
- Examination of peripheral blood films for bacilli within or adherent to erythrocytes.

Management

- *Oroya fever:* ciprofloxacin 500mg po bd for 10d.
- *Verruga peruana:* rifampicin or streptomycin may reduce size and pain of large lesions

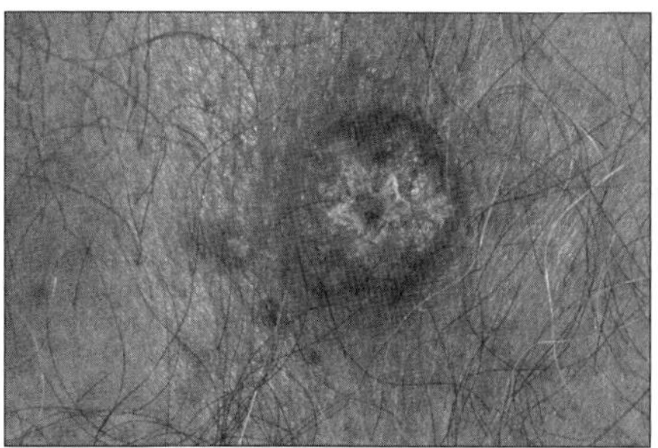

Fig. 18.5 Cutaneous lesion of bacillary angiomatosis (*Bartonella henselae*)

Ehrlichia

Human ehrlichioses are tick-borne zoonoses caused by intracellular bacilli. The organisms are found in vacuoles within leukocytes where they divide to form a cluster (morula). *Ehrlichia chaffeensis* infects monocytes whilst *E. ewingii* and *Anaplasma phagocytophilum* infect neutrophils.

- *E. chaffeensis* and *E. ewingii* are transmitted from a variety of vertebrates (particularly deer and dogs) to humans by the *Amblyomma americanum* tick in the southern USA.
- *A. phagocytophilum* is transmitted from vertebrates (particularly ruminants and rodents) to humans by *Ixodes* spp. ticks in the USA and Europe.

Clinical features

Ehrlichiosis presents with an acute flu-like illness, which may be accompanied by rash, vomiting, and meningoencephalitis. Leukopenia, thrombocytopenia, and ↑ liver enzymes levels are common. Illness caused by *E. chaffeensis* is generally more severe, with a 3% fatality rate. *E. ewingii* generally causes disease in immunocompromised patients.

Diagnosis

- Serology or PCR, in reference laboratories.
- Examination of Giemsa-stained peripheral blood films for morulae within neutrophils or monocytes.

Management

Doxycycline 100mg bd po or IV for 7–10 days.

Paediatric note

Rifampicin may be useful for ehrlichiosis in pregnancy or in children.

Public health note

Control or avoidance of the vectors: delousing of clothing and body with powder; preventative measures against tick bites.

- *Lice:* apply residual insecticide powder (e.g. 1% permethrin, 30–50mg/adult) to clothes and persons in situations favouring infestation; re-apply regularly. Provide facilities for bathing and washing clothes and bedclothes. In epidemic situations, apply residual insecticide to all contacts or the entire community.
- *Ticks:* look for and remove attached or crawling ticks after exposures. De-tick dogs. Use tick repellents and protective clothing to avoid contact.
- *Fleas:* apply residual insecticides to rat burrows or harbourages. Wait until flea populations have been d before instituting rodent control measures (to avoid human exposure to fleas).

Cat scratches and bites should be thoroughly cleaned and cat fleas controlled to prevent cat scratch disease.

Coxiella

Coxiella burnetii is an intracellular coccobacillus that causes *Q fever*. It infects a wide variety of animals (especially cattle, sheep, and goats), including ticks. Animals shed *C. burnetii* in milk, faeces, urine, and, particularly, birth by-products. Hides and wool may be contaminated with tick faeces containing concentrated organisms. Humans acquire infection through inhalation of infected aerosols (which may be air-borne over considerable distances), ingestion of unpasteurized dairy products, or contact with contaminated clothing. Person-to-person spread is rare.

Clinical features

Q fever may be asymptomatic or present as an acute flu-like illness with varying severity of hepatitis and pneumonia. Aseptic meningitis or encephalitis is more common in some areas. Culture –ve endocarditis is an important chronic presentation, usually on a background of previous valve damage or replacement. *C. burnetii* can recrudesce in pregnancy → abortion. It may also cause a chronic fatigue-like syndrome.

Diagnosis

- *Acute Q fever:* serology on acute and convalescent samples. Phase II antibodies higher than phase I.
- *Chronic Q fever:* phase I antibodies higher than phase II.
- PCR, immunostaining or EM of liver biopsy or heart valve in reference labs.

Management

Doxycycline 100mg oral bd for 7–10d. *C. burnetii* endocarditis requires 18mths doxycycline plus hydroxychloroquine.

Paediatric note

- Co-trimoxazole or the newer macrolides (e.g. azithromycin) are useful for the treatment of Q fever in children.
- Erythromycin 10–15mg/kg qds for 7–10d may also be used to treat Q fever in children.

Public health note

Persons at risk of Q fever (abbatoir workers, farmers, researchers) should be educated on sources of infection and safe disposal of infected materials (especially birth products). Milk should be pasteurized. Q fever vaccine is available for those at high risk in some countries.

Relapsing fevers

These are acute febrile illnesses caused by *Borrelia* spirochaetes. Untreated infections relapse repeatedly with afebrile intervals of 5–9d. As well as the usual arthropod vectors (see Fig. 18.6) *Borrelia* can be transmitted by blood transfusion.

Louse-borne relapsing fever (LBRF)

Transmission

Epidemic louse-borne relapsing fever, caused by *Borrelia recurrentis*, is transmitted by human body lice (*Pediculus humanus corporis*) (see Fig. 18.6). Lice are infected by feeding on human blood. They transmit *B. recurrentis* to a new human host not by bites, but by inoculation through broken skin, or intact mucosae by scratching. Humans are sole host and reservoir. LBRF is now confined to Northeast Africa. In the cold, rainy season when people wear more clothes and crowd together for warmth, conditions encourage louse infestation and transmission ↑. Historically, LBRF caused massive pandemics in Africa, the Middle East, and Europe (1903–36, 50 million cases with 5 million deaths; 1943–6 10 million cases), exacerbated by wars, crowding, floods, famines, and forced migration.

Clinical features

- Incubation is 4–17d (average 7d).
- Symptoms start with sudden high fever, chills/rigors, headache, confusion, myalgias, arthralgias, fatigue, dizziness, cough, anorexia, nightmares, and prostration.
- Examination reveals bleeding (epistaxes, subconjunctival haemorrhages, petechiae), tender splenomegaly and hepatomegaly, jaundice, and chest signs.
- The first attack ends dramatically with a febrile crisis, either spontaneously on about the 5th day if untreated or with a Jarisch–Herxheimer reaction (see Box 18.9) precipitated by antibiotic treatment.
- Inadequately treated patients may suffer their 1st relapse about 1wk later. Subsequent attacks tend to be less severe.
- *Complications:* pregnant women are at high risk of abortion. Death is due to myocarditis, liver failure, severe bleeding due to thrombocytopenia, DIC, and hepatic dysfunction; ruptured spleen, splenic infarctions, and bacterial superinfection (dysentery, salmonellosis, typhoid, typhus, malaria, TB). During the Jarisch–Herxheimer reaction, patients may die from hyperpyrexia, hypovolaemic shock, or pulmonary oedema. Untreated case fatalities of 40% or higher have been reported during epidemics. Treatment can reduce this to <5%.

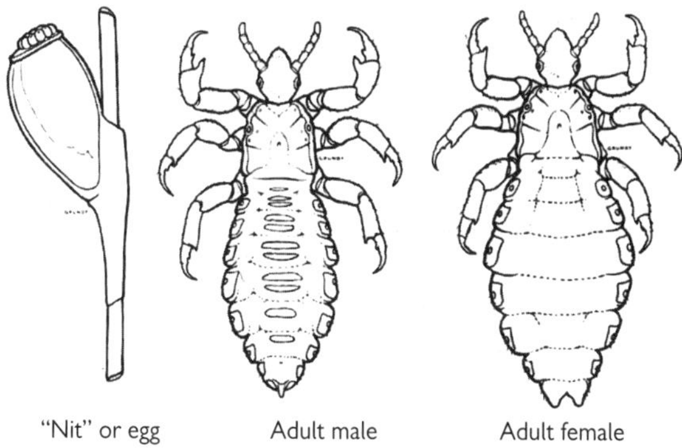

Fig. 18.6 Human body lice (*Pediculus humanus corporis*), the vector of louse-borne relapsing fever and epidemic typhus. Adult body lice are 2.3–3.6mm in length. Body lice live and lay eggs on clothing and only move to the skin to feed. Body lice infestations are spread by close person-to-person contact, especially under conditions of crowding and poor hygiene. Improved hygiene and access to regular changes of clean clothes will cure body lice infestations. Animals do not play a role in the transmission of human lice.

Drawing by J H Grundy, courtesy of D A Warrell.

Box 18.9 Jarisch–Herxheimer reactions in spirochaete infections

Acute inflammatory exacerbation of symptoms and pathology following treatment is most frequent (33–100%) and severe in LBRF, although it also occurs in syphilis and other spirochaetal infections.

Within a few hours of treatment, patient becomes restless, then develops violent rigors with soaring temperature, respiratory, and pulse rates, high BP, and associated vomiting, diarrhoea, coughing, and delirium.

This is followed by the flush phase during which there is profuse sweating and vasodilatation, sometimes complicated by hypovolaemic shock or acute pulmonary oedema attributable to myocarditis.

Treatment

For the severe Jarisch–Herxheimer reactions precipitated by antibiotics:

- Control pyrexia by physical cooling.
- Prevent hypovolaemia with IV fluids.
- Nurse in bed for 48–72h to prevent fatal postural hypotension.

Treat acute pulmonary oedema and myocarditis with digoxin. No effective antibiotic regimen has been shown to cause less Jarisch–Herxheimer reactions.

Tick-borne relapsing fever (TBRF)

Endemic TBRF is caused by >15 *Borrelia* spp. and transmitted by soft (argasid) ticks (genus *Ornithodoros*) (see Fig. 18.7). TBRF is widely distributed in tropical and temperate countries especially in Africa, but not Australasia and Pacific islands.

Transmission

Ticks are infected by feeding on animal or human blood or acquire spirochaetes congenitally (trans-ovarially). They transmit *Borrelia* to a new animal or human host via their saliva while taking a blood meal or by contaminating the bite wound with their coxal gland secretion. They are reservoirs as well as vectors. Peri-domestic rodents are the main vertebrate reservoir. Ecology and species of *Borrelia* and tick vary geographically. Only classic East African TBRF (*B. duttonii* transmitted by *O. moubata* complex) is anthroponotic (not a zoonosis). Risk of infection is associated with sleeping in tick- and rodent-friendly thatched or mud houses or log cabins. Tick bites are painless. They feed for only a few hours at night and then drop off, so exposure is usually unsuspected.

Clinical features

After incubation of 2–18d, presenting symptoms are similar to those in LBRF, but usually milder and less protracted, although ARDS and severe Jarisch–Herxheimer reactions have been reported.

- Epistaxis, abdominal pain, diarrhoea, and cough are described.
- Splenomegaly and splenic infarction are common; hepatomegaly and jaundice are unusual.
- Transient neurological problems occur in 5–10% of patients: paraesthesiae, cranial nerve palsies (especially VII), visual symptoms, hemiparesis or paraparesis, lymphocytic meningitis.
- Erythematous and petechial rashes may appear.
- Fever may recur up to 13 times, separated by gaps of a few days to 3wks in untreated patients.
- Pregnancy is aborted in up to one third of cases.

Diagnosis of the relapsing fevers

LBRF is easily diagnosed by finding spirochaetes (sometimes in vast numbers, e.g. >500 000/mm^3) in Giemsa-stained blood films (see Fig. 18.8 and Colour plate 24). However, in TBRF, spirochaetaemia may be scanty and intermittent, making microscopy insensitive. Serology is not useful.

Management of tick- and louse-borne relapsing fever

Single-dose antibiotic therapy is curative for LBRF:

- Adults: doxycycline 100mg or tetracycline 500mg, oral (for sick patients, tetracycline 250mg IV) stat.
- Pregnant women or children: erythromycin adult 500mg, children 10mg/kg oral (for sick patients, erythromycin IV) stat *or*
- For mixed infections with louse-borne typhus (adults): doxycycline 100–200mg oral stat.
- Benzylpenicillin and chloramphenicol are also effective.

For TBRF, longer courses of the same drugs are required (e.g. adults: tetracycline 500mg qds oral for 10d).
- Treat complicating bacterial infections (typhoid etc.).
- For treatment of Jarisch–Herxheimer reactions see Box 18.9.

Public health note: control of relapsing fever
- *LBRF:* delouse infested clothes (heat, insecticide); bathe patients (*soap and 1% Lysol [Cresol]**); decontaminate using 10% DDT, 0.5–1% malathion, 2% temephos, 1% propoxur, or 0.5–1% permethrin. This is essential to control an epidemic.
- *TBRF:* kill or deter ticks with residual insecticides in dwellings, repellents (DEET), improved house construction, rodent control.

* Cresol requires precautions to prevent absorption through skin.

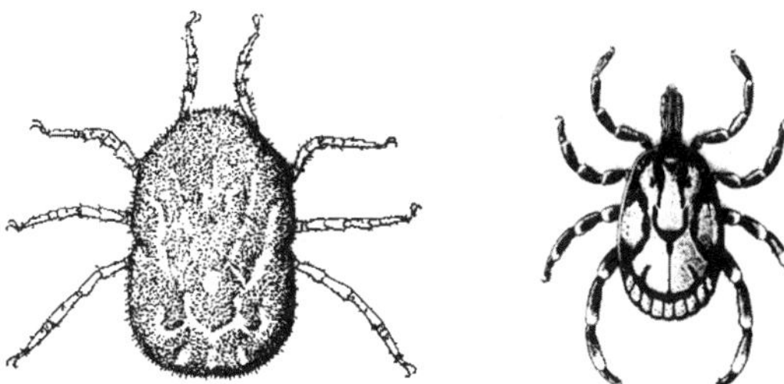

Fig. 18.7 Left: soft tick (genus *Ornithodoros*) vector of tick-borne relapsing fever. Right: hard tick (genus *Ixodes*). Hard ticks are the vectors of Lyme disease, rickettsial infections, and tick-borne encephalitis.

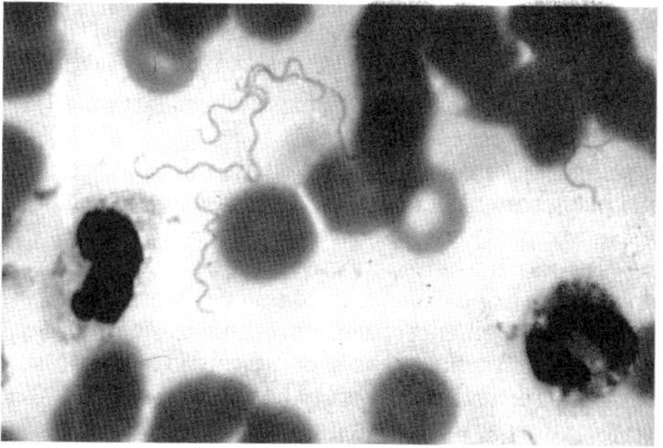

Fig. 18.8 Blood film showing several *Borrelia duttonii* spirochaetes in a patient with untreated TBRF.

Leptospirosis

Zoonotic disease caused by *Leptospira* spp., which are spirochaetes excreted in urine of wild and domestic animals into water sources. Leptospires survive for days in warm, damp conditions especially fresh water and damp soil. Exposure can cause self-limiting or serious disease.

Epidemiology and transmission

Leptospirosis is a global disease, but in tropical regions it is endemic and there are epidemic risks, e.g. after flooding and hurricanes.

- *Leptospira* spp. can be divided by phenotyping into 25 serogroups and >250 serovars, and by genotyping into >17 genomospecies. However, their characterization does not appear to correlate to disease severity.
- Wild and domestic animals excrete *Leptospira* spp. in their urine in large numbers, for long periods.
- *Leptospira* spp. enter the body through cuts or abrasions of skin or mucous membranes after immersion in contaminated water (pools, canals, rivers), or through close animal contact.
- In resource-poor regions the commonest source of infection is rats, but leptospirosis can also be associated with exposure to livestock and domestic animals, e.g. dogs.
- High risk groups include those undertaking outdoor recreational activities on fresh water lakes, rivers and canals (particularly in tropical regions) and those exposed to animals or contaminated water via occupation (e.g. veterinarians, sewer-workers, rice farmers).

Clinical features

Spirochaetes spread to multiple organs as leptospiraemia develops after exposure. Clinical manifestations of leptospirosis reflect organ dysfunction resulting from direct effects of leptospires and/or host immune responses to infection. There are three clinical categories:

- *Subclinical infection:* common in endemic areas (seroprevalence ~5–10%).
- *Self-limiting:* 1–3wks post-infection there is sudden onset fever, headache, severe myalgia, nausea and vomiting, and conjunctival suffusion or haemorrhage.
- *Severe disease:* potentially lethal multi-system illness with jaundice, renal failure, and pulmonary haemorrhage (Weil's disease). Patient may have high fever, be prostrate, and have haemoptysis, dyspnoea, and/or jaundice. May be a 2-d remission after 4–7d, but may → 2nd immunopathological phase and patient's condition worsens with persistent high fever, meningo-encephalitis, myocarditis, widespread haemorrhage, renal failure, jaundice, and shock. Death in leptospirosis due to multi-organ failure. Severe pulmonary haemorrhage (2° to endothelial damage, rather than consumption of clotting factors) has been reported as important cause of death in recent epidemics in Central America and Southeast Asia.

Diagnosis Early diagnosis difficult due to non-specific presentation, similar to other infections that present as undifferentiated febrile syndrome (e.g. malaria, dengue, and rickettsial infections). Usually proteinuria with RBC and WBC in urine. Blood tests usually show neutrophilia +/– thrombocytopenia; muscle enzymes (creatine phosphokinase (CPK)) often elevated. Commonly renal impairment. Hepatic impairment is common: ↑ bilirubin, but only modest elevations of ALT/AST.

Culture Leptospires can be isolated from blood or CSF during first 7–10d of illness, and from urine during weeks 2–3 of illness. Culture difficult, requires several weeks of incubation, and has low sensitivity. Molecular methods to detect leptospires are in development.

Serological Micro-agglutination is the standard serological diagnostic test for leptospirosis IgM, comparing acute and convalescent samples. Several rapid tests are now available. Suitable for preliminary diagnosis. However, because IgM antibodies only appear after 5–7d of illness, all of these have low sensitivity (39–72%) during the acute phase of illness.

Molecular If available and validated, PCR can be a useful tool for the early diagnosis of leptospirosis.

Management

It is important to ↑ awareness among clinicians to include leptospirosis in the differential diagnosis. Antibiotics should be used at any stage of leptospirosis, but rapid diagnosis is essential since antibiotic therapy provides greatest benefit early in the illness. Other measures include supportive treatment of sepsis and organ failures.

- *Mild disease:* doxycycline 100mg bd for 7d, started <3d of onset of symptoms, will hasten recovery.
- *Moderate or severe disease:* benzylpenicillin 1.2–2.4g IV qds for 5–7d (even if patient has been ill for several days). Alternatives for severe disease: ampicillin 1g IV qds or cefotaxime 1–2g IV q12h or ceftriaxone 1–2g IV od. Chloramphenicol is *not* effective.
- Triage of patients is critical since complications require monitoring and aggressive intervention (if available), such as haemodialysis for renal failure and ventilatory support for acute pulmonary complications.

The Jarisch–Herxheimer reaction may occur 4–6h after initiation of IV antibiotics in some patients.

Public health note: control of leptospirosis

- ↓ *Exposure:* education of high risk groups.
- ↓ *Animal transmission:* control of rodent populations and vaccination of domestic animals.
- *Prevent disease:* consider empirical doxycycline therapy in patients with acute, undifferentiated febrile illness presenting to the heath-care facilities soon after flooding or natural disasters. Consider chemoprophylaxis in very high-risk groups. Doxycycline 200mg weekly has been shown to ↓ clinical disease in populations with very high risk of exposure over a limited time.
- There is no currently available human vaccine.

Brucellosis

A zoonosis of worldwide distribution caused by the Gram –ve bacillus, *Brucella*. There are ~500 000 cases/yr in humans. Responsible species are: *Brucella melitensis* (sheep, goats, camels), *B. abortus* (cattle, buffalo, yaks, camels), *B. suis* (pigs, hares, rodents, caribou, reindeer), *B. ovis* (sheep), and *B. canis* (dogs). *B. melitensis* is the commonest. The organism lives and multiplies within phagocytes in the reticulo-endothelial system. The cellular immune response, in particular the interferon-gamma pathway, is important in pathogenesis.

Transmission

Infected animals shed large numbers of bacilli in milk, urine, and products of conception. Humans infected either by:

- Sporadic cases occur by direct contact with infected animals (entry is through breaks in skin or inhalation of aerosols in stables, abattoirs and laboratories).
- Sporadic cases and outbreaks occur by ingestion of unpasteurized milk, soft cheese (see Fig. 18.9), yoghurt, butter, and ice-cream.

Clinical features

Variable incubation period (usually 2–4wks, may be months), followed by acute or insidious onset of fever (may be rigors), and non-specific constitutional symptoms (sweating, anorexia, malaise, headache, back pain). Lymphadenopathy and hepatosplenomegaly may be present. Complications can affect virtually any organ system, including:

- Osteo-articular (spondylitis, peripheral arthritis, sacroiliitis).
- Reproductive (epididymo-orchitis, spontaneous abortion).
- Hepatitis, peritonitis.
- CNS (meningitis, encephalitis, abscess).
- Endocarditis (responsible for most mortality).

Diagnosis

The serum agglutination test is most widely used (single titre >1:160 or rising titre), but cross-reacts with other Gram –ves. ELISA (IgG, IgM, IgA) has ↑ sensitivity and specificity. Rapid (dipstick-type) serological tests are commercially available. PCR is promising. Culture from blood or tissue is confirmatory, but is relatively insensitive and requires prolonged incubation. When cultured, it is readily transmitted to laboratory staff.

Management

Optimal treatment Is with 6wks of doxycycline 100mg oral bd plus 6wks of rifampicin 300mg oral bd plus an aminoglycoside for 2–3wks: either streptomycin 15mg/kg IM daily or gentamicin 5mg/kg IM od.

Alternative Doxycycline plus rifampicin (as above) for 6wks, but relapse rate is greater than regimens including an aminoglycoside. Ciprofloxacin/ofloxacin may be added as an alternative 3rd agent. Rifampicin plus co-trimoxazole are useful in pregnancy. HIV+ individuals respond to the same regimens used for HIV–ve individuals.

Paediatric note: paediatric doses

Children aged >9yrs may be treated as adults. For younger children, combine 2 of the following:

- Rifampicin 15mg/kg (max 600mg) oral od for 6wks.
- Co-trimoxazole: sulfamethoxazole 20mg/kg + trimethoprim 4mg/kg (max 800 + 160mg) oral bd for 6wks.
- Gentamicin 2.5mg/kg IV or IM tds for 2wks.

Public health note: prevention and control

- Pasteurize (or boil) milk products.
- Personal protective equipment (masks, gloves, etc.) for those at occupational risk, e.g. vets.
- Screen livestock by serology or by testing cow's milk and eliminate infected animals.
- Vaccinate animals in high prevalence areas; vaccinate animals using live attenuated vaccine (no human vaccine is available; the vaccine strain may cause disease in humans if accidentally inoculated).
- Identify source of outbreaks (usually milk or milk products from infected herd); recall all affected products.
- Laboratory exposures: give prophylactic rifampicin + doxycycline for 3–6wks.

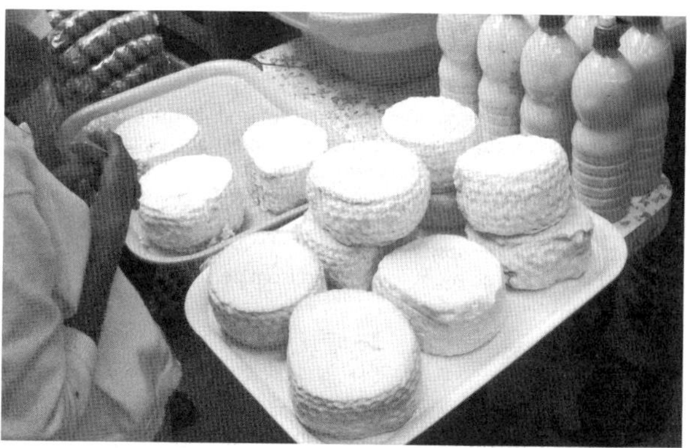

Fig. 18.9 Unpasteurized goat cheese, Canta valley, Peru. Unpasteurized cheese may transmit brucellosis.

Picture courtesy of D A Warrell.

Plague

An acute illness caused by the Gram –ve coccobacillus, *Yersinia pestis*, that can be rapidly fatal unless treatment is started early. Empirical antibiotic therapy is thus essential when clinical suspicion is high. It is enzootic among animals (mainly rodents) in many countries in Africa, Southeast Asia and the Americas (including Southwest USA). It occasionally infects humans. Plague has had a profound effect on the course of human history, mainly through the impact of three pandemics. Although another pandemic is unlikely, plague remains a threat due to high case fatality rates and the potential for epidemic spread. Most human plague cases are reported from rural, underdeveloped areas. Since 2000, >95% of ~22 000 cases reported to the World Health Organization have been from countries in sub-Saharan Africa and the island of Madagascar (see Fig. 18.10).

- The commonest clinical form is *bubonic* plague, in which bacteria spread to lymph nodes. Bubonic plague has a 1–15% death rate in treated cases and a 40–60% death rate if not treated.
- Primary *pneumonic* plague occurs after inhalation of bacteria in droplets coughed from a patient with pneumonic plague → fulminant pneumonia and sepsis, which is uniformly fatal if not treated within 24h. Pneumonic plague might also occur as a result of biological warfare or terrorism. 2° pneumonic plague may complicate septicaemic plague.
- *Septicaemic* plague may be 1°, or occur as a complication of bubonic or pneumonic plague. Infection may spread to every organ including the lungs, liver, spleen, kidneys, and, rarely, CSF causing meningitis. The mortality is ~40% in treated cases and ~100% in untreated cases.

Transmission

Bubonic and 1° septicaemic plague are transmitted via the bite of infected rodent fleas or through direct contact with infectious tissues. Domestic rodents (e.g. *Rattus rattus*, *R. norvegicus*) are the most common reservoirs for human infection as they amplify and bring the infection in closer proximity to humans during an epizootic. Although many flea species can transmit infection, *Xenopsylla cheopis* is a 1° source of transmission to humans. Pneumonic plague is transmitted from person to person through respiratory droplet spread.

Clinical features

Bubonic plague

The first specific sign is usually local lymphadenitis in the nodes draining the site of the flea bite, most commonly in the inguinal, axillary, or cervical region. After 2–7d (always <15d), a 'bubo' forms in these nodes. There is typically a short prodrome of fever, malaise, headache, and, in some cases, a dull ache in the nodes for up to 24h before the bubo is apparent. The enlarged nodes are extremely painful and swollen, and the mass is non-fluctuant and immobile. The overlying skin may be warm, red, oedematous, and adherent (see Fig. 18.11).

Pneumonic plague
Initially, intense headache, malaise, fever, vomiting, prostration with rapidly evolving tachypnoea, dyspnoea, chest pain, cough, haemoptysis (blood tinged or grossly haemorrhagic), ↓ consciousness. CXR shows multilobar consolidation or bronchopneumonia. Paucity of chest signs compared with the CXR is characteristic. This picture needs to be distinguished from ARDS, which may occur in bubonic and septicaemic forms of plague. Rapid deterioration and death from multi-organ/respiratory failure is common.

Septicaemic plague Presents with fulminant sepsis, multi-organ failure, and skin bleeding.

Diagnosis

Fever plus localized lymphadenopathy in endemic area; aspiration of a bubo for culture and Giemsa/Gram-stained smear (bipolar coccobacillus); blood, sputum, CSF for culture; acute and convalescent serology. Antigen detection directly on primary clinical samples (i.e., bubo aspirate, sputum), if available, may give rapid diagnosis.

Management

For severe disease: antibiotics must be started without delay and continued for 7–10d:

- Most clinical experience is with streptomycin 15mg/kg (max 2g) IM bd.
- Alternatives when streptomycin is not available or contraindicated: doxycycline 200mg oral loading dose followed by 100mg oral bd; or tetracycline 2g oral loading dose followed by 500mg oral qds (consider risks vs. benefits of tetracyclines in children); or chloramphenicol 25mg/kg (max 750mg) IV/oral qds (treatment of choice for meningitis).
- Alternatives with good activity in vitro, but comparatively little clinical experience include: gentamicin 5mg/kg (max 500mg) IV/IM od; ciprofloxacin 15mg/kg (max 750mg) IV/oral bd.

Public health note: prevention and control of plague

- Use preventive measures against rodents and fleas (e.g. removing rodent food and harbourage near households, using repellents).
- Flea control must occur before rodent control during outbreaks.
- Notify all suspected cases to local health authorities and pneumonic cases to WHO.
- Conduct case finding in affected and nearby households.
- Isolate pneumonic plague patients under respiratory droplet precautions until at least 48h after starting antibiotics and clinically improving.
- Consider post-exposure prophylaxis (doxycycline 100mg bd for 7d) for close contacts (2–3m) of pneumonic plague patients (e.g. 1° caregivers) and medical staff.
- Vaccination currently not generally available.

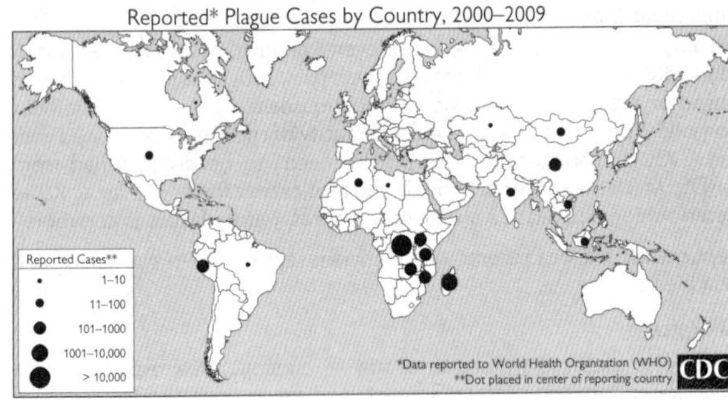

Fig. 18.10 Reported plague cases by country 2000–2009. CDC, Atlanta, GA, USA.

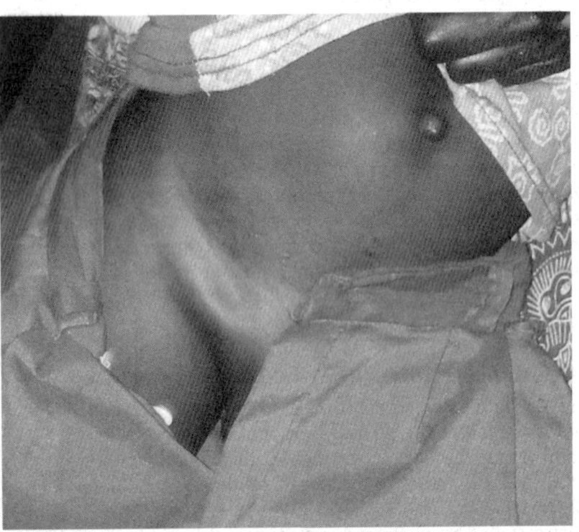

Fig. 18.11 Enlarged inguinal lymph node (bubo) in child with bubonic plague. CDC, Atlanta, GA, USA.

Melioidosis

A disease caused by the Gram –ve bacterium *Burkholderia pseudomallei* that is endemic in South and Southeast Asia, northern Australia, the Caribbean, and probably elsewhere including areas of Africa and South America. It is a major cause of septicaemia in Northeast Thailand. The bacterium is present in mud and surface water (e.g. rice paddies), and infection occurs following inoculation, inhalation or ingestion. The time from exposure to illness ranges from 1d to >60yrs. Overall case fatality is 43% in Northeast Thailand (20–30% in children) and 14% in Australia. *Glanders* is a similar disease of horses caused by *Burkholderia mallei*, with very rare cases in man. Diagnose and treat as for melioidosis.

Clinical features

These are very variable, and range from fulminant sepsis and rapid death to a chronic illness characterized by fever, weight loss, and wasting. The most frequent clinical picture is a septicaemic illness, often with bacterial dissemination leading to pneumonia (50%) and/or abscess formation, most commonly in the liver and spleen (30%) (see Fig. 18.12). Infection may occur in bone, joints, skin, soft tissue, parotid gland, testis, prostate and central nervous system. Severe sepsis and its complications are the usual cause of death if it occurs.

Diagnosis

- Consider melioidosis in febrile patients with a history of one or more of:
  - residency in an endemic region or relevant travel history
  - any contact with soil or water containing *B. pseudomallei*
  - risk factors for melioidosis, e.g. diabetes mellitus or renal disease.
- Diagnostic confirmation relies on culture. *B. pseudomallei* colonization is extremely rare and isolation of even a single colony from any clinical sample can be diagnostic.
- Culture blood, urine, throat swab, and respiratory secretions from suspected patients, together with pus and wound swabs where relevant. Site of culture positivity may not necessarily relate to clinical features (e.g. urine may be +ve without features of UTI).
- *B. pseudomallei* is a hazard group 3 biological agent and requires safe handling during culture, so tell your diagnostic laboratory if you suspect melioidosis.
- *B. pseudomallei* grows on most routine culture media, but as an oxidase +ve Gram –ve rod may be disregarded as an environmental pseudomonad, so be alert to the diagnosis in the right clinical and epidemiological setting. *B. cepacia* agar is often available in Western laboratories (it is used to culture sputum from cystic fibrosis patients) and is a good selective agar for *B. pseudomallei.*
- *B. pseudomallei* can be identified using biochemical tests and susceptibility pattern (resistant to gentamicin and colistin, susceptible to amoxicillin-clavulanate), commercial kits or automated systems.

- Consider sero-diagnosis in cases of suspected melioidosis who are culture –ve, but interpret with caution. It is common for the healthy population living in regions where infection is endemic to be seropositive, possibly due to exposure to closely-related environmental bacteria, and serology may be falsely –ve in definite cases.

Management

- Start appropriate antibiotics as soon as possible—immediately after culture, or even before culture, if sampling is going to be delayed.
- Treatment is divided into IV and oral phases and is required for at least 12wks. Recommendations are given in Box 18.10.
- Use imaging (where available) to detect abscesses in the liver, spleen, and elsewhere. Drain collections of pus wherever feasible.
- Fever clearance is often slow (median 9d), and is not an indication for a change of antimicrobials unless associated with clinical deterioration.
- If blood culture is +ve at presentation then repeat again at 1wk; if still +ve, this is a poor prognostic sign. Review antimicrobial therapy and re-image for pus collections.
- There is no clinical benefit in repeating cultures from other sites. Sputum and draining abscess cultures can be culture +ve for several weeks, but this is not associated with ↑ mortality in a patient who is otherwise responding to treatment.
- Infection is not thought to be easily transmitted person-to-person, but infection control measures may be recommended.
- Recurrent melioidosis is common (6% in 1st year and 13% by 10yrs) and is usually due to relapse following failure to eradicate the infecting organism.

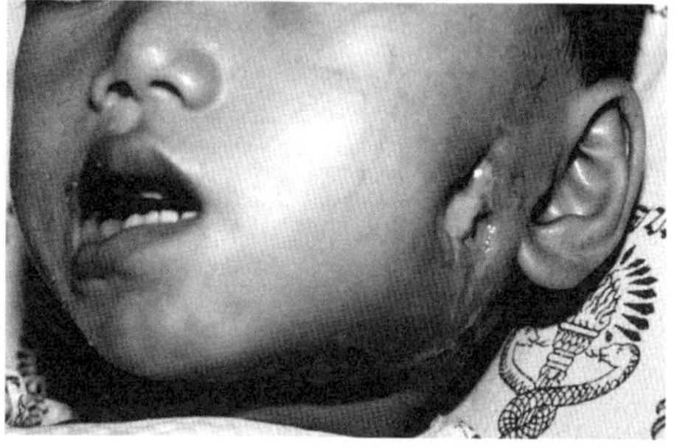

Fig. 18.12 Thai child with melioidosis leading to a parotid abscess, which is discharging pus, and a left VII nerve lesion.

Picture courtesy of S Looareesuwan and D A Warrell.

Box 18.10 Antimicrobial therapy for melioidosis

Initial parenteral therapy

Give IV therapy for at least 10d and extend to 4–8wks for deep-seated infection.

- *1st line:* ceftazidime 50mg/kg per dose (up to 2g) every 6–8h, or meropenem 25mg/kg per dose (up to 1g) every 8h.
- *2nd line:* amoxicillin/clavulanate 20/5mg/kg every 4h; this gives equivalent mortality to 1st-line drugs, but a higher rate of treatment failure.

Oral eradication therapy Duration of oral therapy, 12–20wks.

Adults

Trimethoprim/sulfamethoxazole using a weight-based dosing schedule:

- if <40kg give 2 × 480mg tablets bd.
- if 40–60kg give 3 × 480mg tablets bd.
- if >60kg give 4 × 480mg tablets bd.

+/– Doxycycline 2.5mg/kg per dose up to a max. 100mg every 12h.

Children ≤8yrs and pregnant women

Children: amoxicillin/clavulanate 20/5mg/kg oral tds.

- For adults <60kg, amoxicillin/clavulanate 1000/250mg oral tds .
- For adults >60kg, amoxicillin/clavulanate 1500/375mg oral tds.

Anthrax

Anthrax is a zoonosis from infection with the spores of the Gram +ve rod *Bacillus anthracis*. Anthrax is a disease of a variety of grazing animals (sheep, cattle, goats) in parts of Asia, Africa, South and Central America, southern Europe, Caribbean, and Middle East. The hardy spores may remain viable in soil or animal products for many years.

Transmission

Anthrax is primarily an occupational disease of workers who process hides, hair, bone products, and wool and those who handle infected animals (veterinarians, wildlife workers). Spores may be dispersed by wind, water, scavengers, or transport of animal products. Outbreaks can occur following ingestion of contaminated meat. Since anthrax spores are resistant and can be aerosolized, they have been used as agents of bioterrorism.

Clinical presentation

Cutaneous anthrax

Accounts for 95% of naturally occurring cases. Spores are inoculated into the skin through abrasions or cuts. A short incubation period (typically 1–5d) is followed by an itchy papule which progresses to a vesicle, ulcer, and, finally, a painless black eschar (see Fig. 18.13) with extensive local oedema and surrounding purple vesicles. This heals spontaneously in 1–3wks; however, bacteraemic spread and overwhelming septicaemia may occur. Neck lesions may → airway obstruction (consider early tracheostomy).

Inhalational anthrax

Usually occurs 1–4d following exposure, but may be delayed for up to 43d. This biphasic illness presents with symptoms of a viral upper respiratory tract infection followed by sudden onset of haemorrhagic mediastinitis with fever, hypoxia, dyspnoea and shock. Treatment in the late stages is usually unsuccessful, with mortality up to 90%.

Gastrointestinal anthrax Follows ingestion of contaminated meat. Severe abdominal pain, bloody diarrhoea, massive ascites, and sepsis occur. Mortality is >50%.

Other forms

Include meningitis (which may complicate any of the other forms) and oropharyngeal anthrax. A newly recognized disease form is injection anthrax, associated with skin-popping (injection into sub-cutaneous and muscle tissues) of heroin contaminated with spores of *B. anthracis*. An outbreak in Scotland resulted in 47 proven cases with 13 deaths.

Diagnosis

Rapid diagnosis is by demonstrating Gram +ve bacilli in smears from fluid from under the eschar, or other site-of-disease samples (or using newer methods such as PCR, direct immunofluorescence). Blood should always be cultured; and lymph nodes/CSF when appropriate (see Box 18.11).

Management

- Early, high dose antibiotic therapy is vital: give benzylpenicillin 2.4g IV 4 hourly for 10d. Naturally (or genetically-modified) penicillin-resistant mutants can occur, so some authorities recommend substitute (or add) ciprofloxacin 400mg IV bd followed by 500mg oral bd. Doxycycline 100mg bd is an alternative.
- Surgical debridement of the black, necrotic eschar is contraindicated. Eschar becomes sterile in <2d.
- *Infection control:* little evidence of patient to patient transmission; standard barrier precautions are all that is necessary with use of gloves, gowns/aprons.

Duration of therapy

- *Cutaneous:* 7–10d.
- *Inhalational:* at least 14d after symptoms abate.
- *GI:* at least 14d after symptoms abate.

Post-exposure prophylaxis Should be considered following possible deliberate aerosol release—ciprofloxacin 500mg oral bd, doxycycline 100mg bd, for 60d.

Box 18.11 Differential diagnosis of eschar

Infective causes

- Staphylococcal skin infection.
- Tularemia.
- Scrub typhus.
- Rickettsial spotted fevers.
- Rat bite fever.
- Ecthyma gangrenosus.

Non-infective causes

- Spider bites.
- Vasculitides.

Paediatric note: paediatric doses

- Ciprofloxacin 10–15mg/kg (max 400mg) IV bd followed by 10–15mg/kg (max 500mg) oral bd.
- If penicillin susceptible, use IV benzylpenicillin 150mg/kg daily in 4 divided doses.
- For children >12yrs, use adult doses.

Public health note: prevention of anthrax

- Disinfection: spores are resistant to dessication, heat, UV light, gamma irradiation, and many disinfectants. For disinfection of discharge from lesions or soiled materials use hypochlorite, hydrogen peroxide, peracetic acid, or gluteraldehyde (or burn or autoclave where possible).
- Vaccination: immunize high-risk persons with cell-free, supernatant-derived vaccine (regular boosters required).
- Veterinary public health measures: disposal of infected carcasses (incinerate at site, do not bury or transport if possible); vaccination of all domestic animals at risk (with annual re-immunization).
- Control occupational exposure: control dust; ventilate work areas; wear protective clothing; disinfect wool, hides, and bone prior to processing.

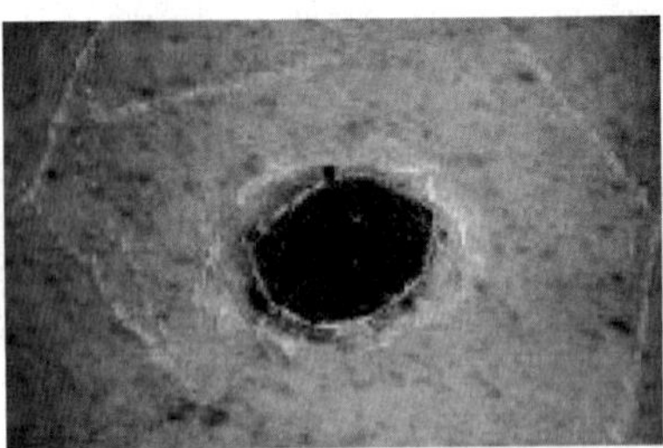

Fig. 18.13 Typical eschar of cutaneous anthrax.

African trypanosomiasis

Human African trypanosomiasis (HAT), 'sleeping sickness', is a protozoan disease caused by *Trypanosoma brucei* spp. confined to sub-Saharan Africa. Two forms of HAT exist, *T.b. gambiense* and *T.b. rhodesiense.*, both transmitted by tsetse flies (genus *Glossina*) (see Fig. 18.15), but epidemiological (Table 18.6) and clinical features (Table 18.7) differ.

Epidemiology

Incidence of *T.b. gambiense* HAT has been decreasing since 2000 (<10 000 cases 2009), but areas of high or unknown disease prevalence remain. *T.b. rhodesiense* HAT is sporadic, but in Uganda, is expanding northwest towards the *T.b. gambiense* endemic area. Geographical overlap would cause a significant problem in diagnosis and treatment. Travellers to game parks in East Africa also have a significant risk of *T.b. rhodesiense* HAT (see Table 18.6).

Table 18.6 Summary epidemiology and transmission of HAT

	T.b. gambiense	*T.b. rhodesiense*
Geography (Fig. 18.14)	Central and West Africa	East Africa
Transmission areas	Waterholes, rivers	Savannah, recently cleared bush
Reservoir	Humans	Game animals, cattle
Disease pattern	Endemic	Sporadic (occasional epidemics)

Table 18.7 Summary clinical features of HAT

	T.b. gambiense	*T.b. rhodesiense*
Clinical time course	Chronic, insidious (after asymptomatic phase)	Acute, sometimes fulminant
Inoculation site	Rarely chancre	Often chancre
Symptoms	*Early:* non-spec. fevers, pruritus, arthralgia *Late:* CNS symptoms	Fever, malaise, headache, myalgia, arthralgia, cardiac symptoms *Late:* CNS symptoms
Signs	*Early:* LNs *Late:* CNS signs	*Early:* rash, LNs, dysrhythmia, heart failure *Late:* CNS signs
Outcomes untreated	Fatal (months–years)	Fatal 1–3mths

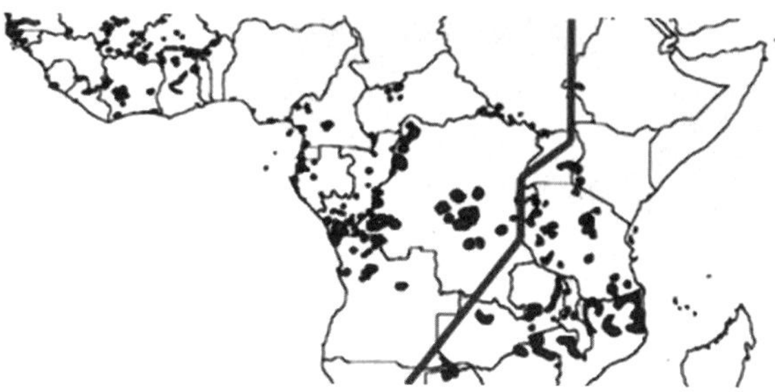

Fig. 18.14 Distribution of human African trypanosomiasis. The area southeast of the line = *T.b. rhodesiense* and northwest of the line = *T.b. gambiense*.

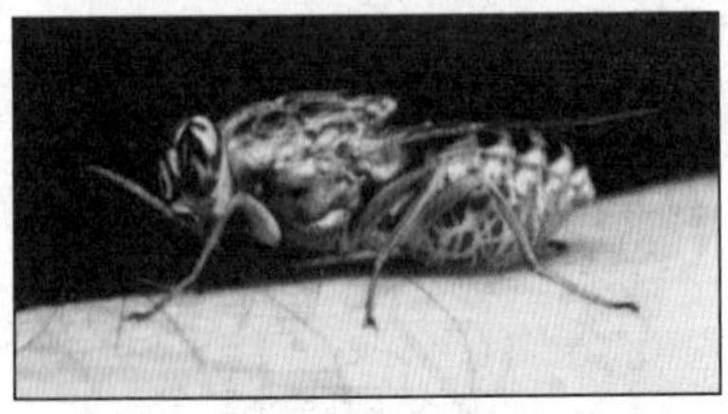

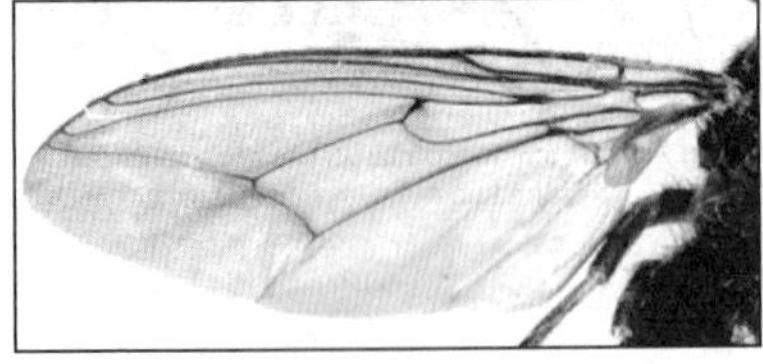

Fig. 18.15 Female tsetse fly (*Glossina morsitans*) engorged with blood after feeding: All Glossina flies can be identified by the pattern of 'cells' on their wings. Between the 4th and 5th veins of the wing is the 'hatchet cell'—looks like a butcher's cleaver.

Clinical features

T.b. gambiense HAT is chronic, but *T.b. rhodesiense* HAT is an acute, sometimes fulminant disease. Both forms usually fatal if untreated. After inoculation, a local inflammatory reaction results in an itchy, painful chancre (*T.b. rhodesiense*) and regional lymphadenopathy (both types). Invasion of bloodstream and lymphoreticular system follows—the haemolymphatic (early) stage. Trypanosomes then invade CNS, producing meningo-encephalitic (late) stage of the disease. Trypanosomes escape host immunological responses by changing surface antigens (antigenic variation; see Table 18.8).

Gambian trypanosomiasis

After asymptomatic phase (months–years), early stage characterized by irregular fevers, fatigue, arthralgia, myalgia, pruritus, headache. Lymphadenopathy, often in post-cervical triangle (Winterbottom's sign), is common; LNs soft and non-tender; splenomegaly rare. CNS symptoms including headache, change in personality, apathy, forgetfulness; psychosis (abnormal behaviour, agitation, delusions). CNS signs including pyramidal (focal motor weakness), extra-pyramidal (resting tremor common), and cerebellar (ataxia). Late features including daytime somnolence, coma, and seizures. Patients die of starvation, intercurrent bacterial infection, or convulsions.

Rhodesian trypanosomiasis

1° chancre at bite site, subsides 2–3wks. After 1–3wks, acute severe illness with high fever, chills, malaise, severe headache, weight loss, myalgia, arthralgia. Erythematous rash (macular, papular or circinate) may occur. Disease often runs a fulminant course with multiple-organ failure and early

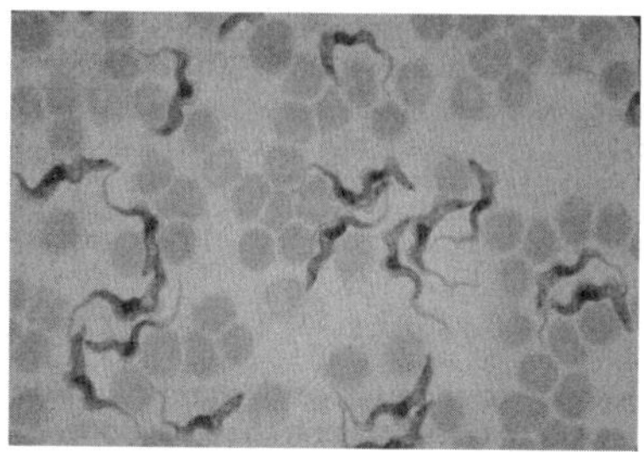

Fig. 18.16 Trypomastigote forms of *T.b. rhodesiense* on a peripheral thin blood smear.

death. CNS involvement (meningo-encephalitis) progresses rapidly and is fatal <1–3mths untreated. Myocarditis causing atrial or ventricular dysrhythmia, or heart failure, may precede meningo-encephalitis.

Diagnosis

Screening for Gambian HAT is by card agglutination trypanosoma test (CATT), a sensitive, practical serological test. No serological assay exists for Rhodesian HAT. Direct microscopic observation of trypanosomes in LN aspirates, blood (Giemsa-stained thick smear, quantitative buffy coat, haematocrit or mini-anion exchange centrifugation techniques) or CSF (single centrifugation) confirms diagnosis. Sensitivity of blood examination is greater in *T.b. rhodesiense* as ↑circulating trypanosomes (Fig. 18.16).

Staging disease by LP is mandatory. CSF findings indicating trypanosomalmeningo-encephalitis:

- Trypanosomes.
- ↑ Leukocytes (>5 per mm^3) *and/or*
- ↑ Total or specific (anti-trypanosomal) IgM.

Treatment

- Depends on stage of disease and if Gambian or Rhodesian. *Note:* following renewed agreement between pharmaceutical industry and WHO, drugs for HAT are being donated to WHO.

Gambian HAT

- Early stage: pentamidine isetionate 4mg/kg IM od for 7d.
- Late stage (first choice): eflornithine 200mg/kg IV bid for 7d, diluted in normal saline and infused over 2h, and nifurtimox 5mg/kg oral tid for 10d.
- Late stage *(alternative if nifurtimox N/A or CI):* eflornithine 100mg/kg IV qid for 14d.
- Late stage *(alternative only if eflornithine N/A or for treatment of relapse after eflornithine-based regimen):* melarsoprol 2.2mg/kg/d slow IV injection with prednisolone 1mg/kg oral od for 10 consecutive days. Use a glass syringe, or draw up and inject with a plastic syringe as soon as possible, since melarsoprol binds to plastic; very irritant, avoid

extravasation (risk soft tissue necrosis). Melarsoprol is more toxic than eflornithine-based regimen and associated with up to 30% treatment failure in parts of Angola, Uganda, Central African Republic, DRC, and Sudan.

Rhodesian HAT

- Early stage: suramin 5mg/kg by slow IV injection on day 1 (test dose), followed by 20mg/kg on days 3, 10, 17, 24, and 31.
- Late stage: melarsoprol sequential regimen (i.e. 3 cycles of 3 daily injections of 3.6mg/kg with resting period of 7–10d between each cycle) or 2.2mg/kg/d for 10 consecutive days (recently showed a similar efficacy and toxicity profile). Eflornithine is thought to be ineffective.

See Box 18.12 for adverse effects of drugs.

Paediatric health note

HAT in neonates and infants can be due to mother-to-child transmission or early exposure to tsetse fly bites. Delayed diagnosis is common in young children due to non-specific symptoms and signs. Chronic neuro developmental disorders are common sequelae of late stage HAT. Treatment regimens are similar to adults.

Public health note: prevention and control of HAT

- *Screening:* Gambian HAT control programmes rely on active case finding through systematic screening of communities and treatment of all those infected (human beings are the only significant reservoir). In areas of low prevalence of Gambian HAT, the integration of disease management within existing health structures is a challenge.
- *Vector control:* by tsetse fly trapping is cumbersome but effective, particularly in Rhodesian HAT control programmes.
- In outbreaks of Rhodesian HAT, a combined programme of vector control, treatment of infected cattle, and active detection and treatment of human cases should be implemented.
- *Challenges:* improved diagnostic tools and drugs and simplified diagnosis-treatment algorithms are urgently needed.

Box 18.12 Adverse effects of drugs used for HAT

- Eflornithine: leukopenia, anaemia, thrombocytopenia, soft tissue infections, and convulsions.
- Nifurtimox: anorexia, nausea, vomiting, insomnia, mood change, psychosis, convulsions.
- Melarsoprol: encephalopathic syndrome (see below), polyneuropathy, severe (sometimes bloody) diarrhoea, and rash.
- Pentamidine isetionate: hypoglycaemia (frequent), hypotension, sterile abscess, and pancreatitis (rare).
- Suramin: anaphylactic shock, fever, neurological, haematological, and/or renal toxicity.

Melarsoprol-induced encephalopathic syndrome (ES)

Occurs in 5–15% of treated patients, producing status epilepticus and coma. Mortality is ~50%. May be partially prevented by oral prednisolone 1mg/kg oral od in Gambian HAT. Onset of fever, tachycardia, headache, tremor, and conjunctival suffusion during melarsoprol treatment should be considered as a warning. Melarsoprol treatment should be stopped immediately; it can be restarted once symptoms subside. Some authorities recommend the use of high-dose dexamethasone IV (e.g. 30mg loading dose followed by 15mg every 6h for adults) for treatment of ES or impending ES.

American trypanosomiasis

American trypanosomiasis or Chagas' disease (CD) is endemic in Latin America, caused by the protozoa *Trypanosoma cruzi*, and transmitted by triatomine bugs of the reduviid family.

Pathogenesis

Parasites invade mesenchymal tissues (especially heart muscle and intestinal smooth muscle) where they persist as amastigotes, without necessarily re-entering the bloodstream, making detection and chemotherapy difficult. In ~70% of adults, an adequate immune response controls infection, producing a benign chronic phase ('indeterminate form'). Persistent infection and immune dysregulation causes chronic disease in ~30% → destruction of autonomic ganglia → chronic dilatation of hollow viscera (GI tract) and heart arrhythmias (see Fig. 18.17).

Epidemiology and transmission

Approx. 8–15 million people are infected by *T. cruzi* in 15 endemic countries of Latin America. 1.8 million individuals have chronic Chagas' cardiomyopathy. Social determinants of CD are very important: poor housing and working conditions, and malnutrition are directly linked to CD. Risk of acquiring CD while travelling is very low, but travellers should avoid poor-quality housing.

Transmission routes

- *Vector transmission:* via >150 spp. of triatomine bugs (reduviid family). Parasites from insect faeces enter via human nose and mouth mucous membranes, conjunctivae, or damaged skin—especially where the insect bite is scratched and rubbed. Transmission by insect vectors → >40 000 cases/yr.
- *Transplacental transmission:* >14 000 cases/yr.
- *Ingestion of accidentally infected food or beverage:* including fruit juice, → occasional outbreaks of disease.
- *Blood transfusion, organ transplantation:* ~1% blood infected.
- Occupational exposure in laboratory and forest workers.

Reservoirs

- Domestic and wild animals are reservoirs for the parasite.
- Repeated infection of humans can occur in the absence of animal hosts, when triatomine bugs are not controlled by insecticides.

Distribution

- CD is a global disease, and individuals infected in the endemic area (Fig. 18.18) may be diagnosed years later in other countries. Non-endemic countries (USA, Canada, Spain, France, Switzerland, Italy, Japan, and emerging countries in Asia and Australasia), receive migrants infected with *T. cruzi*, requiring diagnosis and treatment. In the USA, ~300 000 individuals are infected with *T. cruzi*, and 30 000–45 000 have clinical manifestations.
- In the Americas the epidemiology is divided into four country groups according to transmission cycle (see Table 18.8).

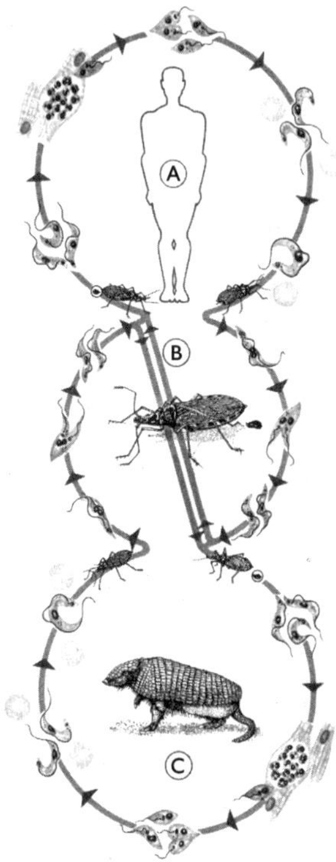

Fig. 18.17 Life cycle of *T. cruzi* . Reduviid bug (B) transmits infection via faeces when taking blood meals from animal reservoirs such as the armadillo (C) or humans (A).

Clinical features

CD is classified into acute phase; indeterminate or latent phase; and chronic phase.

Acute

This phase lasts 6–8wks following 1° or congenital infection. Infection may be subclinical, with non-specific symptoms. Local inflammation at bite site causes chagoma and lymphadenopathy. There may be conjunctivitis and if inoculation site close to eye, unilateral eyelid oedema may occur (Romaña's sign, see Colour plate 9c). This characteristic feature remains ~2mths (c.f. bacterial conjunctivitis which usually only persists max. ~10d).

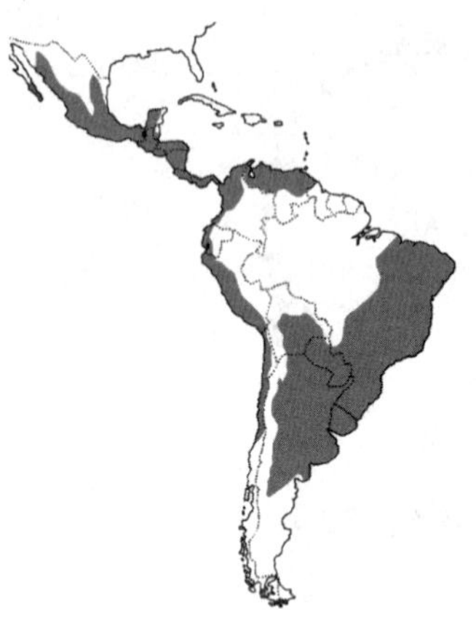

Fig. 18.18 Distribution of American trypanosomiasis. *T. cruzi* infections of animals occur over a much wider range than Chagas' disease in man.

Table 18.8 Grouping of countries by American trypanosomiasis transmission cycle

Countries	Argentina, Bolivia, Brazil, Chile, Ecuador, Honduras, Paraguay, Peru, Uruguay, Venezuela	Colombia, Costa Rica, Mexico	El Salvador, Guatemala, Nicaragua, Panama	Caribbean, Bahamas, Belize, Cuba, USA, French, Guiana, Guyana, Haiti, Jamaica, Suriname
Transmission cycle	Domestic Peri-domestic Sylvatic	Domestic Peri-domestic	Domestic Peri-domestic Sylvatic	Sylvatic
Chagas' cardiomyopathy	Common	Occurs	Limited data	Limited data

Fever occurs after an incubation period of 2–4wks post-infection, coinciding with parasite entry into blood. Rash (non-pruritic) is sharply defined with small macules on trunk, which fade after 7–10d. There is oedema, particularly of the face. Other features include hepatosplenomegaly, cardiac dysrhythmia, or insufficiency, meningo-encephalitis (often mild, but fatal in ~10% children). Congenital infection may be associated with jaundice, hepatosplenomegaly, cutaneous haemorrhage, and neurological signs, especially in premature neonates.

Indeterminate/latent
Serology and/or parasitological tests are +ve for *T. cruzi*, but no symptoms, physical signs or evidence of organ damage (cardiac or extracardiac). Normal ECG, CXR and bowel imaging. Rigorous and sophisticated testing may detect mild changes, but no established evidence of prognostic value.

Chronic Affects ~30% of those infected, often after decades of latent infection.

Cardiac

Pathology includes frequent arrhythmias, ventricular aneurysms, thromboembolic events, progressive dilated cardiomyopathy, cardiac failure +/– valvular incompetence in late stages. Some patients with chronic Chagas cardiomyopathy have normal ventricular function with only arrhythmias and conduction disorders. Ventricular arrhythmias indicate poor prognosis. Patient c/o weakness, rather than dyspnoea. Chest pain (usually atypical angina) is common. Dilated ventricles with aneurysms are important sources of mural thrombi, → systemic, pulmonary and cerebral emboli. Heart failure is exacerbated by AF; prognosis worsens as the disease progresses and arrhythmias ↑.

Five stages of chronic cardiac involvement are recognized:

- *A:* normal echo, no heart failure.
- *B1:* normal overall ventricular function with ventricular ejection fraction > 45%, no clinical heart failure; but echo abnormalities of regional contractility
- *B2:* ventricular ejection fraction < 45%, but no clinical heart failure.
- *C:* abnormal echo findings, treatable and clinically compensated heart failure (LV dysfunction and symptoms of heart failure—NYHA I, II, III and IV).
- *D:* abnormal echo findings, severe heart failure refractory to maximal medical therapy (NYHA IV) requiring specialized and intensive interventions.

Gastrointestinal

Symptoms of dysphagia, regurgitation of food, chronic constipation, abdominal pain.

Pathology Oesophagitis, mega-oesophagus, megacolon, and (rarely) large bowel obstruction.

Mixed (cardiac and GI) Includes features of both cardiac and GI associated disease.

Diagnosis

In acute phase parasites may be detectable in fresh preparations of buffy coat or stained peripheral blood specimens. Serology (>2 tests) for anti-*T. cruzi* IgG +ve is the main diagnostic tool in chronic infection. Parasites may sometimes also be detected directly in wet mount or Giemsa-stained blood films (see Fig. 18.19 and Colour plate 9b) or CSF precipitate; parasite DNA may be detected by PCR. *T. rangeli*, which is not a cause of human disease, may be mistaken for *T. cruzi*. Seropositive individuals should be evaluated for symptoms and signs of cardiac and GI disease.

Management

Acute phase

Give either:

- *Benznidazole 5–7mg/kg/d (children 10mg/kg/d):* orally in two divided doses for 60d; max recommended daily dose is 300mg. For adults >60kg, calculate the total and extend treatment period >60d. Common side effect is urticarial dermatitis (30% in 1st week of treatment), with good response to antihistamines or corticosteroids. If fever and adenopathy occurs, discontinue treatment. Other adverse effects include polyneuropathy (usually towards end of treatment) with pain and/or tingling in the legs, anorexia); *or*
- *Nifurtimox (not available in Brazil) 8–10mg/kg:* oral in three divided doses (children 15mg/kg oral in four divided doses) for 90d; side effects: anorexia (most intense and common), abdominal pain, nausea, vomiting and weight loss.

Chronic phase

Benznidazole is used, but may be ineffective and trial data awaited.

- *Symptomatic treatment:* for complications, such as CCF, arrhythmias (see 📖 Cardiac arrhythmias, p. 384), AV block, and sick-sinus syndrome or anticoagulation for systemic emboli.
- *Pacemakers:* implanted in patients with severe bradyarrhythmias.
- *Surgery:* may be required for mega-oesophagus or megacolon.
- *Heart transplantation:* is frequent in severe heart patients (CD is the 3rd major cause of heart transplantation in Brazil).

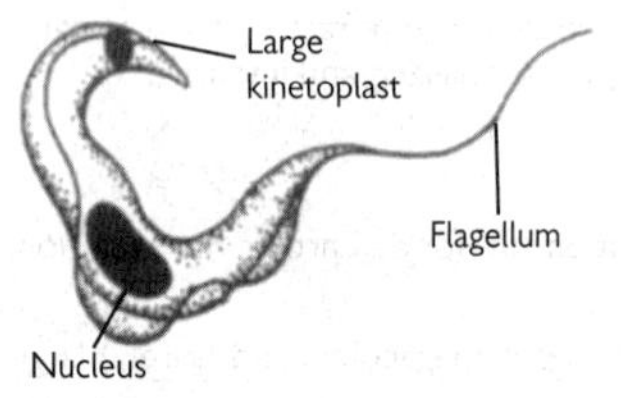

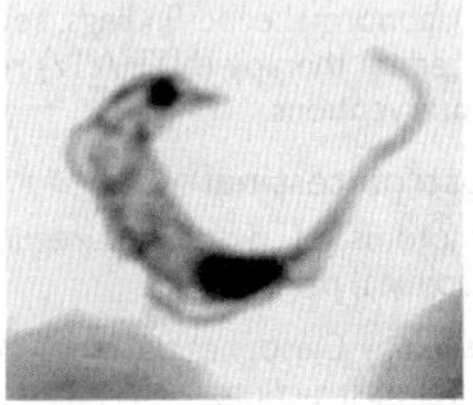

Fig. 18.19 *T. cruzi* as seen in a blood film.

Paediatric note: congenital *T. cruzi* infection

Transmission from infected mother to newborn children varies from 1% to 12% in different Latin American countries and should be evaluated in seropositive mothers. Congenital infection is confirmed by identification of parasites in the infant's blood and/or detection of infant anti-*T. cruzi* IgG 6–9mths after birth (assuming vector and other modes of transmission excluded). Congenital Chagas' disease is considered acute and requires trypanocidal treatment. Notification is mandatory.

Public health note: prevention and control of Chagas' disease

- Limit exposure to the vector: improved housing, insecticide spraying of houses.
- Promote the use of mosquito nets.
- Screen blood for transfusion.

Chagas' disease is a clear example of public policy success, with 5 separate large-scale vector control programmes with modern pyrethroid insecticides being implemented in last few decades in different Latin American countries. Mandatory notification of acute cases for intense epidemiological surveillance. Micro-epidemics of acute cases due to oral transmission through contaminated food, such as meat, sugar cane juice, or açaí (*Euterpe oleracea*) fruit juice, have been described, especially in Amazon Region and in South Brazil.

Visceral leishmaniasis (kala-azar)

A severe systemic protozoal disease, caused by *Leishmania donovani* or *L. infantum* (called *L. chagasi* in S America) and spread by sandflies (see Fig. 18.20). VL is increasing in incidence and causes major epidemics with high mortality. The disease is seasonal and geographically focal (see Fig. 18.21).

Pathogenesis

At infection, promastigotes (flagellate form) invade macrophages, becoming amastigotes (rounded form) which spread within spleen, bone marrow, liver, lymph nodes, and other tissues. Infection may be subclinical, controlled by an efficient cell-mediated immune response. Latent infections are reactivated during immunosuppression, especially HIV. In clinical disease, the immune response is ineffective and the parasite continues to multiply, → pancytopenia and profound immunosuppression (see Fig. 18.22).

Transmission

Is by the nocturnal bite of female *Phlebotomus* and *Lutzomyia* sandflies. In southern Europe, Brazil, etc. dogs are the major reservoirs of *L. infantum*/*L. chagasi*, a zoonotic form of VL which affects humans rarely (mainly infants and those with HIV). Humans are the hosts of highly endemic Indian and East African *L. donovani* parasites, sandflies spreading infection human to human. Patients with post-kalar dermal leishmaniasis (PKDL) can be long-term reservoirs of infection.

Clinical features

Usually ~2–6mths incubation period (asymptomatic) and 1–4mths symptoms have elapsed by the time the patient presents. Initially, patient may appear relatively well, is ambulant, and has a good appetite. Afternoon fevers (without rigors) and night sweats develop, lasting weeks–months. Dry cough and epistaxis are common. The patient notices wasting, weakness, and abdominal distension or pain due to the splenomegaly. The spleen enlarges and can reach the RIF, though a modest splenomegaly is more common. Anaemia and cachexia → fatigue. Diarrhoea, moderate hepatomegaly, ~1–2 cm lymphadenopathy (in Africa), pedal oedema, darkened skin, and zoster are also seen, as well as neurologic signs (confusion, ataxia, convulsions, deafness) in some. Dysentery, pneumonia, and TB may develop due to immunosuppression; malaria, measles, or influenza can be severe or fatal. Death is almost inevitable if untreated; it may follow sepsis, epistaxis, or anaemic heart failure.

During treatment

In Africa, 3–10% of patients will die from complications, or suddenly from antimonial-induced arrhythmias. The risk of death during treatment is much higher in those aged >45yrs or <4yrs, or with the following: severe anaemia (Hb<8g/dL), severe malnutrition (BMI <13kg/m^2), inability to walk unaided, and symptoms for >5mths.

Diagnosis

Serology

Most patients (>90%) have very high anti-*Leishmania* antibody titres on the direct agglutination test or a +ve rapid dipstick test (rK39) using recombinant *Leishmania* antigen. Diagnosis is confirmed by PCR or microscopy - finding parasites in Giemsa-stained smears of spleen aspirates (95% sensitive, but requires training) or lymph node/bone marrow aspirates (60–80% sensitive). Culture of aspirate improves diagnostic yield; cultures on other media can eliminate differential diagnoses (e.g. typhoid, brucellosis, miliary TB). In HIV+ individuals, parasites are often numerous in skin, gut, liver, and on bronchoalveolar lavage.

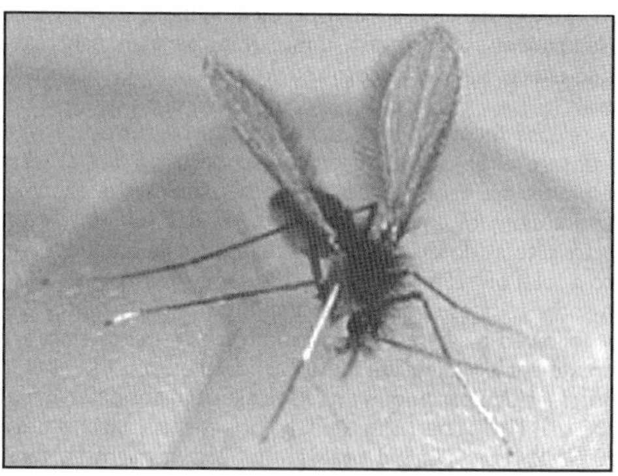

Fig. 18.20 The female phlebotomine sandfly is about half the size of a mosquito and feeds nocturnally. Several species transmit visceral or cutaneous leishmaniasis (Courtesy WHO/TDR).

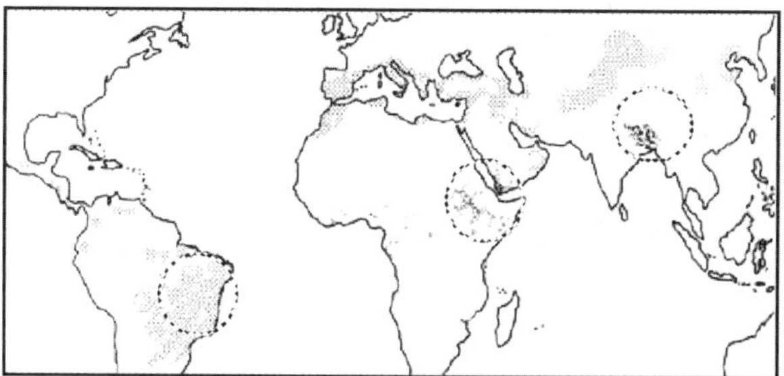

Fig. 18.21 The global distribution of visceral leishmaniasis (kala-azar). The species are *L. infantum*/*L. chagasi* (dotted area) and *L. donovani* (hatched area). 90% of all VL cases occur in Bangladesh, Brazil, India, Nepal, and Sudan. Up to 500 000 cases of kala-azar occur during an epidemic year.

Prevention

Spraying to ↓ sandfly vectors (in urban areas) and culling canine/rodent reservoirs. Insecticide-treated bed nets ↓ risk of VL by 50%. Deltamethrin-impregnated dog collars ↓ transmission of *L. infantum/L. chagasi*. In areas of human to human spread, case identification and treatment of visceral leishmaniasis and PKDL cases ↓ transmission.

Management

VL is usually responsive to IM or IV pentavalent antimony (Sb^v)—20mg/kg IM od for 30d. Meglumine antimoniate (85mg Sb^v/mL) or sodium stibogluconate (100mg Sb^v/mL) are equivalent; good-quality generic stibogluconate is as effective as brand-name preparations. There is no upper limit on the daily dose. 1° Sb^v resistance is a major problem in India; 2° resistance occurs in relapsed patients. Cardiac arrhythmias (may be fatal), pancreatitis, and other side-effects are well-recognized with antimonials, especially in HIV+ individuals.

Patients who relapse following the 1st course can be retreated with the same daily dosage of Sb^v for a longer course, ensuring that at least 2 test-of-cure aspirates are parasite-free before the patient is discharged. Alternative: give infusions of amphotericin 0.5mg/kg/day (or 1mg/kg on alternate days) to a total dose of 15mg/kg, or liposomal amphotericin 2–4mg/kg/day to a total of >20mg/kg over 7–10d.

In India, ultra-short courses of liposomal amphotericin 5mg/kg/day × 2 doses, alone or followed by a week of paromomycin or miltefosine, are effective. This treatment is inadequate in Africa, however.

2nd choice drugs include paromomycin (also called aminosidine) 15mg/kg/day IV/IM for 21d. Miltefosine 2.5mg/kg/day (for patients weighing 8–20 kg); 50mg/d (20–25 kg); or 100mg/d (>25kg), for 28d. It might be teratogenic; do not give to women of childbearing age unless pregnancy can be prevented during treatment and for 2mths thereafter; unsafe in lactating mothers.

Drug combinations are logical developments for the future, to prevent resistance. Sb^v 20mg/kg/day plus paromomycin 15mg/kg/day, both for 17 days, is a safe combination.

Clinical improvement should be evident in 7–10d. Response can be monitored by ↓ fever, ↑ haemoglobin, and ↓ spleen size. A parasitological response is shown by a –ve test-of-cure splenic aspirate (bone marrow or lymph node if spleen impalpable) at the end of treatment. Clinical follow-up is important during next 6mths to detect relapse; by 12mths, the patient can be considered cured. Relapse rates should be <5%, except in HIV +ve individuals, most of whom will relapse unless antiretroviral treatment started early; even on ART, many will have repeated relapses and the VL becomes drug-resistant.

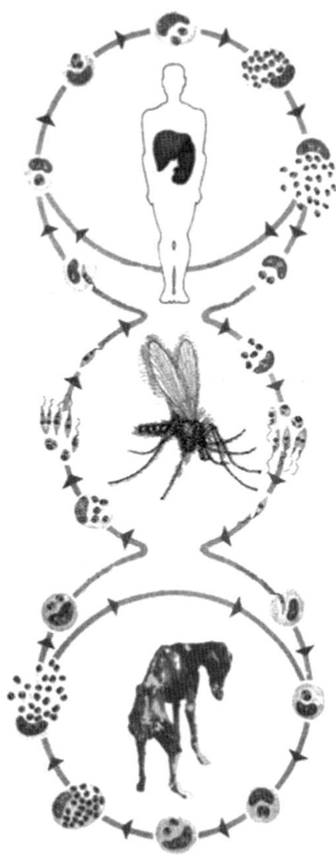

Fig. 18.22 Leishmaniasis (kala-azar) life cycle. The female sandfly inoculates flagellate forms (promastigotes) into man or animals whilst feeding. *L infantum*/ *L. chagasi* are zoonotic, with a canine reservoir. *L. donovani* has no known animal reservoir in India and several (unproven) animal hosts in Sudan.

Infectious mononucleosis

Infectious mononucleosis (glandular fever) is classically caused by 1° infection with EBV infection. A glandular fever-like illness is also caused by acute HIV, CMV, and *Toxoplasma gondii* infection.

Transmission

EBV (human herpes virus 4) is usually transmitted orally via saliva. It establishes infection in the oropharynx and circulating B cells. Latent EBV infection persists, with intermittent viral shedding, which occurs spontaneously and during febrile illnesses, e.g. malaria. In resource-poor regions, >90% children are infected with EBV by 5yrs, but show little clinical illness. The clinical picture of infectious mononucleosis is common in adolescence/adults, of whom ~50% develop the illness when infected.

Clinical features

Symptoms/signs Classically fever, pharyngitis and lymphadenopathy. Splenomegaly/hepatosplenomegaly, hepatitis, thrombocytopenia, palatal petechiae and morbilliform rash may occur.

Complications

Uncommon emergencies, which are sometimes fatal, occur with splenic rupture (spontaneously or after minor trauma) and upper airway obstruction (due to massive tonsillar and adenoidal enlargement). Encephalitis, hepatitis, haemophagocytosis, myocarditis, pericarditis, pneumonitis, haemolytic anaemia and nephritis are rare.

Latent EBV may → malignancy, including:

- Burkitt's lymphoma (childhood endemic type), common in tropical Africa and Papua New Guinea, linked to intense malaria transmission.
- Nasopharyngeal carcinoma, especially in Southeast Asia, China and parts of North and East Africa, linked to environmental/dietary factors.
- Hodgkin's lymphoma.
- B cell lymphoproliferative disease in the immunocompromised.
- Oral hairy leukoplakia in HIV+.
- CNS and other lymphomas in HIV+.

Diagnosis of InfM

- Lymphocytosis with atypical cells, mild thrombocytopenia, ↑ transaminases (typically ALT and ALP both elevated).
- IgM heterophil antibody tests (Paul Bunnell, Monospot) commonly used. IgM Ab against EBV viral capsid antigens can confirm diagnosis.

Management

- *Supportive:* hydration, analgesia, mild non-steroidals.
- Avoid contact sports in case of splenic enlargement.
- A short course of corticosteroids, e.g. prednisolone 0.5–1mg/kg/d may be useful for complications, such as acute respiratory obstruction (no formal evidence).
- Amoxicillin is contraindicated in infectious mononucleosis, it precipitates rash in ~90%.
- Aciclovir is of no proven clinical benefit.

Measles

Measles is a highly infectious, vaccine preventable, viral (paramyxovirus) disease, which predominantly affects children.

Epidemiology

Childhood global mortality from measles has ↓ from 733 000 in 2000 to 164 000 in 2008 as a result of increased immunization. Resource-poor countries (especially in Asia and Africa) with inadequate immunization programmes account for >95% of all measles deaths. There is ↑ risk of resurgence worldwide if immunization coverage is insufficient (<90% coverage).

Transmission

- Airborne by droplet spread.
- Direct contact with secretions from nose or throat of an infected person.
- Indirect contact with secretions (occasional).
- 15min contact with an infected person is sufficient for transmission.
- A person is infectious ~4d before rash to ~4d after rash. Humans are the only reservoir.
- >90% of non-immune people (unvaccinated children or non-immune adults) become infected if exposed.
- ↑risk of severe disease or complications in immunocompromised patients (HIV+), malnutrition (protein-calorie and vitamin A deficiency), pregnant women, and young age (<5yrs), with up to 20% case fatality in those aged <1yr.

See Table 18.9 for clinical features.

Table 18.9 Clinical features

Phase	Incubation	Prodrome	Exanthem	Recovery
Onset		10–14d from exposure	4–5d after symptom onset	4–5d after rash onset
Duration	7–14d	2–5d	4–6d	1–3wks
Clinical features	Asymptomatic	Fever, malaise, ↓ appetite, then conjunctivitis, coryza, cough Koplik spots appear day 2–3, 24–48h before rash	Maculopapular rash Lymphadenopathy High fever	Cough 1–3wks Fever lasting beyond day 3 of rash suggests complications

Rash

Distinctive, non-pruritic maculopapular rash appears on days 4–5 of fever. As well as having rash, patient looks ill, miserable, with conjunctival injection and URTI. Rash begins on face and behind ears, within 24–36h rash spreads down trunk and to extremities (palms and soles rarely involved). Begins to fade 3–5d after first appears, initially to a purplish hue and then brown/black lesions with fine scales.

Koplik spots Greyish white spots surrounded by erythema on the buccal mucosa (pathognomic for measles) appear on days 2–3, 24–48h before rash.

Diagnosis

Usually clinical. WHO defines measles as an illness with:

- Generalized maculopapular rash.
- Fever.
- *One of:*
  - cough
  - coryza
  - conjunctivitis.

In presence of distinctive clinical symptoms (see Table 18.9) and history of exposure, laboratory diagnosis seldom required. May be more important in atypical infection and immunocompromised patients. Can include:

- *Serology:* measles-specific IgM or 4-fold ↑ in measles IgG antibody titres between acute and convalescent phase.
- *Microscopy:* detection of multinucleate giant cells with inclusion bodies in nasopharyngeal secretions during prodrome.
- *Immunofluorescence:* can be used to demonstrate measles virus in cells from nasopharyngeal specimens and urine.
- *Virus isolation:* measles virus can be isolated from throat or conjunctival washings, sputum, urine, and lymphocytes.
- *PCR:* from throat or nasopharygeal swabs or urine samples.

Complications of measles

In resource-poor countries, at least 1 complication is expected in ~3/4 of measles cases and one child may have several complications.

↓ Immunity following measles infection predisposes to infection and this effect persists for ~6–8wks after the acute illness. Pneumonia and diarrhoea are the most common complications and account for ↑ case-fatality.

Lower respiratory tract infection

- Respiratory symptoms are characteristic of measles and assumed to be 1° viral pneumonitis. In minority, (especially immunocompromised) this progresses to severe giant cell pneumonia, which can be a chronic, severe condition.
- 2° bacterial infection occurs ~7–10d after rash onset. Predominant bacteria are *Staph. aureus, Strep. pyogenes, Strep. pneumoniae, H. influenzae, E. coli, Pseudomonas* spp.

Gastrointestinal complications
Diarrhoea occurs within 4d of rash, and is associated with ↑ case fatality and exacerbates malnutrition.

Neurological complications
Encephalitis occurs in ~1/1000 cases. ~25% of children have neurodevelopmental sequelae, with a 15% case fatality.

- Acute disseminated encephalomyelitis is an acute demyelinating disease occurring ~2wks after exanthem (also associated with other infections).
- Sub-acute sclerosing panencephalitis (SSPE) is a fatal, neurodegenerative disease which occurs in ~1/100 000 cases, 7–10yrs after the primary illness
- *Eye complications:* conjunctivitis, keratitis, may → blindness.
- *Other common complications:* include malnutrition, mouth ulceration, and otitis media.

Management

- Ensure adequate nutrition, hydration, and support, including education about complications.
- Give vitamin A (dose and regimen, 📖 Vitamin A deficiency, p. 716): this corrects vitamin A deficiency, ↓ severity of illness and ↓ case fatality.

If specific symptoms/signs or conditions are present:

- Give symptomatic relief from high fever with paracetamol.
- Treat eye infection (cornea cloudy or pus draining from eyes) with topical antibiotics.
- Manage diarrhoea/dysentery and dehydration as on 📖 General management of dehydration, p. 272.
- Broad-spectrum antibiotics for treatment of pneumonia.
- The role of antibiotic prophylaxis for 2° bacterial pneumonia has not been established.

Prevention

All children should be immunized:

- Give 1st dose of measles vaccine at the age of 9mths or shortly thereafter. If HIV+ve give first dose at 6mths (📖 Immunization of HIV-infected persons, p. 902).
- A 'second opportunity' for measles immunization should be provided to all children. This assures measles immunity in children who failed to receive an earlier dose of measles vaccine, as well as in those who were vaccinated but failed to develop immunity (10–15% of children vaccinated at 9mths of age).
- Providing measles vaccine to displaced persons living in temporary settings within a week of entry should be a public health priority.
- Measles surveillance enables prompt recognition and investigation of outbreaks, and provides information on programme impact.

Arboviruses and viral haemorrhagic fever

Arbovirus is a virus transmitted to man by arthropod vector, e.g. mosquito, tick, and midge. Most are zoonoses (infections of animals that spill over into humans). Collectively, they occur worldwide, although individual viruses have a limited geographical range. Most arboviruses can cause a mild self-limiting fever; however, infection can become severe and in some cases life-threatening. Disease caused by arboviruses can be broadly classified into three overlapping syndromes:

- Fever, arthralgia and rash (FAR).
- CNS involvement, especially encephalitis.
- Haemorrhagic fever (HF).

There is some overlap between these presentations. Dengue, for example, typically causes FAR, but may cause HF and can occasionally directly infect brain to cause encephalitis. HF most commonly caused by arboviral infection with yellow fever or dengue virus. Rift Valley and Crimean-Congo HF viruses are transmitted by arthropod vector, but can be transmitted directly by contact with infected blood. Some HF viruses have no arthropod vector (e.g. Ebola, Marburg, and Lassa, hanta, and South-American HF viruses). Table 18.10 outlines the geographical distribution, vector, mode of transmission and clinical syndromes associated with arboviruses and HF viruses.

Table 18.10. Classification of arbovirus infections and viral haemorrhagic fevers

Family/genus, disease	Geographic distribution	Vector/mode of transmission	Natural host	Clinical syndrome
Flaviviruses				
Japanese encephalitis	Asia	***Culex*** mosquito	Birds, (pigs amplifying host)	E, (flaccid paralysis)
St Louis encephalitis	Americas	***Culex*** mosquito	Birds	E
Murray Valley encephalitis	Australia, Papua New Guinea	Mosquito, mainly ***culex***	Birds	E
Yellow fever	Africa, South and Central America	***Aedes*** and jungle mosquitoes	Primates	HF with jaundice
Dengue (serotypes 1–4)	Asia, Central and South America, Africa, Australasia	***Aedes*** mosquito	Humans (and non-human primates)	FAR, HF, E
Kyasanur forest disease	South Asia	***Ixodid*** (hard) ticks	Small forest mammals	HF, E
Kunjin	Australia, Indonesia, Asia	***Culex*** mosquito	Birds	FAR, E
West Nile	Africa, Europe, Asia, Middle East, North/Central America	***Culex*** mosquito	Birds	FAR, E
tick-borne encephalitis	Russia, Asia, Europe, Scandinavia	***Ixodid*** (hard) ticks	Small mammals	E
Alphaviruses				
Chikungunya	Africa, India, Asia	***Aedes*** mosquito	Humans, primates	FAR, E
O'nyong nyong	Africa	Anopheline mosquito	Humans (other unknown)	FAR

(Continued)

Table 18.10 (*Continued*)

Family/genus, disease	Geographic distribution	Vector/mode of transmission	Natural host	Clinical syndrome
Venezuelan equine encephalitis	North and South America	Mosquito	Horses	E
Eastern equine encephalitis	North and South America	Mosquito	Horses	E
Western equine encephalitis	North and South America	Mosquito	Horses	E
Ross River fever	Australasia, South Pacific	***Culex*** and ***Aedes*** mosquitoes	Kangaroos, wallabies, other mammals	FAR
Coltiviruses				
Colorado tick fever	Western USA, Canada	Wood tick	Rodents and small mammals	FAR, (E, HF)
Bunyaviruses				
Rift Valley fever	Africa, Middle East	Contact with animal blood. Mosquito (mostly ***Aedes***).	Domestic livestock	HF, E, ocular disease
La Crosse encephalitis	USA, Canada	***Aedes*** mosquito	Small forest mammals	E
HF with renal syndrome (hantaviruses*)	Far East, Europe	Rodent bite/urine/faeces	Rural rodents	HF with renal syndrome
Crimean-Congo HF	Eastern Europe, Asia, Africa	***Ixodid*** (hard) ticks/contact with infected blood (animal, human)	Small wild mammals and domestic livestock	HF

(*Continued*)

Family/genus, disease	Geographic distribution	Vector/mode of transmission	Natural host	Clinical syndrome
Arenaviruses				
Lassa fever	Western Africa	Rodent urine/faeces, human-human	Mastomys rodent	HF
South American HFs**	South America	Rodent saliva/urine (human-human)	Rodents	HF
Filoviruses				
Ebola and Marburg	Sub-Saharan Africa	Human-human through contact with bodily fluids	Unknown	HF

FAR, fever, arthralgia, rash; HF, haemorrhagic fever; E, encephalitis.

*Hantaan, Seoul, Dobrava, and Puumala viruses.

**Argentine, Bolivian, Venezeuelan and Brazilian HF, caused by Junin, Machupo/Chapare, Guanarito, and Sabia viruses, respectively.

Fever, arthralgia and rash

Viruses that cause FAR affect every part of world. Overall, dengue causes more illness and death than any other arboviral infection. Chikungunya causes outbreaks of FAR in sub-Saharan Africa and much of Southeast Asia. Locally, other viruses such as O'nyong nyong, Ross River fever, and West Nile virus may be more important.

Clinical features

Typically begins a few days following exposure from infected bite. Fever and constitutional symptoms such as headache, nausea and myalgia often precede polyarthralgia. Most commonly affected joints are wrists, elbows, knees, and small joints of hands and feet. Occasionally, back, neck, or jaw may be involved. Joints are painful, with or without joint swelling and morning stiffness. Those affected often feel systemically unwell with myalgia and fatigue. Arthralgia usually lasts days or a few weeks, but may be prolonged. Some have pain and stiffness for months or years, particularly alphavirus infections (such as chikungunya and o'nyong nyong), which can cause symptoms lasting months or longer in up to 25% of cases. Rash variable; may not be present early in the illness. Most commonly, rash generalized and maculopapular, but may be mottled or flushing.

Diagnosis

- Identifying virus by PCR or viral antigen detection is unreliable and usually only possible within the first few days of infection.
- Antibody detection by IgM ELISA is more useful, however antibody may be –ve early in infection. A second test may be needed to demonstrate ↑ titres to exclude recent exposure unrelated to the presenting illness.
- Often these laboratory tests are not available in the areas affected; however there are now rapid bedside card tests for dengue.

The differential diagnosis is broad and depends on geographical area. Febrile arthralgia, with or without rash, may be caused by parvovirus B19, acute hepatitis B, rubella and HIV seroconversion illness. Non-infectious causes include chronic arthritides, such as rheumatoid arthritis and systemic lupus erythematosus, and vasculitides, such as HSP.

Management

Treatment is symptomatic with analgesics and gentle mobilization. No specific antiviral therapy. NSAIDs are mainstay of treatment. Steroids are usually not effective.

Encephalitis

For clinical features, management and aetiology of arboviral encephalitis, see 📖 Arboviruses and viral haemorrhagic fever, p. 804.

Haemorrhagic fever

HF occurs in most parts of the world and is caused by RNA viruses; Flaviviridae, Arenaviridae, Filoviridae, and Bunyaviridae (see Table 18.10) Few diseases cause as much fear as HF, however some viruses causing HF have low case fatality rates and not all have the potential for direct person-to-person spread.

Transmission

- Dengue and yellow fever viruses are transmitted by urban *Aedes aegypti* mosquitoes that breed in standing water in man-made containers. Yellow fever also has a sylvatic cycle via jungle mosquitoes (see Figs 18.25 and 18.26).
- Most Rift Valley fever virus transmission is through contact with infected animal blood (slaughtering, butchering, assisting births, etc.); however, some human infections result from bite of infected mosquitoes.
- Crimean-Congo HF is primarily spread by ticks, but transmission can occur when slaughtering animals. Human-to-human transmission has been described after contact with infected bodily fluids.
- Other HF viruses are not arthropod borne, but are transmitted by human-to-human spread (Ebola and Marburg), by contact with rodent excreta (various hantaviruses) or both (Lassa and some South American HF viruses). Lassa has a long incubation period (5d–3wks). This makes it the most likely directly transmissible viral HF in a returning traveller.
- South American HF viruses are transmitted from contact with rodent excreta but, as with Lassa, human-to-human spread is possible during close contact. They are: Junin virus →Argentine HF, Machupo and Chapare viruses →Bolivian HF, Guanarito virus →Venezuelan HF, Sabia virus →Brazilian HF.

Clinical features

All viral HFs, by definition, are characterized by fever and some form of bleeding tendency. In addition, can be varying degrees of ↑ vascular permeability, frank haemorrhage, hepatic failure, renal failure, and encephalopathy.

- Most early symptoms are non-specific, e.g. fever, myalgia, and malaise.
- Within a few days, illness → ↑ prostration, specific organ involvement, and evidence of vascular damage.
- May be petechial haemorrhages, mucosal bleeding, conjunctival injection, pharyngitis, retrosternal chest pain, vomiting and diarrhoea.
- Severe cases → shock, renal failure, encephalopathy and extensive bleeding.

Clinical features and disease severity varies with pathogen (see Table 18.11). Some HF viruses cause relatively mild illnesses and haemorrhagic manifestations may not be obvious. Look for bleeding from gums, microscopic haematuria and petechiae only visible in the skin folds and axillae, (for tourniquet test see Box 18.13). In contrast, Ebola and Marburg viruses typically → severe, life-threatening disease with extensive haemorrhage, organ failure, and shock. Case fatality rates can be up to 90% and there is no antiviral treatment.

Haemorrhagic fever with renal syndrome is caused by four hantaviruses from the family Bunyaviridae: Hantaan, Seoul, Dobrava and Puumala. Classically there are five phases:

- Febrile.
- Hypotensive (with haemorrhage).
- Oliguric.
- Diuretic.
- Convalescent.

Dengue HF and yellow fever are discussed separately in 📖 Dengue fever, p. 814 and 📖 Yellow fever, p. 818, respectively.

Diagnosis

Virological confirmation generally only available in specialist laboratories with biocontainment facilities. Otherwise, diagnosis by IgM/IgG serology.

There may be leukopenia, thrombocytopenia, ↑ prothrombin and activated partial thromboplastin times, ↑ transaminases, and proteinuria. Haematocrit is usually ↑ due to plasma leakage.

The differential diagnosis includes falciparum malaria and acute bacterial infections, especially meningococcal disease, leptospirosis and rickettsial infection, which require specific treatment.

Management

Management of HF involves intensive supportive care with fluid resuscitation to prevent shock due to capillary leak and haemorrhage. Platelet and coagulation factor replacement should be used with caution due to risk of exacerbating established disseminated intravascular coagulation.

Antiviral therapy with ribavirin should be used in Lassa, Crimean–Congo HF, hantaviruses, Rift Valley fever and South American HF, but is not effective in Ebola, Marburg, yellow fever or dengue HF. Convalescent serum from survivors may help, and a number of experimental treatments are in development.

Table 18.11 Clinical features of VHFs*

Disease	Incubation period (days)	Case infection ratio	Case fatality rate	Features of severe disease
Arenaviridae				
South American HFs	7–14	>50%	15–30%	Overt bleeding and shock; CNS involvement (dysarthria, intention tremor) common
Lassa fever	5–16	Mild infection common	2–15%	Prostration and shock; fewer haemorrhagic or neurological manifestations c.f. South American HF
Bunyaviridae				
Rift Valley fever	2–5	1%	50%	Bleeding, shock, anuria, jaundice; encephalitis and retinal vasculitis occur but are distinct from HF syndrome
Crimean–Congo HF	3–12	20–100%	15–30%	Most severe bleeding and bruising of all the HFs
HF with renal syndrome (Hantavirus)	9–35	>75%	5–15%	Febrile stage followed by shock and renal failure; bleeding at all stages
Filoviridae				
Marburg or Ebola	3–16	High	25–90%	Most severe of HFs; marked prostration; maculopapular rash common
Flaviviridae				
Dengue	See 🕮 p. 814			
Yellow fever	See 🕮 p. 818			
Kyasanur forest disease	3–8	Variable	0.5–9%	Typical biphasic illness—fever and haemorrhage followed by CNS involvement

*Adapted from Peters and Zaki, in *Tropical Infectious Diseases* (eds. Guerrant, Walker, and Weller)

Public health note

If a case of HF with potential for human-to-human spread is suspected, infection control measures to protect personnel should be instituted until more information is available. Consult local experts, the WHO, or Centers for Disease Control (CDC) immediately to advise on infection control and to help with diagnosis. An infection control manual for VHFs in Africa is available at: http://www.cdc.gov/ncidod/dvrd/spb/mnpages/vhfmanual.htm.

Infection control precautions for a suspected case of viral HF with potential for human-to-human spread

- Determine index case's places of residence and activities over last 3wks, search for unreported or undiagnosed cases.
- Establish surveillance for individuals at risk—all close contacts <3wks of onset of illness and laboratory staff handling specimens. Surveillance comprises body temperature measurement twice daily until 3wks after last possible exposure. If oral temperature >38.3°C, the contact should be hospitalized immediately in strict isolation.
- Reinforce and ensure the use of universal precautions in non-isolation areas of the health facility.
- Isolate the patient.
- Wear protective clothing (use two sets of gloves, two sets of clothing, plastic apron, boots, eyewear, bonnet, and mask) in the isolation area, cleaning and laundry area, laboratory, or when in contact with the patient. (Because of experimental infection of primates by aerosols, the observed high mortality among health care workers, and the desire to provide the maximum protection, use masks which meet the US HEPA or N series standards.)
- Handle needles and other sharp instruments safely. Do not recap needles. Dispose of non-reusable needles, syringes, and other sharp patient-care instruments in puncture-resistant containers. Use oral rather than IV medicine where possible.
- Avoid sharing equipment between patients. Designate equipment for each patient, if supplies allow. If sharing equipment is unavoidable, make sure it is not reused by another patient until it has been cleaned, disinfected, and sterilized properly.
- Disinfect all spills, equipment, and supplies safely. (Use disinfectant sprayers and 0.05% hypochlorite solutions.)
- Dispose of all contaminated waste by incineration or burial (including safe disposal of corpse).
- Provide appropriate information to the families and community about the prevention of VHF and the care of infected patients.

Dengue

Infection with dengue virus may be subclinical, or may cause dengue fever (DF), also known as breakbone fever. A small proportion of cases DF → life-threatening dengue haemorrhagic fever (DHF) with bleeding, thrombocytopenia and plasma leakage. Severe cases have circulatory failure (dengue shock syndrome; DSS). Without treatment, mortality is high in patients with DSS, but this is reduced to 1–5% by careful supportive care. Dengue virus can occasionally infect the brain to cause encephalitis.

Epidemiology

The most intense transmission occurs in Southeast Asia, but in recent years there has been dramatic ↑ in dengue transmission in the Indian subcontinent and the Western hemisphere (see Fig. 18.24). ~50–100 million people are infected with dengue each year. In established areas of intense dengue transmission almost all infections occur in children, and adults are immune to locally circulating serotypes of dengue virus. In contrast, if a particular serotype of dengue is newly transmitted in a geographical area, both adults and children will become infected. There is currently no vaccine. Vector control is effective but difficult to sustain.

Transmission

Dengue is transmitted from infected humans by day-biting *Aedes* mosquitoes—domestic mosquitoes that breed in human-made containers. There are four viral serotypes (1, 2, 3, and 4). Infection with one serotype produces only short-term protection against the others. If a person is infected again (especially if infected with a different dengue serotype) they are at risk of the severe complications of DHF and DSS. This is thought to be due to a process called antibody dependent enhancement.

Dengue is not transmitted directly from person to person and therefore no special infection control measures are required for suspected cases in hospital.

Dengue haemorrhagic fever

Clinical features

DHF usually begins in the same way as DF, but after 2–7d (usually on the day fever subsides) signs of bleeding and ↑ vascular permeability become apparent. The most severely ill patients have evidence of circulatory failure known as dengue shock syndrome.

Diagnosis

In order to be classified as DHF there must be fever, haemorrhagic tendencies, thrombocytopenia and evidence of plasma leakage (haematocrit >20% above average, a drop in haematocrit >20% after fluid replacement, or clinical signs e.g. pleural effusion/ascites). However there may be some degree of bleeding and vascular leak in DF and it can sometimes be difficult to differentiate DF from DHF clinically. More recently, WHO have recommended distinguishing DF from severe DF (including DHF and DSS), and identifying those with warning signs requiring strict observation (see Fig. 18.23).

Management

Prompt restoration of circulating volume is the cornerstone of therapy. The vascular leak syndrome typically resolves within 24–48h, and careful monitoring is required to avoid fluid overload during the recovery phase. Pulmonary oedema 2° to fluid overload can contribute to mortality.

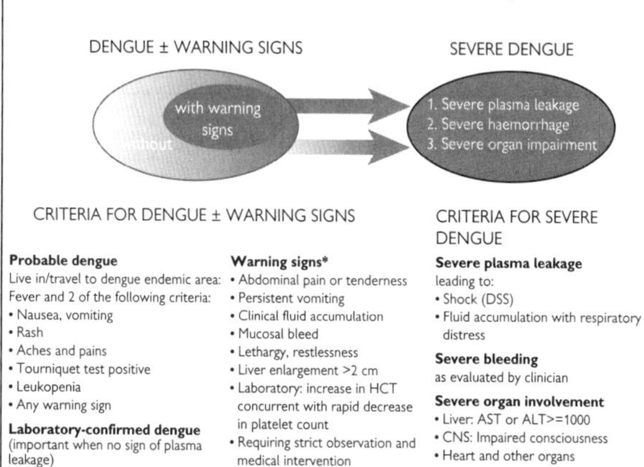

Fig. 18.23 WHO suggested dengue case definition and levels of severity.

Reproduced with permission from the WHO dengue guidelines for diagnosis, treatment, prevention and control (2009).

Dengue fever

Clinical features

DF begins abruptly 3–15d (usually 5–8d) after infected mosquito bite. Fever accompanied by severe headache, retro-orbital pain, and intense myalgia and arthralgia ('break bone fever'). A blanching rash typically appears after a few days and is a useful clue to diagnosis if present. Presence of vascular leak and bleeding are key features that distinguish DHF from DF, but some degree of vascular leak and bleeding may be present in DF. Tourniquet test is measure of capillary fragility and is often +ve in DF and DHF (see Box 18.13); DF usually lasts for 4–7d, followed by complete recovery, but some patients have ongoing symptoms.

Laboratory diagnosis Dengue viraemia correlates well with temperature, thus virus can be isolated (or confirmed by PCR or viral antigen detection) in a febrile patient with dengue. Once the fever has resolved, serology (using IgM capture ELISA) is more useful. Rapid bedside tests for dengue are now available.

Management No specific antiviral therapy and treatment is symptomatic. Arthralgia may respond to NSAIDs, but aspirin should be avoided due to bleeding risk.

Box 18.13 Tourniquet test

BP cuff is inflated to halfway between systolic and diastolic blood pressure for 5min. Test is +ve if this produces ≥20 petechiae in a 2.5cm^2 area of forearm.

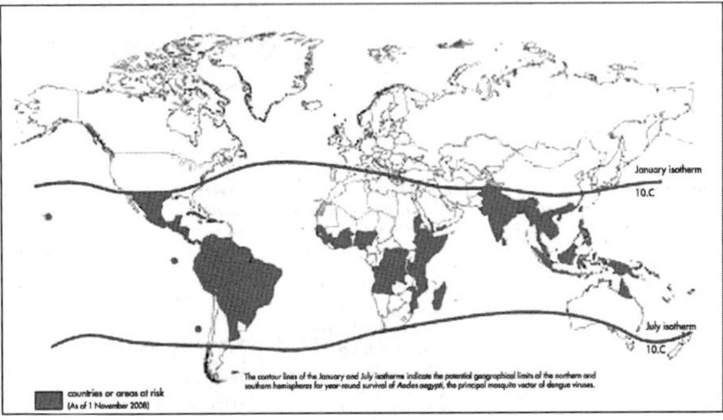

Fig. 18.24 Countries/areas at risk of dengue transmission, 2008 (shaded areas). Lines represent January and July isotherms, which indicate potential geographical limits of northern and southern hemispheres for year-round survival of *Aedes aegypti*, principal mosquito vector of dengue viruses.

Adapted with permission from the WHO dengue guidelines for diagnosis, treatment, prevention and control (2009).

Yellow fever

Yellow fever (YF) is caused by a mosquito-borne flavivirus. The 'yellow' in the name refers to jaundice, although this is not always present. There are ~200 000 cases causing ~30 000 deaths/yr worldwide, most in sub-Saharan Africa, with far fewer in Central and South America (Fig. 18.25). Although disease has never been reported in Asia, the region is potentially at risk because conditions required for transmission are present there.

Transmission

Jungle (sylvatic) YF infects non-human primates who are asymptomatic and maintain the reservoir of infection. Humans entering tropical rain forest are occasionally infected when they are bitten by an infected mosquito. Localized outbreaks can occur in humid savannah regions of Africa where mosquitoes infect both monkeys and humans (intermediate/savannah YF). If a viraemic person enters an urban environment, *Aedes aegypti* mosquito can spread the virus from human-to-human with the potential for explosive epidemics in unvaccinated populations. The urban cycle is extremely rare in South America, where almost all infections are in persons living or working in tropical rainforest areas (Fig. 18.26).

Clinical features of YF

Illness begins abruptly 3–6d after the bite of an infected mosquito. Characteristic features are fever, chills, headache, backache, nausea, vomiting, widespread myalgia, and infected conjunctiva. In most patients this 'acute phase' resolves spontaneously within 3–4d. However, in ~15% of patients, a 'toxic phase' develops within 24h of the initial remission with ↑ fever, jaundice, abdominal pain, diarrhoea, and renal failure. Thrombocytopaenia and coagulopathy can → frank bleeding from gums, nose, eyes and GI tract. May be relative bradycardia in relation to fever (Faget's sign). Up to 50% with severe disease will die within 2wks without treatment. The rest recover without significant organ damage.

Diagnosis

Diagnosis is usually made by detection of IgM by capture ELISA. Virus can be isolated from blood in the first few days of illness. Virus can be identified in post-mortem liver tissue. Differential diagnosis includes malaria, rickettsial infection, viral hepatitis, leptospirosis, dengue or other VHF. Non-infectious causes include hepatobiliary disease and poisoning.

Management

No specific anti-viral therapy and treatment is supportive. Direct human-to-human transmission has not been reported, but insecticide spraying and bed nets should be used to prevent the patient being bitten by a mosquito vector. All YF cases should be notified to the WHO.

Prevention

Vaccination is most important preventive measure; YF vaccine is safe, affordable and highly effective, although in recent years adverse events following vaccination have been described. One dose of live-attenuated YF vaccine provides effective immunity within 1wk and protection is

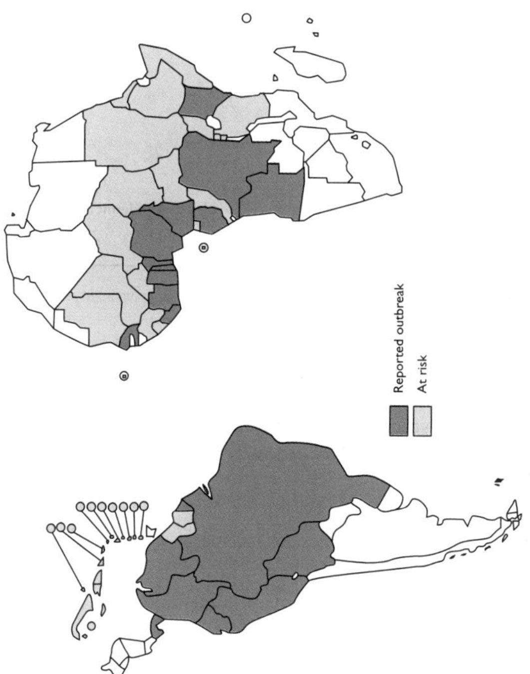

Fig. 18.25 Countries at risk from yellow fever (shaded) and reported cases from 1985–2004 (dark shading). Reproduced with permission from WHO.

probably life-long, although international travel regulations require evidence of immunization within 10yrs prior to arrival in endemic countries 📖 Expanded programme on immunization recommended vaccines, p. 904. Vector control can be effective but is difficult to sustain. In the case of an epidemic outbreak, infection control measures should be taken (Box 18.14).

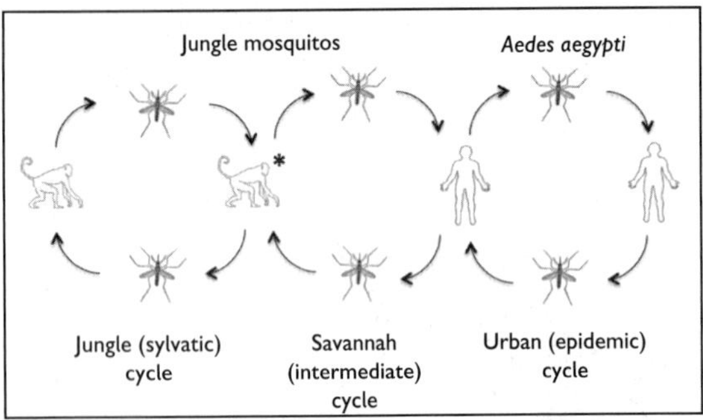

Fig. 18.26 Transmission cycle of yellow fever virus in Africa (savannah YF does not occur in South America, and the urban cycle is rare).

*Humans entering jungle environments can be incidentally infected at this point.

Box 18.14 Public health note

Management of a yellow fever (urban) outbreak

- Notify WHO of any confirmed YF case (required under international health regulations).
- *Mass immunization:* if resources limited, target children 9mths–14yrs old.
- ↓ *Aedes* mosquito breeding sites. Refill domestic water containers and cover. Remove receptacles that collect water, e.g. discarded tyres, tins, and jars.
- In an expanding outbreak, consider widespread insecticide spraying.
- *Local surveillance of epidemic:* collect specimens for laboratory diagnosis from any new suspected cases (post-mortem if necessary).

Longer-term prevention measures

- Include YF vaccine in routine childhood EPI schedule (can give at 9mths with measles vaccine).
- *Provide health education messages:* domestic water containers should be covered with a lid or screen. Waste items that can collect standing water should be buried or disposed of in a safe manner.

Chikungunya

Chikungunya is a mosquito-borne alphavirus with a wide geographical range: sub-Saharan Africa, India, Indian Ocean islands and much of Southeast Asia. In recent decades mosquito vector has spread, and it was reported in Europe for first time in 2007.

Clinical features

The illness begins abruptly 4–8d after bite of an infected mosquito. Joint pain is prominent, and accompanies fever, chills, myalgia, headache, photophobia, vomiting, lymphadenopathy, and a predominantly truncal rash. Minor haemorrhagic phenomena can occur. Symptoms usually subside within 5–7d. However, in some cases, joint pain may persist for months or years, and can be very debilitating. 12% of patients have chronic arthralgia 3yrs after onset of illness.

Infection is not usually life-threatening, unless there are significant co-morbidities, but some outbreaks may be due to more virulent strains. Confirmed cases of meningo-encephalitis in neonates and the elderly.

Diagnosis

Symptoms are often misdiagnosed as dengue. Diagnosis is by antibody detection with IgM-capture ELISA. Viral isolation by PCR may be +ve with acute samples.

Management

Treatment is symptomatic, aimed in particular at relieving joint pain. There is no commercial chikungunya vaccine.

Japanese encephalitis

Japanese encephalitis (JE) is a mosquito-borne flavivirus. Most common viral encephalitis worldwide causing ~50 000 cases and ~10 000 deaths/yr across Asia, mostly among children. For details of Japanese encephalitis see 📖 p. 448.

Further reading

Useful website

Infection control manual for VHFs in Africa. Available at: http://www.cdc.gov/ncidod/dvrd/spb/mnpages/vhfmanual.htm.

Chikungunya

Chapter 19

Mental health

Invited authors **Charlotte Hanlon**
Vikram Patel

Introduction

Mental illnesses account for >10% of the global burden of disease; this proportion is likely to ↑ as populations age and other health problems are controlled. Common mental disorders (depression, anxiety), alcohol use disorders, psychoses (schizophrenia, bipolar disorder) and intellectual disabilities are the leading psychiatric causes of disability.

In most communities, mental illnesses are equated with psychoses. Depression, anxiety, and substance abuse, which account for most mental morbidity, are seen as social problems, with physical symptoms being the typical clinical presentations. Mental illnesses are more common in people with physical illnesses, e.g. diabetes or HIV/AIDS, and may complicate the treatment of physical disorders, e.g. mothers with depression are more likely to have LBW babies and malnourished infants. When people with HIV/AIDS have a mental disorder, this may interfere with their HIV care. Mental disorders are associated with ↑ mortality, through suicide, physical disease (e.g. liver damage from alcohol abuse), and worsening of outcome of co-morbid physical health problems (See Box 19.1 for terminology.).

Most mental disorders can be treated effectively using cheap and relatively simple interventions, delivered by primary or community HCWs. Yet most mental disorders are not recognized by HCW, and treated inappropriately or not treated at all. Lack of knowledge and skills, not having enough time, and the stigma attached to mental disorders (especially psychoses) are major obstacles.

Box 19.1 Terminology: making sense of mental illness

Terms used for mental disorders are heavily influenced by language, e.g. if very few patients complain of 'depression', then the term 'depression' has limited meaning for doctors or patients. However, in all languages, one can find locally meaningful words to describe emotional and behavioural states that doctors may diagnose as a mental disorder. Find out what the most appropriate words are for the descriptions below and use these to help communicate with your patients and other health workers (HWs) more effectively.

- A condition where the person thinks too much, cannot sleep, and is tired all the time (*probable diagnosis:* common mental disorders = anxiety and/or depression).
- A condition where the person gets very scared or frightened for no reason (*probable diagnosis:* panic disorder or post-traumatic stress disorder (PTSD)).
- A condition where the person behaves in a strange way, says strange things, holds strange beliefs or hears things that are not really there (*probable diagnosis:* severe mental disorders = psychoses).
- A health problem where the person drinks too much alcohol or uses drugs (*probable diagnosis:* alcohol or drug use disorder).
- A condition in which a child does not learn as well as others in school (*probable diagnosis:* intellectual disability).

Suicide and deliberate self-harm

Deliberate self-harm may take many forms, e.g. deliberate overdosing with medication, self-poisoning with pesticides, self-cutting, hanging, or burning. The motivations can vary widely and several may play a role simultaneously. There are large variations between countries in the rates and methods used depending on socio-cultural and economic conditions. In most cases, the patient is likely to be suffering from a mental illness, typically depression or alcohol use, or a chronic and debilitating physical illness (e.g. HIV/AIDS). Major risk factors include social factors (especially financial difficulties and violence) and, in young people, educational pressures and conflict with parents or partners. The lethality of suicide attempts varies considerably between the sexes and populations, both due to method used, and availability and access to emergency medical care.

Management of self-harm

- 1st treat medical consequences of suicide attempt (📖 Acute pesticide poisoning, p. 874).
- Try to see person quickly, or offer a place to wait that minimizes distress.
- Decide whether there is an imminent risk of suicide (Box 19.2). Remove dangerous/sharp objects and ensure constant monitoring to maintain safety.
- Suicide is a sensitive and personal matter. Talk to the patient in private. Give the patient enough time to feel comfortable and share their reasons frankly.
- Do not make judgements about patient's character; do not make reassuring statements without fully understanding patient's situation because this may make patient feel even more hopeless
- Talk to family or friends for their version of patient's recent life situation and health.
- Assess mental state (look for common mental disorders, alcohol or drug dependency, and psychotic disorders) and offer appropriate treatment.
- Optimize management of any painful or debilitating conditions.
- Help patient address the main problems. These may be psychological, social (e.g. financial problems, relationship difficulties), or physical (e.g. chronic illness); see Box 19.5.
- Explore reasons to live and ways to stay alive.
- Enlist the help of others (e.g. relatives or friends, social workers, counsellors), with the consent of the patient, to provide close monitoring while at high risk of suicide and provide social support. Support caregivers too.
- If prescribing, give least dangerous medications and only small amounts of medication at any one time.
- If high risk of suicide, consult a specialist mental health worker.
- Ensure you give a follow-up appointment within 1wk.

Box 19.2 Assessment of suicide risk

Consider suicide risk in all patients with mental illnesses. Patients are rarely embarrassed, and often very relieved, to be asked tactfully about suicide. Asking about suicidal thoughts does not increase risk for suicide. Simple questions you might ask are:

- 'Feeling as you've described recently, have you felt that life was a struggle? Have you felt as if there was no point in living anymore?'
- 'Patients with similar difficulties to you sometimes tell me they feel like ending their life. Have you felt like that?'

Is there imminent risk of suicide?

- Current thoughts or plan to commit suicide *or*
- History of suicidal thoughts/plans in last month or act of self-harm in past year in a person who is now extremely agitated, violent, distressed, or uncommunicative.

What is the future risk of suicide?

- *Intention of act:* what was their motivation? Ask about associated actions and thoughts; go through what led up to act and afterwards. Was there planning/preparation?
- *Method chosen:* how lethal or dangerous was method chosen? Why did they choose this method, and did they consider alternatives? Did they make any 'final acts' (e.g. writing a suicide note)? Did they take precautions to avoid discovery?
- *What did the act represent:* a wish to die/for help/something else? Did they seek help or tell anyone? Was medical attention willingly sought or were they coerced?
- *Precipitation*: what problems led to the act? Are these likely to recur or persist? What can be done about them?
- *Resources*: what resources are available (self/friends/family/community/health services)? Is the patient isolated? How can this be addressed?
- *Present feelings and intentions*: do they regret or feel guilty about the act or being discovered? Have they changed how they feel? If they go home, will they cope? What do they want now: to die or get help? Will they accept treatment or help?
- *Mental state*: is the patient severely depressed or psychotic? Do they feel hopeless? Are they agitated, violent, distressed or uncommunicative?
- *Protective factors*: do they have hope for future improvement? Do they have supportive children/partner/family/friends or strong convictions or religious beliefs that would prevent them from committing suicide?
- *Personal history:* previous attempts, chronic pain or illness, social isolation, unemployment, older age (all ↑ risk of eventual suicide).

Acute behavioural disturbance

In most cases, persons with mental illness are not violent, and, indeed, are more likely to be victims than perpetrators of violence. Having said that, risk of disturbed behaviour (including violence) can be ↑ in persons with untreated psychosis, especially when accompanied by substance misuse. In acutely disturbed behaviour, it is critically important to exclude medical or traumatic causes that can cause delirium.

- *Safety first:* do not see patient alone. Ensure clear path to the exit.
- *Try to de-escalate the situation:* respect patient's rights and dignity, irrespective of how disturbed they may be. Avoid confrontation or argument. Where it is necessary to intervene, do it calmly and firmly.
- *Look for evidence of severe medical illness:* ask for any history of medical illness or drug use.
- If possible, check pulse, BP, temperature and blood glucose and look for any indicators of acute confusion or delirium (📖 Acute confusional state and delerium, p. 430) or drug intoxication (📖 Disorders due to substance abuse, p. 842). Treat underlying cause.
- If cause of behavioural disturbance not immediately reversible, and person is a potential danger to themselves or others, administer sedative medications (see Box 19.3).
- Acutely disturbed patients, especially those with acute manic episodes, may need to be admitted to hospital and require intensive nursing. If this is not available, try to arrange a safe environment with adequate supervision (e.g. from a family member or nurse).

Box 19.3 Rapid tranquillization of the acutely disturbed patient

- *Start by offering oral medication:* if already taking an antipsychotic medication, offer diazepam 10mg po (avoid benzodiazepines in delirium) or promethazine 50mg po. If not already taking antipsychotic medication, then consider chlorpromazine 25–50mg po or risperidone 1–2mg po, or haloperidol 1.5–5mg po (use haloperidol with caution if history of IHD; avoid if ↑ QT interval).
- If refusing oral medication give lorazepam 1–2mg IM (if available) or promethazine 50mg IM. Avoid IM diazepam as absorption is erratic. Consider haloperidol 5mg IM as a last resort (acute dystonia is common).
- If insufficient improvement with either po or IM sedation, repeat after 30–60min, up to 2×.
- IV treatment with diazepam 10mg can be used as an alternative if it can be administered safely. Give over at least 5min. Wait 5–10min for a response and repeat up to 3×.
- Monitor temperature, pulse, BP, and RespR several times in the first hour, and regularly thereafter, until the patient is walking around again.
- If RespR drops <10breaths/min after administration of diazepam or lorazepam, give flumazenil to reverse benzodiazepine.

Common mental disorders

Common mental disorders are depressive and anxiety disorders, most often seen in 1° care. Although psychiatric classifications deal with depressive disorders and anxiety disorders separately, many patients have symptoms of both disorders, both have similar risk factors, and both respond to similar treatments. Hence, the broader term of 'common mental disorders' is often used when describing the practical, clinical approach to these disorders.

Common mental disorders are amongst the most important causes of morbidity in 1° care and are the leading mental health cause of disability worldwide. However, these disorders are often missed, because few patients complain of psychological symptoms. Moreover, there is a tendency to prescribe benzodiazepines or placebo treatments (e.g. vitamins) when specific and efficacious treatments exist: antidepressants and brief psychological treatment.

Clinical features

Although the terms 'depression' and 'anxiety' imply a sad mood or feeling fearful, few patients complain of emotional or cognitive (thinking) symptoms. Patients classically have physical complaints (see Box 19.4). That said, on inquiry you can readily elicit emotional and cognitive symptoms. Sometimes, relatives may misinterpret these symptoms as signs of laziness. Physical symptoms with no medical cause can also occur in the absence of depression or anxiety, understood to be a sub conscious way of coping with psychosocial stressors (so-called 'somatization'). In some individuals, irritability or severe symptoms of anxiety may dominate, e.g. panic attacks and phobias (see next section). Panic attacks may present as an emergency, e.g. with acute chest pain.

Diagnosis

Anxiety and depression are normal human experiences in certain situations, e.g. to feel miserable when a relative dies, or a student before an examination will feel anxious and tense. Depression/anxiety is diagnosed as an illness if lasting >2wks and interfering with daily life. Suspect a common mental disorder when physical complaints do not fit into the pattern of common physical illnesses. Remember that common mental disorders are more frequent in persons with chronic physical health problems; always assess depression and anxiety in such patients. Also at ↑ risk are those using drugs or alcohol, tobacco users, women, and people facing severe economic or social difficulties.

In all patients, inquire about drug and alcohol misuse (alcohol/drugs may be used to self-treat anxiety, or anxiety and depression may be the consequence of dependence). Prescribed medications can cause depression and/or anxiety, e.g. steroids, beta-blockers, ART (e.g. efavirenz and nevirapine), oestrogens, anticonvulsants, statins, ciprofloxacin, calcium-channel blockers and others. Rarely, anxiety and depression may be the presenting symptoms of another medical disorder, e.g. hypothyroidism.

Box 19.4 Clinical features

Depression

Presenting complaints

- Tiredness, fatigue, and weakness.
- Vague aches and pains all over the body.
- Crawling or burning sensations.
- Disturbed sleep (usually worse, but occasionally too much sleep).
- ↓ Appetite (sometimes ↑ appetite).

Complaints on inquiry

- Feeling sad and miserable.
- Feeling a loss of interest in life, social interactions, work, etc.
- Feeling irritable.
- Feeling guilty.
- Feeling hopeless about the future.
- Difficulty making decisions.
- 'Thinking too much'.
- Thoughts that one is not as good as others (low self-esteem).
- Thoughts that it would be better if one was not alive.
- Suicidal ideas and plans.
- Difficulty in concentrating.

Anxiety

Presenting complaints

- Palpitations.
- A feeling of suffocation.
- Chest pain.
- Dizziness.
- Trembling, shaking all over.
- Headaches.
- Pins and needles (or sensation of ants crawling) on limbs or face.
- Poor sleep.
- Nausea, non-specific abdominal complaints.

Complaints on inquiry

- Feeling as if something terrible is going to happen.
- Feeling scared.
- Worrying too much about one's problems or one's health.
- Thoughts that one is going to die, lose control, or go mad.

Common management principles

- Use a stepped care approach, i.e. give advice to all patients and reserve medication or psychological treatment for those who do not recover or are moderate/severely depressed (e.g. actively suicidal).
- Rule out medical disorder or medication side effects.
- After confirming diagnosis, assess suicide risk (see Box 19.2). There is no evidence that asking about suicide 'puts ideas into their head'.
- Reassure patient and relatives that just because there are no physical signs or diagnoses, this does not mean that patient is 'making it up'.

- *Counter stigma:* a common problem that can happen to anybody.
- *Instil hope:* explain that effective treatment is possible.
- Identify and ↓ substances that predispose to depression and/or anxiety (e.g. cigarettes, chewing khat (*Catha edulis*), alcohol).
- Identify and discuss ways of ↓ work pressures, disabilities, or conflict at home. Speak with the spouse or relatives.
- Encourage the patient to stop concentrating on –ve ideas or acting on them (e.g. leaving work).
- *Avoid the 'pull yourself together' or 'there is nothing wrong with you' approach:* patients are caught up in guilt and feelings of failure, and do not need to be blamed for their symptoms.
- Recommend a regular sleep cycle and physical activity.
- Behavioural activation and re-activation of previous social networks and activities can be simple but effective ways to improve mood (see Box 19.5).
- A problem-solving approach can also help (see Box 19.5).
- Identify supportive family members and involve them in the patient's care.
- Refer the person to appropriate agencies for social problems, e.g. economic difficulties or intimate partner violence.
- Medication is useful for moderate and severe depressive episodes with 70–80% patients showing an improvement (see Box 19.6).
- Offer regular follow-up.
- *If patient does not respond:* review diagnosis, ensure treatment adherence, check for co-morbid alcohol or substance misuse, and consider ↑ drug dose or changing to an alternative class of drug.

When medically unexplained symptoms are the main complaint

- Only carry out indicated medical investigations.
- Avoid placebo treatments.
- Acknowledge that the patient's symptoms and suffering are real.
- Communicate test results clearly. Reassure that no dangerous disease has been identified, but that it is important to treat distressing symptoms.
- Identify psychosocial stressors and ask about links to physical symptoms.
- Explain how stress can ↑ health problems, including physical complaints, e.g. physical sensations experienced when a person is very scared.
- Explain that stress can make pain worse and needs to be treated too.
- Emphasize the importance of a gradual return to normal activities.
- Advise the person to consult you first if symptoms worsen or new symptoms appear, so that they do not waste money on ineffective treatments.
- Arrange regular follow-up.

Box 19.5 Psychosocial interventions for common mental disorders

Relaxation training

These techniques need to be practised, ideally daily, to develop the ability to relax before and during stressful situations.

- *Progressive muscle relaxation:* in a quiet environment, close eyes, tensing then relaxing muscles, starting from feet, then legs, then thighs, etc., up to the head. Concentrate on the relaxed feelings.
- *Controlled breathing:* close eyes; breathe in and out to a slow count of 4 or 5. Continue for 5min. Patient can say in his/her mind a religious or calming word while exhaling.
- *Imagery:* visualize a scene that is calm, safe, and relaxing. Concentrate on the details—smells, sounds, and feel of the place.
- *Distraction:* focus attention away from anxious thoughts and sensations and on to something relaxing and absorbing.

Problem-solving

Common mental disorders are often consequence of practical problems patient is facing in their daily lives. Unfortunately, disorders ↓ ability of patient to take steps necessary to overcome their problems. Problem-solving aims to empower the patient to regain control over their lives.

- Explain treatment.
- Define problems (what are different problems faced by patient).
- Summarize problems (how are these problems related to patient's symptoms).
- Select one problem and choose goals (why should patient overcome problem).
- Define solutions (small, defined actions to be taken to overcome problem).
- Review the outcome of the actions taken at follow up: did it make the problem less; did it help improve the patient's mood, what were the barriers experienced and how can they be addressed.

Behavioural activation

Aim of this psychological treatment is to ↑ exposure to potentially pleasurable activities which the patient may have stopped due to depression, e.g. playing with grandchildren, meeting friends. Identify these previously enjoyed activities. Set an achievable goal (e.g. meet up with friend twice a week), encourage perseverance even when not immediately enjoyable, and build up from there.

Reactivating social networks

Social withdrawal → loss of social support can make common mental disorders worse and interfere with recovery. Identify previous social networks and activities and encourage person to re-engage with these.

Specific presentations

Recurrent depression

Some patients suffer from repeated episodes of depression. Consider long-term follow up (e.g. monthly) to discuss personal and social issues, and continue antidepressants for 2yrs or more. In addition to an antidepressant, consider a long-term mood-stabilizing medication (e.g. lithium).

Phobic disorder

A phobia is a fear of a specific situation that is out of proportion to the objective risks, beyond voluntary control, and not responsive to reasoning. It results in avoidance of situations in which the trigger might occur (e.g. crowds, open spaces, travelling, social events). Patients may become confined to their house. Phobias can be managed by relaxation training techniques to help them to 'face their fear' (see Box 19.5). Use graded exposure (e.g. to feared situation e.g. crowds) to ↓ avoidance and escape the cycle of reinforcement. Antidepressants may also be effective.

Panic disorder

Panic disorder is characterized by recurrent, frequent, unexpected panic attacks in which the patient experiences severe, acute anxiety accompanied by chest pain, breathlessness, or dizziness that are typically the result of hyperventilation. Panic attacks are best managed using relaxation training techniques in combination with preventing reinforcement of the anxiety through avoidance (e.g. of going out) or escape (running out of the shop when anxiety symptoms appear). Antidepressants are also effective and benzodiazepines can be used for short-term relief.

Obsessive-compulsive disorder

Obsessional thoughts are recurrent thoughts, ideas, or images that are distressing to the patient who makes efforts (often unsuccessful) to get rid of them, e.g. thoughts of being dirty or blasphemous or ugly. Compulsions are behaviours that are repeated (e.g. cleaning or counting rituals), even though patient recognizes that this is irrational, but is unable to resist urge to carry them out. Management involves psychological treatments (e.g. cognitive behavioural techniques) or antidepressants (e.g. fluoxetine, clomipramine, usually requiring treatment at high end of the therapeutic range, and for a longer period than for depression).

Box 19.6 Medicines for common mental disorders

Antidepressants

There are two major classes:

- *Tricyclic antidepressants (TCAs):* e.g. imipramine or amitriptyline, initially 50mg po nocte, ↑ by 25–50mg/wk. Min. effective dose is 75mg; max. daily dose 200mg, given as a single dose at night time.
- *Selective serotonin reuptake inhibitors (SSRIs):* e.g. fluoxetine, initially 20mg po od (also min. effective dose), max. daily dose 60mg given as a single dose in the morning with or after food.

Choice of antidepressant is influenced by:

- *Toxicity:* if risk of overdose is high, avoid TCAs.
- *Side-effect profile:* avoid TCAs in patients with heart disease.
- *Age:* avoid TCAs in adolescents and the elderly; in adolescents, fluoxetine is the antidepressant of choice, but should be used only if psychosocial treatments are not feasible or ineffective.
- Symptoms: consider more sedative medication (e.g. amitriptyline, imipramine) in anxious or sleep-deprived patients.

Regimen

- Explain that antidepressants are not addictive.
- Build up to the minimum effective dose within the 1st week.
- Use lower doses if patient is adolescent, elderly or medically ill.
- Explain side-effects usually fade after 2–3wks and that max benefit builds up over 3–6wks, provided medication taken daily.
- Regularly review side-effects, adherence and suicidal ideation.
- As long as the medication can be tolerated and is at a therapeutic dose, do not ↑ the dose or change class until there has been a proper 'therapeutic trial' (6wks).
- Do not prescribe 2 antidepressants at same time, except briefly if swapping from TCA to SSRI (but not from SSRI to TCA).
- In patients with bipolar disorder, antidepressants should only be prescribed in combination with a mood stabilizer (or antipsychotic if a mood stabilizer is not available).
- If psychotic features present, outcome better if antipsychotic medication prescribed (see 🕮 Antipsychotic drugs for severe mental disorders, p. 838) in addition to antidepressant.
- Once improved continue antidepressant for at least another 6mths (and preferably up to 1yr) to minimize risk of relapse.
- Withdraw gradually to avoid discontinuation syndromes.

Anxiolytic medications

- When using antidepressants to treat anxiety, use a lower starting dose and explain that anxiety may get worse temporarily.
- Benzodiazepines (e.g. diazepam 2mg po tds, ↑ as necessary to 5–10mg tds) should only be used for short-term (<2 wks) relief of severe and disabling anxiety symptoms. Dependence and reinforcement of anxiety may occur with longer use. See 🕮 Management of specific withdrawal states, p. 845 for advice on withdrawing benzodiazepines in cases of dependency.

Severe mental disorders (psychoses)

This group of disorders consists of schizophrenia, bipolar disorder (manic-depressive disorder), and other psychotic disorders (e.g. delusional disorder, brief psychotic episode, schizoaffective disorder). Psychoses are relatively rare and characterized by marked behavioural problems, and strange or unusual thinking. Most patients in psychiatric hospitals have psychoses. Most cultures equate mental disorders with the psychoses but it is critically important to differentiate severe mental disorders from organic psychosis or delirium (see Box 19.7).

Clinical features of psychoses

- *Delusions:* false beliefs, not in keeping with the patient's cultural or educational background, e.g. body or mind are under external control, or that thoughts are being inserted, withdrawn, or broadcast from their mind, or persecutory or grandiose delusions, or other very bizarre beliefs.
- *Hallucinations:* experience of their thoughts being spoken aloud, or other persistent auditory, visual, olfactory, or somatic hallucinations.
- *Thought disorder:* inability to communicate coherently, with thinking and speech becoming illogical and irrelevant.
- *Disturbed behaviour:* both aggressive or agitated; withdrawn or apathetic behaviour may be seen.
- *Insight* (awareness of being ill and needing treatment) is often seriously impaired.

Distinguishing bipolar disorder and other psychoses

- *Affective/mood symptoms:* if there are marked depressive or manic features, most likely diagnosis is psychotic depression or bipolar disorder.
- *Chronicity:* if symptoms have been continually evident for >6mths, likely diagnosis is schizophrenia.
- *Episodic course:* with periods of relatively normal health in between, is more typical of bipolar disorder.
- *Presence of a trigger:* although any psychoses may be precipitated by a trigger, these are the hallmark of acute or brief psychoses.

Schizophrenia

A severe mental disorder that usually begins before the age of 30. Apart from the usual symptoms of psychoses, patients may also show catatonic behaviour (stupor, mutism, posturing), –ve symptoms (unexplained apathy, not speaking, incongruous affect), and marked social withdrawal. Schizophrenia is often a long-term illness that may last years and require long-term treatment. Often a family history of mental illness.

Box 19.7 Features suggestive of organic psychosis or delirium

- Acute onset for 1st time within the preceding month.
- Assume new onset 'psychosis' in the elderly is organic unless proven otherwise.
- ↓ Level of consciousness.
- Disorientation to time, place, and person, worsening at night.
- Presence of medical illness (see Box 19.7).
- Medications with CNS action, e.g. efavirenz, steroids, opioids.

Bipolar disorder or manic depressive illness

Characterized by episodes of 'high' mood or mania, and 'low' mood or depression. Usually begins in adulthood and is generally diagnosed because of the manic phase, characterized by agitation, inappropriate behaviour (e.g. spending money excessively or sexually inappropriate behaviour), ↓ sleep, ↑ levels of energy, irritability, suspiciousness, rapid thinking and speech, and grandiose delusions (e.g. believing one has special powers). Depressed phase is similar to depression in common mental disorders, but it is usually more serious. A typical feature of this condition is that it is episodic. There are months to years when person is completely well, even off treatment. Often family history of mental illness. Bipolar disorder diagnosis requires ≥1 manic episode. Differential diagnosis of manic episodes includes alcohol or drug misuse, and acute psychoses.

Acute or brief psychoses

Usually start suddenly. Characterized by florid or marked psychotic symptoms. Most patients recover completely within a month and do not need long-term treatment. Typically caused by sudden severe stressful event, e.g. death of a loved person, or may be induced by illegal drugs, e.g. amphetamines or cannabis, or prescribed drugs, e.g. mefloquine, chloroquine. Sometimes, acute psychotic episode may be presenting event heralding schizophrenic illness. Important to rule out delirium or organic psychosis.

Management of severe mental disorders

- If acutely disturbed, see Box 19.3.
- Treatment should be started as soon as possible.
- Screen for risk of suicide (Box 19.2) and/or harm to self or others.
- Treat with antipsychotic medication (for schizophrenia, manic episodes or acute psychoses) or mood-stabilizing medication (for bipolar disorder—see 📖 Antipsychotic drugs for severe mental disorders, p. 838). These medications are usually needed for extended >12mths, and often for several years, depending on the response.
- Develop a therapeutic relationship with the patient.

- Review regularly to assess mental health and provide medication.
- Maintain realistic hope.
- If there is no or incomplete response, ↑ dose.
- *Assess adherence:* discuss reasons for non-adherence (e.g. poor insight, intolerable side-effects) and address these reasons (e.g. switch antipsychotic drug to an alternative with fewer side-effects).
- *Family intervention:* discuss the illness with supportive family members, and counsel them to ↓ levels of stress and hostility in the family. A sympathetic explanation that the patient is suffering from an illness that can be treated may help allay fears about the cause and implications of the illness. Emphasize that schizophrenia and bipolar disorder need long-term treatment.
- Advocate for persons with severe mental disorder to be brought for treatment if they relapse, rather than being restrained at home.
- Explain to family that covert administration of medication (e.g. hidden in food) may have long-term –ve effects on the patient's trust, and ultimately cause more harm than good.
- Encourage inclusion of patient in social activities and life of community.
- Once patient has recovered from acute symptoms, encourage participation in sheltered work or appropriate training to help develop occupational and self-care skills.
- Activity or distraction may ↓ severity or burden of symptoms, e.g. hallucinations.
- Especially in bipolar disorder emphasize importance of routine and avoid sleep deprivation, to ↓ risk of relapse.
- Discuss with the patient and their family about early symptoms of relapse and the importance of seeking treatment promptly.
- Counsel patient regarding cessation of substance abuse, especially cannabis, amphetamine, and khat, which can exacerbate psychoses.

Antipsychotic drugs for severe mental disorders

Antipsychotic drugs can be conveniently grouped into:

- *Conventional ('typical') drugs:* e.g. chlorpromazine, trifluoperazine, haloperidol. These drugs are older and more widely available, but have more extrapyramidal and anticholinergic side-effects.
- *Atypical drugs:* e.g. risperidone, clozapine. These are newer, have fewer extrapyramidal and anticholinergic side-effects, but ↑ risk of metabolic syndrome (diabetes, hypercholesterolaemia, hypertriglyceridaemia, obesity); clozapine can → potentially serious bone-marrow suppressive side-effects.
- *Depot medication:* long-acting, injectable formulations (conventional or atypical), e.g. flupentixol decanoate and haloperidol decanoate.

Starting dose

Start drug-naïve patients on a low dose and ↑ based on clinical response (e.g. haloperidol 0.5–3mg po bd (3–5mg bd or tds if severe)) ↑ to 15mg bd max.; or chlorpromazine 75mg po nocte ↑ to 300mg max.; or risperidone 2mg nocte (4mg if severe), ↑ to max. 8mg nocte). Benefit should become apparent within 2wks and continued improvement occurs for 3–6mths. Consider depot medication if oral drug adherence is poor and relapses are frequent; always give a test dose (e.g. 12.5mg of fluphenazine decanoate, 25mg of haloperidol decanoate).

Length of treatment

For first-onset psychosis, antipsychotic drugs may be gradually ↓ after the patient has been well for >12mths. For schizophrenia, the medication may need to be continued, sometimes for many years. Depot medication may be especially useful for these patients; a test dose of a depot must always be administered the first time these drugs are being used.

Side effects

Warn patient about likely side-effects. Acute and chronic movement disorders and anticholinergic effects for conventional drugs, ↑ appetite and ↑ weight, hyperglycaemia/diabetes, sedation, and hyperprolactinaemia (gynaecomastia, galactorrhoea, dysmenorrhoea, and sexual dysfunction).

Movement disorders

Include acute dystonia, which may occur within hours (e.g. painful ocular deviation, neck twisting, or muscle spasms); Parkinsonism (tremors and rigidity); and akathisia (severe motor restlessness). Movement disorders should be managed by:

- ↓ Dose.
- Switching from a conventional to an atypical antipsychotic.
- Treat acute dystonias with an anticholinergic drug, e.g. procyclidine 5–10mg IM (repeated if necessary after 20min; max 20mg daily).
- Treat Parkinsonism with an anticholinergic, e.g. procyclidine 2.5mg po tds, ↑ gradually to max. 30mg in divided doses.
- Akathisia can be managed with a benzodiazepine or beta-blocker.

Issues with treatment of schizophrenia

Most patients with schizophrenia respond to an antipsychotic; however, the majority will relapse within 2yrs if they stop medication. 25% of patients do not respond adequately, despite being compliant. They should be switched to an alternative drug, ideally from a different class. Patients who remain psychotic despite adequate trials of antipsychotics are often termed 'treatment resistant'. The diagnosis should be reviewed. If the diagnosis is schizophrenia, a trial of clozapine is warranted (2/3 of patients will respond to clozapine). Withdraw other antipsychotics and commence clozapine 12.5mg po od or bd initially, gradually ↑ to 300mg daily over 2–3wks in 25–50mg increments (and thereafter up to max. 900mg daily). Monitor FBC weekly for 4mths initially, and monthly, thereafter (causes agranulocytosis). Monitor temperature, pulse and BP daily during 1st week of treatment.

Mood stabilizers

These are drugs used to prevent episodes of mania or depression in people with bipolar disorder, as well as to treat acute relapse. Lithium and sodium valproate are most effective. Both must be taken regularly and require monitoring, especially lithium. Lithium is not recommended in absence of monitoring facilities. Maintenance with antipsychotic drug, e.g. risperidone may be necessary where mood stabilizers not available.

Lithium carbonate

Start at 400mg od and titrate dose (sometimes up to >1g/d) to achieve a serum lithium concentration 0.4–1.0mmol/L 12h after a dose 4–7d after starting treatment. *Note:* doses depend on preparation used. Preparations vary widely in bioavailability and dose. Blood levels should be measured weekly until stable, and then at least 6-monthly. Warn patients about signs of toxicity: coarse tremor, nausea, diarrhoea, confusion, seizures; can → congenital malformations if taken by pregnant women. If preparation changed same precautions required as initiation of treatment. Seek mental health specialist advice if patient considering pregnancy or is pregnant.

Sodium valproate

Is an effective mood stabilizer and has the advantage of being effective for epilepsy, being less toxic in overdose, and requiring less blood monitoring. Start with 750mg daily in 2–3 divided doses and ↑ according to clinical response up to 1–2g/d in divided doses. The risk of teratogenicity is high, so should not be the 1st choice in women of reproductive age: if you do prescribe, give folate and advise contraception.

Disorders due to substance abuse

The most common substances of abuse/dependence are alcohol and tobacco. Others include:

- Inhaled glue or benzene.
- Heroin; cocaine.
- Amphetamines.
- Khat.
- Cannabis.
- Benzodiazepines.

The origin of benzodiazepine abuse is often iatrogenic. Alcohol and drug abuse is rarely the main reason for seeking health care. Instead, the HCW has to be alert to the possibility of substance abuse (e.g. repeated unexplained injuries or absence from work). Substance abuse ↑ risk of common mental disorders and suicide. Psychoses can occur—both during intoxicated and withdrawal states.

Intoxication and overdose

See 📖 Acute confusional state and delerium, p. 430 and 📖 Acute behavioural disturbance, p. 828 for medical management of acute confusional states and acute behavioural disturbance, and 📖 Acute poisoning with pharmaceuticals/chemicals p. 878.

Alcohol intoxication

Characterized by smell of alcohol on breath, slurred speech and uninhibited behaviour. If ↓ level of consciousness, assess airway and breathing; place person on their side to prevent aspiration in case they vomit, and observe until effects of alcohol have worn off. If delirium, consider hypoglycaemia, head injury, sub dural haematoma, infection (especially pneumonia), Wernicke's encephalopathy, delirium tremens (alcohol withdrawal), hypoxia, hepatic encephalopathy, cerebrovascular accidents, and post-ictal confusion (see Box 19.8).

Sedative drugs

Overdose may ↓ level of consciousness, slow respiratory rate and pinpoint pupils (in opioid overdose). See 📖 Acute poisoning with pharmaceuticals/chemicals, p. 878, for emergency medical management.

Stimulants

Look for dilated pupils, ↑ pulse, and BP, excited or disordered thoughts, paranoia, aggressive, erratic or violent behaviour, and a history of recent consumption of cocaine or other stimulants.

- Give diazepam 5–10mg IV every 20–30min until calm and lightly sedated; monitor carefully and have flumazenil available to reverse benzodiazepine effect if over-sedated.
- If psychotic symptoms, and the patient does not respond to diazepam, give parenteral or oral antipsychotic medication.
- Monitor pulse, BP and temperature every 2–4h.
- Chest pain may indicate tachyarrhythmias.
- Observe carefully for suicidal thoughts or actions post-intoxication.

Box 19.8 Assessing alcohol abuse: CAGE questionnaire

Alcohol dependence or harmful use is likely if ≥2 +ve answers:
- Have you ever felt you should *cut* down your drinking?
- Have people *annoyed* you by criticizing your drinking?
- Have you ever felt bad or *guilty* about your drinking?
- Have you ever had a drink first think in the morning to steady your nerves or get rid of a hangover (*eye-opener*)?

Dependence and harmful use

Dependence

Is defined as the presence of ≥3 of the following:
- Strong desire/compulsion to take the substance.
- Difficulties controlling substance-taking behaviour in terms of onset, termination, or levels of use.
- *Withdrawal:* a physiological state when the substance has been stopped or reduced; the patient may use the substance to relieve or avoid withdrawal symptoms.
- *Tolerance:* ↑ doses are required to achieve a given effect.
- *Neglect of alternative interests:* obtaining and taking the substance gradually dominates the individual's life.
- Continued use despite user being aware of harmful consequences.

Dependence → great damage to individuals, their families, and the community, e.g. alcohol not only → physical harm to the drinker, but also ↑ suicide rates, marriage problems and domestic violence, road traffic crashes, and worsening economic circumstances.

Harmful use

Is substance abuse → significant damage to mental or physical health but not fulfilling the above criteria. Harmful use may be defined by the quantity consumed (e.g. >2 standard alcoholic drinks/day over an extended period of time) or the pattern of use (e.g. >5 standard drinks/day at any time in the past year).

Management of dependence

There is increasing evidence that dependent patients have ↓ ability to control substance use; it is not just 'a lack of willpower'. Ask 'open' questions and use 'reflective listening', clarify concerns, convey empathy and, using these techniques, motivate patients to reach their own conclusions about adverse effects of substance use and the need to change their behaviour. Advise that dependence is an illness with serious health effects, and stopping or ↓ use will ↑ mental and physical health, social, and economic benefits. Explain symptoms of withdrawal. Abstinence should be goal in most cases.

Brief interventions can ↓ harmful and dependent use. Clearly explain the link between the patient's level of alcohol or drug use, their health (and other) problems, and short-term and long-terms risks of continuing use. For patients willing to stop or control their use, help them:

- Set a definite day to quit/begin controlled use.
- Enlist the help of a buddy not using the substance to provide support.
- If reducing use, agree a clear goal for reduction (e.g. no more than 4U of alcohol/day and 2 alcohol-free d/wk).
- Agree strategies to control use (e.g. slow down drinking to <1U/h, introduce alternative behavior, e.g. interspersing alcoholic drinks with non-alcoholic drinks, chewing gum, exercise).
- Remove substances from the home.
- Identify high-risk situations (social or stressful occasions) and strategies to avoid or cope with these.
- Make plans to avoid substances (e.g. ways to respond to friends who are using substances).
- Discuss symptoms and management of withdrawal (see 📖 Withdrawal states, p. 845).
- Medicines may be available for withdrawal from opiates (e.g. methadone); these need specialist assessment and monitoring.
- Minimize risk of harm due to substance abuse, e.g. advise not to drive after drinking, never to share needles, safe sexual practice.
- Prevent iatrogenic abuse by using benzodiazepines cautiously, and never for more than four weeks running.

If the attempt is successful consider medicines to ↓ risk of relapse:

- *Acamprosate:* ↓ craving for alcohol. Start immediately following withdrawal (weight ≥60kg, 666mg tds; <60kg, 666mg at breakfast followed by 333mg at midday and at night), continue for 12mths. Adverse effects occur in 20% of patients, most commonly GI disturbance and rash.
- *Disulfiram:* causes an unpleasant and potentially dangerous reaction when taken with alcohol. Fear of this reaction helps motivated individuals to abstain from alcohol. Prescribe 200mg daily and, with patient's consent, enlist caregivers to ensure adherence.

Relapse is common and often occurs because the person is not able to deal with life difficulties. Once drug use is stopped, discuss ways in which the person could cope. Identify different things a person can do to ↓ risk of taking drugs e.g. giving up friends who use drugs; getting back to work, school, other enjoyable activities; learning relaxation and problem-solving; joining community groups which help substance abusers (e.g. Alcoholics Anonymous).

If the attempt is unsuccessful or relapse occurs:

- Praise any areas of success (e.g. cut down use for a period).
- Discuss situations/triggers for relapse; how can changes be made?
- Try again.

Withdrawal states

Physical effects common to many substances include anxiety, tremor, fever, sleep disturbance, tachycardia, GI disturbance. In addition, following symptoms may occur during withdrawal:

- *Opiates:* hypertension, tachycardia, dysphoria, agitation, insomnia, diarrhea, and vomiting, shivering, sweating, lacrimation, rhinorrhoea, dilated pupils, piloerection ('gooseflesh'), muscle aches.
- *Alcohol:* seizures, confusional states incl. delirium tremens (severe confusion with visual/auditory hallucinations and paranoia); risk of Wernicke's encephalopathy (confusion, ataxia, nystagmus, ophthalmoplegia due to thiamine deficiency, 🕮 Vitamin B1 (thiamine) deficiency, p. 716).
- *Benzodiazepines/barbiturates:* ↓ weight, vivid dreams (rapid eye movement (REM) sleep rebound), tinnitus, irritability, ↓ memory and concentration, perceptual disturbance (hypersensitivity to sound, light and touch, derealization and depersonalization), confusion and seizures.

Withdrawal usually begins 4–12h after the last dose, peaks at 48–72h, and lasts 7–10d. Benzodiazepine withdrawal begins later, usually 1–14d after the last dose and lasting for a few weeks (longer in a minority). The confusional states (delirium) following alcohol, benzodiazepine, and barbiturate withdrawal are potentially life-threatening and should be managed as described elsewhere (🕮 Acute pesticide poisoning, p. 874). Seizures occurring in the context of withdrawal of alcohol or benzodiazepines should be managed with diazepam; do not start prophylactic anticonvulsant therapy. Minimize risk of withdrawal by a gradual reducing regime and treat withdrawal rapidly when identified.

Management of specific withdrawal states

Alcohol withdrawal

- Consider admission, especially if there is a history of previous severe withdrawals (e.g. confusion, fits), poor physical health (e.g. liver failure), or mental health (e.g. suicidal ideation).
- Give a benzodiazepine at reducing dose over 5–10d. Initial dose depends on alcohol intake and withdrawal symptom severity, e.g. chlordiazepoxide 10–40mg po qds or diazepam 10mg po qds. Higher doses may be required. For inpatients dose and dosing interval may be adjusted according to symptoms.
- For patients with significant liver failure a short-acting drug may be used instead (e.g. lorazepam 1mg od or bd), or give an initial dose of diazepam 5–10mg stat and determine duration of action before prescribing further doses.
- Give thiamine 100mg tds po (IV in delirium tremens) for 5d to prevent/treat Wernicke's encephalopathy (🕮 Vitamin B1 (thiamine) deficiency, p. 716).

Opiate withdrawal

Withdrawal is more successful if linked to a residential rehabilitation programme. 1st-line medical management for acute opiate withdrawal is as follows:

- *Buprenorphine:* 0.8–4mg sub-lingual on 1st day, ↑ if necessary by 2–4mg daily to usual dose 12–24mg (max. 32mg) daily. Withdraw gradually over 3–14d. 1st dose should not be given until experiencing withdrawal symptoms (8h after last heroin dose, 24–48h after last methadone dose) due to risk of precipitating withdrawal.
- *Methadone:* initial dose 15–20mg po, ↑ to 30mg/d and tapered over 3–10d.
- *Clonidine:* 0.1–0.15mg tds; or *lofexidine* 0.2mg bd (max.1.2mg bd); withdraw over 2–4d; max. duration 10d. Side effects include lightheadedness and sedation.
- Take care with all these drugs if also taking sedative medications.
- Do not give opiate substitutes if the patient has been away from the ward and you suspect illicit drug use.
- Treat nausea, aches, and pains symptomatically. Monitor BP.

Most require maintenance opioid substitution therapy with buprenorphine or methadone. Take care when helping a patient to withdraw from opiates; following withdrawal, tolerance to opiates will ↓ and the patient can overdose if they resume use at the previous level.

Benzodiazepine withdrawal

Withdrawal is most common with short-acting agents, e.g. lorazepam.

- Change to an equivalent dose of a long-acting benzodiazepine, e.g. diazepam (lorazepam 0.5–1mg is equivalent to diazepam 5mg).
- Then gradually ↓ dose every 2–3wks in steps of diazepam 0.5–2.5mg depending on initial dose and duration of treatment.
- If withdrawal symptoms occur, maintain dose until symptoms improve. Thereafter ↓ dose further, in smaller steps if necessary.
- If dependency is chronic, this may take months.

Adjustment disorders and bereavement

A state of emotional disturbance and impaired social functioning may develop shortly (<3mths) after or during a stressor. There may be affective, cognitive, and behavioural symptoms. Stressors may be, e.g. disasters or traumatic events, bereavement, diagnosis of a major illness, e.g. HIV/AIDS, migration. Adjustment disorders are common in people with physical disorders, and should be considered if rehabilitation is slower or poorer than expected.

Bereavement

May be abnormal in form and/or severity compared with cultural norms. Four stages have been described:

- Shock and numbness.
- Preoccupation (yearning or anger, etc.).
- Disorganization (loss is reluctantly accepted).
- Resolution.

These may not necessarily occur in this order. Bereavement is considered abnormal when symptoms are not related to the loss e.g. feelings of worthlessness or inappropriate guilt or if the symptoms last beyond a reasonable period of time and → significant social impairment. Abnormal perceptions involving the lost person (e.g. hearing them whispering) can be a feature of normal bereavement, but hallucinatory phenomena not involving the lost person are indications of abnormal (or pathological) bereavement.

Management

- Allow (but do not push) individual to talk about loss and its circumstances, and to discuss feelings provoked, especially guilt and anger.
- Support culturally appropriate mourning.
- Involve others in family, and aim to ↑ social support/reactivate social networks.
- Identify steps that can be taken to modify causes of stress.
- Medication should be avoided unless there is depression or psychosis. If there is severe insomnia, hypnotics may be used for <2wks, e.g. diazepam 10mg nocte, promethazine 25mg nocte.

Post-traumatic stress disorder

An incident that makes a person fear for their life or causes extreme distress is a traumatic event, e.g. rape, war, major disasters. Many persons affected by trauma will experience some emotional reaction—feelings of being numb or in a daze, fear, insomnia, repeated thoughts of the event, irritability, nightmares, and ↓ concentration. This is a normal response and lasts typically 2–4wks. In a few people, however, these experiences continue for months or years after the trauma, interfering with daily life and → alcohol abuse or problems in relationships. This is called post-traumatic stress disorder (PTSD).

Clinical features

- Experiencing trauma again and again through intrusive and distressing visions of incident, nightmares, and 'flashbacks'.
- Avoiding situations that remind him/her of traumatic incident.
- He/she is unable to remember things related to trauma and feels emotionally distant from people.
- ↑ *Arousal:* sleep is disturbed, patient feels irritable, has difficulty concentrating, and is easily startled or scared.
- Panic attacks may occur.
- Many patients with PTSD feel depressed and lose interest in daily life, feel tired, or suffer aches and pains, and have suicidal feelings.

Management

- Allow, but do not push, patient to talk about what happened and assess their needs and concerns.
- Ensure physical needs are met, and that patient is protected from further harm.
- Support culturally appropriate adjustment to what happened.
- Reassure that emotional reactions are normal, not a sign of madness.
- Encourage patient not to avoid situations that remind them of event. As far as possible, encourage normal routine and getting back to usual activities.
- Victim should not be left alone for some days. Make sure that they are staying with caring relatives or friends.
- For panic attacks, follow steps suggested earlier.
- For acute severe symptoms, use benzodiazepines for up to 2wks.
- A course of antidepressants may help some patients.

Intellectual (learning) disability

Intellectual disability (ID) is a developmental disability, not a mental illness. Child's mental abilities are slower/delayed compared with other children, with impairment in cognitive, social, language, and motor development. Prevalence of moderate to severe ID varies from 1–20/1000 worldwide. Persons with ID are often brought to HCWs by concerned family members for many reasons, e.g. self-care, school difficulties, and behavioural problems, e.g. aggression.

Clinical features

- Delays in milestones, e.g. sitting, walking, speaking.
- Difficulties in school, e.g. coping with studies and repeated failure.
- Difficulties in relating to others, especially other children of same age.
- In adolescents, inappropriate sexual behaviour.
- In adults, problems in everyday activities, e.g. cooking, managing money, finding and staying in a job.

There are degrees of intellectual disability:

- *Mild ID:* may → difficulty in schooling but no other problems.
- *Moderate ID:* may → failure to stay in the school system and difficulties in self-care, e.g. bathing.
- *Severe ID:* often requires help for simple activities, e.g. feeding.
- Persons with mild ID may spend entire lives without being 'detected', those at severe end are diagnosed in early childhood because of obvious severity of disability. People with mild ID may be able to live alone and work in certain jobs; however, severely affected people need close supervision and care.

Assessment

- An informant, e.g. a parent, is essential.
- Record nature and extent of intellectual disability—take developmental history and assess delay in communication and social interaction; motor function and self-care; and functional academic skills.
- Identify problems, e.g. self-harm or harm to others; impulsive or dangerous behaviour.
- Determine aetiology, see Box 19.9. In most cases, no definite aetiology will be identifiable.
- Identify co-existing psychiatric diagnoses e.g. psychoses. Prevalence is 2–4-fold higher in people with ID than the general population.

Box 19.9 Causes of moderate to severe ID

- *Prenatal (50–70%):* genetic (e.g. Fragile X; Down's syndrome), congenital infections (e.g. HSV, rubella, HIV, toxoplasmosis, syphilis, CMV), exposure to toxins, e.g. alcohol, maternal disorder, e.g. pre-eclampsia.
- *Perinatal (10–20%):* LBW, extreme prematurity, birth asphyxia or brain trauma, neonatal sepsis, encephalitis, kernicterus.
- *Postnatal (5–10%):* brain damage due to trauma, infections, toxic agents (e.g. lead poisoning), iodine deficiency, malnutrition.

Management

- Be certain that the child has ID. This implies that child has incurable and life-long disability. It is a label that can cause great unhappiness, so use it with care. If in doubt, get 2nd opinion from specialist.
- Once you are confident that child has ID, determine its severity. The abilities a child has will be an important indicator of how much progress child is likely to make in years ahead.
- Screen for contributory medical problems, e.g. hypothyroidism, sensory impairment, seizures, chronic infection, malnutrition.
- Other than these rare situations, there are no indications for using medicines to treat ID. Do not use 'brain tonics' and other medicines supposed to help 'mental function'. Use antipsychotics or antidepressants to treat psychoses or common mental disorders. Do not use medication to treat behavioural disturbance.
- Reassure family that, even though child has limited mental abilities, he/she will achieve many milestones in life. They must be prepared to accept a delay in these milestones and be realistic in what they expect their child to achieve. Explain that there is no cure and that they should not waste money on false claims of cures.
- Teach the parents how to help child in daily activities, e.g. in toileting and feeding, by breaking down activities into smaller bits.
- Use reward and praise whenever child succeeds in any activity, however small. Find activities that can help parent spend time with child, and yet allow other household activities to be done, e.g. child could learn to help with daily chores in house.
- Never ignore child's educational needs. Some parents feel like giving up on child's education when they discover that child has ID. Explain that their child needs education, just as any other child. Refer family to local schools for children with special needs. Avoid institutionalization.
- Provide information about any special schemes to help families with children with ID, either through financial or educational help.
- Stay in regular touch with family. Children with ID often need guidance about their reproductive and sexual health, when they become adolescents. Some families go through a lot of stress because of caring for a child with ID, especially when severe. Caring can → stress and mental health problems. Refer parents to support groups and offer treatment for common mental disorders *if needed*.

Disorders in children and adolescents

In younger children, most common and disabling disorders are developmental. If child has behavioural problems or difficulties in school, take a developmental history first to rule out ID. Once ID has been ruled out, consider the possibility of:

- *Autism and other pervasive developmental disorders:* characterized by delays or loss of language abilities and marked impairment in social relationships; typically present in early to mid-childhood. These disorders require a similar approach to that described for ID.
- *Attention deficit and hyperactivity disorder:* marked by impulsivity, hyperactivity, and poor concentration; typically presents in primary school. Children with this disorder may benefit from parent and teacher guided behavioural treatments and medication (methylphenidate—only to be used by experienced child or mental health practitioners).
- *Specific learning disabilities:* impairment(s) in specific learning and cognitive abilities, e.g. reading and writing (dyslexia); typically presents when child is in secondary school. Remedial education within mainstream schools is 1° intervention.

In adolescents, emotional and behavioural disorders linked to difficulties in school or at home are common. The most common mental disorders are depression, substance abuse, psychoses, and conduct disorders (antisocial behaviours). Mental health problems in adolescents may be managed similar to adults.

Child abuse

Child abuse is present in most societies, and more widespread than thought previously, although prevalence is not known. Children can be abused physically, emotionally, or sexually, affecting their health and development. Both boys and girls can be abused, most often by someone they know well. Abused children may have problems with:

- *Physical health:* bruises or cuts, fractures, cigarette burns; severe cases can → death.
- *Sexual health:* injuries to the sexual organs, pregnancy, and STIs.
- *Mental health:* fear, aggression, ↓ concentration, bed-wetting (having previously had control), depression, antisocial behaviour, self-harm.
- *School performance:* ↓ school performance.

Diagnosis

- *Ask family:* few adults will openly report that they feel a child they know is being abused. If child abuse suspected, it is essential that you ask adult in a frank and open way whether they think child is being physically, emotionally, or sexually hurt.
- *Ask the child:* interview child with the mother, or another adult who is definitely not a suspected abuser, whom child trusts. Do not ask questions about abuse until you have established a rapport with the child. This may require spending more time. Ask: 'Sometimes, children can get hurt by a grown-up person. Has anyone grown-up hurt you recently?' Do not force the child to answer.

- *Examine the child:* a child who has been abused is likely to be very sensitive to being examined physically. Respect child's privacy. Explain what you are doing and why. Have a trusted family member present during examination. Document findings in detail. These may be needed in a police investigation. A thorough examination of the child should include weight and height, injuries on body, and injuries or inflammation of sexual organs, including anus.

Management

- *Your priority is health and safety of the child:* if you suspect child's life is in danger, refer immediately to a place of safety.
- *Talk to the family members:* explain why you suspect abuse. Many parents are not aware that their actions can be so damaging to the child's health. Just telling them about the dangers of beating a child or neglecting emotional needs may → change in their behaviour.
- It is unlikely that the family will accept sexual abuse easily, especially if abuser is someone close to family. Do not accuse anyone. Instead, share your concerns openly with family and stress that if abuse continues, the child's health will be even more seriously affected.
- *Teach child how to ensure their safety:* explain that the abuse is not their fault and they should not feel guilty for having spoken out about it. Important to make sure this never happens again. Some suggestions on how to prevent abuse from recurring are:
  - to tell the abuser firmly not to touch her
  - to run away from the abuser
  - to be with another adult who can protect her.
- *Put the family in touch with community supports:* e.g. child support groups, family violence groups, legal support, child protection agencies, the police, or specialist health professionals.
- If the child abuse persists or is very serious, refer to specialist team.
- Keep in close touch with child and family at regular intervals for at least 6mths. Very often, abuse stops once it has been openly discussed. If it does not, you may need to encourage family to take action to stop it. Talk to child each time; many children do recover from the trauma, but some children will develop mental health problems.

Further reading

World Health Organization, mhGAP intervention guide for mental, neurological and substance use disorders in non-specialized health settings: mental health Gap Action Programme (mhGAP). 2010, WHO: Geneva. Available free at: http://www.who.int/mental_health/evidence/mhGAP_intervention_guide/en/index.html

Chapter 20

Trauma

Invited authors **Douglas A Wilkinson**

Jenny Thompson

Primary assessment of trauma: ABCDE

The ABCDE system allows rapid systematic assessment and simultaneous treatment of life-threatening injuries.

- Do not move on to next system until current problem is treated.
- If the patient deteriorates, go back to the beginning and assess again.
  - *Airway*—can the patient talk to you and breathe freely? Give supplemental O_2 if available.
  - *Breathing*—is the patient breathing (look, listen, and feel)? Is breathing adequate?
  - *Circulation*—can peripheral or central pulses be felt? Is capillary refill <3s?
  - *Disability*—use AVPU (see 📖 AVPU Scale, p. 7).
  - *Exposure*—undress the patient and look for injury.

The following should prompt a full trauma assessment:

History

- Fall > 3m.
- Motor vehicle accident (MVA) at net speed >30km/h.
- Throw from vehicle/trapped in vehicle.
- Death of a person in accident.
- Patient is a pedestrian involved in MVA.
- MVA involving car/cycle or car/unrestrained occupant.

Examination

- Airway problem or respiratory distress.
- BP <100mmHg.
- GCS <13/15.
- >1 area injured.
- Penetrating injury.

Further reading

Further detailed guidance on trauma management and the resources required in low resource settings are given in the following publications, available to download free from their respective websites:

Wilkinson DA, Skinner MW. *Primary Trauma Care: A Manual for Trauma Management in District and Remote Locations*. Oxford: Primary Trauma Care Foundation 2000. Available at: www.primarytraumacare.org/wp-content/uploads/2011/09/PTC_ENG.pdf

WHO. *Guidelines for Essential Trauma Care*. Geneva: WHO 2004. Available at: http://whqlibdoc.who.int/publications/2004/9241546409.pdf

Airway

Assessment

If the patient can speak clearly, they have a patent airway and are breathing. Signs of airway obstruction include:

- Snoring or gurgling.
- Using accessory muscles of respiration.
- Stridor.
- Cyanosis.
- Agitation.

Management

- *Simple airway management (**remember be aware of possible cervical neck injury**):* chin lift/jaw thrust; suction; insert adjunct oral or nasopharyngeal airway. If these manoeuvres do not help or patient is apnoeic, hypoxic, unconscious, or has severe head, chest or neck trauma, *move onto*
- *Advanced airway management:* includes tracheal intubation (with neck immobilization); surgical access — cricothyroid puncture or tracheostomy depending on equipment, skill, and resources. While tracheostomy is not a difficult procedure, training is required as complications of bleeding and false passage can be fatal.

Breathing (ventilation)

Assessment

Once airway is patent, the next priority is adequate ventilation.

- *Inspect:* for signs of respiratory difficulties including ↑ respiratory rate, use of accessory muscles, and irregular breathing pattern; cyanosis; chest injury (e.g. penetrating injury, flail chest, or a sucking injury).
- *Palpate:*
    - for tracheal shift
    - broken ribs
    - subcutaneous emphysema.
- *Percuss:* for resonance or dullness.
- *Auscultate:* for pneumothorax (decreased breath sounds on side of injury); abnormal sounds in chest.

Management

See 📖 Chest trauma, p. 861.

Circulation

Assessment

- Inspect patient for signs of major bleeding, skin condition, temperature, and pallor.
- Assess pulses and capillary refill time.
- While instituting emergency management (see next paragraph) continue to monitor heart rate and BP.

Management

Goal is to stop bleeding and restore O_2 delivery to tissues. Fluid resuscitation essential; usual problem is blood loss. Insert two large bore (14–16G) cannulae. Interosseous access (in children) or peripheral cut down may be necessary if IV access difficult. Take blood samples (including for cross-match). Control any haemorrhage (see Box 20.1) and start warmed crystalloid infusion (warm bags of fluid in a bucket of warm water). Benefit of aggressive fluid resuscitation depends on controlling any bleeding.

Volume replacement and warming

- *Warm fluid replacement:* hypothermic patients do not clot well. Even in hot climates, trauma patients quickly become hypothermic, especially when being treated outside. IV and oral fluids should have a temperature of 40–42° C.
- *Hypotensive fluid resuscitation:* if haemostasis is not complete, aim to maintain a relatively low systolic BP of 80–90mmHg until definitive haemostasis can be achieved. This will help limit further blood loss.
- *Blood transfusion:* consider transfusion when there is persistent haemodynamic instability despite fluid resuscitation or when Hb is <7g/dL with ongoing bleeding. Use type O –ve packed red cells if cross-matched or type-specific blood is not available. Remember patients' family or friends may be able to donate blood for them, but beware of incompatibility and blood-borne infections.
- *Per-oral fluid resuscitation:* safe and efficient if patient has gag reflex and is without abdominal injury. Use appropriate rehydration fluid (see 🕮 General management of dehydration, p. 272).

Causes of shock following trauma

Inadequate organ perfusion → inadequate tissue oxygenation. Often due to haemorrhage and hypovolaemia in the trauma patient, but can occur from other causes. Urine output is a useful marker of intravascular volume status and response to resuscitation. Expect an output of >0.5mL/kg/h if resuscitation is adequate.

Haemorrhagic (hypovolaemic) shock Due to acute loss of blood or fluids. Easy to underestimate blood loss (see Table 20.1). *Remember*, large volumes may be hidden in abdomen or pleural space and following femoral or pelvic fracture (latter may → loss of >2L). In young, fit patients, signs of blood loss may not be obvious until >1L has been lost.

Treatment Fluid resuscitate and control bleeding.

Cardiogenic shock Due to inadequate cardiac function. May be due to myocardial contusion; penetrating wound to heart; cardiac tamponade; myocardial infarction; tension pneumothorax (preventing venous return). Assessment of JVP and ECG may be helpful.

Treatment Treat cause.

Neurogenic shock Classically presents as hypotension with no reflex tachycardia or skin vasoconstriction. Cause is loss of sympathetic tone 2° to spinal cord injury.

Treatment Fluids, vasoconstrictors, spinal stabilization +/– surgery. Exclude other causes of shock.

Septic shock Rare in early phase of trauma, but common in days or weeks following injury. Most commonly seen in penetrating abdominal injuries and burns patients. Common cause of late death in trauma patient.

Treatment Treat sepsis early (see 📖 Sepsis, p. 734), support organs.

Box 20.1 Strategies to stop bleeding

- *Limb injuries:* place gauze packs under fascia, manually compress proximal artery, apply compressive dressing to entire injured limb.
- *Chest injuries:* chest wall arteries are most common source of bleeding. Place intercostal chest drain and give pain relief. Expanded lung should tamponade bleeding.
- *Abdominal injuries:* damage control laparotomy is required as soon as possible if fluid resuscitation fails to achieve a systolic BP of 80–90mmHg. It is not a surgical procedure, but a resuscitative one, involving gauze packing of bleeding abdominal quadrants and temporary closure of abdominal wound with towel clamps. The procedure should be observed before being done, but with training should be within the capabilities of a doctor or nurse; carry out under ketamine anaesthesia. Done properly, damage control laparatomy can save lives.
- *Pelvic fractures:* stabilize the pelvis, by tying a sheet around pelvis.

Table 20.1 Cardiovascular parameters associated with blood loss in an adult

Blood loss	Up to 750mL	750–1500mL	1500–2000mL	>2000mL
Heart rate	<100	>100	>120	>140
BP	Normal	Systolic normal	↓	↓
Capillary refill	Normal (≤2s)	Prolonged	Prolonged	Prolonged
Respiratory rate	Normal	20–30/min	30–40/min	>40/min
Urine volume	>30mL/h	20–30mL/h	5–15mL/h	<10mL/h
Mental state	Normal	Mild concern	Anxious or confused	Coma

Secondary survey

The 2° survey is only done when patient's ABCDE is stable. If any deterioration occurs during this part of assessment, a second 1° survey should be performed to find and treat the problem before continuing with the 2° survey. 2° survey comprises a head-to-toe examination.

Head examination

Scalp and ocular abnormalities; external ear and tympanic membrane injury; periorbital soft tissue injuries.

Neck examination

Penetrating wounds; subcutaneous emphysema; tracheal deviation; neck vein appearance.

Neurological examination

Assess using the GCS (📖 Glasgow coma scale, p. 433); spinal cord motor activity; sensation and reflex.

Chest examination

Clavicles and all ribs; breath and heart sounds; ECG monitoring (if available).

Abdominal examination

Surgical exploration is required for penetrating wound. Blunt trauma → insert NGT(except in presence of facial trauma); rectal examination; insert urinary catheter (check for urethral meatal blood before insertion).

Pelvis and limbs

- Fractures.
- Peripheral pulses.
- Cuts, bruises, and other minor injuries.

X-rays (if possible and where indicated)

Note Chest, lateral neck, and pelvis X-rays may be needed during 1° survey; cervical spine films (important to see all 7 vertebrae); pelvic and long bone X-rays; skull X-ray (SXR) may be useful to search for fractures when head injury is present without focal neurological deficit, but is seldom indicated. Document all procedures undertaken.

Chest trauma

~25% of trauma deaths are due to thoracic injury.

Rib fractures

May damage underlying lung → lung bruising or puncture. Ribs usually become fairly stable within 10–14d. Firm healing with callus formation occurs after ~6wks.

Flail chest

Unstable segment moves separately and in opposite direction from the rest of thoracic cage → severe respiratory distress. Medical emergency—treat with +ve pressure ventilation + analgesia.

Tension pneumothorax

Air enters pleural space, but cannot leave → progressively ↑ intrathoracic pressure in affected side → CVS instability, extreme pain, and death. Urgent needle decompression is required: insert large bore needle in 2nd intercostal space (ICS) in mid-clavicular line on tension side to decompress. Hiss of decompressed air may occur, but is not always present. Definitive chest drain in fifth ICS, mid-axillary line essential.

Haemothorax

Common in penetrating injures to chest; requires large chest drain. Haemothorax of 500–1500mL that stops bleeding after insertion of intercostal drain can generally be treated in this way; haemothorax of >1500–2000mL or with continued bleeding >200–300mL/h may require thoracotomy.

Pulmonary contusion (bruising)

Common after chest trauma; onset of symptoms can be slow. Most likely following high-speed crashes or falls from a great height. Clinical features include shortness of breath, hypoxaemia, tachycardia, absent breath sounds, rib fractures, and cyanosis. Presents like pneumonia and ventilatory support may be needed.

Open, 'sucking' chest wounds of the chest wall

Lung on affected side collapses; a seal (e.g. a square of plastic taped down on 3 out of 4 sides) is often sufficient to stop sucking and allow re-expansion; intercostal drains and intubation may be required.

Other thoracic injuries

Carry a high mortality, e.g. myocardial contusion, pericardial tamponade, injuries to thoracic great vessels, rupture of trachea or major bronchi, trauma to oesophagus, and diaphragmatic injuries.

Abdominal trauma

Commonest organ injured by penetrating trauma is liver, and in blunt trauma spleen is often torn and ruptured. Suspect abdominal injury in any patient involved in serious accident—unrecognized abdominal injury remains frequent cause of preventable death.

There are two basic categories:

- *Penetrating trauma:* e.g. gunshot, stabbing.
- *Non-penetrating trauma:* e.g. compression, crush, seat belt, acceleration/deceleration injuries.

~20% of trauma patients with acute haemoperitoneum (blood in abdomen) have no signs of peritoneal irritation at the 1st examination and require repeated 1° survey. Blunt trauma can be very difficult to evaluate, especially in unconscious patients. Complete examination of abdomen includes rectal examination (sphincter tone, integrity of rectal wall, blood in rectum, prostate position). Check for blood at external urethral meatus. Catheterize (cautiously if pelvic injury) to decompress bladder and monitor urine output. In women, exclude pregnancy. Best treatment of fetus is resuscitation of mother; however, sometimes a pregnant mother at term may require delivery of baby to ensure she is adequately resuscitated (see 🕮 Pregnant trauma patients, p. 870).

Diagnostic peritoneal lavage (DPL)

A quick USS by a trained operator can reliably assess free fluid in the abdomen. DPL involves putting a peritoneal catheter in abdomen through a small incision in umbilicus, then passing 1L warmed fluid into abdomen. After short period, fluid drains out by gravity, and may be visually assessed for presence of blood or bowel contents. Relative contraindications for DPL include pregnancy, previous abdominal surgery, operator inexperience, and if result will not change management. If doubt, laparotomy is still gold standard.

Pelvic fractures

Often complicated by massive haemorrhage and urological injury. Examine rectum for position of the prostate, the presence of blood, and rectal/perineal laceration.

Management Resuscitation and immobilization, analgesia, transfusion, +/– surgery.

Head trauma

Early assessment and treatment of head-injured patients is essential to ↑ survival and outcome. Hypoxia and hypotension double mortality. The following two conditions are potentially life-threatening, can usually be diagnosed clinically, and require urgent surgical decompression by burr-hole (see 📖 How to do a burr hole, p. 467):

- *Acute extradural haematoma:* typically a rapid ↓ in consciousness following a lucid interval. A middle meningeal artery bleed → acute ↑ ICP → contralateral hemiparesis and ipsilateral dilated pupil.
- *Acute subdural haematoma:* tearing of a bridging vein between cortex and dura → clotted blood in the subdural space → severe contusion of the underlying brain.

The conditions below should be treated conservatively—neurosurgery usually does not improve outcome:

- Base-of-skull fractures: suggested by bruising of eyelids (raccoon eyes) or over mastoid process (Battle's sign), or CSF leak from ears/nose.
- Cerebral concussion: → temporary altered consciousness.
- Depressed skull fracture: impaction of fragmented skull that may penetrate underlying dura and brain.
- Intracerebral haematoma: may result from acute injury or progressive damage 2° to contusion.

Management

Basic medical management for severe head injuries

- ABCDE primary survey with cervical spine control.
- Intubation + moderate hyperventilation to achieve a low/normal pCO_2 (4.5–5kPa), which temporarily ↓ intracranial blood volume and ICP.
- Sedation with paralysis as necessary.
- Moderate IV fluid input with diuresis i.e. avoid fluid overload.
- Nurse head up 20%.
- Prevent hyperthermia.
- Record the GCS (📖 Glasgow coma scale, p. 433): severe head injury = GCS <8; moderate head injury = GCS 9–12; minor head injury = GCS 13–15.

Deterioration may occur due to bleeding

Unequal or dilated pupils may indicate ↑ ICP, with bradycardia, hypertension, ↓ respiratory rate. Brain injury is never the cause of hypotension.

Spinal trauma

Injuries to the cervical spine and T12–L1 are common injuries, as is damage to brachial plexus and nerves to legs and fingers. In addition to sensory and motor loss, **spinal shock** (due to sympathetic loss to limbs and internal viscera) can → hypotension and bradycardia.

1st priority: 1° survey and ABCDE evaluation

Always examine spinal injury patients in the neutral position (i.e. without flexion, extension, or rotation) and without any movement of the spine. The patient should be log-rolled to move (i.e. moved by several people, working together to keep neck and spine immobilized); their neck immobilized with a stiff cervical neck collar or sandbags; and transported in a neutral position (i.e. supine) (see Box 20.2).

Vertebral injury

May → spinal cord injury. Search for local tenderness, deformities for a posterior 'step-off' injury, and swelling.

Cervical spine injury

Look for difficulties in respiration (diaphragmatic/paradoxical breathing); flaccid muscle tone; absent reflexes (check rectal sphincter); and hypotension with bradycardia (without hypovolaemia).

C-spine X-ray

AP and a lateral X-ray (showing all seven cervical vertebrae) with a view of the atlas-axis joint.

Box 20.2 Neurological assessment of spinal trauma

Assess sensation and ask patient to make small movements.

Motor response	Level	Sensory response	Level
Diaphragm intact	C3, C4, C5	Anterior thigh	L2
Shrug shoulders	C4	Anterior knee	L3
Biceps (flex elbows)	C5	Anterolateral ankle	L4
Extension of wrist	C6	Dorsum big + 2nd toe	L5
Extension of elbow	C7	Lateral side of foot	S1
Flexion of wrist	C7	Posterior calf	S2
Abduction of fingers	C8	Perianal sensation	S2–5
Active chest expansion	T1–T12		
Hip flexion	L2		
Knee extension	L3–L4		
Ankle dorsiflexion	L5–S1		
Ankle plantar flexion	L1–S2		

Note If no sensory or motor function is exhibited with complete spinal cord lesion, chance of recovery is small.

Limb trauma

Examine

- Skin colour and temperature.
- Distal pulses.
- Grazes and bleeding sites.
- Limb alignment and deformities.
- Active and passive movements.
- Unusual movements and crepitation.
- Pain caused injury.

Management Maintain peripheral blood flow; prevent infection, skin necrosis and damage to peripheral nerves.

Special issues relating to limb trauma

Beware tourniquets Stop active bleeding by direct pressure, rather than tourniquet (that may be left on by mistake → ischaemic damage).

Compartment syndrome

Cause

- ↑ Pressure in fascial compartments.
- Common in intramuscular haematomas, crush injuries, fractures, or amputations.
- ↑ Pressure → local circulatory collapse by compression of local vessels and peripheral nerves.
- Tissue perfusion becomes limited and ischaemic; necrotic muscles with restricted function can result if the perfusion pressure (systolic BP) is low.
- Forearm and lower leg compartments are at particular risk.

Clinical features

- Pain out of keeping with injury.
- Tense compartments.
- Passive stretch test—pain on moving foot or lower limb.
- Paraesthesia.
- Pulse lost—a late sign.

Damage on reperfusion often serious. If there is local hypoxaemia (high IM pressure, low BP) for >2h, reperfusion can → extensive vascular damage.

Management Decompress early by fasciotomy.

Traumatic amputation

Traumatically amputated body parts should be covered with moistened sterile gauze towels and put into a sterile plastic bag. Non-cooled amputated part may be re-attached <6h later; cooled one within 20h of injury.

Paediatric trauma

Trauma is a leading cause of death in children. Survival depends on early resuscitation. Initial assessment is identical to that of adult, following ABCD, and finally exposing child, without losing heat. Blood volume is 80mL/kg in child, 85–90mL/kg in neonate. ↑ Physiological reserves of child mean that vital signs may be only slightly abnormal despite up to 25% of blood volume loss. Tachycardia is an early response, and useful tool for monitoring, but can also be increased by fear or pain.

Fluid management

Give 20mL/kg of fluid initially to a child showing signs of Class 2 hypovolaemia or worse (see Table 20.2), repeated up to 2× (up to 60mL/kg total) depending on the response. Children with little or no response require further fluids and blood transfusion: initially 20mL/kg of whole blood or 10mL/kg of packed red cells over ~30min.

Heat loss occurs rapidly and a child who is hypothermic may become refractory to treatment. Keep warm.

Acute gastric dilatation (gastroparesis) is common in a seriously ill or injured child. Decompress stomach by inserting an NGT.

Analgesia e.g. morphine 50micrograms/kg IV bolus, followed by 10–20 micrograms/kg at 10-min intervals until adequate response is achieved.

Table 20.2 Classification of hypovolaemia in children

	Class 1	Class 2	Class 3	Class 4
Blood lost	<15%	15–25%	25–40%	>40%
Pulse rate	↑	>150	>150	↑ or ↓
Pulse press	↔	↓	↓↓	Absent
Systolic BP	↔	↓	↓↓	Unrecorded
Capillary refill	↔	↑	↑↑	Absent
Respiratory rate	↔	↑	↑	↓, Sighing
Mental state	↔	Irritable	Lethargic	Coma
Urine (mL/kg/h)	<1	<1	<1	<1

Burns

The source of the burn is important (e.g. fire, hot water, paraffin, kerosene, electric shock) as this may point towards associated problems such as inhalational injury. Electrical burns are often more serious than they appear. Damaged skin and muscle can → acute renal failure.

Management

- Remove source of burning, and cool.
- ABCDE, then determine burn depth and area (rule of 9's see Box 20.3).
- Obtain good IV access and give early fluid replacement (see Box 20.4).
- Keep burns clean.
- Indications for hospital admission include:
  - >10% in child
  - >15% in adult
  - burns in very young, elderly, or infirm patients
  - full thickness or circumferential burns
  - burns with inhalation
  - burns of face, hands, feet, perineum.
- Consider possible inhalation injury in patient with facial burns, singed facial or nasal hair, hoarseness, and circumferential full thickness burns of the chest or neck. Patients with inhalation injury often require early intubation or tracheostomy before laryngeal oedema makes it impossible!
- Look for and treat any associated trauma or pre-burn illness.
- Be aware of the risk of sepsis in burns patients. Use of routine prophylactic systemic antibiotics is controversial although a recent review suggested there may be some benefit. There are limited data from resource-poor regions, but risks are likely to be higher in such settings. Decisions should be made based on the burn severity, risk factors in the patient (such as young age, elderly, nutritional status, HIV status), and the patient's environment. Early recognition and systemic treatment of secondary infection in all cases is essential.
- Check tetanus immunization status; give tetanus booster if needed.

Box 20.3 Calculating % of body surface area involved by burns

Adults 'Rule of 9's'—head 9%, front and back of torso 18% each, arms 9% each, legs 18% each, genitalia 1%.

Children Use palm of the child's hand to represent 1% surface area.

Depth of burn

- *1st degree:* red, pain, no blisters.
- *2nd degree:* red or mottled, pain, blisters.
- *3rd degree:* dark and leathery, no pain, dry.
- Common to find all three depths within the same burn.

Box 20.4 Fluid resuscitation

Adults

Give 2–4mL/kg/% surface area burned in the first 24h (give half in first 8h and half in next 16h), e.g. an 80kg adult with 25% burns:

80 × 25 × 2–4mL in 24h = 4000–8000mL over 24h

Give 2–4L over 1st 8h, then 2–4L over the subsequent 16h.

Children

Give 4mL/kg/% surface area burned in the first 24h (plus maintenance fluids, see 📖 Calculating maintenance fluids in children, p. 7). Give half this volume in the first 8h and half in next 16h. Suitable fluids are 0.9% saline with 5% glucose, or Ringer's lactate with 5% glucose, e.g. an 18kg child with 25% burns:

Total fluid in first 24h: (maintenance) + resuscitation volume
(56mL × 24h) + 4mL × 18kg × 25 = 1344mL + 1800mL = 3144mL.

Give 1572mL in first 8h and another 1572mL in the next 16h.

Further reading

For further information on the management of burns of various depths see:

Papini R. *ABC of burns: management of burn injuries of various depths*. Br Med J 2004; 328: 158–60. Free download available at: www. bmj.com/highwire/filestream/375538/field_highwire_article_pdf/0/158

Pregnant trauma patients

The ABCDE priorities of pregnant patients are the same, but anatomical and physiological changes in pregnancy are important.

Anatomical changes

Uterus is vulnerable to damage. By 12wks gestation, fundus is at symphysis pubis; by 20wks, it is at umbilicus; by 36wks it is at xiphoid. Fetus in 1st trimester is well protected by thick-walled uterus, pelvis, and large amounts of amniotic fluid.

Physiological changes

↑ Tidal volume and respiratory alkalosis; ↑ increased heart rate; 30% ↑ cardiac output; usually 15mmHg lower BP when lying flat.

Special issues in the injured pregnant patient

Blunt trauma may → uterine irritability and premature labour. Beware of partial/complete rupture of the uterus; partial/complete placental separation (up to 48h later); severe blood loss after pelvic fracture.

Management

- Assess mother according to the ABCDE.
- *Resuscitate in left lateral position to avoid aorto-caval compression.*
- Perform vaginal examination with a speculum to look for vaginal bleeding and cervical dilatation.
- Mark the fundal height and assess tenderness.
- Monitor the foetal heart rate.
- Resuscitation of mother may save baby. However, there are times when only option to save mother is to deliver baby by Caesarean section.

Chapter 21

Poisoning and envenoming

Invited authors **Michael Eddleston**

David Warrell

Acute poisoning

Most deaths from acute poisoning are due to deliberate self-poisoning. Although drug poisoning is common in urban areas of resource-poor regions, the majority of deaths occur in rural areas after ingestion of pesticides. While outcome seems to be determined purely by the amount ingested for some pesticides, good management for poisoning by other agents can reduce the death rate.

General management

- *Resuscitate and stabilize (see* *Life support algorithms, inside front cover)**:* in particular, take care of the airway, intubating any patient unable to protect their own airway (check the cough and gag are intact).
- *Give high-flow O_2:* except for paraquat poisoned patients.
- Place patient on their left side to reduce the risk of aspiration and passage of poison; it will also help keep their airway open.
- *If the patient has taken a pesticide:* determine whether he/she needs atropine (see next bullet point). This therapy can be life-saving.
- Suck out secretions as necessary (however, in organophosphate poisoning, patients will require atropine to control secretions).
- *Get a history:* what has been taken? How much and when? Have a handbook available that lists pesticides by both their chemical class and trade name since many people will only know the latter.
- *Calm the patient:* agitated poisoned patient makes management difficult and increases risk of aspiration; consider diazepam.
- *Watch out for and control convulsions:* first-line therapy is diazepam; second-line is phenobarbital (see Coma and convulsions, p. 14).
- *Give antidotes according to the poison ingested:* poison identity can come from history or recognition of a 'toxidrome' (see Box 21.1).
- Finally, consider value of performing gastric emptying or decontamination once everything else is done.

Gastric lavage and induced vomiting

Are no longer recommended in routine management of the poisoned patient. Studies have shown little return of poison, even when performed in ideal circumstances. Gastric lavage is associated with increased rate of ICU admission and aspiration pneumonia. Only consider within an hour of the poisoning and only if it can be done safely, in a consenting or intubated patient. Gastric lavage performed in a non-consenting struggling patient has a high risk of aspiration and death.

Activated charcoal Administered orally. Recommended form of GI decontamination as it offers a large surface area for poison to bind to, reducing absorption into the body. Give 50–100g (1g/kg for children) dissolved in 200–300mL water.

Multiple doses of activated charcoal Some poisons are excreted in bile or diffuse across the intestinal wall into the lumen. In this situation, regular repeated administration of activated charcoal q4h may enhance elimination.

Osmotic cathartics are no longer recommended. They increase the risk of electrolyte abnormalities with no evidence of benefit.

Box 21.1 Toxidromes

Patients are often unable or sometimes unwilling to state which poison they have ingested. Treatment in these situations is based on clinical signs and locally the most likely poison ingested. Toxidromes are collections of signs that may assist in diagnosis (such as cholinergic or anti-cholinergic syndromes). See Box 21.2 for classification of common pesticides.

Box 21.2 Classification of common pesticides

Insecticides

- *OPs:* poisoning is often serious, requiring treatment with atropine, ventilation, diazepam, and close monitoring.
- *Carbamates:* similar to OPs, but acetylcholinesterase (AChE) inhibition is briefer. However, poisoning may still last 2–4d and patients require ventilation. Both OPs and carbamates are associated with aspiration.
- *Organochlorines:* e.g. dichlorodiphenyltrichloroethane (DDT) are little used now due to environmental persistence. Major clinical problem is status epilepticus.
- *Pyrethroids:* low toxicity, but may cause anaphylaxis-like features.

Herbicides

- *Chlorophenoxy compounds:* in large overdoses, cause reduced consciousness and rhabdomyolysis resulting in acute kidney injury.
- *Paraquat:* no proven treatment is available. Management appears not to alter clinical course.
- *Chloroacetanilides:* in large overdoses cause hypotension and coma.
- *Propanil:* causes methaemoglobinaemia; few other signs.
- *Glyphosate:* low toxicity unless pesticide and solvent is aspirated.

Rodenticides

- *Aluminium phosphide:* very toxic. Consider giving severely poisoned patients magnesium 1g IV stat, then 1g q1h for 3h, then 1g q6h.
- *Zinc phosphide:* less toxic. Treat supportively.
- *Coumarin derivatives:* long-acting warfarin-like compounds. Active bleeding requires vitamin K 1mg; patients without bleeding can often be simply monitored via their INR.
- *Thallium:* highly toxic. Banned in many countries.
- *Carbamates:* highly toxic carbamate, aldicarb, is widely used as a rodenticide.

There are many other, often newer, pesticides. None have specific antidotes; conservative management with airway support, close observation and monitoring, and diazepam for seizures is probably best. Some toxicity appears to be due to the solvent in which pesticides are formulated. Aspiration of pesticide and solvent/surfactant co-formulants can cause severe lung injury.

Acute pesticide poisoning

Early careful resuscitation and supportive care of pesticide-poisoned patients, with correct use of antidotes, will reduce deaths. Most pesticides are dissolved in organic solvents, which can cause fatal pneumonia if aspirated; other additives, such as methanol, can cause additional toxicity. Beyond 1h, gastric lavage is futile because of a high risk of complications; forced vomiting *should not be performed*. Activated charcoal should be adminstered orally or by NGT (Box 21.3).

Organophosphates/carbamates See 📖 Organophosphates/carbamates, p. 876.

Organochlorine poisoning Pesticides, e.g. endosulfan, endrin, and less toxic lindane, cause status epilepticus after large ingestions.

Management With diazepam; give phenobarbital and then general anaesthetic if no response. Many organochlorines are banned worldwide.

Pyrethroids are synthetic derivatives of the plant-derived pyrethrin. Low toxicity but may cause anaphylaxis-like signs. *Manage* conservatively.

Chlorophenoxy herbicides

Include MCPA; 2,4-D; 2,4,5-T (latter two appear more toxic). Cause coma, oxidative uncoupling, and rhabdomyolysis after large overdose. Observe for black urine (indicates myoglobinuria) and muscle pain.

Management Keep high urine output with IV fluids. Give sodium bicarbonate 3 mMol/kg if urine is black. Normally has a good outcome if renal failure can be averted.

Paraquat

Uniformly fatal if taken in large amounts due to multi-organ failure. Smaller doses may result in fatal lung fibrosis. Patients often have marked ulceration of mouth, since they may just take it into their mouth, then spit it out; oesophageal damage indicates that paraquat was swallowed and is a poor prognostic sign. Intensive haemofiltration may offer some slight benefit; high-dose immunosuppression (cyclophosphamide 15mg/kg IV od for 2d; methylprednisolone 1g IV od for 3d, followed by po dexamethasone) may prevent lung fibrosis, but definite evidence is not available.

Management Conservative. Activated charcoal should be given early. Gastric lavage risks oesophageal perforation. O_2 may exacerbate lung fibrosis.

Propanil Causes methaemoglobinaemia. Patient looks cyanosed, but is asymptomatic if metHb levels are <20%; headaches and low GCS occur as metHb level rises. Death occurs with metHb >70%.

Management Give methylthioninium chloride (methylene blue) 1–2mg/kg IV over 5min, repeated after 30–60min as necessary, and/or exchange transfusion.

Glyphosate Causes ulcerative damage to oesophagus, but little else. Do not perform lavage since complications may occur after aspiration.

Box 21.3 Gastric lavage for pesticide poisoning

- Lavage must not be performed in combative, conscious patients or in patients with reduced GCS unless intubated.
- Lavage should only be considered when patients present <1h after ingestion of a potentially life-threatening amount of pesticide (usually organophosphate, organochlorine, or carbamate).
- Use an 18G NGT for pesticides. A larger bore tube has a higher rate of complications.

Poisoning with corrosives

After ingestion, acids cause an immediate mucosal burn that scabs over, limiting damage. In contrast, alkalis produce a liquifactive necrosis that produces much deeper tissue damage.

Clinical features Pain in mouth, throat, and abdomen; dysphagia; drooling. Complications include perforation, haemorrhage, and systemic complications of the particular corrosive (e.g. acidosis). Patients with severe poisoning are at high risk of strictures in oesophagus or stomach.

Management Give O_2 and obtain IV access for fluid resuscitation. Watch for signs of airway obstruction or GI perforation. GI decontamination is not indicated. Careful endoscopy is recommended soon after admission to assess damage to GI tract and manage strictures. Patients with alkali ingestions and circumferential oesophageal burns may benefit from early steroids (hydrocortisone 100mg bd), although evidence is weak.

Poisoning with hydrocarbons

- Hydrocarbon toxicity occurs after pulmonary aspiration or after systemic absorption. The compounds can be grouped by volatility/viscosity and systemic toxicity.
- Poisoning with *non-volatile, non-absorbed* hydrocarbons, such as motor oil does not require treatment. The risk of aspiration is low.
- Poisoning with more *volatile, but non-toxic* hydrocarbons, such as kerosene, is very common. Aspiration pneumonia is the main complication so treat conservatively without inducing vomiting or gastric lavage.
- The management of *volatile and toxic* hydrocarbons such as phenol is difficult. Lavage may be indicated in hope of preventing systemic toxicity if the patients have taken a very big dose and been admitted <1 h after ingestion. Beware of causing aspiration pneumonia.
- Care for these patients is supportive with very careful protection of the airway. There is no general antidote; steroids are not indicated.

Organophosphates/carbamates

These pesticides inhibit AChE at autonomic, neuromuscular, and central synapses, causing acetylcholine (ACh) to accumulate and overstimulate receptors. AChE reactivates quickly in carbamate poisoning; the process is much slower in OP poisoning causing a more prolonged poisoning. Atropine antagonizes ACh at muscarinic receptors, reversing parasympathetic features. Oximes, such as pralidoxime reactivate inhibited AChE; however, whether oximes offer benefit to patients is currently unclear (Cochrane review, 2011).

Clinical features

Result from accumulation of ACh at *muscarinic* synapses (salivation, bronchorrhoea, urination, diarrhoea, bradycardia, small pupils); *nicotinic* synapses (muscle fasciculation, weakness, tachycardia, large pupils); *CNS* synapses (agitation, confusion, drowsiness, coma). Inhibition of AChE over hours to days may → failure of the neuromuscular junction and the intermediate syndrome (initially neck flexion weakness, sometimes cranial nerve palsies, respiratory muscle weakness and sudden respiratory arrest). Some OPs cause delayed peripheral motor neuropathy after several weeks.

Diagnosis Is normally clinical, based on typical features. Plasma butyrylcholinesterase levels may support the diagnosis.

Management

- Resuscitation and supportive care is the major initial priority. Decontamination should only be considered *after* the patient is stable.
- Give oxygen: intubate early—as soon as patient's GCS drops <12–13. Give diazepam 10mg IV slowly over 2–3min as required.
- Simultaneously, give atropine 1.2–2.4mg rapidly as a bolus.
- Watch for a response in the markers of atropinization (see Box 21.4).
- If no response at 5–10min, double dose of atropine.
- Continue giving doubling doses of atropine until the chest is starting to clear of wheeze or crackles (beware sounds of aspiration) and pulse is >80/min. Large amounts of atropine may be required.
- Once patient is atropinized (see Box 21.4), set up an infusion giving 20–40%/h of the total bolus dose of atropine required.
- For OPs and where agent is unknown, consider give pralidoxime chloride 2g IV slowly over 5–30min (fast injection causes vomiting, tachycardia). An infusion is not currently recommended; repeat qds.
- Treat convulsions with diazepam 10mg IV slowly over 2–3min; repeated as necessary. Intubate and ventilate if required.
- Observe carefully to ensure that (i) the required amount of atropine is being given—increase or decrease as required—and (ii) detect neck weakness (= early intermediate syndrome; ask patient to lift head off bed against resistance) early so that a patient can be intubated and ventilated before a respiratory arrest. Monitor tidal volume regularly when any weakness is detected.

Box 21.4 Markers

Atropinization

Sufficient atropine has been given when all the following are attained:

- Chest clear (no wheeze or crackles).
- Pulse >80bpm.
- Systolic BP >80mmHg with urine output >0.5mL/kg/h.

Other signs of atropinization include:

- Pupils no longer pinpoint.
- Axillae (or oral mucosa) are dry.

Notes

- Aspiration may complicate chest criteria. Try to differentiate between localized crackles of aspiration and generalized crackles/ wheeze of OP poisoning.
- The pupils may dilate late—after 30min or so.
- There is no need to continue to give atropine until heart rate is 120–140 or pupils widely dilated. The aim is to reverse poisoning, not to induce atropine toxicity.

Markers of over-atropinization

Too much atropine is being given if:

- Bowel sounds are absent.
- Patient is in urinary retention.
- Patient is confused (not alcohol-related).
- Patient is febrile due to atropine.

Atropine-induced fevers These are a particular problem in patients agitated by alcohol withdrawal and in hot environments. They risk causing cardiac arrest.

Agitation Can be decreased with oral or IV benzodiazepines. Lower the temperature by sponging the patient and using a fan.

Sustained tachycardias Of 120–140/min can → myocardial infarction in patients with alcohol cardiomyopathy or ischaemic disease.

Acute poisoning with pharmaceuticals/ chemicals

Relatively few pharmaceuticals have specific antidotes. For most patients management will be supportive. There is no evidence of benefit from lavage, forced vomiting, or activated charcoal.

Benzodiazepines

Cause drowsiness, slurred speech, ataxia, rarely coma (small pupils/ hyporeflexia), or respiratory failure, due to the drugs′ inhibitory effect on the CNS. Most patients can simply be observed if left in the left lateral position. In cases of respiratory failure (often with newer, short-acting drugs), intubate/ventilate. Severe poisoning can be briefly reversed with flumazenil 0.2mg IV over 15-s repeated with doses of 0.1mg at 60-s intervals if required, up to a maximum of 1mg. Flumazenil must not be used if pro-convulsant drugs have been co-ingested.

Cardiac glycosides

Can be due to overdose of digoxin medication or ingestion of a source of natural glycoside (e.g. oleander seeds–*Nerium oleander*). Main effects are on the heart—dysrhythmias and conduction block. Atropine 0.5mg IV for bradycardia is frequently used, but is unlikely to prevent severe dysrhythmia. Temporary cardiac pacing can tide the patient through 3rd degree AV heart block, but risks inducing ventricular arrhythmias in an irritated myocardium. Anti-digoxin antibodies, where available/affordable, can reverse DC-shock resistant VF or cardiogenic shock in severe poisoning.

Isoniazid May cause reduced consciousness, convulsions, coma, respiratory arrest, metabolic acidosis. If severe, give pyridoxine by slow IV injection (quantity equal to the quantity of isoniazid taken; if quantity unknown, give 5g). Can repeat at 5–20-min intervals.

Lithium carbonate

Affects CNS, heart, and kidney. Acute lithium poisoning with normal renal function generally requires only supportive care. In patients with poor renal function and severe poisoning, haemodialysis is the best method to remove lithium. Check serum electrolytes 6–12-hourly; if hypernatraemia is present, give 5% glucose until plasma Na^+ returns to normal. Since most patients will be on chronic lithium therapy and have nephrogenic diabetes insipidus, they will require high fluid maintenance rates. Monitor carefully.

Opiates Found in analgesics and recreational drugs. Cause respiratory depression, ↓ consciousness, and pinpoint pupils. Give repeated boluses of naloxone 0.4–2mg IV; if there is a response, set up a naloxone infusion to counter long-acting or sustained-release opioids. Starting dose is 20–50% of the total initial bolus each hour. The major indicator of naloxone response is reversal of respiratory depression. Response time is several minutes to increase respiratory rate to >10/min. If more than 2mg naloxone is required, review the diagnosis. Has more than one drug been taken?

Paracetamol

For ingestions of >150 mg/kg, give acetylcysteine IV (or orally) unless paracetamol blood levels can be measured and shown to be safe. Dose = 150mg/kg in 200mL of 5% glucose or 0.9% sodium chloride over 15–60 min, followed by 50mg/kg in 500mL over 4h, and then 100mg/kg in 1L over 16h. If liver failure develops, continue as it may improve outcome. If acetylcysteine is unavailable, give methionine 2.5g orally repeated 4-hourly for a total of 4 doses. Check liver and kidney function. Closely monitor blood glucose levels, watching for hypoglycaemia.

Salicylates

Severe aspirin poisoning may cause CNS depression, haematemesis, hyperthermia. However, lethal doses may not affect consciousness. Lesser poisoning → GI pain, N&V, tinnitus. A mixed metabolic acidosis/respiratory alkalosis is common. Metabolic acidosis occurs in young children, respiratory alkalosis more commonly in older patients. Give charcoal and correct electrolyte imbalances. If there are neurological signs, give 50mL of 50% glucose IV; repeat if necessary. Any metabolic acidosis should be corrected (even if there is respiratory compensation) with sodium bicarbonate infusion; patients commonly require K^+ supplementation. The goal of bicarbonate treatment is to restore normal systemic pH and make the urine alkaline (urine pH >7).

Tricyclic antidepressants

May cause CNS toxicity (convulsions, ophthalmoplegia, muscle twitching, delirium, coma, respiratory depression), anticholinergic effects (dry mouth, blurred vision, mydriasis), cardiotoxicity (QRS duration and QT prolongation), hypothermia, pyrexia. Control convulsions; monitor heart and correct arrhythmias; control acidosis. Give IV sodium bicarbonate for cardiotoxicity or for seizures with an initial dose of 3mmol/kg. This dose can be repeated and titrated against clinical response. The pH should be assessed, if possible, after a total dose of 6mmol/kg and should not exceed pH 7.55.

Cyanide

Late presentations include dyspnoea, cyanosis, or unconsciousness. Altered mental status, tachypnoea (in absence of cyanosis), unexplained anion gap metabolic acidosis, and bright red blood are earlier signs. Adminster O_2; correct acidosis; give amylnitrite by inhalation over 30s/min until other drugs are prepared. Then give: sodium nitrite 300mg by IV injection over 5–20min followed by sodium thiosulfate 12.5g IV over 10min (alternative: dicobalt edetate 300mg IV over 1min followed by 50mL of 50% glucose. Repeat ×2 if required).

Metal ions (e.g. gold, mercury, zinc, lead, copper) Acute poisoning can → coma, convulsions, and death, or affect multiple organ systems. Anticipate and treat shock, renal, or hepatic failure. Give penicillamine 1–2g oral od divided into 3 doses (2h before meals, if possible) for 2–4wks. Get a senior opinion. An alternative option (preferred in mercury poisoning) is dimercaprol (British anti-Lewisite) 2.5–3mg/kg q4h for 2d; then qds on the 3rd day; and bd for days 4–10 or until recovery.

Mushroom poisoning

Mushrooms cause a variety of toxic affects on the CNS, kidney, liver, muscle, and GI tract. Clinical features are separated into those appearing early (<6h) or late (>6h) after ingestion.

Clinical features

Early symptoms

Start within a few hours: gastroenteritis, cholinergic (muscarinic) effects, confusion, visual hallucinations, or disulfiram-like reactions to drinking alcohol, according to the species ingested.

Delayed symptoms

Starting 6h to many days later suggest more dangerous poisoning:

- Gastroenteritis with hepato- and nephrotoxicity (amatoxin poisoning) is caused by death cap mushroom (*Amanita phalloides*) and others from *Amanita*, *Galerina*, and *Lepiota* genera. Abdominal pain, vomiting, and watery diarrhoea start after 6–24h (usually 12h) resulting in dehydration. Hepatic and renal failure evolve over next few days or weeks.
- Gastroenteritis with neurological symptoms (gyromitrin poisoning) caused by false morel (*Gyromitra esculenta*). Gastroenteritis, bloating, severe headache, vertigo, pyrexia, sweating, diplopia, nystagmus, ataxia, and cramps followed by delirium, coma, hepatic and renal damage, hypoglycaemia, and haemolysis.
- Renal damage may develop 2–17d after eating *Cortinarius* spp. (orellanine poisoning). Fatigue, intense thirst, headache, chills, paraesthesiae, tinnitus and abdominal, lumbar, and flank pain → polyuria, oliguria, and anuria.
- Rhabdomyolysis occurs after ingestion of *Tricholoma* spp. due to a myotoxin.

Management

- Give activated charcoal 50g q2h for at least 48h.
- Correct hypovolaemia, acid-base disturbances, hypoglycaemia, and renal failure.
- Give atropine (adult 0.6–1.8mg IV) for cholinergic features.
- Give physostigmine (adult 1–2mg IV) or diazepam (adults 5–10mg IV) for anticholinergic hallucinations.
- For amatoxic fungal poisoning, give silibinin/silybin milk thistle (*Silybum marianum*) extract (bolus dose of 5mg/kg IV over 1h, followed by continuous infusion 20mg/kg/24h for 3d post-ingestion). Alternatively, give large doses of benzylpenicillin (2.4g qds). Acetylcysteine may be beneficial. Liver transplantation may become necessary.
- Gyromitrin fungal poisoning is treated with pyridoxine 25mg/kg over 30min, 5% glucose IV, and diuresis.

Prevention

Discourage the ingestion of any wild fungi, especially those with white gills. Cooking does not destroy their poisons.

Methanol poisoning

A common form of poisoning globally, resulting from drinking illegal contaminated forms of alcohol, that results in large epidemics and many deaths. Diagnosis is very difficult due to the lack of distinctive clinical characteristics and to the lack of laboratories able to measure methanol or its metabolite formate.

Clinical Features

Early symptoms include intoxication, headache, dizziness, diarrhoea, and vomiting. Delayed features include poor or blurred vision, coma, seizures, hyperventilation, and mixed metabolic acidosis/respiratory alkalosis as the formate metabolite is formed.

Diagnosis

Methanol and its metabolite formate can be measured in the blood. Other markers of poisoning include an early raised osmolar gap (before the methanol is metabolized into formate) and a later raised anion gap metabolic acidosis (after the formate has been produced).

Management

Treatment aims to prevent the formation of formate so that the methanol can be eliminated by the kidneys. Ethanol and fomepizole inhibit the responsible enzyme, alcohol dehydrogenase.

Ethanol can be given to maintain a blood ethanol concentration of around 100 mg/L (loading dose of 2.5 mL/kg of 40% ethanol [spirits eg whisky, vodka] orally or 10 mL/kg of 10% ethanol by intravenous infusion over 30 min; in the absence of laboratory ability to measure blood ethanol, maintenance doses are typically from 0.25 mL/kg/hr [non drinker or child] to 0.6 mL/kg/hr [heavy drinker] of 40% ethanol; 1 to 2.5 mL/kg/hr of 10% ethanol by intravenous infusion). Complications of ethanol treatment are inadequate dosing and intoxication.

Fomepizole is easier to administer and does not require monitoring. Loading dose: 15 mg/kg IV diluted to a final volume of 250–500 mL saline or dextrose over 30 minutes. Maintenance: 10 mg/kg IV diluted to a final volume of 250–500 mL saline or dextrose over 30 minutes every 12 hours (starting at 12 hours after the loading dose is given) for a maximum of 4 doses; followed by 15 mg/kg IV diluted to a final volume of 250–500 mL saline or dextrose over 30 minutes every 12 hours thereafter.

Dialysis: if neither antidote is available, haemodialysis to remove methanol and its metabolite may be life-saving.

Fish and shellfish poisoning

Ciguatera fish poisoning

Due to accumulation of toxins from the flagellate *Gambierdiscus toxicus* in muscles of carnivorous fish at the top of the food chain. >50 000 cases occur each year. In some Pacific islands >1% are affected/year, case fatality 0.1%. The toxins activate Na^+ channels. Gastroenteritis develops 1–6h after eating warm-water shore or reef fish (groupers, snappers, parrot fish, mackerel, moray eels, barracudas, jacks). GI symptoms resolve within a few hours, but paraesthesiae (reversed hot-cold sensation), pruritus, and myalgia may persist for a week to months. Rare complications include cardiotoxicity and respiratory paralysis.

Tetrodotoxin poisoning

Scaleless porcupine, sun, puffer, and toad fish (order: *Tetraodonitiformes*) become poisonous seasonally. Puffer fish ('fugu') is relished in Japan. Neurotoxic symptoms develop 10–45min after eating the fish and death may ensue from respiratory paralysis 2–6h later.

Scombroid poisoning (histamine-like syndrome)

Histamine is released by bacterial contamination and decomposition of, e.g. dark-fleshed tuna, mackerel, bonito, and skipjack, and of canned fish. Soon after ingestion buccal tingling, smarting or peppery flavour is followed by flushing, burning, sweating, urticaria, pruritus, headache, abdominal colic, nausea, vomiting, diarrhoea, asthma, giddiness and hypotension.

Paralytic shellfish poisoning Bivalve molluscs (mussels, clams, oysters, cockles, and scallops) become toxic when there is a 'red tide' of algal blooms. Within 30min of ingestion, paralysis begins and, in 8% of cases, progresses to fatal respiratory paralysis within 12h.

Management (of all types of fish/shellfish poisoning)

- Scombroid poisoning responds to antihistamines, bronchodilators, and adrenaline.
- Assisted ventilation is required in severe paralytic poisoning.

Prevention

Marine poisons are not destroyed by cooking or boiling.

- Seek local advice about what is safe to eat.
- Prohibit eating shellfish when there is a 'red tide' (toxic plankton bloom).
- Prohibit eating very large reef fish (ciguatera poisoning), especially any parts of the fish other than muscle.
- Prohibit eating especially notorious species such as Moray eels (ciguatera), parrot fish (palytoxin) or puffer fish (tetrodotoxin).

Leech bite

Land leeches infest rainforest floor, attaching to legs or ankles. After a painless bite, they ingest blood, then drop off, but the wound continues to bleed and the clot is fragile. Aquatic leeches are swallowed in river or pond water, or they attack bathers, entering mouth, nostrils, eyes, vulva, vagina, urethra, or anus.

Clinical features

Main effect is blood loss. Other symptoms include 2° infection (by *Aeromonas hydrophila* with medicinal leeches), itching, and phobia. Ingested aquatic leeches attach to the pharynx, producing a sensation of movement at back of throat, cough, hoarseness, stridor, breathlessness, epistaxis, haemoptysis, haematemesis, or upper airway obstruction, or they penetrate bronchi or oesophagus. Via anus, they may reach rectosigmoid junction, causing perforation and peritonitis.

Treatment

Apply salt, a flame, alcohol, turpentine, or vinegar to the leech to encourage detachment. Control local bleeding with a styptic, such as silver nitrate, or a firm dressing. Penetrating aquatic leeches must be removed endoscopically. Spray with 10% tartaric acid or 1:10 000 adrenaline (nasopharynx, larynx, trachea, or oesophagus) or irrigate with concentrated saline (GI tract and rectum).

Prevention

Trousers, socks, and footwear should be impregnated and skin anointed with DEET. Discourage children from bathing in leech-infested waters. People should not drink from natural water sources. Drinking water must be boiled or filtered.

Snake bite

Most parts of world have venomous snakes. In India, 45 000 people/yr die from snake bite. Other hot spots are West Africa, New Guinea, and Latin America. Medically important groups are elapids (e.g. cobras, mambas), vipers, pit vipers, burrowing asps, and a few species of back-fanged colubrids. Do not be discouraged by the 100s of different species; you need only know about the few dangerous ones where you live and work.

Clinical features (depending on the species involved)

- Local swelling, bruising, blistering, regional lymph node enlargement, and tissue damage (necrosis). Occur with vipers, pit vipers, burrowing asps, and some cobras.
- Incoagulable blood, shown by 20min clotting test (see Box 21.5), spontaneous bleeding from gums, nose, skin, gut, GU tract; persistent bleeding from wounds. Occurs with vipers, pit vipers, South African boomslang and vine snake, and Australasian elapids.
- Shock (hypotension) and arrhythmias. Occur with vipers, pit vipers, burrowing asps and Australasian elapids.
- Descending paralysis (ptosis, external ophthalmoplegia, bulbar and respiratory muscle paralysis, generalized flaccid paralysis). Occurs with elapids, a few vipers and pit vipers.
- Generalized rhabdomyolysis (myalgia, myoglobinuria—black urine which is dipstick +ve for blood). Occurs with sea snakes, some kraits, Australasian elapids, a few vipers and pit vipers.
- Acute kidney injury. Occurs with sea snakes, some other elapids, vipers and pit vipers.

Hospital treatment

First aid—see Box 21.5. Assess and observe patients carefully for ≥24h.

- *Antivenom:* only specific antidote is indicated for any signs of systemic envenoming listed in 📖 Clinical features, p. 884, *or* for local envenoming that is rapidly spreading *or* involvesb more than half the bitten limb or digits. Give an appropriate antivenom (check package insert for species covered) by slow IV injection or infusion.
- Give prophylactic sc adrenaline (0.1%; adult 0.25mg, child 5micrograms/kg). Watch for early signs of anaphylactic reactions and treat with IM adrenaline (adult 0.5mg, child 10micrograms/kg) and IV H_1 antihistamine and hydrocortisone 200mg. Do not do time-wasting, non-predictive hypersensitivity tests.
- Give tetanus toxoid booster.
- Give antibiotics (penicillin, erythromycin or chloramphenicol) only if local necrosis, interference with, or contamination of bite site, or abscess formation.
- Bulbar/respiratory paralysis requires intubation and ventilation.
- Correct hypovolaemia (extravasation/bleeding into swollen limbs).
- Treat acute kidney injury with dialysis.
- Nurse swollen limbs in the most comfortable position.
- Debride necrotic tissue, but avoid fasciotomy unless intra-compartmental pressure is consistently >40mmHg and only after haemostasis has been restored.

Box 21.5 Snake bites prevention and treatment

First aid

- Reassure patient (only ~50% of bites by venomous snakes cause envenoming, which usually takes hours to become serious).
- Do not interfere with bite site in any way (e.g. do not attempt to suck out or aspirate poison).
- Immobilize person as far as possible, especially bitten limb.
- Transport patient to medical care by vehicle, boat, stretcher, etc.
- Treat pain with paracetamol or codeine (not for children) tablets (not aspirin or NSAIDs).
- Never attempt to catch or kill the snake.
- Never use traditional methods (tourniquet, incision, suction, herbs, etc.).

20-min whole blood clotting test

Put 2mL of venous blood into a new, plain glass test-tube. Leave undisturbed for 20min, then tip once. If blood runs out (no clot), consumption coagulopathy has occurred and antivenom is indicated. Repeat 6h after giving antivenom. If blood remains incoagulable, give another dose. If the blood clots initially, the test can be repeated hourly if envenoming is suspected. Recovery will take 6h after effective administration of antivenom since the liver must restore coagulable levels of clotting factors.

Pressure-immobilization methods

Elapid venoms can cause rapid paralysis. Unless an elapid bite can confidently be excluded, bind the bitten limb firmly with long elasticated bandages, from digits to axilla/groin, incorporating a splint or firmly apply a 6 x 6 x 3cm pad of cloth immediately over the bite wound, using a non-elastic bandage. Loosen if the limb becomes painful or if peripheral pulses are occluded.

Prevention of snake bites

- Avoid all snakes and snake charmers.
- Never disturb, corner, attack, or handle snakes, dead or alive.
- If a snake is cornered, remain motionless until it has escaped.
- Never walk in undergrowth or deep sand without proper leg/footwear.
- Always carry a light at night.
- Be careful collecting firewood with bare hands.
- Never put a hand or push sticks into burrows or holes.
- Avoid climbing trees or rocks covered with dense foliage.
- When climbing, do not put hands on ledges that cannot be seen.
- Never swim in vegetation-matted rivers or muddy estuaries.
- Avoid sleeping on the ground—use a hammock or camp bed, a tent with sewn-in ground sheet, or a mosquito net tucked under the sleeping bag.

Scorpion sting

The most dangerous scorpions (Fig 21.1) inhabit deserts or hot dusty terrains in North Africa, Middle East, South Africa, the Americas, and South Asia. They probably cause >100 000 medically significant stings each year. Most deaths occur in children.

Clinical features

Stings are excruciatingly painful. Systemic symptoms reflect release of autonomic neurotransmitters: acetylcholine (causing vomiting, abdominal pain, bradycardia, sweating, salivation) and then catecholamines (causing hypertension, tachycardia, pulmonary oedema, and ECG abnormalities).

Management

For pain, infiltrate local anaesthetic at the site, ideally by digital block if the sting is on a finger or toe. Powerful opiate analgesia may be required. For systemic envenoming (difficult to distinguish from pain and fear in children), antivenoms are available for dangerous African/Middle Eastern, Indian, and American species. Hypertension, acute left ventricular failure, and pulmonary oedema may respond to vasodilators such as prazosin (0.5mg oral q3–6h).

Prevention

Scorpions hide in cracks, crevices, and under rubbish. Encourage people to not walk around in bare feet, to sleep off the ground under a permethrin-impregnated bed net, and to always shake out boots and shoes before putting them on.

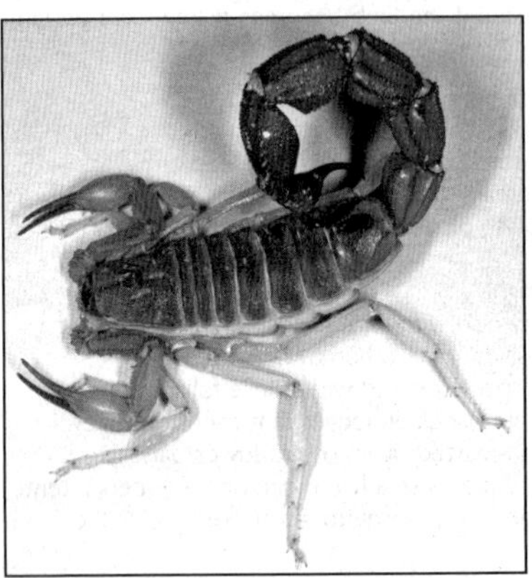

Fig. 21.1 Granulated thick-tailed scorpion (*Parabuthus granulatus*) from South Africa: a large (adults ~12cm long) brown-coloured scorpion; its venom is extremely potent and causes respiratory paralysis.

Picture courtesy of Professor David Warrell.

Spider bite

The most dangerous spiders are:
Black/brown widows (*Latrodectus*) in the Americas, southern Europe, southern Africa, and Australia.
Wandering, armed, or banana spiders (*Phoneutria*) in Latin America.
Funnel web spiders (*Atrax* and *Hadronyche*) in Australia.
Brown recluse spiders (*Loxosceles*) in the Americas and elsewhere.

Spiders cause few deaths (see Fig. 21.2).

Clinical features

Bites happen when people brush against a spider that has crept into clothes or bedding. *Latrodectus*, *Phoneutria*, and *Atrax* are neurotoxic causing cramping abdominal pains, muscle spasms, weakness, sweating, salivation, gooseflesh, fever, nausea, vomiting, alterations in pulse rate and BP, and convulsions. *Loxosceles* is necrotic. Rarely, *Loxosceles* cause systemic effects such as fever, scarlatiniform rash, haemoglobinuria, coagulopathy, and acute kidney injury.

Management Mostly symptomatic. Antivenoms available in South Africa, Australia, and Brazil where bites are an important medical problem.

Hymenoptera sting anaphylaxis

Stings by bees (*Apidae*), wasps, hornets and yellow jackets (*Vespidae*), and ants (American fire ants *Solenopsis*, Australian jumper ants *Myrmecia*) are a very common nuisance in most countries. However, 2–4% of the population becomes allergic, developing massive local swelling or potentially lethal anaphylaxis if stung. In tropical countries, mass attacks by bees and wasp-like insects are not uncommon. In the Americas, Africanized 'killer' bees have killed many people.

Clinical features

Symptoms of anaphylaxis including urticaria, angioedema, shock, bronchospasm, and GI symptoms.

Management

Give adrenaline.

Prevention

Desensitization is effective but time-consuming. Self-injectable adrenaline is the best first aid.

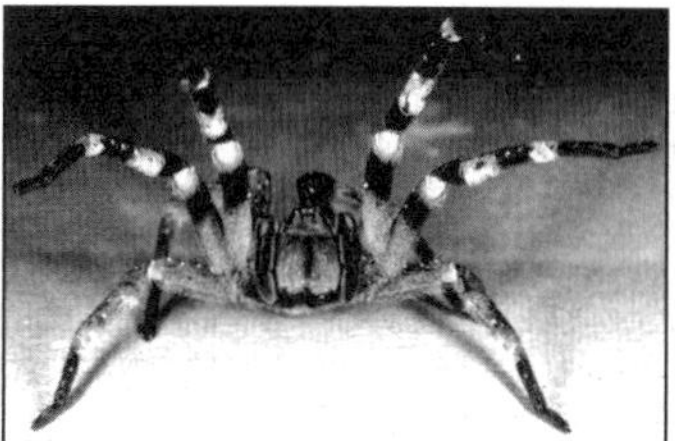

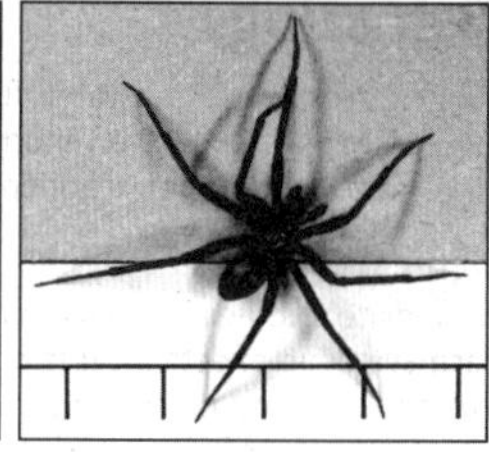

Fig. 21.2 *Left*: Brazilian wandering or armed spider (*Phoneutria nigriventer*) from São Paulo: 3–5cm in body length with a leg span of 13–15cm. Bite causes neurotoxic araneism—autonomic symptoms. Sometimes exported in bunches of bananas and has caused bites in western countries. *Right*: Chilean brown recluse spider (*Loxosceles laeta*) specimen from Brazil: small peri-domestic spiders (see centimetre scale in picture; leg span ~4cm) whose bites can cause extensive local necrosis and, sometimes, life-threatening systemic symptoms.

Pictures courtesy of Professor David Warrell.

Fish stings

Stinging fresh- and saltwater fish (stingrays, cat fish, weevers, scorpion fish, stone fish, etc.) have venomous spines on gills, fins, or tail. Most commonly, they sting when trodden upon on the ocean or river bed.

Clinical features

Immediate excruciating pain, followed by local swelling and inflammation. Rare systemic effects include vomiting, diarrhoea, sweating, dysrhythmia, hypotension, and muscle spasms. Stingrays' barbed spines can inflict fatal trauma (pneumothorax, penetration of organs). Spines left embedded in wound with their venomous integument will cause infection.

Management

First aid Agonizing local pain is dramatically relieved by immersing stung part in hot (<45°C), but not scalding water, which will cause a full thickness scald. Local anaesthetic can also be infiltrated or applied as digital block for pain relief.

Antivenom Australia produces an antivenom for the most dangerous species—stone fish (genus *Synanceia*).

Infection All fish wounds can become infected with lethal marine pathogens including *Vibrio vulnificus*.

Prevention Advise people to shuffle or prod sand ahead of them with a stick to disturb ground-lurking fish, to avoid handling dead or live fish, and to keep clear of fish in the water, especially in vicinity of tropical reefs. Footwear protects against most species except stingrays.

Jelly fish stings

Common stinging jelly fish (*Cnidarians/Coelenterates*) include: Portuguese men o'war (blue bottles), sea wasps, box jellies, cubomedusoids, sea anemones, and stinging corals. Tentacles are studded with millions of stinging capsules (nematocysts) that fire venomous stinging hairs into skin on contact. Lines of painful blisters and inflammation result. Allergy may cause recurrent urticarial rashes over many months. The notorious Northern Australian and Indo-Pacific box jellyfish (*Chironex fleckeri* and *Chiropsalmus* spp.) and *Irukandji* (*Carukia barnesi*) can kill.

Clinical features Severe musculoskeletal pain, anxiety, trembling, headache, piloerection, sweating, tachycardia, hypertension, and pulmonary oedema may evolve or anaphylaxis in those sensitized by previous stings.

Management

Remove victim from water (to prevent drowning). Inhibit nematocyst discharge by applying commercial vinegar or 3–10% aqueous acetic acid (*only Chironex* spp. and other cubozoans including *Irukandji*) or a slurry of baking soda and water (50% w/v) (*Chrysaora* spp.). Do not use sun tan lotion or alcoholic solutions! Immersion in hot water (see 📖 Fish stings, p. 890) relieves pain. Antivenom for *C. fleckeri* is available in Australia.

Sea urchin stings

Long, sharp, venomous sea urchin (*Echinoderm*) spines become deeply embedded in skin, usually of sole of foot, when animal is trodden upon.

Management

Immersion in hot water (see 📖 Fish stings, p. 890) relieves pain. Soften skin with salicylic acid ointment and then pare down the epidermis to a depth at which spines can be removed with forceps. Most sea urchin spines are absorbed rapidly provided they are broken into small pieces in skin. If they penetrate a joint or become infected, surgical removal may be necessary.

Jelly fish stings

[illegible]

[illegible]

[illegible]

[illegible]

Management

[illegible]

Chapter 22

Immunization

Invited author **Matthew D. Snape**

Introduction

Both the achievements and shortcomings of vaccines in preventing disease in tropical countries are extraordinary. Over 100 million children per year are immunized, and ~2.5 million deaths per year are prevented. However, many children receive incomplete immunizations. If immunization coverage ↑ to >90% by 2015, ~2 million additional childhood deaths per year could be prevented. Many vaccines require a cold chain and IM injection, with the challenging infrastructure these demand. Due to the enormous potential of vaccines these issues need to be addressed. Initiatives such as the Global Alliance for Vaccine and Immunization (GAVI) (see 📖 Funding initiatives below) offer hope that populations most in need will benefit from the potential that vaccinology offers.

Expanded programme on immunization

Guidelines of the EPI for childhood vaccination are given in Table 22.1. (Recommended booster doses are given in Table 22.2). Epidemiology of diseases EPI aims to combat differs between countries, thus immunization policy needs to be made at national or regional level. National policies take precedence over EPI guidelines presented here. See Box 22.1 for common abbreviations, and Box 22.2 for space to list your national/regional recommendations. See Fig 22.1 and 22.2 for sites for injection.

A summary of national guidelines can be accessed at the WHO website and is available at: 🖱 www.who.int/immunization_monitoring/en/globalsummary/scheduleselect.cfm/

Funding initiatives

As a result of ↑ recognition of the cost effectiveness of vaccine programmes, new funding initiatives have been developed. Most prominent is the Global Alliance for Vaccines and Immunizations (GAVI). This alliance between key immunization stakeholders such as developing and donor governments, the World Bank, WHO, UNICEF, the pharmaceutical industry, research institutes, NGOs, and the Bill and Melinda Gates Foundation, has brought focus and unprecedented resources to the goal of optimizing immunization uptake and development of new vaccines.

Further reading

Available at: 🖱 http://www.who.int/immunization_financing/about/en/

Table 22.1 Expanded programme on immunization

Age[1]	Vaccines	Scheme I[2]	Scheme II
Birth	BCG, OPV-0[3]	HepB-1	HepB-1
6wks	DTP-1, OPV-1, Hib-1, PC-1, Rota	HepB-2	HepB-2
10wks	DTP-2, OPV-2, Hib-2, PC-2, Rota		HepB-3
14wks	DTP-3, OPV-3, Hib-3, PC-3, Rota[4]	HepB-3	HepB-4
9mths	Measles[5] , Rubella +/- Yellow fever[6]		
Variable	Japanese encephalitis[7] Tick-borne encephalitis		

[1]Babies born prematurely should be vaccinated at exactly the same times after birth as babies born at term.

[2]The monovalent HepB vaccine should be used at birth; subsequent immunization can be with either a monovalent vaccine or in combination with combination diphtheria toxoid, tetanus toxoid and pertussis vaccine (DTP) +/– Hib. While three doses of HepB are considered sufficient (Scheme I), a 4 doses schedule (Scheme II) can be used for pragmatic reasons (e.g. if HepB being administered in a combination vaccine with DTP +/- Hib).

[3]In polio-endemic countries.

[4]Although vaccine manufacturers recommend that the maximum age of administration of the last dose be 32 weeks, the WHO advise that rotavirus vaccines can be administered with DTP vaccine up until 2 years of age.

[5]Where there is a high risk of mortality from measles under the age of 9mths (e.g. HIV+ infants), measles vaccination should be carried out at both 6 and 9mths.

[6]In countries where yellow fever poses a risk (see p. 818).

[7]In endemic countries (📖 p. 985); variable schedules from 9mths (📖 Japanese encephalitis vaccines, p. 905).

Updates and further details are available at the WHO website: http://www.who.int/immunization/policy/Immunization_routine_table1.pdf

Table 22.2 Booster doses recommended for the following vaccines

Vaccine	Recommended boosting schedule
Tetanus[1,2]	Further doses to be given at:
	2–7yrs of age (DTP or dT according to local policy)
	12–15yrs of age (dT)
Pertussis	1 further dose at 1–6yrs
Measles	1 further dose, either as part of routine schedule or in mass immunization campaigns

[1]Maternal immunization is a highly effective method of controlling neonatal tetanus. Recommendations vary according to previous immunization status and are outlined (📖 Tetanus immunization schedules in adults and pregnant women, p. 909).

[2]EPI for children has total of 5 doses of tetanus-toxoid vaccine, but a dose in early adulthood is recommended for long-term protection.

Box 22.1 Abbreviations for vaccines

- *BCG:* Bacille Calmette–Guérin vaccine.
- *dT:* combination tetanus toxoid and low dose diphtheria toxoid vaccine for use in individuals >7yrs.
- *DT:* combination diphtheria toxoid and tetanus toxoid vaccine for use in children <7yrs.
- *DTP:* combination diphtheria toxoid, tetanus toxoid, and pertussis vaccine.
- *DTaP:* combination diphtheria toxoid, tetanus toxoid, and acellular pertussis vaccine.
- *HepB:* hepatitis B vaccine.
- *Hib: Haemophilus influenzae* type b vaccine.
- *MMR:* combination measles, mumps, and rubella vaccine.
- *MR:* combination measles and rubella vaccine.
- *IPV:* injected polio vaccine (Salk vaccine).
- *OPV:* oral polio vaccine (Sabin vaccine).
- *PC:* pneumococcal conjugate vaccine.
- *Rota:* rotavirus vaccines.
- *TetT:* tetanus toxoid vaccine.

Box 22.2 National/regional recommendations[1]

Age	Vaccines
Birth	
6wks	
10wks	
14wks	
6mths	
9mths	

[1]National/regional recommendations for infant immunization may be written here. See Table 22.1 for WHO recommended infant immunization schedule.

Immunization strategies and schedules

Immunization schedule design

Timings of vaccines recommended by EPI are a compromise between:

- Desire to immunize as early as possible, protecting the child before exposure to the infectious agent.
- Requirement to wait for the infant's immune system to mature and for maternally-derived antibodies that crossed the placenta prenatally to ↓, so immunization will be effective.

In general, vaccines are recommended for the youngest age group at risk for developing the disease able to receive vaccine safely and develop an adequate response. Many vaccines require >1 dose and it is recommended these doses be separated by ≥4wks. ↑ intervals between doses, as recommended in many resource-rich countries, ↑ immune response to vaccines, but results in the child being susceptible to the disease for a longer period of time.

Optimization of vaccine uptake

The most common reason for children dying from a vaccine preventable disease is that they have not received the vaccine. ↑ vaccine uptake is crucial and can be facilitated by:

- Offering immunizations as often as possible.
- Administering all vaccines for which a child is eligible at one visit.
- Routine screening of immunization status of all women and children.
- Awareness of true and false contraindications for immunizations (📖 Contraindications to vaccination, p. 901).
- Maintenance of adequate vaccine delivery.
- Appropriate utilization of multi-dose vials (📖 Transport and storage of vaccines, p. 898).

Transport and storage of vaccines

Most EPI vaccines need an adequate 'cold chain' to ensure vaccine transport at optimum temperatures from manufacture to point of use. This is essential for an effective immunization programme. The following innovations have been introduced:

- *Cold chain monitor:* detects excessive temperatures during shipment.
- *Vaccine vial monitor* (VVM): for the cumulative heat exposure of an individual vial.
- The 'shake test' to detect the effects of freezing on vaccines.
- *Freeze watch™ monitor:* for exposure of vaccine shipments to temperatures below freezing point.
- *Stop!Watch™:* combining the indicators from the cold chain monitor and the Freeze watch™ monitor.

Guidance on the use of these devices and the maintenance of cold chain is available at: http://www.who.int/immunization/documents/WHO_IVB_06.10/en/index.html

To ↓ vaccine wastage use, it is acceptable to use already-opened multi-dose vials at subsequent immunization sessions for: OPV, DTP, TetT, DT, HepB and liquid formulations of Hib. Multi-dose vials of these vaccines can be used for up to 4wks after the opening of the vial provided that:

- Cold chain has been maintained, the VVM has not reached the 'discard point', and vaccines are within their 'use by' date.
- The rubber vaccine vial stopper has not been submerged in water (e.g. by melting ice).
- Aseptic technique has been used to withdraw all doses.

Needle use and disposal

>1 billion immunizations/yr are injected in resource-poor countries. Without adequate safety systems, each one of these episodes creates the potential for transmission of blood borne infections to both vaccinees (through re-use of needles) and health-care workers (through needle-stick injuries). To ↓ these risks:

- All immunizations requiring injection be administered via single use auto-destruct (AD) needles.
- Must have access to safety boxes to dispose of used needles.
- Safety boxes should be sealed when ¾ full.
- Disposable syringes can be used to reconstitute lyophilized vaccines, but must not be recapped.

Disposal of safety boxes remains problematic in many areas and is most commonly by incineration.

Administration of vaccines

Data from resource-rich countries has highlighted the importance of:

- Using appropriate needle length (i.e. 25mm) when administering intramuscular vaccines in order to ↓ reactogenicity and, potentially, ↑ immunogenicity. Data addressing this question in resource-poor countries are not yet available.
- Administering IM vaccines to infants in the lateral aspect of the thighs, while children >12 mo should receive vaccines in the deltoid muscle.
- Separating vaccines administered on the same limb by at least 2.5cm.
- If 2 live vaccines (📖 Transport and storage of vaccines, p. 898) are to be administered (with the exception of OPV) they should be administered either at the same time or at least 1 mo apart.
- Due to ↑ risk of lymphadenopathy, no vaccine should be administered into an arm used for BCG administration for 3 mo after BCG.
- If an immunization schedule is interrupted, the schedule should proceed as if no interruption had occurred, i.e. there is no need to 'restart' an immunization schedule.

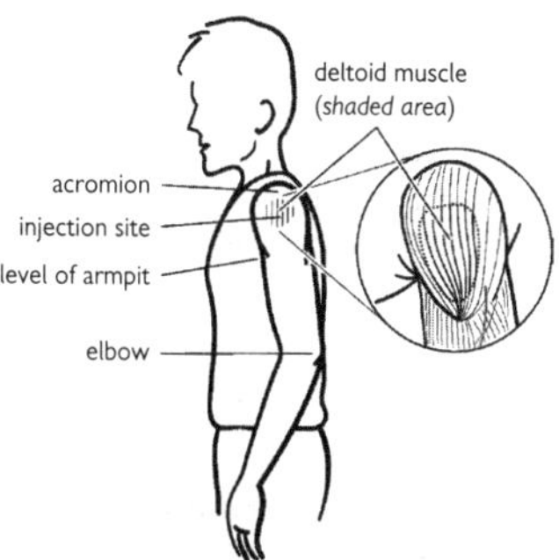

Fig. 22.1 Site of injection for children >1yr and adults.

Reproduced from, Salisbury, D, Ramsay M, and Noakes K, Immunisation against infectious disease, Fig 4.1, (2006) (http://immunisation.dh.gov.uk/category/the-green-book), with permission from WHO.

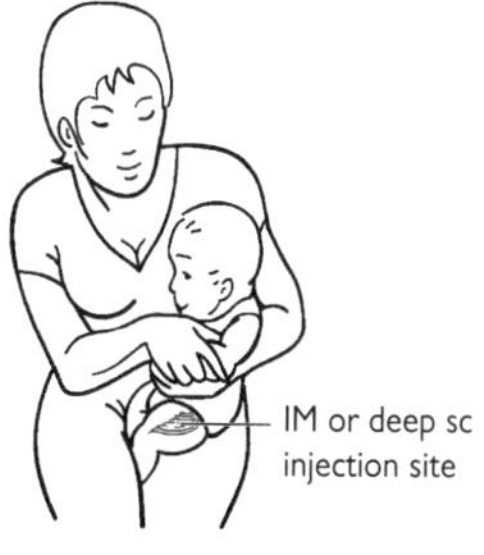

Fig. 22.2 Site of injection for infants <12mths.

Reproduced from, Salisbury, D, Ramsay M, and Noakes K, Immunisation against infectious disease, Fig 4.2, (2006) (http://immunisation.dh.gov.uk/category/the-green-book), with permission from WHO.

Adverse reactions

Although modern vaccines are extremely safe, some vaccines may lead to adverse reactions. Population studies are required to investigate possible associations between vaccines and adverse events (e.g. clustering of cases after immunization or a ↑ incidence in vaccinated vs. unvaccinated groups). Obtaining accurate data on these 'Adverse Events After Immunization' has been aided by, e.g. EU Vaccine Adverse Event Surveillance and Communication network and WHO Global Advisory Committee on Vaccine Safety.

Adverse reactions may be caused by either

- *Inappropriate administration:* e.g. abscesses after use of non-sterile needles or syringes; disseminated disease in immunocompromised patients after inappropriate administration of BCG or measles vaccines (see position papers for these vaccines at www.WHO.int).
- *Properties of the vaccines:* e.g. reactions caused by either the immunizing agent itself or by other components of the vaccine, e.g. antibiotics, adjuvants, or preservatives.
- *The immune response to the vaccine:* e.g. allergic reactions.

Mild adverse events

Are common (20–50% of DTP recipients experience mild local reactions, while 5–15% of measles vaccine recipients experience fever and rash 6–12d after immunization). These are not contraindications to further immunization.

Severe adverse reactions

Are extremely rare, reports of association of DTP with many adverse events have been made, but comprehensive studies have failed to link it to almost all of these. Reactions such as febrile convulsions or anaphylaxis occasionally occur; however, for all EPI recommended vaccines, any vaccine-associated adverse events are much less common than the severe complications caused by the diseases prevented by the vaccines.

Misconceptions about vaccines

There have always been concerns about the safety of immunization programmes—this is understandable because a biologically active agent is given to large numbers of healthy children. Unfortunately, even after a vaccine's safety has been demonstrated, some beliefs may persist, such as the erroneous suggestion of a link between MMR and autism. Recent examples include concerns that OPV → infertility or → spread of HIV. The resurgence of polio in regions rejecting OPV as a result of these erroneous beliefs demonstrates how misinformation undermines immunization programmes.

More information about common vaccine misconceptions and information that can be used to reassure parents and community leaders can be obtained at: www.who.int/immunization_safety/aefi/immunization_misconceptions/en/

Contraindications to vaccination

There are few absolute contraindications to vaccination. Every opportunity to vaccinate a child or woman of childbearing age should be taken. There is high risk that delaying vaccination until the child has recovered from a mild inter-current illness will result in that child not getting fully immunized.

True contraindications to immunization include

- Illnesses severe enough for the child to be hospitalized—if the child is vaccinated, but dies from the pre-existing illness the vaccine may be thought (erroneously) to have contributed to the child's death. Immunize as soon as the child's general condition improves.
- For live vaccines (see Box 22.3), immunodeficiency diseases or immunosuppression due to malignant disease, therapy with immunosuppressive drugs or irradiation. HIV/AIDS is a special case—see 📖 Immunization of HIV-infected persons, p. 902.
- A severe adverse event (anaphylaxis, collapse or shock, encephalitis, encephalopathy, or non-febrile convulsions) to a vaccine contraindicates further doses of that vaccine. If the adverse reaction occurred following a dose of DTP vaccine, either omit the pertussis component and continue with the DT vaccine or use a vaccine containing acellular pertussis (if available).
- For vaccines prepared in egg (e.g. influenza, yellow fever) a history of anaphylaxis following egg ingestion. Vaccines prepared in chicken fibroblast cells (e.g. measles, MR, MMR) are safe for such individuals.

In general, live vaccines should not be given to pregnant women and pregnancy should be avoided for >1mth following immunization. Immunization in pregnancy may be considered where there is a high risk of exposure and need for vaccination outweighs any possible risk to the fetus (e.g. yellow fever vaccine and OPV).

Conditions which are *not* contraindications and *must not* prevent a child from being vaccinated

- Minor illnesses such as URTI or diarrhoea, with fever <38.5°C.
- Allergy, atopic manifestations, asthma, hay fever, or 'snuffles'.
- Prematurity, small for dates infants or jaundice after birth.
- Malnourished child, or child being breastfed.
- Family history of convulsions.
- Treatment with antibiotics, limited corticosteroid treatment (i.e. prednisolone 2mg/kg/day for <1wk, or 1mg/kg/day for <1mth or equivalent doses of other steroids) or locally acting (e.g. topical or inhaled) steroids.
- Dermatoses, eczema, or localized skin infection.
- Chronic diseases of heart, lung, kidney, and liver.
- Stable neurological conditions, e.g. cerebral palsy/Down's syndrome.

Immunization of HIV-infected individuals

Immunization of HIV+ individuals needs special consideration because of:

- ↑ Susceptibility to severe illness from infections such as TB and measles.
- ↓ Response to vaccines in the advanced stages of AIDS. Note: most HIV+ adults and children mount a good vaccine response.
- Potential risk of live vaccines (e.g. disseminated BCG infection following administration of BCG vaccine).

With the exception of BCG, asymptomatic HIV+ individuals should receive all recommended EPI vaccinations at usual ages. The recommendations for children with symptomatic HIV infection are outlined in Table 22.3. As for any severely ill child, severely ill HIV+ children should not be vaccinated.

Table 22.3 WHO/UNICEF recommendations for the immunization of HIV-infected children

Vaccine	Asymptomatic HIV infection	Symptomatic HIV infection
BCG	No[1]	No[1]
DTP	Yes	Yes
OPV[2]	Yes	Yes
Measles[3]	Yes	Yes[4]
Hepatitis B	Yes	Yes
Hib	Yes	Yes
PC	Yes	Yes
Rotavirus	Yes	?[5]
Yellow fever	Yes	No
TetT	Yes	Yes

[1]In regions with high rates of TB, BCG vaccine should be given to all infants, for whom there is no known contraindication, including well children whose HIV status is unknown due to limited diagnostic resources (even if mother is HIV+). However, in view of reports of disseminated BCG in HIV+ children, the vaccine should be avoided in those who are known to be HIV+. Where possible, infants of unknown status born to HIV+ mothers should be tested to exclude HIV infection before BCG vaccine is administered.

[2]IPV can be used as an alternative in symptomatic HIV+ children.

[3]Because of the risk of severe early measles infection, HIV+ infants should receive measles immunization at 6mths and as soon after 9mths as possible.

[4]WHO guidelines suggest measles immunization can be considered in children with symptomatic HIV infection if they are not severely immunosuppressed.

[5]Physicians to assess potential benefits and risk on individual basis

Box 22.3 Live vaccines

- BCG
- Measles
- Mumps
- Rotavirus
- Rubella
- MR
- MMR
- Varicella
- OPV
- Yellow fever
- Oral typhoid

Expanded programme on immunization recommended vaccines

Always consult manufacturer's data sheet for detailed information on indication, dose, and reactions. See 📖 Contraindications to vaccination, p. 901, for general contraindications.

BCG

A freeze-dried preparation of a live attenuated strain of *Mycobacterium bovis* given as a single ID injection.

- Early administration is recommended as it is most effective in preventing TB meningitis and miliary TB in infants.
- Duration of protection >10–15yrs is uncertain; booster doses are not recommended.
- Hypersensitivity should be excluded by a –ve tuberculin skin test if BCG is administered after the neonatal period.
- BCG also protects against leprosy.

Contraindications HIV+ or other immunocompromise.

Side-effects

A small swelling forms 2–6wks post-vaccination that may → a benign ulcer. Local abscesses may occur, particularly after incorrect administration (e.g. sc rather than ID) and regional lymphadenitis occurs in ~0.5% of recipients.

Hepatitis B vaccines

Use a suspension of inactivated HBsAg adsorbed onto alum given by IM injection at birth and in infancy (📖 Administration of vaccines, p. 899).

- Booster doses are not recommended.
- Both recombinant and plasma derived products are equally safe and effective and can be used interchangeably.
- The vaccine is available either as monovalent HepB or in combination with DTP +/– Hib or DTaP +/– Hib; only the monovalent vaccine should be used for immunization at birth.
- Neonatal vaccination provides immunoprophylaxis against perinatal infection. Use of hepatitis B immunoglobulin at birth for prevention of perinatal transmission is not recommended due to concerns about supply, safety, and cost.
- Infants with birth weight <2000g should be vaccinated at birth and also receive 3 additional doses in infancy. Vaccination is safe in pregnancy, lactation, and HIV+ individuals.
- Following exposure beyond the perinatal period (e.g. after a needle stick injury in unimmunized health workers) a 0, 1, 2mths schedule should be used (plus a 12mths booster dose if ongoing risk).

Diphtheria toxoid vaccine

Is a formaldehyde-inactivated preparation of diphtheria toxin, adsorbed onto alum to ↑ immunogenicity.

- It is normally given IM combined with DTP, but can be given as DT if pertussis is contraindicated.

- The vaccine does not prevent infection, but inhibits diphtheria toxin's effects, preventing systemic illness.
- A low dose vaccine (combined with tetanus: dT) should be used in individuals >7yrs to ↓ risk of vaccine reactions.

Haemophilus influenzae type b (Hib) vaccine

Consists of Hib polysaccharides conjugated to carrier proteins to stimulate a T cell response.

- The vaccine is given IM either alone or with DTP+/– HepB.
- Use of Hib vaccine has ↑ dramatically in the last decade as a result of a GAVI initiative, and 82% of countries now use this vaccine routinely.
- Booster doses of vaccine are currently used in most resource-rich countries, but are not recommended in the EPI schedule.

Japanese encephalitis vaccines

Until the last decade the most widely used vaccine against Japanese encephalitis was an inactivated vaccine derived from infected mouse brain cells. This inactivated vaccine (commonly known as the 'Green Cross' vaccine) remains the only vaccine available for use in the EU for children and is supplied on a 'named patient' basis. Concerns regarding the relatively high rates of allergic reactions to this vaccine (approximately 0.6% of recipients), anecdotal reports of acute demyelinating encephalomyelitis following immunization and difficulties with supply, have led to the development of new vaccines against JE that have been adopted on a regional basis.

- The most widely used in China, India, Cambodia, Sri Lanka, Nepal, and South Korea is the Chinese-manufactured live attenuated vaccine (SA 14-14-2). The vaccine is administered sc, often with the measles vaccine at 9mths.
- An inactivated, vero-cell culture vaccine (Ixiaro®) is licensed in the USA and Europe for use in adults and is administered as 2 doses 28d apart, usually as a 'travel vaccine'.
- A chimeric vaccine (Imojev®) which uses live attenuated yellow fever virus as a vector for protective antigens from SA 14-14-2 has been licensed in Australia for use as a single sc injection from 12mths.

Pertussis vaccines

These are available in 2 forms—whole-cell vaccine (containing killed *Bordatella pertussis* bacteria, commonly used in resource-poor countries) or acellular vaccine (containing inactivated pertussis toxin in combination with 1–4 other immunogenic components).

- Both vaccines are given IM, normally as part of DTP or DTaP.
- Primary immunization in infancy is essential as pertussis mortality occurs predominantly in this age group (📖 Immunization strategies and schedules, p. 896).
- A booster dose is recommended at 1–6yrs.
- Duration of protection following booster is estimated at 6–12yrs.
- Adolescents and adults can ∴ be infected and transmit pertussis to susceptible infants.

Side-effects

10–50% of infants experience mild reactions such as local swelling, fever, and irritability after whole cell vaccine. Prolonged crying occurs in <1%; seizures and hypotonic episodes occur much less commonly. These reactions are less common after acellular pertussis. Following a severe reaction to DTP whole cell pertussis should be omitted from subsequent immunizations, either by using DT or acellular pertussis vaccines. No association has been found between whole cell pertussis and chronic encephalopathy.

Pneumococcal vaccines

There are two types of pneumococcal vaccine: plain polysaccharide vaccine and glyco-conjugate vaccine (PC vaccine). The polysaccharide vaccine contains capsular polysaccharide antigens from 23 serotypes of *Streptococcus pneumoniae*.

Glycoconjugate vaccine (PC vaccine)

There are now 3 licensed PC vaccines. There are 7 and 13-valent PC vaccines; a 10-valent PC vaccine uses a protein ('Protein D') that may provide some protection against non-encapsulated *Haemophilus influenzae* (a common cause of otitis media and lower respiratory tract infection).

- 10 and 13-valent PC vaccines ↑ protection against pneumococcal disease in resource-poor countries vs. the 7-valent vaccine.
- PC vaccines are immunogenic in infancy and induce immunological memory.
- EPI schedule recommends 3 doses in infancy; although most resource-rich countries use a booster dose in the 2nd year of life this is not currently recommended in resource-poor countries.
- It is anticipated that PC vaccine will be routinely used in 40 developing countries by 2015.

Polysaccharide vaccine

- Unfortunately, these antigens do not induce a protective response in children <2yrs and protective immunity in older individuals may be limited or short lived.
- The polysaccharide vaccine is still recommended for those >2yrs at ↑ risk for severe infection: sickle cell disease, chronic renal failure, immunosuppression, CSF leaks, HIV+, asplenia, diabetes mellitus or chronic liver, heart or lung disease. This recommendation may change with further studies on the efficacy of PC vaccines.

Contraindications Pregnancy, breastfeeding, during acute infection.

Side-effects

Hypersensitivity reactions may occur. These are more common following re-immunization within 3yrs.

Poliomyelitis vaccine

After a global eradication campaign wild type polio virus type-2 has not been detected since 1999. The Americas, Pacific region, and Europe have been declared polio free. However, 1604 infections with polio types 1 or 3 were reported in 23 countries in 2009.

- Both oral, live attenuated vaccines (OPV, Sabin vaccine) and injectable, killed virus vaccines (IPV, Salk vaccine) are available.

- EPI recommends OPV because of its low cost, ease of administration, superiority in conferring intestinal protection and potential for boosting immunity in household and community contacts.
- Trivalent OPV vaccine is generally used; however monovalent and bivalent vaccines against strains 1 and 3 are used in mass immunization campaigns.
- Unfounded reports that OPV causes infertility → ↓ immunization coverage, e.g. in Nigeria, with a resultant ↑ in poliomyelitis.
- Vaccine-associated paralytic poliomyelitis occurs in ~1 in 250 000 doses of OPV; many countries in 'polio-free' regions have therefore switched to IPV and this trend may continue as the goal of global eradication is reached.

Cautions Patients with diarrhoea and vomiting require a further dose after recovery. IPV rather than OPV should be administered to immunocompromised individuals *and their household contacts.*

Measles vaccine

This is a live attenuated virus given by IM or sc injection. Measles may be given as a monovalent vaccine or in combination with rubella +/– mumps (MR, MMR).

- Normally given at 9mths, but can be given at 6 and 9mths to those at high risk and offered to susceptible children <2d of exposure to infection.
- All children should receive 2 doses of measles vaccine.
- In areas of high HIV incidence initial vaccination can be at 6mths.
- For high-risk patients in an outbreak setting, post-exposure prophylaxis (measles vaccine within 2d of exposure or, if vaccine contraindicated, measles immune globulin within 3 to 5d, of exposure) will modify/ prevent symptoms.

Side-effects Mild measles-like illness may occur in 5–15% of children 6–12d after immunization. Febrile convulsions occur in approximately 1 in 3000 children.

Rotavirus vaccines

WHO now recommends all infants be immunized against rotavirus. Two live oral vaccines are available against this virus, responsible for up to a half of diarrhoea related hospital admissions in Africa.

- A live attenuated vaccine (RIX 4414, Rotarix®) is given as a 2-dose course.
- A pentavalent bovine-human re-assortant vaccine (Rotateq®) is administered as 3 doses.
- 1st dose of both vaccines should be administered at 6–15wks, subsequent doses are given at least 4 weeks apart. The manufacturers recommend that the last dose is given no later than 32 weeks of age, however the WHO have raised concerns that stringently applying this could mean that vulnerable children may be unnecessarily be deprived of the potential benefits of immunisation. Accordingly the WHO recommend that the rotavirus vaccines being given with DTP vaccines up until two years of age.

- Large scale studies of both vaccines have shown them to be safe and highly effective against severe rotavirus disease. There is a small ↑ risk of intussusception (~1–2/100 000 infants) after the 1st dose of vaccine, but this risk is far outweighed by the benefits of immunization.

Rubella vaccines

These are live attenuated vaccines, mostly based on RA 27/3 strain. They are often given as part of combination vaccine with MR, MMR, and varicella (MMRV) and are administered by IM or deep SC injection.

- The purpose of rubella immunization is to ↓ incidence of 1° infection in pregnant women and thus ↓ incidence of congenital rubella syndrome in their offspring.
- WHO recently recommended that countries that are providing 2 doses of measles vaccine should consider incorporating routine infant immunization against rubella using combination vaccines. This approach (ideally accompanied by an initial immunization campaign targeting a wide range of ages) is preferred to the alternative strategy of immunizing adolescent girls and females of childbearing age, as this may be undermined by ↓ vaccine coverage and on-going circulation of the virus.

Contraindications Although no evidence that vaccine is teratogenic, immunizing women in early pregnancy should be avoided, and women should be advised to avoid pregnancy for 1mth following immunization.

Tetanus toxoid vaccine

This is a formaldehyde-inactivated preparation of TetT adsorbed onto alum given by IM or deep SC injection. Normally administered to infants as part of DTP (but can be administered as DT if pertussis contraindicated).

WHO recommended schedule

- *6 doses of vaccine:* 3 in infancy, a booster at 4–7yrs, another at 12–15yrs and a final dose in adulthood.
- In addition, administration of TetT to a pregnant woman induces antibodies that can cross the placenta and prevent neonatal tetanus.
- Optimal schedule depends on the immunization history of the woman, as outlined in Table 22.4.
- Supplementary mass immunization campaigns are recommended in countries of high risk for neonatal tetanus and aim to immunize all women of childbearing age.

Yellow fever vaccine

A freeze-dried preparation of live attenuated virus strain (17D strain) grown in egg embryos and given by SC injection.

- Yellow fever is endemic in 33 countries in sub-Saharan Africa (where by far the greatest burden of disease lies) and 11 countries in South America. In these countries infant immunization at the same time as measles immunization is recommended.
- Protection from a single dose of vaccine is probably life-long, however, international travel regulations require evidence of immunization <10yrs prior to arrival in endemic countries.

- In order to ↓ risk of YF re-introduction, proof of immunization is also required for travellers from endemic countries to countries at risk for endemic disease.

Contraindications Anaphylactic reaction to egg, immunocompromise and age <9mths, but can be given at 6–8mths if high risk of YF.

Side-effects

Minor reactions (e.g. headache, myalgia), in 10–30% of recipients. Uncommon reactions include vaccine-associated neurological disease, e.g. meningo-encephalitis or peripheral neuropathy. This occurs in ~0.8/100 000 doses (1.8/100 000 in those >60yrs). Vaccine-associated yellow fever-like illness, of variable severity, occurs in approximately 0.4 per 100 000 doses, but is commoner in those >60yrs. A WHO working group has recently published an update of yellow fever vaccine recommendations and risk of disease (Jentes *et al.*, 2011).

Further reading

Jentes ES, Poumerol G, Gershman MD, *et al.* The revised global yellow fever risk map and recommendations for vaccination, 2010: consensus of the Informal WHO Working Group on Geographic Risk for Yellow Fever. *Lancet Inf Dis* 2011; **11**: 622–32.

Table 22.4 Tetanus immunization schedules in adults and pregnant women

History	1st dose	2nd dose	3rd dose	4th dose	5th dose
Adolescents and adults with no previous immunization	As early as possible	>4wks later	>6mths later	>1yr later	>1yr later
Pregnant women with no/uncertain previous immunization	As early as possible in 1st pregnancy	>4wks later	>6mths later, or in next pregnancy	>1yr later	>1yr later
Pregnant women with 3 childhood DTP doses	As early as possible in 1st pregnancy	>4wks later	>1yr later		
Pregnant women with 4 childhood DTP doses	As early as possible in 1st pregnancy	>1yr later			
Supplementary immunization activities in high risk areas	During round 1	During round 2, >4wks after round 1	During round 3, >6mths after round 2	>1yr later, or next pregnancy	>1yr later, or next pregnancy

Other vaccines

Cholera vaccine

Two types of oral cholera vaccines are available. WHO recommends that, along with other preventative measures, cholera vaccines should be used where disease is endemic and considered in areas at risk for outbreaks. Travel immunization is only recommended for relief and disaster workers, or travellers to remote areas in which epidemics are occurring. The parenteral cholera vaccine has poor efficacy and is no longer recommended.

The rCTB-WC vaccine

This is based on killed whole cells of *V. cholerae* 01 combined with a recombinant B subunit of cholera toxin. This vaccine is given with bicarbonate buffer as 2 doses 1–6wks apart in adults and 3 doses 1–6wks apart in children 2–6yrs. The vaccine is not licensed for children <2yrs. The immunization course should ideally be completed 1wk before potential exposure to cholera. If there is an on-going risk of infection WHO recommend a booster dose every 2yrs (for those >6yrs) and every 6mths (for children aged 2–6yrs). rCTB-WC does not protect against *Vibrio cholerae* 0139, a serogroup found in South Asia.

Bivalent oral vaccines

These are based on killed whole cells of *V. cholerae* strains 01 and 0139. These vaccines are administered as 2 doses 2wks apart, and can be given without buffer to children aged >1yr. A booster dose is recommended after 2yrs.

Side-effects: Both types of oral vaccine are well tolerated.

Hepatitis A vaccines

Exist in 6 variations; 4 inactivated and 2 live attenuated (produced and used only in China).

- Antibodies persist for >2yrs after a single dose of inactivated vaccine, and for many years after a 2nd dose. Current recommendations suggest these vaccines are administered as 2 doses 6–12 or 36mths apart.
- No Hep A vaccine is licensed for use in infants <1yr.
- Hep A vaccine is also available combined with Hep B vaccine in a formulation to be administered as 3 doses as a 0, 1 and 6mths schedule.
- High prevalence of Hep A in resource-poor countries → predominance of asymptomatic childhood infections, therefore Hep A vaccines are not yet considered necessary in these settings.
- Travellers from resource-rich countries to these regions should be immunized.
- Clinical trials in outbreak settings have demonstrated effectiveness for post-exposure immunization with Hep A vaccines.

Side-effects Well tolerated; no serious adverse effects reported.

Human papilloma virus

HPV-induced cervical cancer causes ~260 000 deaths worldwide, and immunization against HPV has therefore been introduced in many resource-rich countries. A bivalent (HPV16 and 18) and quadrivalent vaccine (HPV16, 18, 6 and 11) are licensed; both based on inactivated HPV strains and administered in a 3 dose schedule (0, 1–2, and 6mths). Both vaccines are licensed for administration in girls >10yrs of age—ideally prior to the onset of sexual activity.

Influenza vaccines

These may either be inactivated vaccines for intramuscular injection or or live attenuated vaccines for intra-nasal administration. Most vaccines contain three influenza strains (2 influenza A and 1 influenza B), however quadrivalent vaccines (2 A and 2 B strains) have also recently been licensed. The haemagglutinin (H) and neuraminidase (N) antigens used in the vaccines are determined by WHO each year according to the anticipated prevalent strains. The 2009 emergence of novel influenza A H1N1 (swine 'flu) highlighted the challenges in planning for timely, but proportionate vaccine production in response to an influenza pandemic.

Meningococcal vaccines

Two forms of meningococcal vaccines exist.

- The plain polysaccharide vaccines are available either as a monovalent serogroup A vaccine or as combination vaccines, i.e. A and C; A, C and W-135, or A, C, Y and W-135. These vaccines are used in outbreak control, however, protection ↓ after several years and, apart from serogroup A, are poorly immunogenic in infants.
- Glyco-conjugate meningococcal vaccines (in which meningococcal polysaccharide capsules are conjugated to carrier proteins). Monovalent serogroup C glyco-conjugate vaccines are routinely used in many resource-rich countries and a tetravalent meningococcal serogroup A, C, W-135 and Y vaccine is recommended for adolescents in the USA. A monovalent serogroup A meningococcal glyco-conjugate vaccine (MenAfriVac) has been introduced across the 'meningitis belt' into Burkino Faso, Mali, Niger, Cameroon, Chad, Nigeria, Benin, Ghana, Senegal, and Sudan. Meningitis outbreaks continue to be monitored but in 2012/13 levels were at the lowest reported levels in a decade.
- The poor immunogenicity of the meningococcal serogroup B polysaccharide capsule renders this unsuitable for use in a glycoconjugate vaccine. A vaccine (Bexsero) based on sub-capsular proteins has recently been licensed in Europe and Australia, while another vaccine is in late stage development.

Mumps vaccine

Consists of a live attenuated strain of the virus grown in chick embryo cells. It is normally given by IM injection with measles and rubella vaccines in the MMR triple vaccine at 12–15mths with a 2nd dose at 2–6yrs.

Pigbel vaccine

An inactivated preparation of toxin from *Clostridium perfringens* type 3 that is given by IM injection. It is effective in infants and has been given routinely to children in Papua New Guinea at 2, 4 and 6mths since 1980. Protection lasts for 2–4yrs.

Rabies vaccines

Based on inactivated viruses grown using a range of cell-culture or embryonated-egg methods. Vaccines derived from animal nerve tissues are still available, but are not recommended due to high rate of severe neurological complications (~1:1000). The cultured vaccines are safer, but more expensive, however, cheaper ways of administering the vaccine (e.g. by intradermal injection) have been developed. See 🕮 Rabies, pp. 450–3 for prophylactic and post-exposure vaccination schedules.

Typhoid vaccine

Four typhoid vaccines types are currently available:

- Killed parenteral whole cell vaccine (now largely superseded due to its side-effects).
- Plain polysaccharide ('Vi') parenteral vaccine.
- Live attenuated oral vaccine.
- Glyco-conjugate vaccine (in India).

Plain polysaccharide ('Vi') parenteral vaccine

This is administered as a single dose by IM or SC injection, and is immunogenic >2yrs. Duration of protection is uncertain, however, booster doses are recommended every 3yrs.

Live attenuated (Ty21) oral vaccine

This is available in capsule form (for ages ≥5yrs) and a liquid form (ages ≥2yrs); the latter is supplied with a bicarbonate buffer. The vaccine is administered as 3 oral doses given 2d apart (travellers from the USA are advised to have a 4th dose if taking the capsules). Re–immunization is recommended every 3–5yrs for those living in endemic regions. Antibiotics and proguanil should be avoided during the three days before and after vaccination as they will inactivate the vaccine.

Glyco-conjugate vaccine

This consists of the Vi polysaccharide conjugated to a TetT carrier protein (*Peda typh*) is licensed in India from the age of 3mths and offers potential for protection against typhoid from a young age; however, data on immunogenicity and side effects are limited.

Varicella vaccine

Multiple formulations of a live-attenuated varicella vaccine are licensed; all are based on the OKA strain VZV and may either be in a monovalent preparation or in combination with MMR vaccine (MMRV). The latter vaccine is associated with ↑ risk of febrile convulsions and is not recommended for a 1st dose of varicella vaccine in those <2yrs. Routine immunization against VZV is employed in many resource-rich countries, most of which recommend 2 doses of vaccine to reduce the risk of 'breakthrough' infections. Recent studies suggest VZV vaccine is safe and immunogenic in immunocompromised individuals, including those with asymptomatic HIV; however, there are case reports of disseminated OKA strain infections following immunization in these populations.

Chapter 23

Health emergencies in humanitarian crises

Invited Author **Koert Ritmeijer**

Introduction

Annually, >2.5 million people are uprooted due to armed conflict, repression, and natural or manmade disasters, and the total number displaced amounts to >40 million. Refugee and population displacements mostly occur in countries which do not have the resources or capacity to deal with them, creating an enormous economic, social, and ecological burden. Effective aid to refugee and displaced populations in host countries is almost always dependent on a rapid response by the international community.

Mortality rates

- Mass population movements into areas with poor resources → high mortality rates (especially in camp settings) that can be, during the first weeks/months following displacement, ~60× expected mortality rates. Relief programmes must begin promptly to ↓ excess mortality.
- Crude mortality rate (CMR) in stable populations is <0.5 deaths per 10 000/d.
- In the emergency phase CMR is >1 death per 10 000 per day.
- The post-emergency phase (consolidation phase) starts when CMR is <1 per 10000/d and basic needs have been addressed.

Priorities of intervention

In the emergency phase there are 10 priority activities:

- Initial assessment.
- Measles immunization.
- Water and sanitation.
- Food and nutrition.
- Shelter and site planning.
- Healthcare.
- Control of communicable diseases and epidemics.
- Public health surveillance.
- Human resources and training.
- Coordination.

Ideally, these interventions should be carried out simultaneously, which becomes feasible when different teams of relief workers are involved.

Initial assessment

An initial assessment within the first few days is undertaken to:
- Identify health priorities.
- Plan the implementation of these priorities.
- Decide strategies.
- Determine resources needed.
- Work out a time frame.

The assessment includes 6 categories:
- *Geo-political context:*
  - cause and duration of displacement, conditions under which it took place
  - security situation on the settlement site
  - human rights abuses
  - acceptance of the refugees by the host authorities and the local population.
- *Description of the refugee population:*
  - *demography*—estimate of total population and age/sex distribution
  - *socio-cultural characteristics*—ethnic background, type of leadership and community organization, religion, particular customs
  - *vulnerable groups*—unaccompanied children, female-headed households, elderly, disabled, minority groups.
- *Characteristics of environment in which refugees have settled:*
  - *water supply*—availability, quantity, and quality
  - physical characteristics (map), climate, accessibility, roads
  - types of shelter, % of refugees with proper shelters
  - *density*—surface area available per refugee
  - *general hygiene and disposal of excreta*—defecation areas, type and number of latrines
  - presence of vectors transmitting communicable diseases.
- *Major health problems:*
  - *mortality*—rates and causes of mortality
  - morbidity data on the most common diseases
  - diseases with epidemic potential (cholera, shigellosis, measles, meningitis, hepatitis)
  - prevalence of acute malnutrition
  - data on vaccine coverage (especially measles, meningitis).
- *Requirements of human and material resource:*
  - qualified staff among the refugee and host population
  - *food available*—existing food reserves, food rations distributed
  - cooking utensils, water containers, soap, blankets, clothes
  - existing health facilities.
- Operating partners.

Data collection methods are quantitative as well as qualitative, and will be gathered by systematic observation, interviews with key persons, focus group discussions, sample surveys, and mapping. Methods will often be 'quick and dirty', and results may need to be confirmed later with more in-depth methods.

Measles immunization

Measles kills 1 in 10 children affected in resource-poor countries. In refugee emergencies, low vaccination coverage, overcrowding, and poor hygiene in camps are risk factors for the emergence of measles outbreaks, and malnutrition ↑ severity of measles, resulting in ↑ mortality (see 📖 Measles, p. 800).

Mass measles immunization should always be an absolute priority during the 1st week. Target group is all children aged 6mths–15yrs, but all ages can be included if older age groups also affected. Measles immunization is only contra-indicated in pregnant women. Mass vaccination can be conducted together with the distribution of vitamin A (age <6mths 50 000IU; 6–12mths 100 000IU; >1yr 200 000IU).

Water and sanitation

Water supply

Drinking water supply is the priority. Inadequate water supply and sanitation ↑ transmission of diarrhoeal and other diseases. During the first days of the emergency phase a minimum of 5L of water/person/d is required for drinking and cooking. During the next stage of the emergency phase, this must be rapidly ↑ to 15–20L/person/d to allow for personal hygiene and ↓ risk of epidemics.

- Existing water sources must be assessed, and open water sources (e.g. lakes, ponds, wells) protected to prevent contamination.
- Temporary water supply by tanker deliveries may be necessary until a more permanent supply (e.g. boreholes) are set up.
- Plastic tanks are most often used for water storage, treatment, and distribution.
- Water quality should be checked with simple kits, and can be improved by chlorination (disinfection) and/or pre-treatment (sedimentation).

Excreta control

Indicators in regard to water supply and latrines must be monitored in the same manner as disease incidence and mortality rates.

During the first days of the emergency phase, simple and quick community facilities should be organized: defecation areas or fields, shallow trench latrines, collective latrines: 1 latrine or trench per 50–100 persons during the first days of the emergency. This is to be improved as soon as possible to 1 latrine/20 persons or ideally 1/family.

Disposal of the dead A cemetery or burial place should be planned.

Personal hygiene Consider large-scale distribution of soap.

Food and nutrition

Population displacement is generally either the cause or consequence of food shortages. Malnutrition is frequent in refugee populations and is an important cause of mortality. Outbreaks of vitamin deficiencies (e.g. scurvy or pellagra) may occur.

Assessment of food and nutritional situation

- Food availability and accessibility:
  - *information relating to food distributions*—theoretical food ration, ration actually distributed, distributing agency, target group, frequency of distributions
  - *assessment of local market*—type and price of food available
  - estimate the food basket of individual households by a sample survey.
- Nutritional status of the refugee population—prevalence of MAM and SAM are assessed in children 6mths–5yrs by measuring MUAC or W/H (see 📖 Nutrition, p. 683). Global acute malnutrition (GAM) is the sum of SAM and MAM.
- *Other information which influences nutrition:* mortality figures, disease outbreaks, micronutrient deficiencies, water supply, climate and shelter, dietary habits, security situation, provision of health services.

Interventions

Objectives of food intervention programmes:

- To ensure an average of at least 2100Kcal/person/d containing: 10% protein energy and 10% fat energy, micro nutrients.
- To ↓ prevalence of malnutrition and mortality from malnutrition by treating acutely malnourished individuals.
- Preventing malnutrition in other groups at risk.

How to decide on nutrition interventions

Tables 23.1 and 23.2 can be used to help interpret the seriousness of a situation and select the appropriate type of intervention.

- *General food ration available:* when the ration is inadequate, the food supply must be improved. Low rations are also a factor in deciding on selective feeding programmes. General food distribution is a major undertaking and is usually carried out by specialized agencies. Registration and a census of refugees upon arrival are essential for estimating food needs and identifying beneficiaries. It is also essential to monitor the basic food ration by regular random food basket surveys of households.
- *Malnutrition prevalence:* the prevalence of acute malnutrition indicates the level of intervention required. GAM >10% defines a *food crisis*.

- *Aggravating factors:* if present, a higher level of intervention is required:
  - CMR >1/10,000/d
  - inadequate food ration (<2100Kcal/person/d)
  - epidemics of measles, *Shigella*, or other important communicable diseases
  - severe cold and inadequate shelter
  - unstable situation, e.g. caused by a new influx of refugees.

There are three categories of interventions serving different target groups:

- Prevention programmes: general food distribution (GFD) for an entire population at risk, and targeted food distribution (TFD) or blanket supplementary feeding programme (BSFP) for vulnerable households or individuals.
- Nutrition treatment programmes: therapeutic feeding programmes (TFP) and targeted supplementary feeding programmes (TSFP) for treatment of acute malnutrition (see 🕮 Nutrition, p. 683).
- Nutrition during illness to encourage healing and recovery of sick for treatment of acute malnutrition and nutrient deficiencies.

Table 23.1 Food security classification

LEVEL	1	2	3	4	5
INDICATORS FOOD SECURITY	**GENERALLY FOOD SECURE**	**BORDERLINE FOOD INSECURE**	**ACUTE FOOD CRISIS**	**FOOD/ HUMANITARIAN EMERGENCY**	**FAMINE/ HUMANITARIAN CATASTROPHE**
Food access/ availability	Adequate and stable	Borderline adequate and/or seasonal variation	↓ resources; limited food access	Severe ↓ resources, unable to meet food needs	Extreme ↓ resources; starvation
Kcal/person/day	>2100	~2100	<2100	<1600	
Dietary diversity	Constant quality/ quantity, diversity	Chronic and/ or limited dietary diversity	Acute deficit and insufficient nutrient intake	Severe acute deficit and nutrient intake	Negligible
Destitution/ displacement		Seasonal migration, mainly by men	Migration stretches in period and household members	Concentrated, often entire families	Large scale, concentrated
NUTRITION					
GAM WHZ *	<5 %	5–10 %**	10–20 %	20–40 %	>40 %
GAM MUAC *		>7 %	>15 %	>20 %	
SAM WHZ **	<2 %	<2–3 %	3–7 %	>7–10 %	>10 %
SAM MUAC **	<1.5%	1.5–3%	3.5–5%	>5 %	

LEVEL	1	2	3	4	5
INDICATORS FOOD SECURITY	**GENERALLY FOOD SECURE**	**BORDERLINE FOOD INSECURE**	**ACUTE FOOD CRISIS**	**FOOD/ HUMANITARIAN EMERGENCY**	**FAMINE/ HUMANITARIAN CATASTROPHE**
HEALTH					
Morbidity	Under control.	Under control, endemic diseases ↑ (e.g. seasonal)	↑ morbidity, epidemics likely	Epidemic	Epidemic
Crude Mortality***	<0.5	<1	1–2	>2	>5
<5y mortality****	<1	<2	>2	>4	>10
Impact on healthcare system	Stable admission rates	Seasonal ↑ in admissions	Risk of epidemics, nutrition programmes fail to cope	healthcare system overwhelmed.	

* *Global acute malnutrition (GAM):* W/H <-2Z score WHO 2006 and/or bilateral oedema; or MUAC <12.5 cm and/or bilateral oedema

** *Severe acute malnutrition (SAM):* W/H <-3Z score WHO 2006 and/or bilateral oedema; or MUAC <11.5 cm and/or bilateral oedema

*** deaths/10,000 people/day

**** deaths/10,000 children <5 y/day

Table 23.2 Types of food and nutrition programmes

Programmes	Objectives	Rations	Target groups	Food security level
		1. Prevention programmes		
GFD **General Food Distribution**	Meet basic food needs	General food 2100 kcal/person/day + Specific food for <2 years	The entire population	**Levels 4 and 5**
TFD **Targeted Food Distribution**	Increase food availability at household level	Food From 500 to 2100 kcal/person/day + Specific food for <2 years	Vulnerable households (e.g. headed by women or with a child below 5 years	**Levels 3 and 4:** **Level 5: to wait for the GFD coming**
BSFP **Blanket Supplementary Feeding Programme**	Improve diet quality for vulnerable individuals	Rations/needs From 125 to 500 kcal/person/day	Vulnerable individuals (e.g. <3 yrs; pregnant and lactating women)	**Levels 2, 3, 4 and 5**
Infant Feeding in emergency	Strengthen breastfeeding	No food given Referral to BSFP for pregnant and lactating women	Young infant below 6 months and their mothers	**Levels 4 and 5**
		2. Nutrition treatment programmes		
TFP **Therapeutic Feeding Programme**	Treat SAM and its associated medical complications.	Ration/physiological needs Specific food	SAM patients	**At all levels of food insecurity**
TSFP **Targeted Supplementary Feeding Programme**	Treat MAM Prevent SAM	Ration/physiological needs Specific food	MAM patients	**Levels 3, 4 and 5**
		3. Nutrition during illness		
Nutrition during illness	Provide correct calorific, macronutrient and micronutrient needs to encourage healing and recovery	Rations/needs Specific food	Sick patients and hospital patients	**At all levels of food security**

Shelter and site planning

Poor shelter and overcrowding are major risk factors in the transmission of diseases with epidemic potential (e.g. measles, meningitis, typhus, cholera) and outbreaks of disease are ↑ frequent and ↑ severe when population density is ↑. Provision of a secure living space, with protection against sun, rain, cold, and wind, and a sense of privacy is essential for refugee welfare.

Site planning

Security and protection

Settlement must be in a safe area (e.g. free of mines), and at distance from war zones.

- *Water:* must be available on the site or nearby.
- *Space:* ensure $30m^2$ per person.
- *Accessibility:* the site must be accessible during all seasons.
- *Environmental health risks:* no nearby vector breeding sites.
- *Local population:* avoid tensions arising between local community and refugees (e.g. legal and traditional land rights must be respected).
- *Drainage:* terrain should slope to provide natural drainage for rain water.

Basic healthcare

In emergency phase of refugee crises, basic healthcare focuses on 'top 5', common diseases with high mortality: acute respiratory infections, diarrhoeal disease, malaria, measles, malnutrition. Special issues also need to be addressed during emergency phase:

- *Physical trauma:* refugees may have been subject to physical violence → physical trauma requiring wound care or surgery.
- *Mental trauma:* a significant proportion of the refugee population will have suffered psychological trauma, → PTSD. Provide basic counselling services for individuals and groups. Absence of appropriate mental health services → a high burden in the outpatient department (OPD) health services by refugees with psycho-somatic complaints.
- *Sexual and reproductive health:*
  - *prevent and manage the consequences of sexual and gender based violence*—treat physical trauma and STIs, provide emergency contraception, PEP, hepatitis B vaccination, and mental health support
  - guarantee availability of free condoms
  - ensure safe uncomplicated deliveries and organize a referral system for obstetric complications
  - plan provision of comprehensive reproductive health services, e.g. ante-and post-natal care, tetanus vaccination, STI and HIV screening, prevention of mother to child transmission (of HIV) (PMTCT)
  - *HIV and TB*—identify patients requiring ongoing ART or TB treatment, and provide treatment.

Healthcare systems in refugee emergencies

- Provide curative treatment for most common communicable killer diseases.
- ↓ Suffering from other debilitating diseases.
- Able to carry out active case finding.
- Able to cope with a high demand for curative care.
- Easy access to different levels of care, including referrals.
- Deal with the majority of illnesses at a basic level of care.
- Contribute to surveillance activities by routine data collection.
- Combine both curative and preventive services.
- Flexible enough to adapt to changes in situation (e.g. outbreaks of disease).

Levels of healthcare A four-tier healthcare model may fulfil the criteria above:

Referral hospital

Specialized hospital services, e.g. for surgery or major obstetric emergencies. May be provided in an existing hospital near the settlement. In the case of large camps, field hospitals will have to be established on site.

Central health facility (health centre)

Able to deal with most illnesses, offer 24-h services, and possibly basic in patient service.

Peripheral health facilities (health post or health clinic)

Decentralized, easily accessible to the whole population. This basic level deals with only a few killer diseases, e.g. diarrhoea and malaria, and refers serious cases to the health centre. It also provides treatment for a few, non-life-threatening diseases (e.g. scabies, conjunctivitis).

Community health workers

A community outreach programme links the fixed health facilities and the population. Duties: active case finding, surveillance, directly observed TB treatment, health promotion, and community mobilization, e.g. for vaccination campaigns. A network of community health workers based in the population requires training and supervision.

Organizing a decentralized network of healthcare facilities in situations where there are many different operating partners requires good coordination (see Table 23.3). Manuals and guidelines allow standardization among partners in regard to essential drugs and treatment regimens.

Experience has led to the creation of 'kits' of essential drugs and materials. The WHO Emergency Health Kit includes medicines, disposables and instruments, sufficient to support 10 000 people during a 3-mth period.

Table 23.3 Levels of healthcare and activities they can carry out

Level	Population coverage	Activities	Clinical staff per facility
Referral Hospital	Variable	Surgery Major obstetrical emergencies Referral laboratory	Doctors: variable 1 Nurse per 20–30 beds, 8-h shifts
Central Health Facilities (health centre)	1/10 000–30 000 refugees	Triage OPD**(1st level and referral) Dressing and injections ORT Emergency service (24h) Uncomplicated deliveries Minor surgery Pharmacy Basic laboratory tests Blood transfusions Immunizations	Min. 5 medical staff: 1 doctor 1 HW* for 50 consultations/d 1 HW for 20–30 beds, 8-h shifts 1 HW for ORT 1–2 HW for pharmacy 1–2 HW for dressings/injection/sterilization
Peripheral Health Facilities	1/3,000 –5,000 refugees	OPD (first level) ORT Dressing Referral of patients to higher level	Min 1 HW*, based on 1 person for 50 consultations/d 1 non-medical for ORT, dressing, registering
Outreach activities (home-visitors)		Home visits and active screening Referral of patients to facilities Health education, information	1 CHW* per 500–1000 referrals 1 supervisor for 10 CHWs 1 senior supervisor

** OPD, outpatient department; * HW, health worker (includes nurses, health assistants, medical assistants, midwives); * CHW, community health worker (limited training; may not be clinically qualified).

Control of communicable diseases and epidemics

During emergency phase, four most frequent communicable diseases which together are responsible for the highest morbidity and mortality rates are:

- Measles.
- Diarrhoeal diseases.
- Acute respiratory infections.
- Malaria.

Apart from that, frequent epidemics of cholera, *Shigella*, meningococcal meningitis, typhoid may result in very high mortality.

Objectives of epidemic control

- ↓ Transmission.
- ↓ Mortality among cases by early detection and treatment.

The implementation of these control measures should not wait until the epidemic is fully investigated. Control measures vary according to the disease, but fall into 3 major categories:

- *Attack the source:* ↓ sources of infection to prevent the disease from spreading. Depending on the disease, this may involve the prompt diagnosis and treatment (e.g. cholera), isolation (e.g. viral haemorrhagic fevers), and controlling animal reservoirs (e.g. plague).
- *Protect susceptible groups to ↓ risk of infection:* immunization, better nutrition, or chemoprophylaxis of high risk groups (e.g. intermittent presumptive treatment for malaria among pregnant women and children <5yrs).
- Interrupt transmission by improvements in environmental and personal hygiene, health education, vector control, disinfection, and sterilization.

General measures for communicable disease control

- General preventive measures aimed at ↓ cases consist mainly of improving the environment and living conditions of refugees., ↓ overcrowding, providing shelters, ensuring water supplies, excreta disposal, food supply, vector control. Mass immunization against measles must always be given the highest priority.
- Outreach activities by home-visitors to conduct early case finding and active screening, covering the whole population. Suspected cases should be rapidly referred to health facilities.
- A basic health system to ensure early and adequate treatment of the 4 biggest killer communicable diseases (measles, diarrhoeal diseases, acute respiratory infections, and malaria).
- Epidemic control needs a good surveillance system, allowing an early and appropriate outbreak response.
- Prepare contingency plans in advance, e.g. for cholera.

Epidemic preparedness

General contingency plans should be prepared in any refugee emergency in order to enable health teams to react as quickly as possible if an epidemic is declared.

- Gain information on potentially epidemic diseases that already occur in the area or which might be introduced.
- Have a surveillance system ready to detect diseases as soon as they appear. Use standard case definitions, and train health staff in use of case definitions.
- Consult standard protocols for prevention, diagnosis, and treatment procedures for epidemic diseases. Adapt protocols to the local conditions, the level of skill of HWs, local characteristics of the causative agent (drug resistance and serotype), background immunity of the refugee population. Protocols can be worked out with help of experts, and should be agreed upon in health coordination meetings.
- Identify a laboratory for confirmation of cases. Sample material for the most common tests (stools and serum) should be available nearby, and a few rapid diagnostic tests may also be stored locally. A reference laboratory should also be identified, at regional or international level (e.g. for antibiotic sensitivity testing of *Shigella*).
- Identify sources of relevant vaccines for mass campaigns (e.g. measles or meningitis).
- Prepare, and store on site, emergency stocks of material and medical supplies (e.g. oral rehydration salts, intravenous fluids, immunization material, tents, plastic sheeting, cholera kit).
- Identify possible treatment sites (e.g. cholera treatment centre).
- Assess the availability of staff and their level of skills to respond to outbreaks. Upgrade by training in anticipation of an epidemic, in situations where there is a high risk.

Public health surveillance

Epidemiological surveillance measures and monitors the health status of a population, and generates information on a regular basis for use in decision-making. It is based on the daily collection of selected health data and their analysis.

Objectives

- To provide early warning of epidemics.
- To determine the main health problems and trends over time.
- To assist the planning of interventions and ensuring resources are properly targeted.
- To evaluate the coverage and effectiveness of programmes.
- To provide information on the refugee situation (for witnessing).
- To constitute a data bank that might be useful for training or operational research.

Principles

- During the emergency phase, data collection should only focus on the main health problems, i.e. those which produce the highest mortality and morbidity.
- Data collection should be limited to problems that can be effectively prevented or treated.
- The system should be as simple as possible.
- The frequency with which data is transmitted and analyzed should be adapted to the situation, i.e. weekly in the emergency phase and monthly thereafter.
- Responsibility for organizing and supervising the surveillance system should be clearly assigned, and close coordination between all partners (UN agencies, NGOs and the host country's Ministry of Health (MOH)) is essential.
- Data analysis should take place in the field, where it will be translated into action.
- The surveillance system should be flexible in order to respond to new health problems or changes in programme activities.

Data coverage and sources

In general, 5 categories of data are gathered:

- *Demography:* total and <5yrs population, new arrivals and departures; (source: UN agencies, community leaders, home-visitors, rapid household sample surveys).
- *Mortality:* crude and <5yrs mortality rates, cause specific mortality rates; (source: grave counts, hospitals, home-visitors, community leaders).
- *Morbidity:* disease incidence and attack rates (per 1000/wk) (source: OPD and in patient health services, home-visitors).
- *Basic needs:* water quantity, food availability, sanitation, shelter, other needs; (source: agencies in charge of specific services).
- *Programme activities:* No. consultations/wk, attendance rate, no. admissions/wk, hospital mortality rate, measles vaccine coverage. (source: registers of the programmes concerned).

The daily CMR is the most useful health indicator to monitor the health status of a refugee population. The CMR is the number of deaths per 10 000 population per day. A CMR >1 indicates an emergency situation (see Table 23.4). Because high <5yrs mortality (U5MR) may be masked by the CMR, mortality in this age group is monitored separately. Calculating disease-specific mortality rates helps in determining the major killer diseases and establishing priorities.

Table 23.4 Mortality classification

	CMR (deaths/10 000/d)	**<5yrs mortality rate (deaths/10 000/d)**
Stable population in resource-poor countries	< 0.5	< 1
Refugees/displaced		
Under control	< 1	< 2
Emergency	> 1	> 2
Out of control	> 2	> 4
Catastrophic	> 4	> 8

Human resources and training

A refugee emergency response requires large numbers of medical and other staff: public health doctors, sanitation specialists, nutritionists, logisticians, administrators. Home-visitors are a particularly important category of staff required to ensure the link between the refugee community and assistance programmes, and should be recruited rapidly at the start of programmes. They should be chosen from among the refugee or displaced population.

Determining staff requirements

- Establish a list of activities and the tasks to be performed.
- Identify the different categories of personnel required to execute these tasks.
- A job description should be prepared for each category of staff, and an organization chart must be drawn up for every programme and facility.
- The number of staff required may then be calculated, based on the estimated work load (e.g. one HW should not be expected to perform >50 consultations/d). Day-shifts, night-shifts, and days off should be taken into account.

Staff training

Several types of training (formal; on-the-job) are necessary in most refugee programmes, and should be preceded by an assessment of the training needs. It is usually necessary to organize training courses on:

- Conducting mass measles immunization.
- Data collection.
- Essential drugs and standard treatments.
- Conducting surveys.
- Environmental health measures.
- Specific measures to take during epidemics.
- Oral rehydration.
- Active screening for those who are sick and/or malnourished.
- Safe deliveries.

Coordination

- Coordination mechanisms must be established in the early phase of the emergency. Leadership has to be defined. If the initiative has not been taken by United Nations High Commission on Refugees (UNHCR) or the host government, relief organizations must organize a coordination team and, if required, take on the leadership role themselves.
- The host government must be encouraged to participate in the coordination process; govt. ministries (e.g. health and water) should be involved.
- UNHCR plays a major role in the coordination of refugee programmes. Its mandate includes responsibility for ensuring protection and the adequate care of refugees and may also be extended to cover internally displaced populations (IDPs).
- Common objectives should be agreed upon and followed by all involved. Distribution of tasks must be determined among agencies, and formalized in a written agreement.
- Regular meetings and reporting must be formalized to ensure information exchange and facilitate decision-making. Sector meetings are useful for working on technical guidelines and standardization.
- Technical guidelines, standard policies (including standard data collection) will be introduced from the beginning. Their content can be better adapted to the situation after the emergency period.

Post-emergency phase

The post-emergency phase begins when the excess mortality of the emergency phase is under control, and the basic needs (water, food, shelter) have all been addressed through the implementation of the 10 top priorities. During this phase, relief programmes have to be adapted to changing needs and constraints.

Disease patterns become roughly the same as those in any non-refugee population, and diarrhoeal diseases, acute respiratory infections, and malaria are still the major killers. However, refugees are still at ↑ health risk than stable populations, and other diseases, such as reproductive health problems, HIV/AIDS, tuberculosis, mental problems, may account for a significant proportion of morbidity and mortality. In addition, infectious disease epidemics continue to occur. In most post-emergency situations, low levels of malnutrition persist, as refugee populations continue to be dependent on food distributions, and inadequacies in the food rations (in quantity and quality) continue to occur beyond the emergency phase.

Objectives of interventions in the post-emergency phase

- *Consolidating what has already been achieved:* low mortality, good nutritional and health status.
- *Preparing for possible new emergencies:* major disease outbreaks or an influx of new refugees/displaced.
- *Achieving a certain level of sustainability:* ↓ assistance in line with ↓ needs, better use of local resources, training.

Chapter 24

Obstetrics and Gynaecology: emergencies

Invited authors: **Bryn Kemp**
Angela Koech

Introduction

Almost all maternal mortality occurs in resource-poor settings. Reducing maternal mortality and morbidity is an international priority. Emergency obstetric care is an essential part of this, and the focus of this chapter. More broadly, it is an important part of reproductive health, which includes adolescent health, family planning, antenatal care, and postnatal care. Clinical guidelines from WHO on further aspects of reproductive health can be found at: http://www.who.int/reproductivehealth/publications/en/ and on maternal and perinatal health at http://www.who.int/reproductivehealth/publications/maternal_perinatal_health/en/index.html

Remember Suspect pregnancy in any collapsed woman of childbearing age.

Early pregnancy bleeding

Vaginal bleeding, +/– abdominal pain, in the first 22wks of pregnancy.

Management

- Assess ABC (see inside cover leaf) and resuscitate with IV fluids.
- Clinical assessment to determine cause (see Table 24.1).
- Urine human chorionic gonadotrophin (HCG) test and pelvic US where available. Take urine sample using catheter in collapsed patient.
- For inevitable or incomplete miscarriage give a single dose of 600μg misoprostol oral. Immediate manual vacuum aspiration (MVA) may be necessary (where bleeding heavy).
- For septic miscarriage (fever, +/– purulent vaginal discharge), start broad-spectrum IV antibiotics for 24h before uterine evacuation.
- For suspected or confirmed ectopic pregnancy, resuscitate and proceed immediately to surgery to control haemorrhage.
- Suspect molar pregnancy if there is passage of vesicles and a boggy uterus larger than dates.

Table 24.1 Causes of vaginal bleeding (pv) and/or pain in early pregnancy

	Threatened miscarriage	Inevitable miscarriage	Incomplete miscarriage	Ectopic pregnancy
History				
PV bleeding	Light bleeding	Heavy bleeding No POCs* passed	Heavy bleeding POCs passed	Light bleeding
Pain	Cramping, suprapubic	Cramping, suprapubic	Cramping, suprapubic	Severe Often uni-lateral
Examination				
Cervical os	Closed	Dilated	Dilated	Closed
Abdomen		Tender uterus	Tender uterus	Tender adnexal mass Haemo-peritoneum
Size of uterus	Equal to dates	Equal to dates	Small for dates	Small for dates
Investigations				
Pregnancy test	+	+	+	+/-
US	Viable intrauterine pregnancy	POCs in utero	POCs in utero	Empty uterus Adnexal mass

*POCs, products of conception.

Hypertensive emergencies

Severe pre-eclampsia

BP ≥160 systolic or ≥110 diastolic WITH proteinuria ≥2+ on urine dipstick *and/or* severe maternal symptoms (frontal headache, visual disturbance, or epigastric pain) diagnosed after 24wks gestation.

Management

BP needs rapid correction. Aim for systolic <160 and diastolic <110. Use oral nifedipine 10mg oral (modified release) repeat after 20min if necessary, or hydralazine 5mg IV, repeated after 20–30min if necessary. Avoid rapid acting sublingual preparations.

- Definitive treatment is delivery.
- *Measure:* Hb, platelets, creatinine, and LFTs.
- Conservative management *may* be considered at gestations of <34wks. Patient should be managed in a facility offering comprehensive obstetric care.

Indications for immediate delivery in pre-eclampsia

- *Severe maternal symptoms:* frontal headache, visual disturbance, papilloedema, epigastric pain +/– vomiting, clonus.
- Worsening thrombocytopenia (platelet count <100).
- Worsening renal function or liver function.
- Uncontrollable blood pressure.
- HELLP syndrome.
- Eclampsia.

Eclampsia

Occurrence of generalized tonic-clonic seizures in association with pre-eclampsia and in the absence of any other cause.

Eclampsia may be the first presentation of pre-eclampsia and should be considered in all women presenting with seizures in pregnancy. Always exclude alternative pathologies. Women with pre-eclampsia should be observed for >72h post-delivery as 44% of seizures occur in this time.

Management of eclampsia

- Get assistance and resuscitation if needed (ABC, see 📖 inside cover).
- When safe, place in left lateral position and obtain IV access.
- Send blood for FBC, U&E, LFT, and clotting where available.
- Perform bedside clotting test: failure of a clot to form <7min or formation of a soft clot that breaks down suggests coagulopathy.
- Measure and monitor BP, pulse, RR, tendon reflexes.
- Insert urinary catheter and monitor input/output; fluid restrict to 80mL/h IV. Keep nil by mouth.
- Treat as per Box 24.1.

Box 24.1 Treatment

Seizures

Magnesium sulfate is the first line treatment for seizures.

Loading dose

- 4g of 20% $MgSO_4$ IV over 5–15min.
- Follow with 5g of 50% $MgSO_4$ with 1mL of 2% lidocaine IM into both buttocks.
- If further seizures (after 15min), give a further 2g $MgSO_4$ (50%) solution IV over 5min.

Maintenance dose

- 5g of 50% $MgSO_4$ with 1mL of 2% lidocaine in the same syringe every 4h into alternate buttocks.
- Treatment should continue until 24h after delivery or the last seizure, whichever is the latter.

Treat hypertension

If hypertensive (BP >160/110), give nifedipine or hydralazine as for severe pre-eclampsia above.

Treat coagulopathy

Give blood/blood products as available.

For more information (and dosing for magnesium infusion rather than IM, if available): http://www.who.int/reproductivehealth/publications/maternal_perinatal_health/9241545879/en/index.html

If undelivered

Assess foetal wellbeing only once mother is stable. Aim for delivery <12h:

- Cervix favourable artificial rupture of membranes (ARM) and oxytocin.
- Cervix unfavourable and safe anaesthesia available → caesarean section (CS).
- If foetal death confirmed, pre-viable live fetus *or* unsafe anaesthesia induction of labour (IOL) with misoprostol or catheter.
- Continue maintenance $MgSO_4$ (as Box 24.1).

Prophylaxis

Consider administration of $MgSO_4$ to prevent seizures in women with severe pre-eclampsia AFTER a decision to deliver has been made.

HELLP syndrome

A variant of severe pre-eclampsia characterized by **HELLP** and with significant maternal and perinatal morbidity and mortality.

Diagnosis RUQ/epigastric pain (liver capsule swelling) alongside usual symptoms of pre-eclampsia with evidence of HELLP on FBC and LFTs.

Management Delivery. Manage as eclampsia.

Pregnancy-related infection

Maternal adaptation to pregnancy predisposes to many types of infection. Aggressive management is needed to ↓ complications. Chorioamnionitis and puerperal sepsis → significant morbidity and mortality.

Chorioamnionitis

Cause

Bacteria from the perineum and genital tract ascend into the uterus after rupture of foetal membranes, infecting uterine membranes and amniotic fluid.

Diagnosis

Maternal fever, tachycardia, uterine tenderness, offensive vaginal discharge, and foetal tachycardia. Patients with prolonged rupture of membranes are at high risk of chorioamnionitis.

Management

Delivery and broad-spectrum IV antibiotics; e.g. ampicillin 2g IV qds plus gentamicin 5mg/kg IV od plus metronidazole 500mg IV tds. There is no place for conservative management. Inhibiting labour (tocolysis) should be avoided. Steroids (for foetal lung maturation) should be used with caution and delivery should not be delayed until after steroid administration.

Puerperal pyrexia

Maternal temperature ≥38°C within 14d of delivery.

Causes

Endometritis, retained POCs, perineal infection, breast abscess/mastitis, UTI, venous thromboembolism, wound infection.

Management

- Determine likely source and give appropriate antibiotic treatment.
- For genital tract sepsis give antibiotics as for chorioamnionitis.
- For mastitis cover *S. aureus* (e.g. flucloxacillin). Consider surgical drainage if breast abscess.

Preterm prelabour rupture of membranes

- Antibiotic prophylaxis is recommended: erythromycin 250mg qds oral for 10d.
- ✆ http://www.rcog.org.uk/files/rcog-corp/GTG44PPROM28022011.pdf
- Antenatal corticosteroids should be administered.
- Delivery should be considered from 34wks gestation.

Obstetric haemorrhage

Haemorrhage is the leading cause of maternal mortality worldwide. Healthy women can have catastrophic, unpredictable blood loss. Continuous slow bleeding is an emergency as much as sudden haemorrhage.

Management of obstetric haemorrhage

- Stabilize mother (ABC) and provide high flow O_2 via face mask.
- Insert two IV cannulae and resuscitate with IV fluid. Insert urinary catheter—monitor input and output hourly.

If undelivered

- Consider delivery once stable.
- Give blood/blood products as required.
- Consider transfer to a facility able to perform CS.

If delivered

- Massage the uterine fundus and rub up a contraction.
- Remove any clots from the uterus.
- Give 200micrograms ergometrine IV (give IM if IV route difficult).
- Give 20IU of oxytocin in 1L crystalloid IV at 60 drops/min.
- Inspect for causes of bleeding as Box 24.2.
- If blood loss persists, use the following drugs in sequence:
  - repeat ergometrine 200micrograms IV every 15min up to 5 doses (max 1mg),
  - give 10IU oxytocin IV bolus,
  - give 800 micrograms of misoprostol pr,
  - give blood products as available.

Box 24.2 Assessing and managing specific causes of bleeding

Antepartum haemorrhage (APH)

- Placenta praevia (painless bleeding, high presenting part). Resuscitate and immediate transfer to surgical facility.
- Placental abruption (painful bleeding, firm and tender uterus). Resuscitate; expedite delivery or immediate referral to surgical facility.

Intrapartum

- Ruptured uterus (severe pain, maternal shock, loss of presenting part). Resuscitate and immediate transfer to surgical facility.
- Ectopic pregnancy (see 📖 Early pregnancy bleeding, p. 937).

Postpartum haemorrhage (PPH)

Four Ts—exclude these for every case of PPH:

- *Tone:* uterine atony, expel clots, rub contraction, empty bladder, administer uterotonic drugs.
- *Tissue*: retained products. Empty bladder. Examine uterine cavity. Remove tissue, membranes, and clots.
- *Trauma:* perineal trauma/cervical tears. Compress and suture.
- *Thrombin:* DIC. Give fresh, whole blood to replace red cells and clotting factors.
- Surgical treatment (hysterectomy) may be needed: Seek senior help early. Reassess blood loss. Keep systolic BP >100mmHg and urine output >30mL/h.

Intrapartum emergencies

Cord prolapse

Umbilical cord prolapsed below the presenting part after the rupture of membranes. Cord may be visible at the vagina or felt during vaginal examination. Determine cervical dilatation and whether cord is pulsating.

- *Cord pulsating, Cervix not fully dilated:*
  - deliver as soon as possible by emergency CS. Relieve cord compression by keeping patient in knee chest position or pushing presenting part up,
  - for long transfers or delays before surgery, fill bladder with 500–750mL of saline using foley catheter. Clamp catheter once filled.
- *Cord pulsating, cervix fully dilated:* delivery by rapid assisted vaginal delivery: episiotomy and vacuum.
- *Cord not pulsating:* confirm fetal demise. Deliver vaginally unless there is another indication for CS.

Shoulder dystocia

Impaction of the anterior shoulder against the maternal symphysis pubis after the fetal head has delivered (🖱 http://www.rcog.org.uk/womens-health/clinical-guidance/shoulder-dystocia-green-top-42).

Diagnosis

- Head remains tightly applied to the vulva—the 'turtle sign'.
- Chin retracts and depresses the perineum.
- Gentle traction on the head fails to deliver the shoulder.

Management

- Call for **H**elp.
- **E**valuate for Episiotomy and perform one if needed.
- *Legs:* flex thighs, abduct and rotate legs outwards (McRoberts).
- Apply suprapubic **P**ressure using the heel of the hand to push the shoulder down.
- **E**nter—internal rotational manoeuvres—using a finger in the vagina attempt to manipulate the fetus to rotate the anterior shoulder into an oblique plane to deliver.
- **R**elease the posterior arm by grasping the radius, flexing the elbow, and sweeping it across the chest.
- **R**oll the patient over to all fours and repeat the above steps.

Breech delivery

- Fetus presents with buttocks or feet first. Identified on abdominal palpation and confirmed by US or vaginal examination during labour. Significant increase in maternal morbidity and perinatal mortality.
- Consider elective CS if available.
- Pre-requisites for vaginal delivery: complete or frank breech, adequate pelvis, a fetus that is not large for dates and no previous CS.

Vaginal breech delivery

- Confirm full dilatation. Contractions should be regular and strong.
- *Hands off:* await spontaneous delivery of the buttocks. Maintain fetus in sacro-anterior position. Await delivery of inferior border of scapulae.
- Using the index finger, hook down arms at the elbows and bring them down to the chest.
- If the arms are stretched above the chest and cannot be reached, perform *Løvset's manoeuvre*. Place hands around hips with thumb on the sacrum. Rotate baby 180° clockwise to release the arm. Repeat in counterclockwise direction for other arm.
- *Mauriceau-Smellie-Veit manoeuvre:* When nape of neck is visible, place two fingers of right hand over maxilla and two fingers of the left at back of head to flex it.

Obstructed labour

Labour is considered obstructed when there is failure to progress despite strong, regular contractions and is often due to mechanical problems such as cephalopelvic disproportion (CPD), malpresentation, and malposition. Obstruction should be suspected when there is slow cervical dilatation and a presenting part that remains high despite good contractions.

Clinical features

- Prolonged labour (>12h) with maternal exhaustion and severe pain.
- *Maternal examination:* tachycardia and pyrexia are common.
- Strong uterine contractions with formation of a retraction ring (Bandl's ring). Foetal distress or foetal death develops.
- *Vaginal examination*: ruptured membranes, an oedematous cervix, severe moulding and a large caput.

Management

- Insert IV line and resuscitate. Catheterize the bladder (insertion may be difficult).
- Give broad-spectrum IV antibiotics and prepare for urgent delivery.
- Prepare for neonatal resuscitation.
- *Preferred mode of delivery:* CS. Vacuum delivery, symphysiotomy and destructive delivery may be attempted in selected cases if the attendant is competent.
- Exclude uterine rupture.
- *Post-operatively:* bladder catheter should remain for 10d to prevent fistula formation. IV antibiotics should be given as indicated. Appropriate counselling on future pregnancies: early antenatal booking and delivery in healthcare facility.

Appropriate use of the partograph results in early diagnosis and intervention before the development of complications.

Chapter 25

Nosocomial infection, antibiotic prescribing, and resistance

Invited authors **Alexander Aiken**
Susan Morpeth

Nosocomial infection

Nosocomial or hospital-acquired infections (HAI) are a large, under-recognized and largely preventable burden of disease in low resource settings (see Box 25.1). Hospitals bring vulnerable individuals and HCWs into close proximity, with a wide range of potential transmission risks—not least of which are treatments and doctors themselves!

The WHO Patient Safety campaign has led efforts to increase the profile of nosocomial disease as key area for improvement of healthcare in low-resource settings (www.who.int/patientsafety/en/index.html).

Nosocomial infections are often caused by extensively drug-resistant bacteria, for which appropriate diagnostic facilities and antibiotic treatments may not be available (see Rational antibiotic prescribing, p. 954), or only at great expense. Hospitals can serve as a 'breeding ground' for drug resistance and many patients leave hospital with carriage of drug-resistant organisms that may later cause disease. Drug resistance is therefore also potentially 'exported' into the local community and beyond.

Institutional support

Infection prevention and control (IPC) activities are often seen by hospital managers as a low priority in busy healthcare settings, but these can be highly cost-effective interventions: prevention of HAIs can lead to shorter admissions, less use of expensive antibiotics, and healthier staff.

A key step to tackling nosocomial diseases is to gain institutional support for IPC. Further useful steps include the formation of Hospital/Departmental IPC Committees, writing a local IPC Policy, conducting IPC audits and securing a budget for IPC activities within the institution. Many hospitals in resource-poor countries will not have any specialized IPC nurses: 1 full-time IPC nurse/200 inpatient beds should be a minimum, and this will make a cost saving to the hospital.

Prevention of HAI mainly involves 'process' steps (e.g. hand hygiene, use of personal protective equipment, isolation measures, etc.) that do not have an obvious immediate impact in ↓ disease, and without accurate surveillance of HAI outcomes it can be hard to know whether any effect is being achieved. These are very important areas to address in resource-poor settings, and these 'process' steps are straightforward to measure with internal hospital audits.

Hand hygiene

HCWs, hands are the main route of transmission for many nosocomial pathogens—hand washing is therefore the most important IPC activity. Provision of basins, soap, and running water in all clinical areas is essential, though this can be hard to maintain. Drying hands can be tricky; communal towels will remove most of the benefit of hand washing, but disposable paper towels or electric hand-driers are expensive. Most tropical countries are usually warm enough to quickly 'air-dry' hands.

Hands should be washed before and after all clinical activities (see WHO 'Five moments for hand hygiene' in Fig. 25.1). A proper clinical handwash takes ~1min and includes all areas of the hands. Compliance with hand hygiene is notoriously poor—especially amongst doctors—and many

HCWs think they are much better at performing hand hygiene than they actually are. One simple way to tackle this is to use observational audits:

- Ask a member of staff to stand in a clinical area for 20min and record every 'hands washed' and 'hands not washed' by professional cadre.
- Feedback these results at an appropriate time (e.g. morning handover/ward round) with +ve encouragement +/– identification of barriers to hand washing.
- Repeat whole exercise frequently.

Alcohol-based handrubs are as effective as soap + water hand washing for preventing most form of HAI and are more convenient, quicker to use and less irritating to the hands—and do not depend on a reliable hospital water supply. A WHO 'recipe' for local production of handrub is available at www.who.int/gpsc/5may/Guide_to_Local_Production.pdf. Costs can be as low as US$0.40/100mL. Get help from your hospital pharmacy or laboratory.

Box 25.1 Types of HAI

Very common	Surgical Site Infections/Wound infections UTIs – usually catheter-associated Diarrhoeal diseases
Less common but more severe	Ventilator-associated pneumonia Nosocomial TB transmission
Rare but most severe	Bacteraemia – device or transfusion-associated Blood borne viruses – esp. HIV and Hepatitis B Nosocomial disease outbreaks

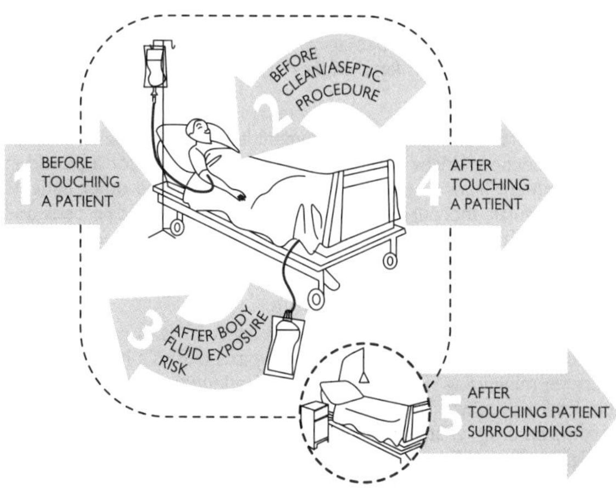

Fig. 25.1 Five moments for hand hygiene.

Reproduced from Sax H, *et al.* 'My five moments for hand hygiene': a user–centred design approach to understand, train, monitor and report hand hygiene. *J Hosp Infect* 2007; 67: 9–21, with permission from Elsevier.

Personal protective equipment (PPE)

Use of gloves, aprons, surgical gowns, boots, and protective eyewear are all important parts of IPC in any healthcare setting. Availability of such equipment is usually limited. However, usage of gloves is no 'substitute' for proper hand washing, and surgical masks provide little protection against TB and some other respiratory pathogens. Even expensive N95 masks offer limited benefit unless perfectly fitted. There is probably more use in getting infectious patients to wear the masks themselves and in designing healthcare facilities to maximize natural ventilation and sunlight.

Isolation measures

Overcrowded, understaffed wards with multiple patients per bed can be the norm for many hospitals in the tropics—it can be very hard to carry out IPC activities in such circumstances. Isolation rooms are a luxury many hospitals cannot afford, so 'cohorting' of patients with similar symptoms is often the best that can be achieved. This, in itself, can bring problems, e.g. putting patients with suspected TB together may mean that the most immunosuppressed HIV+ individuals are then in close proximity to the most infectious smear +ve TB cases. Pragmatic assessment of what is possible for the healthcare facility is the best approach. Consult with your nursing colleagues on this.

Waste disposal

Disposal of needles and other sharps into safety sharps boxes is very important—ensure proper disposal once sharps boxes are ¾ full. Waste should always be segregated to red (highly infectious), yellow (infectious), and black (non-infectious) bags at point of generation. Infectious waste and sharps should be disposed of by local incineration, but >80% of waste generated by hospitals (e.g. packaging, food remains, paper) can go to municipal dumps—which is far cheaper.

Hospital hygiene

Maintenance of a clean hospital environment is also important to limit the spread of infections. Many pathogens are able to survive for a period in the environment from where they may be transmitted to other patients and staff. Regular, thorough cleaning of clinical areas including beds and adjacent surfaces with a suitable disinfectant, and regular laundry of bedding, are therefore important.

Prevention of surgical site infections

Surgical Site Infections (SSIs) are the commonest HAIs in resource-poor countries and pre-operative antibiotic prophylaxis (AP) is a highly effective measure for minimizing SSIs. Many surgeons continue to use post-operative antibiotics for prophylaxis—but this is largely ineffective in preventing SSIs and promotes drug resistance. There are often beliefs amongst HCWs that SSIs originate from 'dirty wards' or 'poor patient hygiene', whereas most SSIs actually result from bacterial contamination at the time of surgery.

AP should consist of a single pre-op dose of antibiotics(s) that cover the locally relevant pathogens and resistance patterns for surgical sepsis, ideally given IV 20–30min before skin incision, with repeat doses for very long procedures. Routine post-operative antibiotics should be avoided.

Use of checklists is also an important element of ensuring safe surgery (see WHO template on this at www.who.int/patientsafety/safesurgery/en/).

Surgical prophylaxis works by ↓ bacterial inoculum in the operation wound, so even if there is some resistance to a drug in the community, that drug may still be a reasonably effective AP agent. Changing long-established post-operative antibiotic dosing habits can be difficult, but this is an effective IPC intervention, a cost-saving measure, and a prudent use of antibiotics which may reduce the burden of resistant infections in the long-term. (see Rational Antibiotic Prescribing, p. 952).

A good choice of surgical AP for most major procedures in adults (including CS and laparotomy) is a single-dose of 1.2g co-amoxiclav; a cheaper alternative is ampicillin 2g +/– metronidazole 500mg.

Transmission of blood-borne infections

Contaminated injections caused an estimated 21 million HBV infections, 2 million HCV infections and 260 000 HIV infections in the year 2000 alone. Other infections (syphilis, viral haemorrhagic fevers, malaria) can also be transmitted by injections. Minimize the number of injections given and ensure needles are never re-used. Many people believe a medicine given by injection is 'stronger' than an oral formulation. HCWs must strive to re-educate patients that injections (especially those given outside of hospitals) are risky for many reasons, and are often unnecessary. Technological advances mean that 'single use only' syringes and IV cannulas are cheaply available—ensure your hospital switches to these where possible.

Use of HIV PEP after needlestick injuries is covered elsewhere (see Post-exposure prophylaxis following needlestick injuries, p. 146). All HCWs and laboratory staff should be fully vaccinated against HBV—this is a far more infectious virus than HIV and almost totally preventable, but it is often seen as a lesser concern.

Blood transfusions

Blood transfusions are likely to be an important source of HAI. The WHO has estimated that 5–10% of HIV infections in Africa are transmitted by this route. Many blood packs in resource-poor countries may have bacterial contamination (found in 9% in one study in Kenya), which probably leads to (frequently undiagnosed) post-transfusion bacteraemia. Balance the infectious risk and the potential benefits of each transfusion—if you ↓ blood transfusions, you are conserving a precious resource and avoiding a serious risk to patients.

Nosocomial disease outbreaks

Hospital outbreaks of Viral Haemorrhagic Fevers (VHFs) and other highly pathogenic viruses (e.g. SARS) or bacteria (e.g. *Vibrio cholera*) are frightening, but relatively rare. See sections on individual diseases for specific advice on outbreak management. Every hospital should have an 'outbreak emergency plan', which should include a method for effectively communicating that an outbreak is taking place in the hospital and knowing when and who to ask for help. More commonly, hospital outbreaks involve drug-resistant bacteria in high-risk patient groups or specialist wards, especially ICUs, burns units, and neonatal care units. Effective control of these outbreaks is best achieved by vigorous enforcement of all the IPC policies described above.

Rational antibiotic prescribing

Rational prescribing limits the use of antibiotics to patients who need them, tailoring therapy towards the likely pathogens and resistance profile, with as little collateral damage to the healthy microbiota as possible, for as short a duration as necessary to attain cure. It aims to reduce side effects and limit the development of antibiotic resistance, and is arguably of greatest importance in resource-poor settings where the choice of available antimicrobial drugs is already limited.

Strategies to improve antimicrobial use include restricting the antibiotics available on the hospital/clinic formulary; requiring senior/specialist approval for prescription of 2nd or 3rd line treatments so they are reserved for patients who really need them; and the use of evidence-based guidelines for management of specific clinical syndromes (e.g. pneumonia, meningitis, soft tissue infections, etc.). WHO and/or national guidelines provide a useful template in many situations, but guidelines should ideally be adapted in the light of local data on the most likely pathogens and their resistance profiles for each clinical syndrome where local data of sufficient quality exists. Where resources allow an antimicrobial stewardship team—including an infectious diseases physician and/or microbiologist and a pharmacist—is helpful in developing and implementing institutional policies for rational prescribing of antimicrobials.

The following are general principles for rational prescribing:

- If possible obtain appropriate specimens for bacterial culture before starting antimicrobial therapy (e.g. blood, urine, pus, pleural fluid, CSF, stool, depending on the clinical presentation). This is usually possible, but should not delay antibiotic administration in patients with severe infection (e.g. meningitis) or sepsis, for whom appropriate antimicrobial therapy should be commenced as soon as possible—ideally within 1h.
- Start empiric antimicrobial therapy guided by the most likely pathogens for the presenting clinical syndrome (e.g. community or hospital acquired pneumonia, meningitis, UTI, sepsis without a focus, skin or soft tissue infections, etc.)—follow local/national/WHO guidelines.
- Give IV antibiotics for severely unwell patients (e.g. severe pneumonia), infections at sites where antibiotic penetration is difficult (e.g. meningitis), and in patients who cannot take or absorb oral medication (e.g. in severe vomiting or severe malnutrition). Give oral antibiotics to patients without a good indication for parenteral therapy (never give an injection just because the patient expects one).
- Always ask about drug allergies (especially penicillins and sulphur drugs) and consider drug interactions, side effects, and how the drug is cleared (is there evidence of renal or hepatic failure?) when choosing antibiotics.
- Adjust or de-escalate antimicrobial therapy according to clinical response and any +ve culture results. If in doubt about how to interpret culture results consult a microbiologist or infectious diseases doctor for advice if available. In most infections it is possible to switch from IV to oral therapy once the patient is improving consistently (e.g. eating, afebrile for 24–48h). Avoid unnecessarily prolonging treatment.

Indications for antibiotics

Indications for antibiotics include the following common clinical syndromes:

- Septic shock or signs of sepsis (📖 Sepsis, p. 734).
- Severe malaria; bacteremia may also be present (📖 Chapter 2).
- Pneumonia (📖 Pneumonia, p. 180), meningitis (📖 Acute bacterial meningitis, p. 440), and symptomatic UTI.
- Severe/complicated diarrhoea.
- Skin and soft tissue infections, including abscesses that cannot be treated with incision and drainage alone—antibiotics are an adjunctive treatment for abscesses and should not be used 'instead of' surgery: if there is pus, let it out! Surgery is always required in addition to antibiotics for necrotizing fasciitis and gas gangrene.

Have a lower threshold for giving antibiotics to an immunosuppressed patient or those at the extremes of age.

Antibiotics are *not* indicated for the following:

- Colds and flu: usually viral.
- Uncomplicated diarrhoea.
- Bloody diarrhoea if haemolytic-uraemic syndrome suspected.
- Non-severe malaria confirmed by slide or rapid antigen test.
- Asymptomatic bacteriuria (except in a pregnant woman).

Antibiotic prophylaxis is rarely indicated—antibiotics do not prevent infections, but will select for resistant organisms so that if infection does occur it may be more difficult to treat. Exceptions include:

- Prevention of opportunistic infections in HIV (see 📖 pp. 83, 110).
- Penicillin prophylaxis against Group A *Streptococci* in rheumatic heart disease (and occasionally for recurrent Group A streptococcal cellulitis).
- Ampicillin or erythromycin or to prevent mother-to-child transmission of Group B *Streptococcus*.
- Penicillin prophylaxis in children with sickle cell disease.

Antibiotics for surgical prophylaxis only work if given as a single dose *immediately pre-operatively* (see 📖 p. 950).

Antimicrobial resistance

Antimicrobial resistance is a global problem, but disproportionately affects low resource settings where the availability and use of antibiotics is frequently unregulated, and amplification of resistance in communities and hospitals is facilitated by poorer standards of sanitation and hygiene. Limited resources, competing public health priorities and under-recognition of the problem due to limited antimicrobial resistance surveillance data together mean the public health response to this increasing problem is often inadequate, further compounding the problem.

Antibiotic exposure selects for resistant organisms, not only among circulating pathogens, but also within the human microbiota, particularly the gut flora. Resistance determinants are often carried on mobile genetic elements so are then easily transmitted from normal flora to pathogenic bacteria, and genes for resistance to different antibiotics are often transmitted together on the same mobile genetic element, meaning that selective pressure by one antibiotic can lead to selection of a multi-drug resistant phenotype (e.g. use of third-generation cephalosporins can lead to selection of *Enterobacteriaceae* with extended-spectrum beta-lactamase (ESBL) activity plus aminoglycoside and quinolone resistance). Once resistance to available antibiotics occurs, serious infections become untreatable. In this instance, prevention is infinitely better than cure.

The following are examples of some of the more important drug resistant organisms of particular relevance to clinical practice:

Meticillin-resistant *Staphylococcus aureus* (MRSA)

MRSA is a widespread problem. Susceptibility testing is needed to diagnose MRSA and inform treatment, which usually requires a glycopeptide (e.g. vancomycin). MRSA prevalence in tropical countries is not well documented, but it is probably on the rise. Local variation in MRSA prevalence means that you need to know your local situation. It is crucially important to prevent transmission of MRSA because glycopeptides are often not available in resource-poor settings.

Glycopeptide intermediate *Staphylococcus aureus* (GISA)

Strains are meticillin resistant, but also have reduced susceptibility to glycopeptides. Prevalence in resource-poor settings unknown, but likely to be low.

Vancomycin-resistant *enterococci* (VRE) Are a widespread problem in countries where glycopeptides are used.

Salmonellae

Multi-drug resistant non-typhi Salmonellae (NTS) resistant to ampicillin, co-trimoxazole and chloramphenicol are common in many parts of the world. Reduced susceptibility to quinolones (e.g. ciprofloxacin) is emerging and ESBL carrying strains have been described.

Salmonella typhi, the causative agent of typhoid fever, has unfortunately developed even more resistance than its NTS cousin (see 🕮 Typhoid and paratyphoid fevers, p. 748).

Extended spectrum beta-lactamase (ESBLs)

ESBL carrying *Enterobacteriaceae* (e.g. *Klebsiella pneumoniae*, *Escherichia coli*) present an increasing problem worldwide. ESBLs confer resistance to 3rd generation cephalosporins such as ceftriaxone, and are easily transmissible between bacteria. They are also frequently linked to resistance to other classes of antibiotics, so that many ESBL strains are resistant to all available agents except carbapenems (e.g. imipenem).

The emergence and spread of Enterobacteriaceae expressing carbapenemases such as *Verona integron-encoded metallo-β-lactamase* (VIM), *Klebsiella pneumoniae* carbapenemase (KPC), and most recently, the NDM-1 metallo-β-lactamase that is carried by a particularly promiscuous plasmid, present a serious threat worldwide. Effective treatment of these organisms often requires agents such as tigecycline (which is only bacteriostatic) or colistin (which may have toxic side effects), and strains also carrying resistance to these agents are essentially untreatable.

❶ Hospitals with resource-limited antibiotic formularies quickly reach the end of their antibiotic armoury in the face of multi-drug resistance, and inadequate or non-existent surveillance for antibiotic resistance allows policy makers to continue to ignore this situation.

Appendix: websites

Chapter 1

Management of the Sick Child

Pocket Book of Hospital Care for Children
🖱 http://apps.who.int/iris/bitstream/10665/81170/1/9789241548373_eng.pdf or 🖱 http://www.who.int/maternal_child_adolescent/documents/child_hospital_care/en/index.html

Integrated management of childhood illness (IMCI)
🖱 http://www.who.int/maternal_child_adolescent/documents/imci/en/index.html

Emergency triage assessment and treatment (ETAT)
🖱 http://whqlibdoc.who.int/publications/2005/9241546875_eng.pdf

Newborn Life Support
🖱 http://www.resus.org.uk/pages/GL2010.pdf

Emergency Triage, Assessment and Treatment: A manual for participants
🖱 http://whqlibdoc.who.int/publications/2005/9241546875_eng.pdf

Adult and Paediatric Life Support Resuscitation Council UK
🖱 http://www.resus.org.uk/pages/GL2010.pdf

Chapter 2

Malaria

Maps of malaria transmission
🖱 www.map.ox.ac.uk

Management of malaria
🖱 http://whqlibdoc.who.int/publications/2010/9789241547925_eng.pdf
🖱 http://www.who.int/malaria/publications/atoz/mal_treatchild_revised.pdf

Protocol for in vivo testing of the efficacy of antimalarial drugs against *P. falciparum* in the field
🖱 http://www.who.int/malaria/en

Resistant malaria
🖱 http://www.rbm.who.int/wmr2005/html/map5.htm

Chapter 3

HIV/AIDS

WHO Consolidated Guidelines on the use of antiretroviral drugs for treating and preventing HIV infection. June 2013
🖱 http://www.who.int/hiv/pub/guidelines/arv2013/en/

UNAIDS Report on the Global AIDS Epidemic, 2010
🖱 http://www.unaids.org/globalreport/global_report.htm

Children's HIV association (UK based)
🖱 http://www.chiva.org.uk/professionals/resources/index.html

Trials in paediatric HIV
www.pentatrials.org/guidelines.htm

Opportunistic infections in children
http://www.cdc.gov/mmwr/preview/mmwrhtml/rr5811a1.htm#tab4

Antiretroviral drug interactions
www.hiv-druginteractions.org

Management of renal impairment in HIV, including ART doses
http://cid.oxfordjournals.org/content/40/11/1559.full.pdf.

Chapter 4

Tuberculosis

TB and HIV drug interactions:
http://www.cdc.gov/tb/publications/guidelines/TB_HIV_Drugs/PDF/tbhiv.pdf

Chapter 5

Chest Medicine

Asthma guidelines (British Thoracic Society)
http://www.brit- thoracic.org.uk/Portals/0/Guidelines/AsthmaGuidelines/qrg101%202011.pdf

Chapter 6

Diarrhoeal diseases

Diarrhoea, dehydration and rehydration – portal for many resources
http://rehydrate.org/

Chapter 7

Gastroenterology

Images of parasites
http://prep4md.blogspot.co.uk/2008/07/parasitology-cestoda-related-free.html

Detailed country maps of schistosomiasis
http://www.who.int/schistosomiasis/epidemiology/global_atlas_maps/en/index.html

Chapter 10

Neurology

WHO advice on surveillance and epidemic control of meningococcal disease
www.who.int/csr/resources/publications/meningitis/whoemcbac983.pdf

Chapter 12

Endocrinology and Biochemistry

Management of DKA in children
http://www.bsped.org.uk/clinical/docs/DKAGuideline.pdf

Chapter 14

Dermatology

Detailed information on head lice detection and management is available at
🖱 www.health.wa.gov.au/headlice

New Zealand Dermatological Society resource:
🖱 http://dermnetnz.org/

Dermatology atlas online:
🖱 http://dermatlas.med.jhmi.edu/derm/
and

Dermatology Information Service (includes atlases and case reports)
🖱 http://dermis.net/dermisroot/en/home/index.htm

Chapter 16

Sexually-transmitted Infections

STI atlas
🖱 http://stiatlas.org/

British Association of Sexual Health and HIV
🖱 http://www.bashh.org/guidelines

Melbourne Sexual Health Centre
🖱 www.mshc.org.au

CDC
🖱 http://www.cdc.gov/std/treatment/

Faculty of Sexual and Reproductive Health
🖱 http://www.fsrh.org/

WHO: Male circumcision for HIV prevention
🖱 http://www.who.int/hiv/topics/malecircumcision/en/index.html

WHO Guidelines for the management of sexually transmitted infections
🖱 http://www.who.int/hiv/pub/sti/pub6/en/

Chapter 17

Nutrition

Reference growth standards and growth charts. Full tables available at:
🖱 http://www.who.int/childgrowth/standards/en/

RUTF production WHO website:
🖱 http://www.who.int/nutrition/topics/backgroundpapers_Local_production.pdf

Severe malnutrition: report of a consultation to review current literature. Geneva, World Health Organization, 6–7 September 2004
🖱 http://www.who.int/nutrition/publications/malnutrition/en/

Valid International, Community Based Therapeutic Care (2006):
🖱 www.validinternational.org

The Lancet series on Maternal and Child Undernutrition (2013):
🖱 http://www.thelancet.com/series/maternal-and-child-nutrition

Use a supplemetary suckling technique to continue to stimulate breast milk production:
http://www.docstoc.com/docs/48486395/UNICEF-IMAM-Publication-pdf-National-Guideline-for--malnutrition

UN SCN Food & Nutrition Resource Portal
http://www.unscn.org/en/resource_portal/index.php?themes=203

Community-based Management of Acute Malnutrition
http://www.cmamforum.org

Chapter 18

Multi-system Diseases and Infections

Images on bacteria
http://prep4md.blogspot.co.uk/2008/07/medically-important-bacteria-images.html

Images on viruses
http://prep4md.blogspot.co.uk/2008/08/medically-important-viruses-images.html

Test yourself on identification of parasites and arthropods
http://www.k-state.edu/parasitology/546tutorials/titlepage.html

CDC's Department of Parasitologic Diagnosis parasite image library
http://www.dpd.cdc.gov/dpdx/html/image_library.htm

Atlas of Department of Parasitology, Faculty of Medicine, Chiang Mai University, Thailand
http://www.medicine.cmu.ac.th/dept/parasite/

Tutorials and images on parasites
http://www.stanford.edu/group/parasites/ParaSites2003

Chapter 19

Mental Health

World Health Organization, mhGAP intervention guide for mental, neurological and substance use disorders in non-specialized health settings: mental health Gap Action Programme (mhGAP). 2010, WHO: Geneva.
http://www.who.int/mental_health/evidence/mhGAP_intervention_guide/en/index.html

Chapter 20

Trauma

Management of burn injuries of various depths
http://www.bmj.com/cgi/content/full/329/7458/158

Further detailed guidance on trauma management and the resources required in low resource settings are given in the following publications, available to download free from their respective websites:

Wilkinson & Skinner, Primary Trauma Care: A Manual for Trauma Management in District and Remote Locations. 2000. Primary Trauma Care Foundation, Oxford.
www.primarytraumacare.org/wp-content/uploads/2011/09/PTC_ENG.pdf

WHO, Guidelines for Essential Trauma Care. 2004, WHO, Geneva.
http://whqlibdoc.who.int/publications/2004/9241546409.pdf

Chapter 22

Immunization

WHO vaccine-preventable diseases: monitoring system. 2013 global summary
http://apps.who.int/immunization_monitoring/globalsummary/schedules

WHO: Immunization financing
http://www.who.int/immunization_financing/about/en/

Summary of WHO Position Papers–Recommendations for Routine Immunization
http://www.who.int/immunization/policy/Immunization_routine_table1.pdf
http://www.who.int/immunization/documents/WHO_IVB_06.10/en/index.html

WHO: Global Vaccine Safety
www.who.int/immunization_safety/aefi/immunization_misconceptions/en/

Chapter 24

O&G emergencies

Clinical guidelines from WHO on further aspects of reproductive health can be found at:
http://www.who.int/reproductivehealth/publications/en/
http://www.who.int/reproductivehealth/publications/maternal_perinatal_health/en/index.html
http://www.who.int/reproductivehealth/publications/maternal_perinatal_health/9241545879/en/index.html

Clinical guidelines from the Royal College of Obstetricians and Gynaecologists (UK) can be found at:
http://www.rcog.org.uk/womens-health/guidelines

Chapter 25

Nosocomial infection, antibiotic prescribing, and resistance

Hand hygiene in healthcare settings
http://www.cdc.gov/handhygiene/index.html

Drug resistance
http://www.who.int/drugresistance/en/

Index

A

D

E

M

P

Q

R

S

T

U

V

Adult Advanced Life Support

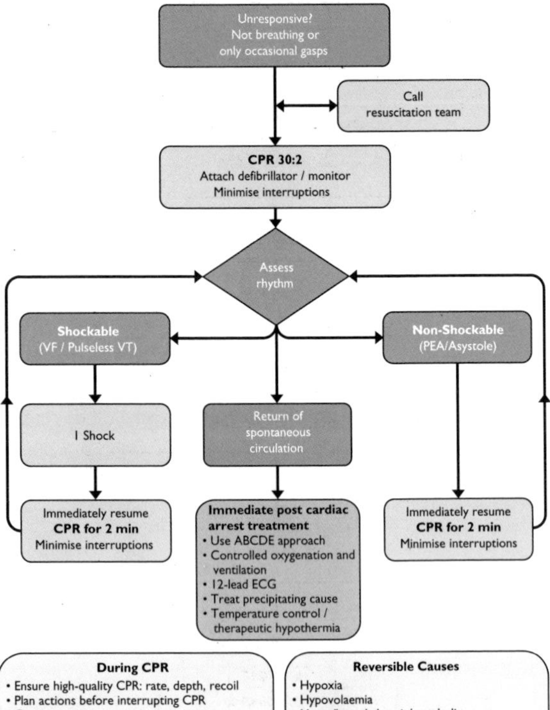

During CPR

- Ensure high-quality CPR: rate, depth, recoil
- Plan actions before interrupting CPR
- Give oxygen
- Consider advanced airway and capnography
- Continuous chest compressions when advanced airway in place
- Vascular access (intravenous, intraosseous)
- Give adrenaline every 3-5 min
- Correct reversible causes

Reversible Causes

- Hypoxia
- Hypovolaemia
- Hypo-/hyperkalaemia/metabolic
- Hypothermia

- Thrombosis - coronary or pulmonary
- Tamponade - cardiac
- Toxins
- Tension pneumothorax